Decision Making *AND* Outcomes *IN* Sports Rehabilitation

Decision Making AND Outcomes IN Sports Rehabilitation

Dinesh A. Kumbhare, MD, MSc, FRCP(C)
Assistant Clinical Professor
McMaster University
Head of Service of Physiatry and Rehabilitation Medicine
St. Joseph's Hospital
Hamilton, Ontario
Canada

John V. Basmajian, MD, LLD, FRCP(C)
Professor Emeritus in Medicine and Anatomy
McMaster University
Chedoke-McMaster Rehabilitation Centre
Hamilton, Ontario
Canada

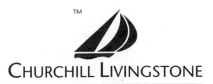

TM

CHURCHILL LIVINGSTONE

A Harcourt Health Sciences Company
New York • Edinburgh • London • Philadelphia

CHURCHILL LIVINGSTONE

A Harcourt Health Sciences Company

The Curtis Center
Independence Square West
Philadelphia, Pennsylvania 19106

Library of Congress Cataloging-in-Publication Data

Decision making and outcomes in sports rehabilitation / [edited by] Dinesh A.
Kumbhare, John V. Basmajian.
    p. ; cm.
  ISBN 0-443-06546-2
  1. Sports medicine. I. Kumbhare, Dinesh A. II. Basmajian, John V.
  [DNLM: 1. Athletic Injuries—rehabilitation. 2. Decision Making. QT 261 D294 2000]
RC1210.D36 2000
617.1'027—dc21

                       99-048218

Acquisitions Editor: Andrew Allen
Senior Editorial Assistant: Suzanne Hontscharik
Production Manager: Donna L. Morrissey

DECISION MAKING AND OUTCOMES IN SPORTS REHABILITATION   ISBN 0-443-06546-2

Printed in the United States of America

Last digit is the print number: 9   8   7   6   5   4   3   2   1

*Dedicated to all who strive to give
the best possible preventive and restorative care
to athletes of all ages, sports, and exercise regimens.*

Contributors

Per-Olof Åstrand, MD, PhD

Professor Emeritus, Department of Physiology and Pharmacology, Karolinska Institute, Stockholm, Sweden
Exercise Physiology in the Mature Athlete

John V. Basmajian, MD, LLD, FRCPC, FRCPS(Glasg), FRCP(Edin), FAFRM-RACP(Austral), FABMR, OC, OOnt

Professor Emeritus in Medicine and Anatomy, Faculty of Health Sciences, McMaster University; Honorary Staff, Hamilton Health Science Corporation; Former Director, Chedoke Hospital Rehabilitation Centre, McMaster University Medical Centre, Hamilton, Ontario
Appraisal of Alternative Treatment Methods in Sports Medicine Rehabilitation; Sports Injuries of the Wrist and Hand; Acute Lower Back Pain: Concise Review of Nonsurgical Treatments; Building on Our Strengths

W. Watson Buchanan, MD, FRCP(Glasg, Edin, and Can), FACP, FACR(Hon)

Emeritus Professor of Medicine, Faculty of Health Sciences, McMaster University; Consultant Rheumatologist, Sir William Osler Health Institute, Hamilton, Ontario
Inflammation: Its Influence and Consequences in Athletes

Bert Chesworth, BA, BScPT, MClSc

Honary Lecturer, University of Western Ontario; Research Analyst, London Health Sciences Centre, Research Incorporated, London, Ontario
Physical Therapy Management of the Injured Athlete

Chong-Hyuk Choi, MD

Clinical Fellow, University of Toronto, Toronto, Ontario
Treatment Modalities for Soft Tissue Injuries of the Ankle

Edward R. Crowther, BA, DC, FCCS

Associate Clinical Professor, Division of Clinical Education, Canadian Memorial Chiropractic College, Toronto, Ontario
Chiropractic Management of the Injured Athlete

Catherine Demers, MD, FRCPC

Clinical Scholar, Heart and Stroke Research Fellow, McMaster University; Cardiologist, Hamilton Health Corporation, McMaster University, Hamilton, Ontario
Cardiovascular Benefits and Precautions of Regular Physical Activity

David W. Dodick, MD, FRCP(C), FACP

Assistant Professor, Mayo Graduate School of Medicine, Mayo Medical School, Rochester, Minnesota; Consultant in Neurology, Mayo Clinic, Scottsdale, Arizona
Concussion in Sports

M. Alan J. Finlayson, PhD

Adjunct Faculty, University of Windsor, Windsor, Ontario; Adjunct Faculty, York University, Toronto, Ontario; Psychologist, Independent Practice, Hamilton, Ontario
Neuropsychology in Sports

Gunnar Grimby, MD, PhD

Professor in Rehabilitation Medicine, Göteborg University; Attending Physician, Sahlgrenska University Hospital, Göteborg, Sweden
Exercise in Neuromuscular Conditions

Jaroslaw P. Grod, DC, FCCS

Professor and Chair, Division of Diagnosis, Los Angeles College of Chiropractic, Los Angeles, California
Chiropractic Management of the Injured Athlete

Anita Gross, MSc, Grad Dip Manipulation Therapy, BScPT

Assistant Clinical Professor, School of Rehabilitation Sciences, McMaster University; Clinical Specialist in Manipulation Therapy, Hamilton Health Sciences Corporation, Hamilton, Ontario
Physical Therapy Management of the Injured Athlete

Liz (Elizabeth) Harrison, PhD, MSc, BPT, Dip PT, Dip Sport PT

Professor, School of Physical Therapy, College of Medicine, University of Saskatchewan, Saskatoon, Saskatchewan
Physical Therapy Management of the Injured Athlete

Lawrence E. Hart, MBBCh, MSc, FRCPC, FACP, FACR, Dip Sport Med

Associate Professor, Department of Medicine, McMaster University; Head of Rheumatology and Director of Rheumatic Disease Unit, Chedoke Division, Hamilton Health Sciences Corporation, Hamilton, Ontario
Evidence-Based Sports Medicine; Arthritis and Exercise

Robert W. Jackson, OC, MD, MS(Tor), FRCSC

Clinical Professor, Orthopaedic Surgery, University of Texas, Southwestern; Chief, Department of Orthopaedic Surgery, Baylor University Medical Center, Dallas, Texas
Hip and Knee Injuries

Sander Koëter, MD

Resident, Erasmus University, Rotterdam, The Netherlands
Hip and Knee Injuries

Kaare Kolstad, MD

Assistant Clinical Professor, Baylor College of Medicine; Attending Orthopedic Surgeon of Sport Medicine, Baylor Sports Medicine Institute, Houston, Texas
Rehabilitation of the Shoulder

Dinesh A. Kumbhare, MD, MSc, FRCP(C)

Assistant Clinical Professor, McMaster University; Head of Service of Physiatry and Rehabilitation Medicine, St. Joseph's Hospital, Hamilton, Ontario, Canada
Appraisal of Alternative Treatment Methods in Sports Medicine Rehabilitation; The Pediatric Athlete; Sports Injuries of the Wrist and Hand; Acute Lower Back Pain: Concise Review of Nonsurgical Treatments

Larry M. Leith, PhD

Professor, Faculty of Physical Education and Health, University of Toronto, Toronto, Ontario
Psychological and Sociologic Factors in Sport

Mark R. Lovell, PhD

Division Head, Neuropsychology, Henry Ford Health System, Detroit,Michigan
Neuropsychology in Sports

Robert S. McKelvie, MD, PhD, FRCPC

Associate Professor, McMaster University; Cardiologist, Hamilton Health Sciences Corporation, Hamilton, Ontario
Cardiovascular Benefits and Precautions of Regular Physical Activity

Michelle F. Mottola, PhD

Associate Professor, Faculty of Health Sciences, School of Kinesiology, and Faculty of Medicine and Dentistry, Department of Anatomy and Cell Biology, University of Western Ontario, London, Ontario
Validation of Guidelines for Aerobic Exercise in Pregnancy

Stephen J. Nicholas, MD

Director, The Nicholas Institute of Sports Medicine and Athletic Trauma, Lenox Hill Hospital, New York, New York
Rehabilitation of the Shoulder

D.J. Ogilvie-Harris, MBChB, Hons, BSc, Hons, MSc(Tor), FRCSC

Associate Professor, University of Toronto; Orthopaedic Surgeon, Toronto Western Hospital, Toronto, Ontario
Treatment Modalities for Soft Tissue Injuries of the Ankle

Anita Symonds Perrigo, BPE, BScPT

Physiotherapist, Hamilton Health Sciences Corporation, Hamilton, Ontario
Physical Therapy Management of the Injured Athlete

Brian D. Roy, MSc, BPE

Post-Doctoral Fellow (MRC), McMaster University, Hamilton, Ontario
Nutritional Strategies, Including Creatine Supplementation, to Promote Muscle Functional Recovery

Neville Suskin, MBChB, FRCPC

Assistant Professor, Medicine, Division of Cardiology, London Health Sciences Centre, University of Western Ontario, London, Ontario
Cardiovascular Benefits and Precautions of Regular Physical Activity

Mark A. Tarnopolsky, MD, PhD, FRCP(C)

Assistant Professor, McMaster University; Department of Neurology/Physical Medicine and Rehabilitation, McMaster University Medical Center, Hamilton, Ontario
Nutritional Strategies, Including Creatine Supplementation, to Promote Muscle Functional Recovery; Caffeine and Carbohydrate Loading in Endurance Exercise

Timothy F. Tyler, MS, PT, ATC

Clinical Research Associate, The Nicholas Institute of Sports Medicine and Athletic Trauma, Lenox Hill Hospital, New York, New York
Rehabilitation of the Shoulder

C. Bruce Wenger, MD, PhD
Research Pharmacologist, Military Performance Division, United States Army Research Institute of Environmental Medicine, Natick, Massachusetts
Exercise and Core Temperature

Dean M. Wingerchuk, MD, FRCP(C)
Assistant Professor, Mayo Medical School, Rochester, Minnesota; Senior Associate Consultant, Department of Neurology, Mayo Clinic Scottsdale, Scottsdale, Arizona
Epilepsy in Sports Medicine

Larry A. Wolfe, PhD
Professor, School of Physical and Health Education and Department of Physiology, Queen's University, Kingston, Ontario
Validation of Guidelines for Aerobic Exercise in Pregnancy

Preface

Sports Medicine in all its sheltered and exposed areas is now being buffeted by a fresh breeze—*evidence-based practice*. Most of its relatively short existence has been dominated by dogmatic approaches aggressively promoted by charismatic trainers and practitioners. These people range from sports greats to side-line clinicians including orthopedists, internists, physiatrists, physical therapists, chiropractors, masseurs, and others. A few have relied on whatever research evidence exists in a few narrow niches, but the majority are still flying by the seat of their pants. Judging by the air of quiet self-satisfaction or stubborn authoritarianism that survives among all too many, the time has come for publishing this book.

After drawing up a list of chapters we felt to be necessary, we invited leading experts who would survey their assigned field with a critical eye and assign as precise a verdict as possible on each of the subsections of chapters. We were guided by the principles and process used in our recent book *Clinical Decision Making in Rehabilitation: Efficacy and Outcomes* (J.V. Basmajian, S.N. Banerjee). That book revealed a wide range of clinical practices, most of which remain untested by evidence-based investigation. As in that book, the authors of this book were asked to grade the available literature supporting or rejecting every approach. They were asked to use firm guidelines and definitions and then to specify, where possible, the level of evidence (I to V) and the recommended grade (A to C) and below (Sackett, Chapter 1 of Basmajian and Banerjee book).

Because sports medicine in its modern form is so new, this book cannot be the final judgment. The literature is being enlarged—and sometimes enriched—daily. Our purpose is to sound a clarion call for more evidence-based practices and for a windstorm of controlled research. Otherwise, everyone in sports activities at every level—from backyard family fun and gymnasium conditioning exercises to the acme of Olympic sports—will be hamstrung. They will be doomed to perpetuating and promoting the bad and doubtful along with the good and useful practices of prevention, soothing, and healing. We cannot and must not permit this to happen.

Dinesh A. Kumbhare
John V. Basmajian

Acknowledgments

This book depends heavily on the chapter authors, and we thank them again with deep appreciation for their work. A book of this nature required enormous preliminary investigations and data filtering, not just a recitation of personal views. We believe that the results are both well balanced and of great and immediate value.

We also wish to thank our private assistants—Verna Johnson and Julie Stockl—whose responses to the added load of work took an enormous load off our shoulders.

Finally, we note with love the tolerance of our families who cheerfully lived with the steady drain on our commitments at home.

Dinesh A. Kumbhare
John V. Basmajian

Contents

BASIC
CONSIDERATIONS

Evidence-Based Sports Medicine

LAWRENCE E. HART

Optimal medical practice depends on the rational interpretation of research evidence and its application in the clinical setting. It follows, therefore, that astute clinicians need to be able to identify relevant and methodologically acceptable studies to address pertinent questions relating to the care of their patients. Sorting through an often overwhelming literature on a topic of interest can be arduous and time consuming. Moreover, despite efforts by most reputable journals to improve their general standards, flawed research still frequently appears in mainstream publications.[1]

Prompted by the assumption that health care, in general, could be improved if practitioners were able to move from an often empiric approach to a more evidence-based model, the proponents of what has come to be known as evidence-based medicine (EBM) have worked to provide clinicians and investigators with comprehensive guidelines to facilitate the practice of EBM. In acknowledging that the effective implementation of EBM depends on the proper identification of sound research, this framework includes comprehensive guidelines[2–13] on how to critically appraise the literature and effectively identify those articles that will most likely be helpful in the clinical environment.

WHAT IS EVIDENCE-BASED MEDICINE?

The philosophy of EBM is thought to date back to the mid–19th century or earlier,[14] but the tenets and practice of this discipline have undergone a renaissance more recently.[15] EBM, as presently described,[14,16] is the conscientious, explicit, and judicious use of current best evidence in making decisions about the care of individual patients. Applying EBM requires the integration of individual clinical expertise with the best available external evidence from systematic research. By merging a sophisticated and thoughtful clinical experience with the results of valid, clinically relevant research, the practitioner strives to adopt the most efficacious therapies that will improve care and positively affect patient quality of life.

The evolution from more traditional medicine to EBM has been explored within the context of a paradigm shift.[17] According to what has been referred to as the "former paradigm," clinical medicine has been guided by the following assumptions[17]:

1. Unsystematic observations from clinical experience are a valid way of building and maintaining knowledge about patient prognosis, the value of diagnostic tests, and the efficacy of treatment.
2. The study and understanding of basic mechanisms of disease and pathophysiologic principles are a sufficient guide for clinical practice.
3. A combination of thorough traditional medical training and common sense are sufficient to evaluate new tests and treatments.
4. Content expertise and clinical experience are a sufficient base from which to generate valid guidelines for clinical practice.

When adapting this framework to the practical setting of patient care, various strategies can be used to address pertinent clinical questions. Dependence on clinical experience or reflection on underlying biologic mechanisms might guide decisions, while reference to textbooks and consultation with local experts are also options.

Reading the introduction and discussion sections of an article might be regarded as sufficient to glean the required information from a selected journal. This paradigm values what has been termed "traditional scientific authority".[17]

In contrast, the assumptions of the new paradigm have been articulated as follows[17]:

1. Clinical experience and the development of clinical instincts (particularly with respect to diagnosis) are a crucial and necessary part of becoming a competent physician. Many aspects of clinical practice cannot, or will not, ever be adequately tested. Clinical experience and its lessons are particularly important in these situations. At the same time, systematic attempts to record observations in a reproducible and unbiased fashion markedly increase the confidence one can have in knowledge about patient prognosis, the value of diagnostic tests, and the efficacy of treatment. In the absence of systematic observation, one must be cautious in the interpretation of information derived from clinical experience and intuition; it may at times be misleading.
2. The study and understanding of basic mechanisms of disease are necessary but insufficient guides for clinical practice. The rationales for diagnosis and treatment, which follow from basic pathophysiologic principles, may in fact be incorrect, leading to inaccurate predictions about the performance of diagnostic tests and the efficacy of treatment.
3. Understanding certain rules of evidence is necessary to correctly interpret literature on causation, prognosis, diagnostic tests, and treatment strategies.

In adhering to these principles, clinicians are required routinely to track and critically appraise the original literature on topics of interest and apply the results of such exercises to clinical problem solving and the provision of exemplary patient care. It also needs to be recognized that definitive answers may not always be forthcoming and that management decisions may therefore need to be made despite relative uncertainty about whether the desired outcome is possible. This new paradigm places a lower premium on "authority" but presupposes, instead, that physicians can learn to make independent assessments of available evidence and thereby judge the credibility of expert opinion. This does not necessarily imply total rejection of traditional scientific authority, since it is a given that much can be learned from colleagues and teachers whose years of experience have provided them with clinical acumen that can never be gained from formal scientific investigation. A final assumption of the new paradigm is that evidence-based practice results in better patient care.[17]

FRAMEWORK FOR CRITICAL APPRAISAL

Critical appraisal has been defined as the ability to read original research, to make a judgment on its scientific value, and to consider how its results can be applied in practice.[18] It requires the application of certain rules of evidence to published data to determine their validity and applicability.[19,20]

The process is directed toward the efficient extraction of relevant and methodologically robust data to address a pertinent clinical or research question. By providing a mechanism for excluding less rigorous (and often anecdotal) studies on the subject of interest, critical appraisal also helps the clinician or researcher reduce the volume of material that might previously have required closer examination.

In the sports medicine literature, as in the broader biomedical literature, most research concentrates on one of four principal themes: causal relationships, risk and prognosis, effectiveness of therapy, and selection of diagnostic tests. Critical appraisal criteria have been developed for each of these.[16,20] In addition, there are guidelines for the qualitative evaluation of systematic reviews and meta-analysis.[11,16,20]

Studies in Causation

Although cause-effect relationships are often inferred in the sports medicine literature, most of these associations lack enough evidence to advance the case for true causation. What is often overlooked is that in sports medicine, as in other areas of clinical investigation, cause-effect relationships may be difficult to prove. Nonetheless, it is possible to increase the likelihood of a cause-effect relationship by gathering empiric data to the extent that, for practical purposes, cause can be assumed. In contrast, evidence against causation can be accumulated until support for a cause-effect relationship becomes implausible.[21]

It is therefore helpful to identify the sort of evidence that, when present, will likely strengthen the case for causation. In most instances, the methodologic rigor of the research design will provide useful clues.[20,22] A good randomized controlled trial is recognized as the best way to determine cause-effect relationships in clinical studies, but for a variety of practical reasons, it is often not possible to utilize this design to explore certain research questions.[23,24] Instead, one or another of the observational study designs, such as cohort studies, case control studies, case series, or descriptive studies, might be used. These provide much weaker evidence for causal relationships.[25]

However, regardless of the one selected, it is important that the strongest possible study design has been used in a given circumstance. Moreover, when cohort or case-control studies are performed, it is essential that the determination of outcomes, in the former, and the clear distinction between cases and controls, in the latter, are free from discernible bias.[20] In general, the case for causation in observational studies needs to be carefully evaluated, and recognized criteria can be applied to facilitate this exercise.[20,21] These criteria include *temporality* (ie, the recognition that cause precedes effect); strength of association (ie, the observation that a large relative risk or odds ratio is better evidence for a causal relationship than a weak association is); the presence of *dose-response relationships* (ie, varying amounts of dose are related commensurately with varying amounts of effect); *reversibility* (ie, a reduction in exposure is associated with a lower rate of a particular condition); consistency (ie, the assertion that causal associations are strengthened when several studies, conducted at variable times and in different settings, all arrive at essentially the same conclusion); *biologic plausibility* (ie, the recognition that cause and effect are consistent with prevailing knowledge of the condition of interest); specificity (ie, a single cause and effect); and *analogy* (ie, cause-effect relationships have been demonstrated for a similar condition).

Establishing causation becomes more complicated when multiple factors might be contributing to an overall effect. For example, if one considers the possible intrinsic and extrinsic factors that have been implicated in one or another of the overuse syndromes, it is evident that a single or more dominant factor is often difficult to identify. To address this issue, Meeuwisse[26] has proposed a model that accommodates a multifactorial assessment of causation in athletic injuries. It is his contention that such an approach will promote better understanding of injury causation and might thereby assist in more rational development of treatment and prevention guidelines.

Studies on Risk and Prognosis

Though risk and prognosis have similar attributes, they occupy different time frames in the natural history of a condition. Risk factors are identified before the onset of the condition, and prognostic factors predict outcome once the condition has been recognized.[19,21]

In addition to predicting the occurrence of disease or injury, risk factors can help with diagnosis and can be applied in recommendations for disease or injury prevention. Identifying a risk factor increases the likelihood that a particular condition is present, and the diagnosis can thus be made earlier and with greater certainty. Moreover, when a risk factor for an illness has been found, its elimination can prevent future occurrences.[21]

It is important to recognize that risk factors need not be, and often are not, causes of disease or injury but may merely be markers of a particular condition. Moreover, by virtue of an association with some other determinants of the same condition, they may be confounded with causal factors. For example, it has been suggested that distance runners who "sometimes stretch" are at increased risk for musculoskeletal injuries.[27,28] However, this does not necessarily mean that "sometimes stretching" *causes* injury. Other factors may potentially provoke the same spectrum of morbidity. In effect, we know relatively little about risk factors for sport-related injuries, with existing data pertaining mainly to running injuries.[28–34]

When scrutinizing articles on prognosis, several factors need to be considered.[9,19–21,35,36] The most important of these is to determine whether an inception cohort was assembled. An inception cohort is a group of study subjects who have been identified at an early and uniform point in the conduct of a study (ie, at zero time). If the study has not identified an inception cohort, the subsequent course will lack precision and the outcome will likely be unpredictable. It is generally considered that the absence of a well-defined inception cohort constitutes a fatal flaw in the methodology of prognosis studies.

It is also essential that the pattern whereby subjects were entered into the study be satisfactorily described. This provides information about the participants and permits a judgment on the generalizability of the results. As well, knowledge of the referral pattern makes it easier to judge whether bias has been avoided.[20,25]

Follow-up is the next requirement of a prognosis study. All members of the inception cohort should be accounted for at the end of the study, and the reasons for any "dropouts" need to be clearly explained. Attrition usually does not occur without good reason, and may be associated with prognostic outcomes that need to be carefully considered when drawing inferences from the study's conclusions.[20]

Objective outcome measures should be developed and used in prognosis studies, and outcome assessments should be blinded. Without blinding, studies are more prone to diagnostic suspicion bias (ie, an investigator who knows that a study subject has an attribute of presumed importance will look much more carefully for the prognostic outcome of interest) or expectation bias (ie, prior knowledge of a particular attribute may influence subsequent clinical judgment). Adjustment for extraneous prognostic factors is another criterion that should be appraised.[25] For example, in the Ontario Cohort Study of Running Related Injuries, it appeared that taller runners may have been more prone to injury than their shorter counterparts. However, once the data were subjected to more robust interpretation (by multivariate, rather than univariate, analysis), the height factor did not feature as a significant risk factor.[28]

Choosing the Best Therapy

Clinicians are constantly required to judge whether a proposed treatment does more good than harm. In this area, perhaps more than in any other, the strength of the studies used to arrive at decisions is of the utmost importance. A well-conducted randomized controlled trial is generally accepted as the gold standard for determining the efficacy of any therapeutic intervention.[20,37] Usually, a large randomized controlled trial with clear-cut results and a low risk for error provides the best evidence for supporting a specific treatment strategy.[35,38] It must be recognized, however, that randomized controlled trials have potential weaknesses that need to be considered when exploring the effectiveness of specific interventions.[25]

When dealing with an article on therapy, three pertinent questions need to be addressed[3,4]:

1. *Are the results of the study valid?* It should be established whether the reported results reflect an unbiased estimate of the treatment effect. Primary and secondary guides have been proposed to assist with this exercise.[3,4]
   a. The primary guides require that the following questions be addressed:
      (1) Was the assignment of patients to treatments randomized?
      (2) Were all patients who entered the trial properly accounted for and attributed at its conclusion?
      (3) Was follow-up complete?
      (4) Were patients analyzed in the groups to which they were randomized?
   b. Questions contributing to the secondary guides are
      (1) Were patients, health workers, and study personnel blind to treatment?
      (2) Were the groups similar at the start of the trial?
      (3) Aside from the experimental intervention, were the groups treated equally?
2. *What were the results?* If the results have been judged as valid, then the second question examines the size and precision (ie, reliability or reproducibility) of the treatment effect. This effect is best represented by the study findings themselves, with superior precision in larger studies. As part of the recommended guides, two questions should be posed to assess the results:
   a. How large was the treatment effect?
   b. How precise was the estimate of the treatment effect?
3. *Will the results help me in caring for my patients?* Questions that address this issue are

a. Can the results be applied to (my) patient care?
b. Were all clinically important outcomes considered?
c. Are the likely treatment benefits worth the potential harm and costs?

Selecting a Diagnostic Test

The pertinent questions for appraising the clinical usefulness of a diagnostic test are similar to those proposed for choosing optimal therapy, and, as with therapy, guidelines have been formulated to enable practitioners to address these questions.[7,8,16,20]

When assessing validity of the study results, the primary guides address the following:

1. Was there an independent, blind comparison with a reference standard?
2. Did the patient sample include an appropriate spectrum of patients to whom the diagnostic test will be applied in clinical practice?

Questions included in the secondary guides are:

1. Did the results of the tests being evaluated influence the decision to perform the reference standard?
2. Were the methods for performing the test described in sufficient detail to permit replication?

When considering what the results are, the most important factor is to ensure that likelihood ratios are presented for the test results or, if not, whether the data necessary for their calculation are provided.[8]

Finally, when determining whether the results would be helpful in caring for your patients, the following questions are relevant:

1. Will the reproducibility of the test result and its interpretation be satisfactory in your setting?
2. Are the results applicable to your patient?
3. Will the results change your management?
4. Will patients be better off as a result of the test?

Assessing Reviews, Overviews, and Meta-Analyses

Review articles have long been regarded as a time-efficient resource for discussing a particular topic of interest, yet it is well recognized that they may vary in quality and completeness. This has prompted redefinition of the traditional review article. In current terms, a *review* can be regarded as any synthesis of the results and conclusions of two or more publications on a given topic. When strategies have been used to comprehensively identify and extract all of the available literature on the topic, the term *overview* is invoked. When the overview also utilizes a recognized statistical technique to bring together the results of several studies into a single estimate, the resulting publication is termed a *meta-analysis*.[20,39] While meta-analyses are still uncommon in sports sciences literature, reviews and overviews appear frequently and often provide a basis for drawing inferences about causation, prognosis, and clinical management.[40,41]

When subjecting a "quality filter" to articles of this sort, the following issues should be addressed[20,35,39]:

1. Were the questions and methods clearly stated?
2. Were the search methods used to locate relevant studies comprehensive?
3. Were explicit methods used to determine which articles to include?
4. Was the methodologic quality of the primary studies evaluated?
5. Were the selection and assessment of the primary studies reproducible and free of bias?
6. Were differences in individual study results adequately explained?
7. Were the results of the primary studies combined appropriately?
8. Were the reviewer's conclusions supported by the data cited?

These criteria have been updated and redefined as users' guides.

Many of these guidelines specifically examine the qualities of the individual articles that contribute to the review, and unless there is confidence that the contributing studies are methodologically sound and free of bias, the message conveyed by the review may lack validity. Moreover, a good review will expand on areas of potential (or real) disagreement between different studies on the same topic and provide enough detail on the primary studies to enable the reader to critically evaluate the rationale for the reviewer's conclusions. Any review that overinterprets the available data or provides a recommendation that lacks supporting evidence should be regarded with scepticism.

A series of the most up-to-date and methodologically robust systemic reviews on a variety of health care topics has been compiled under the auspices of the Cochrane Collaboration and can be accessed through the Cochrane Database.[37,41,42]

Critical Appraisal of Other Types of Studies

Sets of critical appraisal guidelines have also been proposed for studies on screening, quality of care, and economic analyses and can be reviewed through their original sources.[25] As well, users' guides have been published on clinical decision analysis,[12] clinical practice guidelines,[6,13] and the grading of health care recommendations.[5]

QUALITY OF THE SPORTS MEDICINE LITERATURE

To examine the robustness of sports medicine research in general, a study has been reported in which a selection of the literature, for a specified 12-months, was critically appraised.[43–45] Of the 756 papers reviewed according to specific criteria, 606 (80%) were original research studies. Of these, 182 had used an epidemiologic approach, and of those that did, only 8% were randomized controlled trials. Thirty-seven percent used a cohort study design, 35% were cross-sectional studies, 13% were case series, and 7% used case-control methods. The most commonly recorded weaknesses in this literature sample were overinterpretation of numerator-based case series data (implying nonrecognition of the limitations of this design), inadequate attention to power (ie, sample size) considerations in study design, and the frequent lack of randomization or the exclusion of a control group in studies where such elements of methodology were considered essential.

These findings reflect prevailing standards in several other subspecialty literatures, where observational studies inevitably outnumber randomized controlled trials (and even a proportion of the randomized controlled trials are much less rigorous than what might be considered

ideal). Given this reality, we need to be especially aware of the potential strengths and weaknesses of specific study designs and inferences that might safely be drawn from them. For further information on study design, the reader is referred, in particular, to texts by Sackett et al[20] and Fletcher et al[21] and to in-depth review by Casperson[23] and Walter and Hart.[45]

CONCLUSIONS

Since the earliest practice of medicine, physicians have been guided by the necessity to do what is best for their patients. As empiricism has given way to an emerging science, clinical decision making has become easier to defend. Biologic mechanisms, once explored and understood, have provided a foundation for diagnosis and therapy, and new technologies have offered often useful avenues for dealing with obscure or difficult problems.[46]

The information explosion of the past several years has generated a complex and often unwieldy biomedical literature, and it has therefore become increasingly necessary to develop ways of dealing effectively with the literature itself. Principles of critical appraisal have given initial expression to a developing methodology for selecting the best studies as a basis for rationalizing clinical decisions, and by building on these, EBM has added a further level of sophistication to a discipline that is now widely accepted as the yardstick for using the best available evidence as a vehicle for optimizing patient care.[46]

Perhaps the major challenge facing EBM is how to convince the skeptical and the uninitiated to use it in daily patient care. Learning a new set of skills, however useful, can be daunting for already overworked clinicians, and their routine application might require some fundamental changes of habit and pattern of practice. It has been suggested that the acceptance of EBM will increase only when high-quality evidence becomes easier to identify, all published recommendations (eg, guidelines and consensus conferences) include explicit statements about levels of evidence, and systems become more available to access EBM resources in as close to real time as possible.[46–48] The further development of user-friendly electronic modules will be important steps in these directions.

But accept it or not, EBM appears to be here to stay.[46] Conferences and workshops are providing effective forums for learning and applying EBM principles, and Internet sites are also available for those who are interested. Medical institutions and policy makers have embraced the EBM concept and are beginning to work collaboratively toward developing methodologic standards for "evidence-based health care."

REFERENCES

1. Altman DG: The scandal of poor medical research. Br Med J 308:283–284, 1994
2. Guyatt GH, Rennie D: Users' guides to the medical literature. JAMA 270:2096–2097, 1993
3. Guyatt GH, Sackett DL, Cook DJ: Users' guide to the medical literature. Part II. How to use an article about therapy or prevention: A. Are the results of the study valid? JAMA 270:2598–2601, 1993
4. Guyatt GH, Sackett DL, Cook DJ: Users' guide to the medical literature. Part II. How to use an article about therapy or prevention: B. What were the results and will they help me in caring for my patients? JAMA 271:59–63, 1994
5. Guyatt GH, Sackett DL, Sinclair JC, et al: Users' guide to the medical literature. Part IX. A method for grading health care recommendations. JAMA 274:1800–1804, 1995
6. Hayward RSA, Wilson MC, Tunis SR, et al: Users' guide to the medical literature. Part VIII. How to use clinical practice guidelines. A. Are the recommendations valid? JAMA 274:570–574, 1995
7. Jaeschke R, Guyatt GH, Sackett DL: Users' guide to the medical literature: how to use an article about a diagnostic test. A. Are the results of the study valid? JAMA 271:389–391, 1994
8. Jaeschke R, Guyatt GH, Sackett DL: Users' guide to the medical literature: how to use an article about a diagnostic test. B. What are the results and will they help me in caring for my patient? JAMA 271:703–707, 1994
9. Laupacis A, Wells G, Richardson WS, Tugwell P: Users' guide to the medical literature: how to use an article about prognosis. JAMA 272:234–237, 1994
10. Oxman AD, Sackett DL, Guyatt GH: Users' guide to the medical literature. I. How to get started. JAMA 270:2093–2095, 1993
11. Oxman AD, Cook DJ, Guyatt GH: Users' guide to the medical literature. VI. How to use an overview. JAMA 272:1367–1371, 1994
12. Richardson WS, Detsky AS: Users' guide to the medical literature. VII. How to use a clinical decision analysis. JAMA 273:1292–1295, 1995
13. Wilson MC, Hayward RSA, Tunis SR, et al: Users' guide to the medical literature. Part VIII. How to use clinical practice guidelines. JAMA 274:1630–1632, 1995
14. Sackett DL, Rosenberg WMC, Gray JAM, et al: Evidence-based medicine: what it is and what it isn't. Br Med J 312:71–72, 1996
15. Sackett DL: Evidence-based medicine: a new approach to teaching the practice of medicine. JAMA 268:2420–2425, 1992
16. Sackett DL, Richardson WS, Rosenberg W, Haynes RB: Evidence-Based Medicine. Churchill Livingstone, New York, 1997
17. Guyatt GH: The Evidence-Based Working Group: Evidence-based medicine. JAMA 268:2420–2425, 1992
18. Evidence-Based Practice in Primary Care. Silagy C, Haines A (eds): BMJ Books, London, 1998
19. Hart LE: Guidelines for evaluating future research in the epidemiology of sport injuries. In: Caine DJ, Caine CG, Lindner KJ (eds): Epidemiology of Sports Injuries. Human Kinetics Publishers, Champaign, IL, 1996, pp. 448–453
20. Sackett DL, Haynes RB, Guyatt GH, Tugwell P: Clinical Epidemiology: A Basic Science for Clinical Medicine, 2nd Ed. Little Brown & Co, Boston, 1991
21. Fletcher RH, Fletcher SW, Wagner EH: Clinical Epidemiology: The Essentials. 2nd Ed. Williams & Wilkins, Baltimore, 1988
22. Hart LE: Making the case for causation. Clin J Sports Med 4:276, 1994
23. Casperson CJ: Physical activity epidemiology: concepts, methods, and applications to exercise science. Exerc Sports Sci Rev 17:423–473, 1989
24. Horwitz RI: The experimental paradigm and observational studies of cause-effect relationships in clinical medicine. J Chronic Dis 40:91–99, 1987
25. Rosser WW, Shafir MS: Evidence-Based Family Medicine. B.C. Decker, Hamilton, Ont, Canada, 1998
26. Meeuwisse WH: Assessing causation in sport injury: a multifactorial model. Clin J Sports Med 4:166–170, 1994
27. Hart LE, Walter SD, McIntosh JM, Sutton JR: The effect of stretching and warmup on the development of musculoskeletal injuries in distance runners. Med Sci Sport Exerc 21(2)(Suppl):S59, 1989
28. Walter SD, Hart LE, McIntosh JM, Sutton JR: The Ontario cohort study of running-related injuries. Arch Intern Med 149:2561–2564, 1989
29. Blair SN, Kohl HW: Rates and risks for running and exercise injuries: studies in three populations. Res Q Exerc Sports 58:221–228, 1987
30. Hart LE: Exercise and soft tissue injury. Balliere's Clin Rheumatol 8:137–148, 1994

31. Koplan JP, Powell KE, Sikes RK, et al: An epidemiologic study of the benefits and risks of running. JAMA 248:3118–3121, 1982

32. Macera CA, Pate RR, Powell KE, et al: Predicting lower extremity injuries among habitual runners. Arch Intern Med 149:2565–2568, 1989

33. Macera CA: Lower extremity injuries in runners: advances in prediction. Sports Med 13:50–57, 1992

34. Marti B, Vader JP, Minder CE, Abelin T: On the epidemiology of running injuries: the 1984 Bern Grand-Prix Study. Am J Sports Med 16:285–294, 1988

35. Hart LE: The role of evidence in promoting consensus in the research literature. In: Bouchard C, Shephard RJ, Stephens T (eds): Physical Activity, Fitness, and Health: International Proceedings and Consensus Statement. Human Kinetics Publishers, Champaign, IL, 1994, pp. 89–97

36. Hart LE: Preventing prognostic pitfalls. Clin J Sports Med 6:270, 1996

37. Sackett DL: The Cochrane Collaboration. ACP J Club May/June:A11, 1994

38. Sackett DL: Rules of evidence and clinical recommendations on the use of antithrombotic agents. Chest 95(Suppl):2S–4S, 1989

39. Oxman AD, Guyatt GH: Guidelines for reading literature reviews. Can Med Assoc J 138:697–703, 1988

40. Hart LE, Meeuwisse WH: Reviews, overviews, and meta-analyses. Clin J Sports Med 5:206, 1995

41. Hart LE, Meeuwisse WH: Systematic reviews come of age: the Cochrane Collaboration. Clin J Sports Med 6:63, 1996

42. Bero L, Rennie D: The Cochrane Collaboration. JAMA 274:1935–1938, 1995

43. Hart LE, Walter SD: Critical appraisal of a selection of the sports medicine literature. Med Sci Sport Exerc 22(2)(Suppl):S116, 1990

44. Hart LE, Meeuwisse WH: Evaluating methodology in the sport medicine literature. Clin J Sports Med 4:64, 1994

45. Walter SD, Hart LE: Application of epidemiological methodology to sports and exercise science research. Exerc Sports Sci Rev 18:417–448, 1990

46. Hart LE: Putting principles into practice: the evolution of evidence-based medicine. Clin J Sports Med 7:311, 1997

47. Hart LE: Evidence-based medicine. Clin J Sports Med 4:198, 1994

48. Wallace EZ, Leipzig RM: Doing the right thing right: is evidence-based medicine the answer? Ann Intern Med 127:91–94, 1997

2

Cardiovascular Benefits and Precautions of Regular Physical Activity

CATHERINE DEMERS ■ NEVILLE SUSKIN ■ ROBERT S. McKELVIE

All parts of the body which have a function, if used in moderation and exercise in labours in which each is accustomed, become thereby healthy, well-developed and age slowly, but if unused and left idle they become liable to disease, defective growth, and age quickly (Hippocrates).[1]

Over the last 25 years there has been a steady decline in the age-adjusted cardiovascular mortality caused by coronary heart disease (CHD) and stroke.[2] Despite this decrease, cardiovascular disease remains the leading cause of death in North America. Known risk factors related to CHD include smoking, high blood pressure, elevated serum lipid levels, obesity, diabetes, and physical inactivity. Physical inactivity has become an important problem as newer technologies contribute to a more sedentary lifestyle. In the United States, one in four adults, more women than men, were reported to have a sedentary lifestyle with no leisure time physical activity (LTPA).[2]

In this chapter, we review the current data on the benefits and risks associated with regular physical activity in primary prevention. Recommendations for patient evaluation and precautions with exercise are addressed for healthy persons and patients with CHD.

PHYSICAL ACTIVITY, EXERCISE, AND FITNESS

Physical activity is defined as "any bodily movement produced by skeletal muscles that results in energy expenditure."[3] Moderate physical activity is equivalent to a brisk walk, and corresponds to an intensity of 3 to 6 metabolic equivalents (METs; 1 MET = $3.5 \, ml \, O_2/kg/min$). Exercise or exercise training denotes a subcategory of physical activity and is defined as "a planned, structured, and repetitive bodily movement done to improve or maintain one or more components of physical fitness."[3] Physical fitness is "a set of attributes that people have or achieve that relates to the ability to perform physical activity."[3] Physical fitness could also be defined as "the ability to pursue daily activities without fatigue."[4] Finally, physical inactivity is defined as a level of activity that is less than required to maintain good health.

EVIDENCE FOR BENEFITS OF PHYSICAL ACTIVITY

A large amount of evidence from epidemiologic studies supports the health benefits of physical activity. Studies have demonstrated a protective effect of physical activity on cardiovascular morbidity,[5–9] all-cause and cardiovascular mortality,[1,7,10–23] hypertension,[24,25] non-insulin-dependent diabetes mellitus,[26–28] osteoporosis,[29] and colon cancer.[30] Other benefits are also supported by experimental studies and include body composition,[31–33] blood lipid profile,[34] glucose tolerance, and insulin sensitivity.[35]

For more than 30 years, the benefits of physical activity have been evaluated on all-cause and cardiovascular mortality, demonstrating an inverse association between physical activity and CHD mortality.[1,9–16,36,37] These data on the benefits of physical activity come from cross-sectional surveys, case-control, and cohort studies, and have provided large amounts of evidence on the benefits of physical activity in a primary prevention setting. Randomized controlled trials have evaluated the effects of multiple risk factor modification interventions, including physical activity, on surrogate end points, such as changes in plasma lipids and blood pressure, but have not examined cardiovascular morbidity or mortality.[38–41] Conducting randomized controlled trials comparing a long-term exercise intervention to a usual care group and its effect on all-cause and cardiovascular mortality would present some feasibility issues because the intervention would continue over years and a large number of participants would be required to ensure a minimal number of events. Systematic overviews of the literature have provided further evidence of the benefits of regular physical activity on health.[5,42] In this chapter, we present data from prospective cohort studies and systematic overviews, because they represent the highest level of evidence available in the absence of randomized controlled clinical trials evaluating cardiovascular morbidity and mortality.

Effects of Physical Activity on Morbidity and Mortality

Earlier studies have evaluated the role of work-related physical activity and its benefit on reducing all-cause mortality and CHD.[6,21] Morris et al[6] evaluated the incidence of ischemic heart disease in 667 London male bus drivers, ages 30 to 69 years. Physical activity was defined by the occupational classification of the participants as sedentary (drivers) or active (conductors). During the 5-year follow-up, the incidence of ischemic heart disease was 1.8 for the drivers compared with the conductors.

Paffenbarger and Hale[21] evaluated the role of physical activity on coronary mortality in 6,351 longshoremen, ages 35 to 74 years at entry, in a prospective cohort study over 22 years. Work activity levels were classified as light, moderate, and heavy, and CHD deaths were recorded during the follow-up period. "Heavy work" was found to have a protective effect on fatal cardiovascular events. The relative risk (RR) of light to moderate physical activity was 1.8 compared with heavy levels of activity ($P < .001$) in all age groups, 1.7 in the 45- to 54-year age group

($P < .01$), and 2.1 in the 65- to 74-year age group ($P < .01$). Heavy work was protective of sudden death, with a RR of 2.9 for workers engaging in light and moderate work.

With the progressive decline of work-related physical activity, the role of LTPA has been examined in epidemiologic studies.[18,20,23,37] In a prospective cohort study, Morris et al[37] evaluated the relation of LTPA and fatal and nonfatal CHD in 17,994 middle-aged male civil servants over a mean duration of 8.5 years. A 48-hour recall questionnaire was used to determine the amount of physical activity performed by each subject. In this study, vigorous exercise was defined as energy expenditure of 7.5 kcal/min. Men, aged 40 to 65, participating in vigorous exercise had lower rates of fatal (1.1% vs 2.9%, $P < .001$) and nonfatal (2% vs 4%, $P < .001$) CHD events compared with men reporting no vigorous exercise.

Paffenbarger et al[18] evaluated LTPA with questionnaires to assess the role of physical activity and its relation to mortality in 16,936 Harvard alumni men free of documented CHD, ages 35 to 74. Physical activity was inversely associated with total mortality, due mainly to cardiovascular or respiratory causes. Higher levels of the physical activity index (PAI; $>2,000$ kcal) were associated with decreased death rates, with RR of 0.72 ($P < .0001$) compared with lower levels of activity. Clinical attributable risks were calculated, defined as the potential percentage reductions in the risk of death for persons who exchanged the adverse characteristics for more healthy ones, and demonstrated a 24% reduction in the risk of death for sedentary men who became more active.

The Iowa Women's Health Study[23] evaluated the relation between physical activity and all-cause mortality in postmenopausal women in a prospective cohort study with a 7-year follow-up. Women aged 55 to 69 years were randomly selected to fill out a questionnaire evaluating health habits, anthropometric measurements, and LTPA. A total of 40,417 women were eligible for follow-up, and women with baseline disease, such as cancer and CHD, were not excluded from this cohort. Higher levels of the PAI, based on the frequency and intensity of exercise, were associated with decreased all-cause mortality, with a multivariate-adjusted RR of 0.77 (95% confidence interval [CI], 0.69–0.86) for the medium PAI and 0.68 (95% CI, 0.60–0.77) for the high PAI. This study supports the evidence that regular physical activity is also beneficial in postmenopausal women by decreasing the risk for all-cause and cardiovascular mortality.

The Finnish Twin Cohort study[20] evaluated the relationship of LTPA and premature mortality in 7,925 healthy men and 7,977 healthy women. This prospective cohort study included twin pairs free of CHD, diabetes, and chronic obstructive pulmonary disease. Participants were mailed a questionnaire to evaluate physical activity, anthropometric measurements, smoking, and alcohol consumption. Baseline physical activity data were used in the mortality analysis, and data were collected from 1975 to 1994. Participants who reported exercising at least 6 times per month for a mean duration of at least 30 minutes and a mean intensity corresponding to at least vigorous walking to jogging were classified as conditioning exercisers. Participants were considered sedentary if not participating in LTPA. Adjusted odds ratios (for smoking, occupation, alcohol use, hypertension, and body mass index) showed a 30% and a 44% reduction in mortality, respectively, in occasional and conditioning exercisers.

Cardiorespiratory or physical fitness has been assessed with exercise testing in studies to further support the inverse association of physical activity and CVD mortality found in studies using physical activity questionnaires.[13,16] Ekelund et al[13] evaluated the relation between physical fitness and mortality from cardiovascular disease in asymptomatic men (n = 4,276), ages 30 to 69 at entry, in a prospective cohort study, The Lipid Research Clinics Prevalence Survey. Cardiovascular risk factors were assessed and physical fitness was measured, with heart rate at stage 2 of a modified Bruce protocol and the amount of time on a treadmill test. Some participants were excluded from the final analysis because of missing or incomplete exercise test data (n = 308) or use of medications that may affect heart rate (n = 213). The rate of death from CHD in healthy men was 0.26% (95% CI, 0–0.62) in the most fit men, and 1.69% (0.77–2.61) in the least fit men. Men with CHD had a RR of 3.4 for death from CHD, compared with the healthy group. Risk factors (total, low-density lipoprotein [LDL], and high-density lipoprotein [HDL] cholesterol and triglyceride levels, blood pres-

sure at rest and during exercise) were most favorable in men with the highest fitness levels.

Blair et al[16] studied the relation between the risk of all-cause and cause-specific mortality in healthy men (n = 10,224) and women (n = 3,120) who could achieve 85% of age-predicted maximal heart rate during a screening treadmill test. Treadmill time at baseline, and cardiovascular risk factors were recorded. Less-fit subjects were found to be at higher risk for death compared with women and men who were more fit. There was a linear trend in decreasing mortality from the least fit to the more fit quintiles for both men (64–18.6 per 10,000 person-years; slope, −4.5) and women (39.5–8.5 per 10,000 person-years; slope, 5.5).

Effects of Physical Activity/Fitness are Independent of Changes in Cardiovascular Risk Factors

Pekkanen et al[14] observed a group of 636 healthy Finnish middle-aged men for 20 years. Interviews and questionnaires recorded occupational activities and LTPA. At entry, 39% of the men were classified as having high overall physical activity, and 61% were defined as having low overall physical activity (sedentary or moderate occupational activity combined with walking, cycling, or cross-country skiing below the levels given above). Over the 20-year follow-up, men with high physical activity levels lived 2.1 years longer (P = .002) than those with low overall physical activity levels. This survival advantage persisted after adjustment for age, smoking, blood pressure, serum cholesterol, and body composition.

Blair et al[11] evaluated 25,341 men and 7,080 women, with an average follow-up of 8.4 and 7.5 years respectively, in a prospective cohort study quantifying the relation of cardiorespiratory fitness to CHD and all-cause mortality. Fitness was assessed using a maximal treadmill exercise test. Cardiovascular disease and all-cause mortality were significantly associated to low fitness, smoking, increased systolic blood pressure, elevated serum cholesterol level, and poor health status (abnormal electrocardiogram or chronic illness).

In summary, these studies indicate that the benefits of greater levels of physical fitness are independent of the effects of regular physical activity on risk factors for CHD. The mechanism through which physical fitness independently confers a survival benefit has not been determined.

Intensity of Physical Activity/Fitness Required to Alter Morbidity and Mortality

Results from a number of studies suggest that higher levels of physical activity are associated with lower incidence of total and cardiovascular mortality.[7,9,12,17,36] Morris et al[7] enrolled 9,376 healthy male civil servants, ages 45 to 64 at entry, to evaluate the role of LTPA on the incidence of coronary attacks and death rates in a prospective cohort study. A questionnaire was used to assess physical activity levels. Men involved in vigorous sports were found to have less than half the incidence of nonfatal and fatal CHD than the less active men. Nonvigorous exercise did not provide protection against CHD.

In the British Regional Heart Study, Shaper and Wannamethee[36] evaluated the relation between reported physical activity and nonfatal and fatal heart attacks in 7,735 men, ages 40 to 59 at entry. This prospective cohort study included men with preexisting ischemic heart disease, and physical activity was assessed with a questionnaire. Inactive men had significantly higher heart attack rates compared with all other men, with decreasing risk with increasing levels of physical activity ($P <.001$). Men who performed moderate to moderately vigorous activities had lower rates of events than did inactive or occasionally active men. The RR (adjusted for age, body mass index, social class, and smoking status) for myocardial infarction (MI) was only slightly reduced in men without preexisting CHD who were physically active, compared with those who were inactive (0.8; 95% CI, 0.4–1.4). A strong inverse relation remained between the risk for MI and physical activity in men without documented CHD.

In a Finnish cohort of 1,072 middle-aged men, Haapanen et al[17] prospectively evaluated the relation between LTPA, assessed with a questionnaire, with all-cause and cardiovascular mortality. Men with a low physical activity energy expenditure index (<800 kcal/wk) compared with considerably more active participants (>2,100 kcal/wk) were found to have an increased risk for all-cause mortality (RR = 2.74; 95% CI, 1.46–5.14; $P = .002$) and cardiovascular disease mortality (RR = 3.58; 95% CI, 1.45–8.85; $P = .006$).

Lakka et al[9] evaluated the independent relation between the type, duration, and intensity of LTPA assessed with questionnaires and with measured maximal oxygen uptake on a bicycle ergometer with the risk for MI in 1,453 men, ages 42 to 60, free of cardiovascular disease or cancer at baseline in a prospective cohort study. An inverse association between higher levels of both LTPA evaluated by questionnaire and physical fitness was found with the risk for MI. The RR for MI was 0.26 (95% CI, 0.10–0.68; $P = .006$) in the third of subjects with the highest maximal oxygen uptake (>2.7 L/min), compared with the third with the lowest level of conditioning.

Lee et al[12] evaluated the associations of vigorous activity (≥6 METs) and nonvigorous activity (<6 METs) of LTPA with longevity in men participating in the Harvard alumni prospective cohort study. Physical activity level and energy expenditure were estimated with a previously validated questionnaire. An inverse association, which was independent of other confounding factors, was observed between energy expenditure and mortality rate ($P <.001$). Vigorous activity was associated with longevity; nonvigorous activity was not.

Change in Physical Activity/Fitness Level on Morbidity and Mortality

Change in the level of physical activity has also been evaluated, and has been shown to decrease mortality. Paffenbarger et al[15] evaluated changes in physical activity and its association with lower rates of all-cause and CHD mortality in Harvard alumni men with questionnaires estimating energy expenditure. Men starting moderate physical activity levels (intensity ≥4.5 METs) had a 23% lower risk for mortality (95% CI, 4%–42%; $P = .015$) compared with those not participating in moderately vigorous sports. Favorable changes in lifestyle were associated with decreased all-cause mortality. Men who expended higher levels of activity (≥3,500 kcal/wk) had a 50% reduction in death compared with the least active men (<500 kcal/wk).

Blair et al[10] studied 9,777 men in a prospective cohort to evaluate the relationship between changes in physical fitness, assessed with a maximal treadmill test, and risk for mortality. The population was divided between healthy men and unhealthy men. Unhealthy men were defined as having one or more of the following conditions: MI, stroke, diabetes, or hypertension. Those who were initially unfit and became fit had a 44% lower age-adjusted risk for all-cause mortality (95% CI, 41%–75%) and a 52% lower age-adjusted risk for CVD mortality (95% CI, 31%–74%) than their peers who remained unfit. For each age group, men who were fit at both examinations had the lowest death rates.

Results of Systematic Overviews of Physical Activity on Mortality and Morbidity

Powell et al[5] performed a systematic overview of the literature to evaluate the relation between physical activity and the incidence of CHD. Although these authors did not report a pooled RR, the RR of CHD associated with inactivity varied from 1.5 to 2.4 (median, 1.9), and better quality studies, assessed with predetermined criteria, reported a higher RR.

Meta-analysis

Berlin and Colditz[42] summarized studies published until 1990 in a meta-analysis and further confirmed the inverse relation of physical activity and the decrease in all-cause and cardiovascular mortality. The primary analysis was performed by pooling results from work-related studies separately from LTPA studies. Studies that looked at both work and LTPA were included with the leisure activity group. The pooled RR from occupational studies for moderate activity compared with high activity for CHD death was 1.4 (95% CI, 1.2–1.8) in studies reporting both moderate and sedentary comparison groups, and 1.9 (95% CI, 1.6–2.2) for CHD death for sedentary compared with high-activity groups. These findings were similar in the nonoccupational studies, with a RR of 1.1 (95% CI, 1–1.3) for CHD death for the moderate activity group compared with the high-activity group, and 1.7 (95% CI, 1.2–2.3) for the sedentary group compared with the high-activity group.

Similarly to the findings of Powell et al,[5] studies of higher quality scores tended to have higher RR than studies with lower quality scores. The authors concluded that the protective effect of physical activity lay in the prevention of the occurrence of major cardiovascular effects, rather than reduction of the severity of events that occurred.

In summary, the evidence from numerous prospective cohort studies and systematic overviews are consistent with regard to the effects of physical activity on CHD events. The reduction in risk is related to the level of fitness and amount of activity performed. An increase in physical activity anytime in life results in a decrease in the risk of CHD morbidity or mortality. Furthermore, the effects of regular physical activity to decrease CHD event rate are independent of the effects on risk factors for CHD. With the cumulative evidence of the benefits of regular physical activity on CHD events in men and women, the National Institutes of Health Consensus Group[3] has proposed that all persons take part in regular moderate-intensity physical activity (energy expenditure of approximately 200 calories per day), for at least 30 minutes a day, and preferably every day of the week.

EXERCISE PRECAUTIONS

In general, three types of exercise act as stressors to the cardiovascular system: static, dynamic, and resistance (combination of static and dynamic).[43] Unless indicated to the contrary, this discussion is limited to dynamic exercise, which is defined as muscle contraction resulting in movement of the limb through a full range of motion.[43] *Grade of recommendation*[44] concludes each section (see Table 2–1).

Contraindications to Exercise Training

In general, the contraindications to exercise testing apply equally to exercise training, namely, unstable cardiac syndromes, severe noncardiac disease that precludes exercise, or significant locomotor disability (Table 2–2).

Guidelines for Exercise Participation

The American College of Cardiology (ACC) and the American Heart Association (AHA) have

TABLE 2–1. The Relation Between Levels of Evidence and Grades of Recommendations

Level of Evidence	Grade of Recommendation
Level I: Large randomized trials with clear-cut results (and low risk of error)	Grade A
Level II: Small randomized trials with uncertain results (and moderate to high risk of error)	Grade B
Level III: Nonrandomized, contemporaneous controls	Grade C
Level IV: Nonrandomized, historical controls	Grade C
Level V: No controls, case series only	Grade C

From Sackett DL: Levels of evidence and clinical decision making in rehabilitation: efficacy and outcomes. In: Basmajian JV, Banerjee SN (eds): Clinical decision making in rehabilitation. Churchill Livingstone, New York, 1996, pp. 1–4.

recently published guidelines for exercise testing.[45] In asymptomatic persons without known CHD, exercise testing in men older than 45 and women older than 55 who plan to start vigorous exercise is recommended with a Class IIb status (Table 2–3). These recommendations are complemented by those of the American College of Sports Medicine, which recommends that men older than 45, women older than 55, and younger individuals perceived to be at high risk for CHD (Table 2–4) undergo a medical examination and diagnostic exercise test before starting an exercise program at more than low level (>50% peak oxygen consumption).[43,46] In addition, all persons with established CHD should undergo a thorough clinical assessment, including an exercise test, before starting an exercise program.[46] After myocardial infarction, the current ACC/AHA Guidelines for Exercise Testing have assigned class I status to exercise testing for activity prescription and cardiac rehabilitation assessment.[45]

Risks of Exercise Training

Observational, case series, case control, and case-crossover designs have been used to study the risks of exercise training.[47–53] Age, presence of heart disease, and exercise intensity are the three most important factors that influence the cardiovascular risk from exercise. Ventricular fibrillation and myocardial ischemia are the respective causes of sudden cardiac death and myocardial infarction during exercise, with myocardial ischemia not necessarily preceding ventricular fibrillation.[54] Before an exercise program is started, medical clearance should be obtained unless the anticipated activity is low level (<50% of maximal exercise capacity).[43] This medical assessment should class people into three groups: the apparently healthy, unselected or mixed population, and those with presumed or documented cardiac disease.

Apparently Healthy Individuals

Gibbons et al[47] examined the activity records of 2,935 adults (1,001 women) over a 65-month period, with a mean age of 37 years (<30 years, n = 744; >60 years, n = 93). Each participant underwent a brief cardiovascular examination, rest and maximal exercise ECG prior to being entered in the program. In 374,798 person-hours of exercise performed there were two cardiac events. Both of these events involved men and were nonfatal. Adjusting for age, the 95% CI for the maximum risk estimates per 10,000

TABLE 2–2. Some Contraindications to Exercise Training

Less than 5 days after myocardial infarction
Unstable angina
Uncontrolled arrythmia
Severe aortic stenosis
Uncontrolled congestive heart failure
Acute pulmonary embolus
Acute myocarditis or pericarditis
Thrombosis of lower extremity
Acute noncardiac disorder that may be aggravated by exercise (eg, infection, thyrotoxicosis)
Physical disability that precludes safe exercise

Modified from Fletcher GF, Balady G, Froelicher VF, et al: Exercise standards: a statement for healthcare professionals from the American Heart Association. Special Report. Circulation 91:580, 1995

TABLE 2-3. ACC/AHA Guidelines for Exercise Testing

CLASS	GUIDELINE
I	Conditions for which there is evidence and/or general agreement that a given procedure or treatment is useful and effective
II	Conditions for which there is conflicting evidence and/or a divergence of opinion about the usefulness/efficacy of a procedure or treatment
IIa	Weight of evidence/opinion is in favor of usefulness/efficacy
IIb	Usefulness/efficacy is less well established by evidence/opinion
III	Conditions for which there is evidence and/or general agreement that the procedure/treatment is not useful/effective and in some cases may be harmful

Modified from Gibbons RJ, et al, for the ACC/AHA Task Force on Practice Guidelines: ACC/AHA guidelines for exercise testing: executive summary. A report of the ACC/AHA Task Force on Practice Guidelines (Committee on Exercise Testing). Circulation 96:345, 1997

person-hours of exercise were 0.3 to 2.7 for men and 0.6 to 6 for women. The estimates for women were based on the event rate for men and are inflated because of the lower number of exercise hours among the women. Most subjects were healthy, and the major types of activity performed were mainly intensive exercise, eg, running, basketball, and racquetball. As well, given the occurrence of only two cardiac events,

TABLE 2-4. Guidelines for Medical Examination and Diagnostic Exercise Testing Prior to Exercise Training

Workup is suggested for subjects with two or more of these risk factors for coronary artery disease
  Age: men, >45; women, >55
  Current smoker
  History of hypertension or blood pressure ≥140/90 on two separate occasions
  Family history of premature coronary artery disease (age <55 years for male and <65 yrs for female first-degree relative)
  Total serum cholesterol >5.2 mmol/L or high-density lipoprotein (HDL) cholesterol <0.9 mmol/L
  Diabetes, and age >30 years
  Sedentary lifestyle
If HDL >1.6 mmol/L, subtract 1 from the sum of positive risk factors

Modified from Lowensteyn I, Joseph L, Grover S: Who needs an exercise stress test? Evaluating the new American College of Sports Medicine risk stratification guidelines. J Cardiopulm Rehabil 17:253, 1997

the actual event rate is less useful than the message that the risk of exercise is likely low.

Thompson et al[48] investigated the 12 reported deaths that occurred in men while jogging during 1975 through 1980 in Rhode Island. A random digit telephone survey was conducted, which estimated the prevalence of at least twice a week jogging in men aged 30 through 64 years at (mean ± SE) 7.4% ± 2.6%. An annual death rate of 1 per 7,620 male joggers was calculated (95% CI, 1 in 2,000–13,000). From record review, an antemortem diagnosis of CHD was possible in 5 of the 12 deceased; thus, among asymptomatic 30- to 64-year-old joggers, the 95% CI for the annual death rate during jogging was 1 in 4,000 to 26,000 joggers. The authors then made the somewhat arbitrary assumption that each jogger performed 52 hours of jogging annually and so calculated a death rate during jogging of 1 death per 396,000 man-hours of jogging. This rate was seven times that expected during more sedentary activities. This latter comparison lacks validity, given the somewhat arbitrary assumption of the number of hours spent jogging annually.

Siscovick et al[49] were among the first investigators to examine, in a case-control study, whether habitual exercise decreased the risk of sudden death during acute exercise. The wives of previously well men aged 25 to 75 years who had experienced out-of-hospital sudden cardiac arrest were interviewed. The interview included information regarding LTPA over the previous year and CHD risk. Age-matched healthy male controls were randomly selected from the area of residence of the men, and their wives were interviewed in similar fashion. These data were used to calculate the RR for primary cardiac arrest during physical activity compared with during nonphysically active times, according to their physical activity levels. The RR of death during activity for men who were not regularly physically active (<20 minutes of high-intensity exercise per week) was 56 (95% CI, 23–131). The RR of death during activity for men who were regularly physically active (>140 minutes of high-intensity exercise per week) was 4 (95% CI, 2–14). In addition, despite adjustment for a history of hypertension and cigarette smoking, men who performed more than 20 minutes of high-intensity exercise per week had a significantly lower risk for sudden death at any time (RR, 0.4; 95% CI, 0.23–0.67) compared with men who performed less activity than this.

In conclusion, the evidence would suggest that the risk of physical activity in apparently healthy individuals is low (approximately 1 cardiac arrest per 565,000 hours of activity)[43] and that the risk is significantly reduced by habitual physical activity (*grade C recommendation*).

Mixed Populations

Recently, studies have examined the role of physical activity as a trigger for acute MI using a case-crossover design.[52,53] The Myocardial Infarction Onset Study investigators examined the risk of heavy physical exertion[52] and sexual activity[51] as triggers for MI in 1,228 and 1,774 patients, respectively. Approximately one third of these patients had a history of CHD. Patients underwent an extensive interview covering the day preceding the infarction to determine the frequency and level of physical activity and other triggers. Data for this "hazard period" immediately before MI onset were compared with either a "control period" at the same time on the day prior or the usual frequency of the activity.

Strenuous activity (≥6 METs) such as jogging, speed walking, or shoveling snow was reported by 4.4% of patients within 1 hour before MI symptom onset. The RR for MI onset in the hour following strenuous activity was 5.9 (95% CI, 4.6–7.7). The RR for MI decreased markedly with increasing habitual physical activity levels: sedentary individuals 107 (95% CI, 65–171); one or two sessions per week, 19.4 (95% CI, 9.9–38.1); three or four sessions per week, 8.6

(CI, 3.6–20.5); and five or more sessions per week, 2.4 (CI, 1.5–3.7).

Twenty-seven (3% of the 858 subjects who reported sexual activity in the year preceding the MI) reported sexual activity in the 2 hours preceding the MI, yielding a RR of 2.5 (95% CI, 1.7–3.7) for MI within 2 hours after sexual activity. The presence of CHD did not significantly increase this risk. This RR is consistent with the lower average energy expended during sexual activity (3–4 METs) compared with heavy exertion (≥6 METs). Again habitual physical activity appeared protective; the RR for MI onset in the 2 hours following sexual activity decreased from 3 to 1.9 to 1.2, respectively, in patients who engaged in heavy physical exertion once a week or less, twice a week, or three times a week. Despite the increased RR for MI during acute exercise, the absolute risk remained low, at about 1 : 565,000 person-hours of exercise in healthy individuals and only 1 : 60,000 person-hours of exercise for patients with CHD.[55]

The evidence seems to suggest that habitual physical activity reduces the risk for MI associated with acute exertion.

The Triggers and Mechanisms of Myocardial Infarction Study Group,[53] in a combined case-crossover and case-control study, interviewed approximately 1,200 (74% male) patients, ages (mean ± SD) 61 ± 9 years, 13 ± 6 days after MI. Approximately 20% to 25% had a history of previous MI. Cases were compared with themselves at an earlier time, and with age- and gender-matched controls from the same area, to determine the risk of physical activity for MI. The odds ratio (95% CI) for the patients compared with the matched controls of having engaged in strenuous physical activity (≥6 METs) at the onset of MI was 2.1 (1.1–3.6). The case-crossover comparison yielded a similar RR of 2.1 (1.6–3.1) of having engaged in strenuous physical activity (≥6 METs) within 1 hour of the onset of MI. Habitual physical activity significantly reduced these risks; patients exercising fewer than four times a week had a significantly greater RR for MI compared with those who exercised four times a week (6.9 vs 1.3; P <.01). Given that only patients who exerted themselves reasonably often and for whom complete information was available were included in this analysis, these results are compatible with those of the Myocardial Infarction Onset Study.[52]

In summary, physical exertion significantly increases the RR of a MI in mixed populations. This is especially evident in sedentary individuals (RR, 100); however, in those who habitually exercise, this risk is significantly reduced (RR, 2–3). Despite this increase in RR, the absolute risk of MI following activity remains low, from 1:565,000 person-hours of exercise in healthy individuals to 1:60,000 person-hours of exercise for patients with CHD. Sexual activity is associated with a similar increase in the risk for MI in those with and without CHD, with habitual physical activity reducing this risk. Therefore, physical activity is safe for those in whom the diagnosis of CHD is uncertain (*grade C recommendation*).

Presumed or Documented CHD

Haskell[56] obtained information by survey about events occurring from 1960 through 1977 in 30 post-MI cardiac rehabilitation programs. During this period, 13,570 patients had contributed 1,629,634 hours of exercise. Sixty-one major cardiovascular events were reported, including 50 cardiac arrests (eight fatal) and seven MIs (two fatal). This breaks down to one cardiac event per 32,593 patient hours of exercise, and one cardiac event per 271 participants. The risk of death of 1 per 116,000 patient hours of exercise was comparable with that in the general post-MI population (sedentary) at that time.

Van Camp and Peterson[55] updated this database with a retrospective survey from 142 randomly selected cardiac rehabilitation programs from 1980 through 1984. In the majority of patients (no percentage was given), CHD was the primary diagnosis. Patients at both high risk (eg, poor left ventricular function, prior cardiac arrest) and low risk were included. Programs provided target training heart rates based on a percentage of the maximal heart rate at a preparticipation maximal exercise stress test. More than 51,000 patients participated in the rehabilitation programs, performing more than 2.3 million hours of exercise. Twenty-one cardiac arrests (three fatal) and eight MIs (all nonfatal) were documented by the survey. These findings represent event rates of one cardiac arrest per 112,000 patient hours of exercise, one fatal cardiac arrest per 784,000 patient-hours of exercise, and one nonfatal MI per 294,000 patient hours of exercise. The use of ECG monitoring or size

of the program did not have a significant effect on the cardiac event rate.

The authors concluded that adverse cardiac events were rare during prescribed outpatient cardiac rehabilitation exercise training. Critical examination of the data demonstrates that expressing adverse events per hour of patient exercise is less useful from a clinical or statistical perspective than expressing adverse events per patient participating in the program.

Clinically, physicians and patients are interested in the likelihood that a patient will experience an event because expressing events per patient-hour of exercise implies that the longer a patient trains, the more likely he or she will experience an event. This has never been demonstrated, however. Given that multiple events per patient did not occur and no interaction was reported between duration of exercise training and occurrence of events, expressing events per hours of patient exercise may inflate the denominator and falsely decrease the adverse event rate.

However, even expressing the rate of adverse events per patient yields one cardiac arrest per 2,443 patients, one fatal cardiac arrest per 17,101 patients, and one nonfatal MI per 6,413 patients, all very low. Finally, the authors suggest that there has been an approximate 72% decrease in cardiac arrest during exercise from the 1970s (one cardiac arrest per 32,500 patient-hours of exercise)[56] to the 1980s (one cardiac arrest per 112,000 patient hours of exercise),[55] based on events per patien-hours of exercise. Expressing event rates per patient appear to demonstrate this decline even more dramatically (one cardiac arrest per 271 patients vs one per 2,443 patients, an 89% decrease). Advances in medical care over this period may explain some of this improvement in outcome.

In conclusion, the data suggest that the cardiac event rate is low among participants in post-MI rehabilitation exercise programs and that the event rate has substantially decreased over time (*grade C recommendation*).

SUMMARY AND CONCLUSION

Convincing evidence of the cardiovascular benefits of physical activity have been demonstrated in large epidemiologic studies and systematic overviews. Most individuals are at a low risk for fatal events and can take part in moderate-intensity physical activity without consulting a physician or further testing. Individuals with documented CHD, men older than 40, and women older than 50 with multiple risk factors should undergo appropriate evaluation before initiating an exercise program.

Appropriate evaluation and exercise prescription in individuals at high risk may reduce the risk of performing regular physical activity, and these individuals will further benefit from the effects of physical activity. Finally, to further encourage regular physical activity as a primary and secondary prevention tool, we must find new ways of initiating and maintaining lifelong programs in the general population as well as in patients with established CHD.

REFERENCES

1. Leon AS, Connett J, Jacobs DR, et al: Leisure-time physical activity levels and risk of coronary heart disease and death: the Multiple Risk Factor Intervention Trial. JAMA 258:2388, 1987
2. Physical activity and cardiovascular health: NIH Consensus Development Panel on Physical Activity and Cardiovascular Health. JAMA 276:241, 1996
3. Pate RR, Pratt M, Blair S, et al: Physical activity and public health: a recommendation from the Centers for Disease Control and Prevention and the American College of Sports Medicine. JAMA 273:402, 1995
4. US Department of Health and Human Services: Physical activity and health: a report of the Surgeon General. Department of Health and Human Services, Centers for Disease Control and Prevention, National Center for Chronic Disease Prevention and Health Promotion, Bethesda, MD, 1996
5. Powell KE, Thompson PD, Caspersen CJ, et al: Physical activity and the incidence of coronary heart disease. Ann Rev Public Health 8:253, 1987
6. Morris JN, Kagan A, Pattison DC, et al: Incidence and prediction of ischaemic heart-disease in London busmen. Lancet 2:553, 1966
7. Morris JN, Clayton DG, Everitt MG, et al: Exercise in leisure time: coronary attack and death rates. Br Heart J 63:325, 1990
8. Young DR, Haskell WL, Jatulis DE, et al: Associations between changes in physical activity and risk factors for coronary heart disease in a community-based sample of men and women: the Stanford five-city project. Am J Epidemiol 138:205, 1993
9. Lakka TA, Venalainen JM, Rauramaa R, et al: Relation of leisure-time physical activity and cardiorespiratory fitness to the risk of acute myocardial infarction in men. N Engl J Med 330:1549, 1994
10. Blair SN, Kohl HW III, Barlow CE, et al: Changes in physical fitness and all-cause mortality: a prospective study of healthy and unhealthy men. JAMA 273:1093, 1995
11. Blair SN, Kampert JB, Kohl HW III, et al: Influences of cardiorespiratory fitness and other precursors on cardiovascular disease and all-cause mortality in men and women. JAMA 276:205, 1996
12. Lee I-M, Hsieh C-C, Paffenbarger RS: Exercise intensity and longevity in men: the Harvard Alumni Health Study. JAMA 273:1179, 1995
13. Ekelund LG, Haskell WL, Johnson JL, et al: Physical fitness as a predictor of cardiovascular mortality in asymptomatic North American men. The Lipid Research Clinics mortality follow-up study. N Engl J Med 319:1379, 1988
14. Pekkanen J, Marti B, Nissinen A, et al: Reduction of premature mortality by high physical activity: a 20-year follow-up of middle-aged Finnish men. Lancet 1:1473, 1987
15. Paffenbarger RS, Hyde RT, Wing AL, et al: The association of changes in physical-activity level and other lifestyle characteristics with mortality among men. N Engl J Med 328:538, 1993
16. Blair SN, Kohl HW III, Paffenbarger RS, et al: Physical fitness and all-cause mortality: a prospective study of healthy men and women. JAMA 262:2395, 1989
17. Haapanen N, Miilunpalo S, Vuori I, et al: Characteristics of leisure time physical activity associated with decreased risk of premature all-cause and cardiovascular disease mortality in middle-aged men. Am J Epidemiol 143:870, 1996
18. Paffenbarger RS, Hyde RT, Wing AL, et al: Physical activity, all-cause mortality, and longevity of college alumni. N Engl J Med 314:605, 1986
19. Kaplan GA, Strawbridge WJ, Cohen RD, et al: Natural history of leisure-time physical activity and its correlates: associations with mortality from all causes and cardiovascular disease over 28 years. Am J Epidemiol 144:793, 1996
20. Kujala UM, Kaprio J, Sarna S, et al: Relationship of leisure-time physical activity and mortality: the Finnish Twin Cohort. JAMA 279:440, 1998
21. Paffenbarger RS, Hale WE: Work activity and coronary heart mortality. N Engl J Med 292:545, 1975
22. Chave SP, Morris JN, Moss S, et al: Vigorous exercise in leisure time and death rate: a study of male civil servants. J Epidemiol Community Health 32:239, 1978
23. Kushi LH, Fee RM, Folsom AR, et al: Physical activity and mortality in post-menopausal women. JAMA 277:1287, 1997

24. Blair SN, Goodyear NN, Gibbons LW, et al: Physical fitness and incidence of hypertension in healthy normotensive men and women. JAMA 252:487, 1984

25. Paffenbarger RS, Wing AL, Hyde RT, et al: Physical activity and incidence of hypertension in college alumni. Am J Epidemiol 117:245, 1983

26. Helmrich SP, Ragland DR, Leung RW, et al: Physical activity and reduced occurrence of non-insulin-dependent diabetes mellitus. N Engl J Med 325:147, 1991

27. Manson JE, Nathan DM, Krolewski AS, et al: A prospective study of exercise and incidence of diabetes among US male physicians. JAMA 268:63, 1992

28. Manson JE, Rimm EB, Stampfer MJ, et al: Physical activity and incidence of non-insulin-dependent diabetes mellitus in women. Lancet 338:774, 1991

29. Snow-Harter C, Marcus R: Exercise, bone mineral density, and osteoporosis. Exerc Sport Sci Rev 19:351, 1991

30. Lee I, Paffenbarger RS, Hsieh C: Physical activity and the risk of developing colorectal cancer among college alumni. J Natl Cancer Inst 83:1324, 1991

31. Bouchard C, Despres JP, Tremblay A: Exercise and obesity. Obesity Res 1:133, 1993

32. Pavlou K, Krey S, Steffee WP: Exercise as an adjunct to weight loss and maintenance in moderately obese subjects. Am J Clin Nutr 49:1115, 1989

33. Wood PD, Stefanick ML, Williams PT, et al: The effects of plasma lipoproteins of prudent weight-reducing diet, with or without exercise, in overweight men and women. N Engl J Med 325:461, 1991

34. Haskell WL: The influence of exercise training on plasma lipids and lipoproteins in health and disease. Acta Med Scand 711(suppl):25, 1986

35. Koivisto VA, Yki-Jarvinen H, DeFronzo RA: Physical training and insulin sensitivity. Diabetes Metab Rev 1:445, 1986

36. Shaper AG, Wannamethee G: Physical activity and ischaemic heart disease in middle-aged British men. Br Heart J 66:384, 1991

37. Morris JN, Everitt MG, Pollard R, et al: Vigorous exercise in leisure-time: protection against coronary heart disease. Lancet 2:1207, 1980

38. King AC, Haskell WL, Taylor CB, et al: Group-vs home-based exercise training in healthy older men and women: a community-based clinical trial. JAMA 266:1535, 1991

39. Katzel LI, Bleecker ER, Colman EG, et al: Effects of weight loss vs aerobic exercise training on risk factors for coronary disease in healthy, obese, middle-aged and older men: a randomized controlled trial. JAMA 274:1915, 1995

40. Dunn AL, Marcus BH, Kampert JB, et al: Reduction in cardiovascular disease risk factors: 6-month results from project Active. Prev Med 26:883, 1997

41. Stefanick ML, Mackey S, Sheehan M, et al: Effects of diet and exercise in men and postmenopausal women with low levels of HDL cholesterol and high levels of LDL cholesterol. N Engl J Med 339:12, 1998

42. Berlin JA, Colditz GA: A meta-analysis of physical activity in the prevention of coronary heart disease. Am J Epidemiol 132:612, 1990

43. Fletcher GF, Balady G, Froelicher VF, et al: Exercise standards: a statement for healthcare professionals from the American Heart Association: special report. Circulation 91:580, 1995

44. Sackett DL: Levels of evidence and clinical decision making in rehabilitation: efficacy and outcomes. In: Basmajian JV, Banerjee SN (eds): Clinical decision making in rehabilitation. Churchill Livingstone, New York, 1996, pp. 1–4

45. Gibbons RJ, et al, for the ACC/AHA Task Force on Practice Guidelines: ACC/AHA guidelines for exercise testing: Executive Summary: a report of the ACC/AHA Task Force on Practice Guidelines (Committee on Exercise Testing). Circulation 96:345, 1997

46. American College of Sports Medicine: Guidelines for exercise testing and prescription, 5th Ed. Williams & Wilkins, Baltimore, 1995, pp. 18–25

47. Gibbons LW, Cooper KH, Meyer BM, et al: The acute cardiac risk of strenuous exercise. JAMA 244:1799, 1980

48. Thompson PD, Funk EJ, Carleton RA, et al: Incidence of death during jogging in Rhode Island from 1975 through 1980. JAMA 247:2535, 1982

49. Siscovick DS, Weiss NS, Fletcher RH, et al: The incidence of primary cardiac arrest during vigorous exercise. N Engl J Med 311:874, 1984

50. Tofler GH, Mittleman MA, Muller JE: Physical activity and the triggering of myocardial infarction: the case for regular exercise. Heart 75:323, 1996

51. Muller JE, Mittleman MA, Maclure M, et al: Triggering myocardial infarction by sexual activity: low absolute risk and prevention by regular physical exertion: Determinants of Myocardial Infarction Onset Study investigators. JAMA 275:1405, 1996

52. Mittleman MA, Maclure M, Tofler GH, et al: Triggering of acute myocardial infarction by heavy physical exertion: protection against triggering by regular exertion. N Engl J Med 329:1677, 1993

53. Willich SN, Lewis M, Lowel H, et al: Physical exertion as a trigger of acute myocardial infarction. N Engl J Med 329:1684, 1993

54. Cobb LA, Weaver WD: Exercise: a risk for sudden death in patients with coronary disease. J Am Coll Cardiol 7:215, 1986

55. Van Camp SP, Peterson RA: Cardiovascular complications of outpatient cardiac rehabilitation programs. JAMA 256:1160, 1986

56. Haskell WL: Cardiovascular complications during exercise training of cardiac patients. Circulation 57:920, 1978

3

Nutritional Strategies, Including Creatine Supplementation, to Promote Muscle Function Recovery

BRIAN D. ROY ■ MARK A. TARNOPOLSKY

Many diseases and acute trauma injuries are characterized by accelerated muscle proteolysis, which is the primary cause of the loss of lean body mass characteristic of such conditions. The loss of muscle mass and function in such hospitalized patients is multifactorial and includes decreased physical activity, decreased energy and protein intake, and alterations in protein metabolism, all of which contribute to the net loss of muscle mass (atrophy). This catabolic metabolic milieu is further compounded by the fact that many patients are relatively immobile and de-conditioned prior to admission.

The loss of nitrogen from the body is due to an imbalance between protein synthesis and catabolism.[1,2] Net protein balance is a function of synthesis (SYN) and catabolism (CAT), and can thus be negatively influenced under any of the following circumstances:

- ↓ SYN, ↑ CAT
- ↓ SYN, CAT →
- SYN →, ↑ CAT
- ↓↓ SYN, ↓ CAT

It appears that synthesis is the predominant process regulated in response to physiologic stressors and that catabolism usually follows directionally[2-4]; however, under certain circumstances, protein breakdown may be directly regulated.[5] Protein synthesis depends upon the availability of substrate (nutrition)[6,7] and is significantly depressed after surgery[1,4,6] and with immobilization.[8] Therefore, the development of

countermeasures to these possible changes has been a primary focus in an attempt to both prevent and overcome such decreases in lean body mass.

The many factors that can influence protein metabolism include hormonal status, nutritional status or intake, and physical activity, all of which can be manipulated to potentially minimize loss of lean body mass or to maximize gains in lean body mass to maximize rates of recovery. Countermeasures that have been examined to date include physical exercise, nutritional supplements, growth factors, and anticatabolic agents. This chapter reviews the basics of protein turnover, with emphasis on the influence of exercise, hormones, and nutritional supplements. A complete review of these factors would require a dedicated book, and the aim here is to provide an understanding of the basic processes. An attempt is made to suggest strategies that may be beneficial for the patient participating in a therapeutic exercise program. A short section on practical guidelines ends the chapter.

PROTEIN METABOLISM

Skeletal muscle is a tissue that depends on both aerobic and anaerobic energy production pathways. The primary substrates used to produce adenosine triphosphate (ATP) aerobically are fat and carbohydrate. There is a small contribution to ATP production from protein oxidation. For example, during prolonged endurance exercise, ATP derived from protein oxidation represents approximately 3% to 6% of the total energy expended.[9,10] Human skeletal muscle has the capacity to oxidize seven amino acids: alanine, asparagine, aspartate, glutamate, isoleucine, leucine, and valine. Of these, the branched chain amino acids (BCAA) are primarily oxidized with increases in protein catabolism.[11] For oxidation of proteins within skeletal muscle to occur, the amino acids of the proteins must be mobilized via a number of different catabolic pathways. The three main catabolic pathways within skeletal muscle are the lysosomal pathway,[12,13] the ATP-dependent ubiquitin pathway,[5] and the calpain pathway (calcium activated).[14,15] Each of these pathways has the potential to contribute to the free amino acid pool within skeletal muscle.

Each of the three proteolytic pathways is active under different conditions in skeletal muscle. For example, the lysosomal pathway degrades endocytosed proteins; however, its overall contribution to muscle proteolysis is not quantitatively important.[5] Whereas both the ATP-dependent ubiquitin pathway and the calpain pathway have the potential to contribute significantly to the free amino acid pool within skeletal muscle.[5,14] The ATP-dependent ubiquitin pathway appears to be the most active pathway for protein degradation in most catabolic states. It has been observed that blocking of this pathway slows rates of protein degradation during periods of muscle wasting (eg, denervation, starvation, acidosis).[5] The calpain pathway appears to be important when there are increases in intracellular calcium concentrations within the cell. Such increases can occur when sarcoplasmic reticulum is damaged (eg, following eccentric exercise).[14] The ultimate outcome of these pathways is liberation of free amino acids from the proteins that are being degraded. Once in the free amino acid pool, there are three possible fates for the amino acids: oxidation, export from the cell, and direct reincorporation into new proteins (protein synthesis).

Amino Acid Oxidation

Amino acid oxidation involves a number of steps. The amino acid is transaminated to its α-keto acid equivalent by BCAA transferase (BCAAT). The newly formed α-keto acid is then oxidatively decarboxylated by branched chain α-keto acid dehydrogenase (BCKAD) to form acetyl coenzyme A derivative. The subsequent reactions resemble those of fatty acid oxidation, with eventual complete oxidation of the molecule through the tricarboxylic acid cycle (TCA) and the electron transport chain.

Since the activity of BCAAT and BCKAD are both high in skeletal muscle, and the BCAA represent a large percentage (~20%) of amino acids in skeletal muscle, they are generally thought of as the greatest contributor to amino acid oxidation in skeletal muscle.[16,17] It has been observed that BCAAT has the greatest affinity for leucine, isoleucine and, finally, valine.[16] Amino acid oxidation does not contribute a large amount to total ATP production within skeletal muscle at rest, but the overall contribution can increase under certain conditions.

Amino Acid Extrusion

Another fate of amino acids mobilized by proteolysis is export from the cell into the circulation. The primary amino acids exported from skeletal muscle cells are glutamine and alanine.[18,19] It is well established that alanine release from skeletal muscle increases in periods of starvation and serves as a gluconeogenic precursor at the liver.[19] Alanine release is also increased with exercise.[20] This increase in alanine export results from an increase in the transamination of pyruvate via the alanine amino transferase reaction with glutamate (derived from amino acid transamination, predominantly of the BCAAs).[20] The ultimate fate of amino acids exported from skeletal muscle is transamination and exchange with other pathways within the liver.

Protein Synthesis

The third fate of amino acids mobilized from proteolysis is incorporation back into protein (protein synthesis). Many factors are required for this process to occur, including transfer RNA (tRNA), messenger RNA (mRNA), ATP, enzymes, and ribosomes. Proteins are synthesized by the sequential addition of activated precursors (aminoacyl-tRNA) to the carboxyl end of the growing peptide chain. The formation of each precursor molecule (aminoacyl-tRNA) is catalyzed by a corresponding aminoacyl-tRNA synthetase and requires energy in the form of ATP. Each amino acid has its unique tRNA and aminoacyl-tRNA synthetase.[21]

In brief, protein synthesis involves three main steps: initiation, elongation, and termination. Initiation involves the binding of the initiator tRNA to the start signal on the mRNA. Elongation involves the binding of aminoacyl-tRNA to the ribosome and the subsequent linking of the aminoacyl-tRNA to the growing peptide chain. Termination occurs when a stop signal is reached on the mRNA and the polypeptide is released from the ribosome.

Many factors can influence protein synthesis within skeletal muscle, including various hormones, nutritional status, and exercise (all are discussed in more detail later in this chapter). The difficulty in interpreting the influence of these different factors rests in the various methods used in evaluating muscle protein synthesis. Of numerous methods used, each with its own assumptions and advantages, the isotope incorporation technique is most widely used. In this method, tissue (ie, skeletal muscle) is sampled before and after infusion of an isotope-labeled amino acid. The amount of label in each sample is then determined, and from this a fractional synthesis rate (FSR) can be determined. More recently, a method of determining the synthesis rate of specific proteins such as myosin and actin has been described.[22,23] This method allows for the distinct determination of the rate of protein synthesis in the actual functional units of skeletal muscle (ie, contractile proteins).

An overview of protein metabolism is presented in Figure 3–1.

FACTORS THAT INFLUENCE PROTEIN METABOLISM

Endocrine Hormones and Growth Factors

Certain hormones and local growth factors appear to have some control over protein turnover. Many hormones and growth factors have been identified as having significant effects on protein synthesis and protein degradation. Some of the more studied hormones and growth factors with respect to protein turnover include human growth hormone (hGH), insulin-like growth factor-I (IGF-I), testosterone, and insulin, among others. These hormones do not regulate the entire process, but likely contribute to providing an environment that influences the magnitude of various aspects of protein turnover.

Human Growth Hormone

Human growth hormone is a polypeptide hormone secreted by the anterior pituitary gland. It has direct and indirect (via insulin-

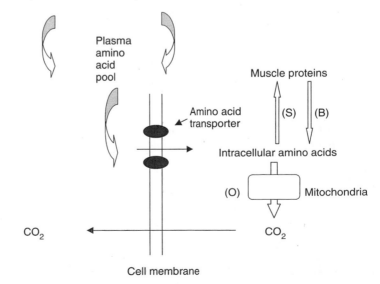

FIGURE 3–1. Overview of protein metabolism. *S*, protein synthesis; *B*, protein breakdown; *O*, amino acid oxidation.

Dietary intake with or without intravenous infusion

Plasma amino acid pool

Amino acid transporter

Muscle proteins

(S)   (B)

Intracellular amino acids

(O)   Mitochondria

CO_2 CO_2

Cell membrane

like growth factors [IGF's]) stimulatory effects on anabolism.

Many stimuli can result in increased hGH secretion, including physical activity, amino acid ingestion, psychological stress, and other hormones.[24,25] hGH administration in healthy young persons results in increased muscle protein synthesis but does not affect whole body protein synthesis.[26,27] Intra-arterial infusions of hGH cause a significant increase in amino acid balance across the forearm.[27] This increase in balance appears to be mediated by an increased uptake of amino acids. Despite the influence of hGH on protein balance across the forearm, hGH does not appear to have a significant effect on whole body protein synthesis.[27]

Administration of hGH in both clinical and healthy populations acutely increases nitrogen balance,[28] suggesting that hGH can increase lean tissue mass. However, it appears that the increase is not maintained with prolonged hGH treatment.[28]

The combined effects of hGH treatment and resistance exercise have been investigated in resistance-trained persons.[29] It was observed that 14 days of hGH treatment had no effect on whole body protein turnover or FSR in the vastus lateralis.[29] It was concluded that resistance exercise may render the muscle unresponsive to the potential anabolic effects of hGH administration. The same group also investigated the effects of resistance training with hGH treatment in previously sedentary individuals.[30] They observed that the hGH administration and exercise led to significant increases in whole body protein synthesis as compared with resistance training alone. However, no significant differences were observed with respect to mixed muscle FSR. These data suggested that increased whole body protein synthesis contributes to lean tissue other than skeletal muscle.[30]

To summarize, it appears that short-term administration of hGH leads to a more positive nitrogen balance; however, conflicting data exist, depending on which method is used to determine protein turnover. Clearly, from whole body estimates of protein turnover and the nitrogen balance data, definite changes in protein turnover occur. It is necessary to isolate the specific sites of this turnover to give a better understanding of interaction of hGH and protein turnover.

Given the expense, the requirement for parenteral injections, and the modest effects on protein anabolism, the routine clinical use of hGH cannot be advocated.

Insulin-like Growth Factor–I

Insulin-like growth factor–I is a polypeptide that is produced primarily in the liver, but has been demonstrated to be synthesized in skeletal muscle cells.[31] One of the possible mechanisms of hGH action is through stimulation of IGF-I release. The entire IGF family has been demonstrated to be important stimulators of many anabolic processes in muscle.[32] The effects of IGF-I on protein turnover are similar to those observed with hGH. Administration of IGF-I increases whole body protein synthesis by about 15% to 20%,[33,34] yet does not alter whole body protein degradation.[33] IGF-I has also been observed to result in a more positive protein balance across the forearm.[35] The more positive balance was due to both an increase in amino acid uptake (protein synthesis) and a decrease in release (protein degradation).[35] It is not clear from the methods used in these studies which specific tissues the changes in protein metabolism occurred in. Therefore, further work is required to determine the specific effects of IGF-I on protein turnover and to isolate the specific sites of these changes (eg, contractile protein vs skin vs connective tissue).

Testosterone

Exogenous testosterone administration increases muscle size, muscle strength,[36] lean body mass,[37] and the FSR of mixed muscle protein.[38]

In a recent study,[36] administration of testosterone plus resistance training resulted in significant increases in body weight (~8%), fat-free mass (~9%), strength (~30%), and muscle cross-sectional area (~14%), whereas testosterone alone resulted in significant increases in body weight (~4%), muscle cross-sectional area (~9%), and strength (leg squats) (~12.6%).

Similar increases in fat-free mass have been observed by others.[37] Forbes et al[37] observed a 12% increase in fat-free mass and 27% decrease in body fat relative to baseline values with 12 weekly injections of testosterone. No control or placebo groups were included in this study, and no strict controls were in place to control for exercise. As a result, it is unclear that these results are due solely to the intervention. However, with the dramatic changes in body composition, it is difficult to dispute that the testosterone had an effect.

Twelve weeks of testosterone administration has also been observed to result in a 27% increase in muscle protein synthesis, but no changes in whole body protein synthesis or indices of protein degradation.[38] Clearly, if muscle protein synthesis had been elevated 27% for the duration of the 12-week study, there should have been much greater increases in body weight and lean muscle mass. There must have been a simultaneous increase in protein degradation, or the increase in muscle protein synthesis did not occur until late in the 12-week protocol.

It is clear that testosterone has a significant effect on protein turnover and lean body mass. As well, with recent indirect evidence, it appears that testosterone also has an effect on contractile protein content, as demonstrated by increased strength.

Insulin

Insulin is a well studied hormone with respect to protein turnover in humans. It has been observed to have varied effects on protein turnover. It can alter FSR,[39,40] muscle protein degradation,[41-43] and whole-body protein degradation.[41-49]

The most consistent effect of insulin on protein turnover, a suppression of whole body protein degradation,[41-49] appears to be related to the insulin concentration. Tessari et al[46] and Fukugawa et al[42] observed a dose-response effect for insulin on whole body protein breakdown. Clearly, insulin results in decreased protein degradation.

Some groups have investigated the specific source of the decreased protein degradation in skeletal muscle. The most common method for assessing the effects of insulin on muscle protein turnover is the A-V balance model, in which it is assumed that the major contributor to protein degradation and synthesis across the limb is skeletal muscle. Skin and fat also contribute to these calculated differences. Decreases in amino acid release have been routinely observed, suggesting a decrease in skeletal muscle protein degradation.[41,43] Similarly, significant decreases in circulating 3-methylhistidine have been ob-

served during insulin infusion, suggesting a decrease in muscle protein degradation.[42]

The exact mechanism of insulin on muscle protein degradation remains unclear; however, insulin inhibits lysosomal protein degradation and can also antagonize the catabolic actions of glucocorticoids (the reader is referred to references 50–54). Furthermore, the ubiquitin protein degradation pathway is attenuated by insulin, and this pathway is active in catabolic disease states.[5] These factors may be mechanisms by which protein degradation is decreased, but further work is required.

Insulin has an anabolic effect by increasing protein synthesis,[39,40] and this anabolic effect is affected by the availability of amino acids in the systemic circulation.[39] There is considerable support for this concept from studies involving insulin infusions with elevated amino acid levels.[40,44,55] Both increases in protein synthesis and decreases in protein degradation have been observed with insulin infusion and simultaneous amino acid infusion.[40,44,55] As previously discussed, many studies have revealed a decrease in protein degradation,[41-49] but few have reported an increase in protein synthesis without simultaneous amino acid infusion.[40,44,55] Increases in muscle protein synthesis associated with insulin infusion are likely a function of the increase in amino acid transport that results from the insulin stimulation[39] and an increase in peripheral blood flow.[56,57]

Insulin has several different effects on protein turnover. Most of the work in the area of insulin and protein turnover has utilized insulin infusions. It is unclear how diet-induced increases in insulin concentration affect protein turnover.

Other Factors

A number of growth factors have been identified in the last few years that may have a role in the regulation of protein turnover. Two of these factors are fibroblast-derived growth factor and tumor necrosis factor. Both of these growth factors have been implicated in influencing different components of protein turnover.[58,59] Further work is required to determine the exact influence and mechanisms of these various growth factors, as well as the interactions of these growth factors and various other hormones, and the overall effects of these interactions on protein turnover.

Summary

The hormonal control of protein turnover is complex and involves a number of factors. Some of the more important factors are endocrine hormones and growth factor. Much is known about how these hormones individually affect protein turnover, but little is known about the complex interactions that are likely occurring. In addition, the literature contains some controversy about the influence of some of these hormones; however, some of these differences are due to the various techniques that are available to investigate protein metabolism. A summary of the effects of various hormones upon protein metabolism is presented in Table 3–1.

Physical Activity and Exercise

Physical activity has a dramatic effect on protein turnover. Endurance exercise increases whole body protein synthesis.[60] In contrast, similar increases in whole body protein synthesis have not been found following resistance exercise in fed humans.[61] It has also been noted, however, that both forms of exercise result in chronic elevation of whole body protein synthesis.[62,63] Exercise is also associated with elevated protein degradation.[64] Both resistance and endurance exercise result in increased muscle protein synthesis.[65–67] Specifically, resistance exercise results in increases in both muscle protein synthesis and muscle protein degradation, but the increased synthesis is greater than the increased degradation.[66] The specific causes for these changes in protein turnover are likely quite different for the different forms of exercise. With respect to resistance exercise, these changes likely occur in the contractile proteins because (1) muscle hypertrophy occurs with resistance exercise, (2) there is increased 3-methylhistidine excretion, and (3) resistance exercise results in disruption of the myofilaments. For endurance exercise, the increased protein turnover is likely due to different factors than in resistance exercise, including increased amino acid oxidation, increased mitochondrial volume, and increased fiber capillary density and myoglobin content. In addition, the actual mechanism of protein degradation may be different between these two forms of exercise.

Nutritional Intake and Supplementation

Macronutrients

Nutritional intake has an important role with respect to protein turnover. From a metabolic standpoint, the provision of either increased nitrogen or energy will promote a more positive nitrogen balance and increase protein synthesis.[6,68,69] In addition to energy and protein, a high carbohydrate intake also promotes a more positive nitrogen balance,[68,70] likely related to the hyperinsulinemia that results from a high carbohydrate intake.[39,55] Hyperinsulinemia results in decreased muscle and whole body protein breakdown and a lesser increase in muscle and whole body protein synthesis.[39,55,70,71] Overall, this leads to a more positive nitrogen balance and protein retention. Therefore, from a practical standpoint, the provision of a high-carbohydrate diet (>60% of energy intake) during exercise training and in rehabilitative exercise is a simple and important dietary suggestion. This also fits in well with guidelines for cardiovascular risk reduction in both Canada and the United States.

Clearly there must be enough dietary protein to support whole body protein turnover, and studies have quantified this, which has formed the basis for governmental protein intake guidelines.[72–74] With respect to protein intake, most requirements for adults are in the range of 0.8 to 0.9 g/kg/d.[73,74] The requirements are higher for children, patients under extreme metabolic stress (eg, burns, sepsis), and for women who are pregnant or lactating.[73,74] The reader should

TABLE 3–1. Summary of Effects of Hormones on Muscle Protein Turnover

HORMONE	PROTEIN SYNTHESIS*	PROTEIN DEGRADATION
Insulin	Increase + to ++	Decrease ++
hGH	Increase ++	Decrease +
IGF-I	Increase ++	?
Testosterone	Increase ++	No change
Most cytokines	Decrease + to ++	Increase + to ++

*Increase is seen primarily with simultaneous amino acid infusion; see text for hormone definition and examples of cytokines.

consult his or her country's nutritional recommendations for more complete details.

Of relevance in this book is the question of whether there is an elevated protein requirement in athletes and those participating in therapeutic exercise. Studies have shown that there is an increased need for dietary protein with very strenuous resistance exercise (ie, 2-hour sessions at high intensity, 5 or 6 days per week).[61,75,76] The amount of protein necessary, however, is only 1.2 to 1.75 g/kg/d, which is covered by the habitual dietary intake of these athletes.[61,75] In fact, most athletes erroneously believe that protein supplements are required for optimal muscle mass accretion. Protein consumed in excess of the requirement is oxidized for energy.[75] From a patient's perspective, more modest resistance exercise, even in the elderly, does not require an appreciable increase in protein requirements.[77] Therefore, it is important that the athlete or patient consume adequate energy to cover his or her needs, and protein intake need be only at a given country's recommended intake level, with a marginal increase for those few who participate in very strenuous exercise programs. Although there are additional protein requirements under periods of extreme metabolic stress, it is not likely that these patients would be participating in therapeutic resistance exercise.

Timing

Interest in the timing of nutrient delivery came from studies in athletes in which it was demonstrated that the consumption of a high-carbohydrate supplement immediately following exercise led to greater rates of glycogen repletion than if the supplement was provided 2 hours later.[78–80] The mechanism for such effect is thought to be via the simultaneous stimulation of the contraction-stimulated and insulin-stimulated glucose transport pathways.[78–80] We have recently shown that glycogen resynthesis is similarly enhanced by administration of a high-carbohydrate supplement following resistance-type exercise.[81] From a perspective of protein turnover, we have demonstrated that provision of a glucose supplement after resistance exercise leads to reduction in protein degradation.[82] Specifically, we showed significant reductions in 3-methylhistine excretion with the consumption of carbohydrate, compared with placebo, after

an isolated bout of resistance exercise.[82] The elevated insulin concentration may also increase protein synthesis to a greater extent than that induced by exercise alone. Increases in whole body protein synthesis have been observed with the consumption of carbohydrate after a bout of resistance exercise.[83] Increases in insulin concentration alone do not appear to be enough to stimulate protein synthesis. It appears that the effect insulin has on muscle is to stimulate amino acid uptake; however, unless exogenous amino acids are supplied or amino acids are mobilized from other areas, this increased rate of uptake may be self-limited.[39] Therefore, if a source of amino acids or protein is included with the carbohydrate, the substrate self-limiting effect that occurs with insulin and protein synthesis may be averted.

Mechanism

The mechanism involved in the action of macronutrients on protein metabolism may be related to cell hydration levels. Cell volume in the liver is well established to have a dramatic effect on protein metabolism.[84–86] It has been observed that a reduction in cell volume is associated with an increase in proteolysis, and an increase in cell volume is associated with an increase in protein synthesis.[84–86] Macronutrient intake results in an increase in plasma insulin, glucose, and amino acid levels, depending on the composition of the supplement. It is established that plasma insulin in physiologic concentrations can stimulate a number of ionic channels within various cells, which translates into net ion movement in and out of cells.[86,87] Such ion movement can translate into significant alterations in cell volume. Therefore, it is possible that one mechanism of insulin on protein metabolism may be alteration in cell volume, thereby resulting in a more positive protein balance due to an increase in protein synthesis and a decrease in protein degradation. The actions of cell volume on protein metabolism are well established in hepatocytes, but much further work is required in skeletal muscle cells.

Cumulative substrate transport has also been associated with alterations in cell volume.[85,87] The transport of amino acids into the cell by the Na^+-dependent amino acid transporter results in an increase in cell volume. For example, glutamine administration in isolated rat muscle preparations was associated with a 35% increase in muscle cell volume.[88] Therefore, inclusion of glutamine with the composition of a macronutrient supplement may be beneficial in terms of increasing muscle cell volume and possibly improving protein balance. Work in this area is limited, and much further research is required.

Hormonal Change

It has been observed that consumption of nutritional supplements after resistance exercise can provide a hormonal environment that may be favorable for muscle growth.[89] It has also been observed that consumption of a beverage of carbohydrate and protein, compared with placebo, after a bout of resistance exercise results in a significant increase in hGH concentration 6 hours later. In addition, a carbohydrate-protein supplement produces an increase in circulating insulin (as previously discussed), which may also have an anabolic effect. No study has measured all the hormonal changes that occur with nutritional intake after exercise and correlated these changes with changes in protein turnover. Therefore, it is unclear whether such changes in the hormonal environment have any influential effects on protein turnover. Based on the literature, nutritional intake (or supplementation) likely provides a suitable hormonal environment to promote protein synthesis and decrease in the rate of protein degradation.

Clearly, further work is required regarding the influence of nutritional intake and supplementation on protein turnover after exercise. It appears that supplementation may lead to a more positive protein balance through changes in the hormonal environment. A summary of practical suggestions for both athletes and patients undergoing therapeutic exercise is presented in Table 3–2.

Creatine Monohydrate

Creatine (Cr), a guanidine-derived compound, is found in most mammalian cells and has an important role in metabolism. Cellular total creatine (TCr) is the sum of free Cr plus phosphorylated creatine (PCr). In many tissues (eg, muscle, brain), PCr functions primarily as a high-energy phosphate donor to rephosphorylate adenosine diphosphate (ADP) to ATP during periods of high energy demand (temporal

TABLE 3–2. Nutritional Suggestions for Enhancing Muscle Mass Accretion

	REQUIREMENT
Basal protein	~0.85 g/kg/d
Additional requirements	
Metabolic stress*	
Very strenuous resistance training	1.2–1.75 g/kg/d
Energy intake	Enough for metabolic needs
Energy intake	>60% carbohydrate, <30% fat, remainder protein

*See definitions and requirements in Food and Agriculture Organization/World Health Organization/United Nations University: Energy and protein requirements. WHO Technical Report Series, no. 74. World Health Organization, Geneva, Switzerland, 1985; and Food and Nutrition Board, Commission on Life Sciences, National Research Council: Recommended Daily Allowances, vol 10. National Academy Press, Washington, DC, 1989, pp. 52–77.

energy buffering) (PCr + ADP → Cr + ATP).[90] Temporal energy buffering occurs in the cytosol and is catalyzed by the enzyme creatine kinase (CK). The Cr-PCr system also functions as a spatial energy buffer between the cytosol and mitochondria, using a unique mitochondrial CK isoform (mtCK).[91-93] The Cr-PCr system also functions as a proton (H⁺) buffer,[94] stimulator of protein synthesis,[95,96] and activator of glycolysis.[97] A recent study demonstrated a role for the Cr-PCr system in the regulation of excitation-contraction coupling in skeletal muscle contraction using site-directed mutagenesis of both the cytosolic and mitochondrial CK isoforms.[98] Limb immobilization has been demonstrated[99] to result in a 50% reduction in CK activity, which correlates with marked atrophy, and both the reduced CK activity and atrophy are attenuated by hGH, which increases creatine synthesis.

Endogenous Cr synthesis occurs in the liver, kidneys, and pancreas from the amino acids arginine and glycine. The rate-limiting enzyme is L-arginine/glycine amidinotransferase (transamidinase), which results in the production of guanidinoacetate, which in turn is methylated by *S*-adenosyl-L-methionine (catalyzed by guanidinoacetate methyltransferase) to produce Cr.[100,101] Creatine downregulates transamidinase mRNA expression, whereas hGH upregulates it.[101] In spite of the upregulation of the trans-amidinase enzyme in response to a low Cr concentration, it appears that this is insufficient to restore muscle TCr concentrations to normal levels in persons with low Cr intake (eg, vegan vegetarians).[102] Vegetarians are likely to have low muscle TCr concentrations.[103] Thus, patient populations with low Cr intake (eg, patients with low energy intake, or who are fasting before surgery, or have low energy and protein intake) would not likely be able to compensate with increased endogenous Cr synthesis.

After production, Cr is transported in the blood to tissues, primarily, skeletal muscle, heart, brain, and peripheral nerves for uptake. Creatine is transported by a sodium-dependent and insulin-sensitive transporter that has been cloned, sequenced, and expressed in COS-7 cells.[104,105] Creatine transport also depends upon the extracellular Cr concentration, with increased concentrations inhibiting Cr transport through a protein synthesis–dependent mechanism (presumably, through production of Cr transporters).[106] This likely explains the observation that there is an upper limit of muscle TCr concentration at about 160 mmol/kg dry mass (dm), with large doses of exogenous Cr.[103] Creatine transport is also enhanced by muscle contraction[103] and glucose feedings.[107]

The concentration of TCr, PCr, and Cr are approximately 120, 75 to 85, and 40 to 45 mmol/kg dm, respectively,[103] and these concentrations are lower in the elderly.[108] In addition, many neuromuscular disorders have also been associated with lower levels of ATP, TCr, PCr, and Cr, and alterations in the PCr/TCr ratio (109–111; and unpublished data from our laboratory). Reductions in ATP and the PCr/TCr ratio have also been demonstrated in 20 patients in an intensive care setting.[112] Immobilization of the triceps brachii muscle in healthy men resulted in a 25% decrease in muscle PCr concentration, and resistance exercise training resulted in an increase in PCr and Cr to levels even greater than for the preimmobilization measurement.[113]

Dietary (exogenous) Cr is found predominantly in meat products. For example, 5 g of creatine is found in about 1.1 kg of beef.[103] A typical North American diet containing some meat products provides about 1 g of creatine per day. Recently, exogenous Cr has also been available as a nutritional supplement in the form of creatine monohydrate. This tasteless white powder is water soluble and commercially available in Canada and the United States. Research has demonstrated that the consumption of 20 g of creatine monohydrate for 4 to 5 days results in an increase in TCr of about 25 mmol/kg dm.[103,114–116] The PCr/Cr ratio is not altered by the consumption of exogenous creatine monohydrate.[115] The majority of the increase in muscle Cr retention in response to supplementation occurs within the first 3 days of ingestion.[103] After a loading protocol, muscle TCr concentrations return to baseline within a month with a normal diet, and can be maintained in the loaded state by consuming 3 g of creatine monohydrate per day.[116] The ingestion of 3 g of creatine monohydrate per day for 1 month results in similar muscle concentrations as those seen with the traditional load described above.[116] Persons with low muscle TCr stores have the greatest potential for loading.[103,115] Therefore, patients with neuromuscular disease, postoperative patients, and critically ill and elderly patients would likely benefit most from strategies aimed at restoring or enhancing intracellular Cr homeostasis.

Synthesis and Balance

The effect of Cr and the PCr/Cr system upon muscle protein synthesis and balance has not been heavily investigated in spite of some interesting observations both in vitro and in vivo that it may have an important role in protein metabolism. The stimulus for an increase in myofibrillar protein synthesis in response to resistance exercise is not known; however, a series of studies by Ingwall et al[96,117] were designed to investigate the hypothesis that protein synthesis is a byproduct of high-intensity muscle contractions, Cr, increased actin, and myosin synthesis. These authors found that Cr increases the rate of actin and myosin synthesis in differentiated myocytes by 100%, does not affect protein degradation, and does not induce differentiation of myotubes, and that these effects were due to creatine per se and not its constituent amino acids, arginine and glycine.[96] Further evidence to support a role for Cr came from the observation that inhibition of the CK enzyme resulted in marked reduction of muscle protein synthesis in rat diaphragm.[95]

A model to study the role of the PCr/Cr pathway in metabolism is to feed rats a creatine antagonist (β-guanidinopropionic acid [β-GPA]), which results in significant reductions in PCr, TCr, and CK activity. β-GPA treatment results in a significant reduction in skeletal muscle weight.[118,119] Furthermore, β-GPA feeding accentuates skeletal muscle atrophy in rats undergoing hind-limb suspension (a model of muscle atrophy).[118] β-GPA feedings also result in skeletal muscle ultrastructural alterations that are commonly seen as nonspecific pathologic findings in neuromuscular disease.[120]

In humans, surprisingly few studies have attempted to measure protein metabolism by any method, and no study has used isotopic tracer methods. One of the earliest reports of a potential beneficial effect of Cr upon whole body protein metabolism was published in 1975 when Crim et al[121] demonstrated an increase in weight and nitrogen balance during a 10-day feeding period of 10 g/d of Cr. Another line of evidence in support of a role for Cr in the regulation of muscle protein balance came from observations in a group of patients with muscle TCr depletion secondary to an inborn error of metabolism in ornithine catabolism (gyrate atrophy), in whom profound type 2 muscle atrophy was reversed with creatine monohydrate supplementation of 1.5 g/d for 1 year and was maintained for 5 years.[122] Muscle fiber atrophy is a common finding in postoperative and immobilized patients.

A number of studies have shown an increase of about 1 kg in body weight in response to a Cr load of 20 g/d for 4 to 5 days that is associated with net water retention.[123] A trend toward an increase in lean mass was found in male resistance athletes in a recent study ($P <.06$).[123] In theory, cellular swelling is considered an important stimulator of protein synthesis, and con-versely, cell shrinkage results in an increase in protein catabolism.[86] Muscle cell hydration status is positively correlated with whole body nitrogen balance in a wide variety of disease states.[86] Furthermore, an increase in oxidative stress, known to accompany muscle atrophy,[99] decreases cellular hydration.[124] Vitamin E deficiency (increased oxidative stress) resulted in myopathy in rats and attenuated Cr uptake, which was diminished with vitamin E administration.[125] A further observation is that testosterone administration in humans directly increases Cr synthesis.[126] A summary of the effects of creatine monohydrate supplementation that may be of benefit to patient populations is presented in Table 3–3.

Given that muscle weakness is a significant cause of disability in many disorders, there may potential therapeutic uses for creatine monohydrate.[115,127,128] A reduction in muscle phosphocreatine has been demonstrated in mitochondrial cytopathies,[109,110] Huntington's disease, inflammatory myopathies, and a variety of other neuromuscular disorders.[109] Creatine may also have favorable effects on cerebral hypoxia, and has antioxidant properties.[127] We recently published the results of a randomized, double-blind trial showing improved muscle performance in seven patients with mitochondrial cytopathies[128]; however, there is a paucity of information about the potential therapeutic efficacy of Cr in humans with neurologic disorders. Another study demonstrated an improvement in muscle function in patients with cardiomyopathy.[115] Finally, a study found that Cr supplementation enhanced muscle strength recovery in a group of patients who underwent outpatient knee surgery.[129]

The potential for Cr to attenuate or reverse the deleterious effects of immobilization and neurologic diseases on protein metabolism re-

TABLE 3–3. Potential Therapeutic Benefits of Creatine

EFFECT	POTENTIAL BENEFIT	REFERENCE
↑ Power	Perform more exercise repetitions	29,53,119
↑ Strength	As above, plus enhance ADL performance	29,53,119
↑ Lean mass	Functional recovery	29,53,60,66–68
↓ Oxidative stress	Long-term cellular protection	81

ADL, activities of daily living.

quires further investigation. In addition, the potential benefits of creatine monohydrate supplementation in patients recovering from surgery also warrants investigation. It is possible that if creatine monohydrate has a positive effect on muscle protein synthesis, it could aid in recovery and rehabilitation, thus shortening the required hospital stay. A typical Cr supplementation protocol is presented in Table 3–4.

SUMMARY AND CONCLUSIONS

It is clear that many factors can influence muscle protein metabolism. Some of these factors are various endocrine hormones and growth factors, physical activity and exercise, and nutritional intake. Although trials have demonstrated improvements in protein status with anabolic hormones, the cost and potential side effects of such agents limit their potential use in patient populations. It is also evident that both physical activity and nutritional intake influence a number of the anabolic endocrine hormones. It is most important that patients and athletes consume adequate energy and protein to meet metabolic needs. Carbohydrates should provide at least 60% of total energy intake. Furthermore, there is evidence to support the use of supplemental nutritional intake immediately after physical activity as a method of preventing increases in protein degradation and possibly increasing protein synthesis. For example, a patient undergoing rehabilitative exercise may not consume any nutrient energy for hours after therapeutic exercise, depending on the time of the session. Hence, the hormonal and nutritive milieu would not promote maximal net protein accretion.

It is, therefore, reasonable that immediately after rehabilitative exercise, patients should consume some form of energy. This may improve protein balance and potentially could shorten the patient's hospital stay. If such a strategy reduced hospital stays by 1 day, the cost savings would be significant. For example, total joint arthroplasty of the knee or hip is performed in patients over the age of 60 years with moderate to severe osteoarthritis that interferes with their functional capacity. In Ontario, Canada, about 60,000 of these procedures are performed each year (~550/100,000 persons). With a conservative in-hospital cost of $750/d, it can be seen that an intervention that reduces this stay by only 1 day could save nearly $43,500,000 (Canadian) per year.

Creatine supplementation is another nutritional intervention that potentially could aid many hospitalized patients or those scheduled for elective surgery. There is enough supportive evidence in the literature to indicate a small but significant increase in muscle power with consumption of this supplement. Such increase in muscle power may enable earlier recovery of independence after surgery, or may aid in weaning patients from ventilator dependence. In addition, the possible increase in muscle cell volume that occurs with Cr supplementation may have anabolic effects and thus help maintain lean body mass. Even if the loss in lean body mass that occurs in most hospitalized patients could be partially prevented, the use of Cr may have a central role in elective surgery or recovery from trauma. Thus, as with nutritional intake following rehabilitative exercise, Cr supplementation has the potential to speed recovery, thereby reducing the hospital stay and, therefore, reducing health care costs. Clearly, much further work on the possible role of nutritional

---

TABLE 3–4. Typical Creatine Monohydrate Supplementation Protocol

Prescreening: Medical history, history of dehydration practices, physical examination and blood pressure, blood work for CK activity, creatinine, and blood urea nitrogen

Exclusion: History of dehydration practices (eg, wrestlers), uncontrolled hypertension, or other medical condition not investigated or under control; preexisting renal disease needs full investigation, and risk-benefit ratio of supplement, with monitoring, is required.

Dosage: 5 g qid for 4 to 5 days; 2.5 g once a day maintenance (consume in carbohydrate-containing cool or warm (not hot) beverage

Patient groups most likely to benefit: Mitochondrial myopathy, muscle atrophy following orthopedic conditions, neuromuscular diseases with muscle wasting, cardiomyopathy (see text for details)

Athletes most likely to benefit: Team sports requiring high power output and weight (eg, rugby, football) and power sports (eg, weight lifting, throwing sports); no evidence of any benefit in endurance activities

intake after rehabilitative exercise and Cr supplementation is required in patient populations.

PRACTICAL GUIDELINES

This review leads to a number of plausible treatment options. Such options are highly dependent on each individual case, and there is potential for some of these interventions to be modified in the near future. For example, protein and carbohydrate supplementation following therapeutic exercise should be mandatory. It is a basic and cost-effective treatment that potentially could aid in recovery by attenuating catabolism or increasing anabolism and thereby shorten hospital stay. In addition to providing protein and energy to meet the metabolic needs of the patient, some strategies may enhance anabolism. Probably the most significant strategy is to administer a supplement containing carbohydrate and protein (250–350 kcal; equivalent to a can of defined or high-energy defined formula) after exercise. Carbohydrate-containing beverages may also be of benefit and may improve endurance.

Administration of creatine monohydrate also has the potential for application. There is definite potential for creatine monohydrate to be of benefit in patients admitted for elective surgery. For example, preloading with creatine monohydrate the week before surgery and then a maintenance dose immediately after surgery may attenuate any decrease in lean body mass and strength and enhance the rate of recovery from surgery. Thus far, creatine monohydrate supplementation in the short term has been well tolerated in both young healthy persons[103,123,130] and patient populations.[115,128] Given the evidence for worsening of renal function in patients with glomerulosclerosis,[131] it would be prudent to use caution when considering the use of Cr supplements in patient populations.

In summary, it is important to consider the unique needs of each patient and athlete when devising a nutritional strategy to maximize muscle mass accretion. This is best done by careful history of activity patterns and nutritional habits. A registered nutritionist can be extremely helpful in obtaining a careful dietary history and in helping to devise an appropriate nutritional strategy. These suggestions must consider the type, frequency, and intensity of the exercise,

as well as age and gender considerations. The physician must carefully screen the patient and consider disease states and medications in the nutritional planning. For example, an athlete or patient who is considering adding creatine monohydrate to their dietary intake should be screened for underlying renal dysfunction. Adequate nutrition and nutrient timing are relatively easy and inexpensive interventions for patients undergoing therapeutic exercise, and should be considered in every patient involved in a rehabilitation program.

REFERENCES

1. O'Keefe SJD, Sendr PM, James WPT: Catabolic loss of body nitrogen in response to surgery. Lancet 2:1035–1037, 1974
2. Rennie MJ, Eden BE, Emery PW, Lundholm K: Urinary excretion and efflux from the leg of 3-methylhistidine before and after major surgical operation. Metabolism 33:250–256, 1984
3. Phillips SM, Tipton KD, Aarsland A, et al: Mixed muscle protein synthesis and breakdown following resistance exercise in humans. Am J Physiol 273:E99, 1997
4. Rennie MJ: Muscle protein turnover and the wasting due to injury and disease. Br Med Bull 41:257–264, 1985
5. Mitch WE, Goldberg AL: Mechanisms of muscle wasting. N Engl J Med 335:1897–1905, 1996
6. Clague MB, Keir MJ, Wright PD, Johnston IDA: The effects of nutrition and trauma on whole-body protein metabolism in man. Clin Sci 65:165–175, 1983
7. Garlick PJ, Clugstone GA, Waterlow JC: Influence of low-energy diets on whole body protein turnover in obese subjects. Am J Physiol 238:E235–E244, 1980
8. Ferrando AA, Tipton KD, Bamman MM, Wolfe RR: Resistance exercise maintains skeletal muscle protein synthesis during bed rest. J Appl Physiol 82:807–810, 1997
9. Phillips SM, Atkinson SA, Tarnopolsky MA, MacDougall JD: Gender differences in leucine kinetics and nitrogen balance in endurance athletes. J Appl Physiol 75:2134–2141, 1994
10. Tarnopolsky MA, Atkinson SA, Phillips SM, MacDougall JD: Carbohydrate loading and metabolism during exercise in men and women. J Appl Physiol 78:1360–1368, 1995
11. Goldberg AL, Chang TW: Regulation and significance of amino acid metabolism in skeletal muscle. Fed Proc 37:2301–2307, 1978

12. Vihko V, Salminen A, Rantamaki J: Exhaustive exercise, endurance training, and acid hydrolase activity in skeletal muscle. J Appl Physiol 47: 43–50, 1979

13. Salminen A, Vihko V: Effects of age and prolonged running on proteolytic capacity in mouse cardiac and skeletal muscles. Acta Physiol Scand 112:89–95, 1981

14. Belcastro AN: Skeletal muscle calcium-activated neutral protease (calpain) with exercise. J Appl Physiol 74:1381–1386, 1993

15. Belcastro AN, Parkhouse WS, Dobson G, Gilchrist JS: Influence of exercise on cardiac and skeletal muscle myofibrillar proteins. Mol Cell Biochem 83:27–36, 1988

16. Boyer B, Odessey R: Kinetic characterization of branched chain ketoacid dehydrogenase. Arch Biochem Biophys 285:1–7, 1991

17. Khatra BS, Chawla RK, Sewell CW, Rudman D: Distribution of branched-chain α-keto acid dehydrogenases in primate tissues. J Clin Invest 59:558–564, 1977

18. Ahlborg G, Felig P, Hagenfeldt L, et al: Substrate turnover during prolonged exercise in man. J Clin Invest 53:1080–1090, 1974

19. Felig P: Amino acid metabolism in man. Ann Rev Biochem 44:933–955, 1975

20. Carraro F, Naldini A, Weber JM, Wolfe RR: Alanine kinetics in humans during low-intensity exercise. Med Sci Sports Exerc 26(3):348–353, 1994

21. Stryer L: Biochemistry, 4th Ed. WH Freeman and Co, New York, 1995

22. Balagopal P, Ljungqvist O, Nair KS: Skeletal muscle myosin heavy-chain synthesis rate in healthy humans. Am J Phsyiol 272:E45–E50, 1997

23. Rooyaciers OE, Adey DB, Ades PA, Nair KS: Effect of aging on in vivo rates of mitochondrial protein synthesis in human skeletal muscle. Proc Natl Acad Sci USA 93:15364–15369, 1996

24. Macintyre JG: Growth hormone and athletes. Sports Med 4:129–142, 1987

25. Guyton AC, Hall JE: Textbook of Medical Physiology, 9th Ed. WB Saunders Co, Philadelphia, 1996

26. Fryburg DA, Louard RJ, Gerow KE, et al: Growth hormone stimulates skeletal muscle protein synthesis and antagonizes insulin's antiproteolytic action in humans. Diabetes 41:424–429, 1992

27. Fryburg DA, Barrett EJ: Growth hormone acutely stimulates skeletal muscle but not whole-body protein synthesis in humans. Metabolism 24:1223–1227, 1993

28. Yarasheski KE: Growth hormone effects on metabolism, body composition, muscle mass, and strength. Exerc Sports Sci Rev 22:285–312, 1994

29. Yarasheski KE, Campbell JA, Smith K, et al: Effect of growth hormone and resistance exercise on muscle growth in young men. Am J Physiol 262:E261–E267, 1992

30. Yarasheski KE, Zachwieja JJ, Angelopolous TJ, Bier DM: Short-term growth hormone treatment does not increase muscle protein synthesis in experienced weight lifters. J Appl Physiol 74:3073–3076, 1993

31. Florini JR, Ewton DZ, Magri KA: Hormones, growth factors, and myogenic differentiation. Ann Rev Physiol 53:201–216, 1991

32. Florini JR: Hormonal control of muscle growth. Muscle Nerve 10:577–598, 1987

33. Russell-Jones DL, Umpleby AM, Hennessy TR, et al: Use of a leucine clamp to demonstrate that IGF-I actively stimulates protein synthesis in normal humans. Am J Physiol 267:E591–E598, 1994

34. Mauras N, Beaufrere B: Recombinant human insulin-like growth factor I enhances whole body protein anabolism and significantly diminishes the protein catabolic effects of prednisone in humans without a diabetogenic effect. J Clin Endocrinol Metab 80:869–874, 1995

35. Fryburg DA: Insulin-like growth factor I exerts growth hormone- and insulin-like actions on human muscle protein metabolism. Am J Physiol 267:E331–E336, 1994

36. Bhasin S, Storer TW, Berman N, et al: The effects of supraphysiological doses of testosterone on muscle size and strength in normal men. N Engl J Med 335:1–7, 1996

37. Forbes GB, Porta CR, Herr BE, Griggs RC: Sequence of changes in body composition induced by testosterone and reversal of changes after drug is stopped. JAMA 267:397–399, 1992

38. Griggs RC, Kingston W, Jozefowicz RF, et al: Effect of testosterone on muscle mass and muscle protein synthesis. J Appl Physiol 66:498–503, 1989

39. Biolo G, Flemming RYD, Wolfe RR: Physiologic hyperinsulinemia stimulates protein synthesis and enhances transport of selected amino acids in human skeletal muscle. J Clin Invest 95:811–819, 1995

40. Newman E, Heslin MJ, Wolf RF, et al: The effect of systemic hyperinsulinemia with concomitant amino acid infusion on skeletal muscle protein turnover in the human forearm. Metabolism 43:70–78, 1994

41. Denne SC, Liechty EA, Liu YM, et al: Proteolysis in skeletal muscle and whole body in response to

euglycemic hyperinsulinemia in normal adults. Am J Physiol 261:E809–E814, 1991

42. Fukagawa NK, Minaker KL, Rowe JW, et al: Insulin-mediated reduction of whole body protein breakdown: dose-response effects on leucine metabolism in postabsorptive men. J Clin Invest 76:2306–2311, 1985

43. Heslin MJ, Newman E, Wolf RW, et al: Effects of hyperinsulinemia on whole body and skeletal muscle leucine carbon kinetics in humans. Am J Physiol 262:E911–E918, 1992

44. Castellino P, Luzi L., Simpson DC, et al: Effects of insulin and plasma amino acid concentrations on leucine metabolism in man. J Clin Invest 80:1784–1793, 1987

45. Flakoll PJ, Kulaylat M, Frexes-Steed M, et al: Amino acids augment insulin's suppression of whole body proteolysis. Am J Physiol 257:E839–E847, 1989

46. Tessari P, Trevisan R, Inchiostro S, et al: Dose-response curves of effects of insulin on leucine kinetics in humans. Am J Physiol 251:E334–E342, 1986

47. Shangraw RE, Stuart CA, Prince MJ, et al: Insulin responsiveness of protein metabolism in vivo following bedrest in humans. Am J Physiol 255:E548–E558, 1988

48. Pacy PJ, Nair KS, Ford C, Halliday D: Failure of insulin to stimulate fractional muscle protein synthesis in type-I diabetic patients. Diabetes 38:618–624, 1989

49. Moller-Loswick AC, Zachrisson H, Hyltander A, et al: Insulin selectively attenuates breakdown of nonmyofibrillar proteins in peripheral tissues of normal men. Am J Physiol 266:E645–E652, 1994

50. Biolo G, Wolfe RR: Insulin actions on protein metabolism. Bailliere's Clin Endocrinol Metab 7:989–1005, 1993

51. Goldberg AL: Influence of insulin and contractile activity on muscle size and protein balance. Diabetes 28(suppl):1, 1979

52. Goldberg AL, Tischler M, DeMartino G, Griffin G: Hormonal regulation of protein degradation and synthesis in skeletal muscle. Fed Proc 39:31–36, 1980

53. Nair KS, Schwenk WF: Factors controlling muscle protein synthesis and degradation. Curr Opin Neurol 7:471–474, 1994

54. Kimball SR, Jefferson LS: Cellular mechanisms involved in the action of insulin on protein synthesis. Diabetes Metab Rev 4:773–787, 1988

55. Bennet WM, Connacher AA, Scrimgeour CM, et al: Euglycemic hyperinsulinemia augments amino acid uptake by human leg tissues during hyperaminoacidemia. Am J Physiol 259:E185–E194, 1990

56. Baron AD: Hemodynamic actions of insulin. Am J Physiol 267:E187–E202, 1994

57. Shoemaker JK, Bonen A: Vascular actions of insulin in health and disease. Can J Appl Physiol 20(2):127–154, 1995

58. Yamada S, Buffinger N, Dimario J, Strohman RC: Fibroblast growth factor is stored in fiber extracellular matrix and plays a role in regulating muscle hypertrophy. Med Sci Sports Exerc 21(5):S173–S180, 1989

59. Evans DA, Jacobs DO, Wilmore DW: Effects of tumour necrosis factor on protein metabolism. Br J Surg 80:1019–1023, 1993

60. Devlin JT, Brodsky I, Scrimgeour A, et al: Amino acid metabolism after intense exercise. Am J Physiol 258:E249–E255, 1990

61. Tarnopolsky MA, Atkinson SA, MacDougall JD, et al: Evaluation of protein requirements for trained strength athletes. J Appl Physiol 73:1986–1995, 1992

62. Tarnopolsky MA, Atkinson SA, MacDougall JD, et al: Whole body leucine metabolism during and after resistance exercise in fed humans. Med Sci Sports Exerc 23(3):326–333, 1991

63. Lamont LS, Patel DG, Kalhan SC: Leucine kinetics in endurance trained humans. J Appl Physiol 69:1–6, 1990

64. Pivarnik JM, Hickson JF, Wolinsky I: Urinary 3-methylhistidine excretion increases with repeated weight training exercise. Med Sci Sports Exerc 21(3):283–287, 1989

65. Chesley A, MacDougall JD, Tarnopolsky MA, et al: Changes in human muscle protein synthesis after resistance exercise. J Appl Physiol 73:1383–1388, 1992

66. Biolo G, Maggi SP, Williams BD, et al: Increased rates of muscle protein turnover and amino acid transport after resistance exercise in humans. Am J Physiol 268:E514–520, 1995

67. Carraro F, Stuart CS, Hartl WH, et al: Effect of exercise and recovery on muscle protein synthesis in human subjects. Am J Physiol 259:E470–E476, 1990

68. Forse RA, Elwyn DH, Askanazi J, et al: Effects of glucose on nitrogen balance during high nitrogen intake in malnourished patients. Clin Sci 78:273–281, 1990

69. Todd KS, Butterfield GE, Howes Calloway D: Nitrogen balance in men with adequate and deficient energy balance intake at three levels of work. J Nutr 114:2107–2118, 1984

70. Sim AJW, Wolfe BM, Young VR, et al: Glucose promotes whole body protein synthesis from infused amino acids in fasting man: isotopic demonstration. Lancet 1:68–71, 1979

71. McNurlan MA. Essen P, Thorell A, et al: Response of protein synthesis in human skeletal muscle to insulin: an investigation with L-[^{2}H$_5$] phenylalanine. Am J Physiol 267:E102–E108, 1994

72. Garza C, Scrimshaw NS, Young VR: Human protein requirements: a long-term metabolic balance study in young men to evaluate the 1973 FAO/WHO safe level of egg protein intake. J Nutr 107:335–352, 1977

73. Food and Agriculture Organization/World Health Organization/United Nations University: Energy and protein requirements. WHO technical report series, no. 74. World Health Organization, Geneva, Switzerland, 1985

74. Food and Nutrition Board, Commission on Life Sciences, National Research Council: Recommended Daily Allowances, Vol 10. National Academy Press, Washington, DC, 1989, pp. 52–77.

75. Tarnopolsky MA, MacDougall JD, Atkinson SA: Influence of protein intake and training status on nitrogen balance and lean body mass. J Appl Physiol 64:187–193, 1988

76. Lemon P, Tarnopolsky MA, MacDougall JD, Atkinson S: Protein requirements and muscle mass/strength changes in novice bodybuilders. J Appl Physiol 73:767–775, 1992

77. Campbell WW, Crim MC, Young VR, et al: Effects of resistance training and dietary protein intake on protein metabolism in older adults, Am J Physiol 268:E1143–E1153, 1995

78. Ivy JL, Katz AL, Cutler CL, et al: Muscle glycogen synthesis after exercise: effect of time of carbohydrate ingestion. J Appl Physiol 64:1480–1485, 1988

79. Ivy JL, Reed MC, Brozinick JT Jr, Reed MJ: Muscle glycogen storage after different amounts of carbohydrate ingestion. J Appl Physiol 65:2018–2023, 1988

80. Zawadzki KM, Yaspelkis BB, Ivy JL: Carbohydrate-protein complex increases the rate of muscle glycogen storage after exercise. J Appl Physiol 72:1854–1859, 1992

81. Roy BD, Tarnopolsky MA: Influence of differing macronutrient intakes on muscle glycogen resynthesis after resistance exercise. J Appl Physiol 84:890–896, 1998

82. Roy BD, Tarnopolsky MA, MacDougall JD, et al: The effect of glucose supplement timing on protein metabolism after resistance training. J Appl Physiol 82:1882–1888, 1997

83. Roy BD, Fowles J, Hill R, Tarnopolsky MA: Macronutrient intake and whole body protein metabolism following resistance exercise. Med Sci Sports Exerc (In press)

84. Haussinger D: The role of cellular hydration in the regulation of cell function. Biochem J 313:697–710, 1996

85. Haussinger D: Regulation of cell function by the cellular hydration state. Am J Physiol 267:E343–E355, 1994

86. Haussinger D, Roth E, Lang F, Gerok W: Cellular hydration state: an important determinant of protein catabolism in health and disease. Lancet 341:1330–1332, 1993

87. Lang F, Busch GL, Ritter M, et al: Functional significance of cell volume regulatory mechanisms. Physiol Rev 78:247–306, 1998

88. Low SY, Rennie MJ, Taylor PM: Modulation of glycogen synthesis in rat skeletal muscle by changes in cell volume. J Physiol 495:299–303, 1996

89. Chandler RM, Byrne HK, Patterson JG, Ivy JL: Dietary supplements affect the anabolic hormones after weight training exercise. J Appl Physiol 76:839–845, 1994

90. Bogdanis GC, Nevill ME, Boobis LH, et al: Contribution of phosphocreatine and aerobic metabolism to energy supply during repeated sprint exercise. J Appl Physiol 80:876–884, 1996

91. Meyer RA, Sweeney HL, Kushmerick MJ: A simple analysis of the "phosphocreatine shuttle." Am J Physiol 246:C365–C377, 1984

92. Wallimann T, Wyss M, Brdiczka D, Nicolay K: Intracellular compartmentation, structure and function of creatine kinase isoenzymes in tissues with high and fluctuating energy demands: the "phosphocreatine circuit" for cellular energy homeostasis. Biochem J 281:21–40, 1992

93. Wyss M, Smeitink J, Wevers RA, Wallimann T: Mitochondrial creatine kinase: a key enzyme of aerobic energy metabolism. Biochim Biophys Acta 1102:119–166, 1992

94. Rossiter HB, Cannell ER, Jakeman PM: The effect of oral creatine supplementation on the 1000-m performance of competitive rowers. J Sports Sci 14:175–179, 1996

95. Carpenter CL, Mohan C, Bessman SP: Inhibition of protein and lipid synthesis in muscle by 2,4-dinitrofluorobenzene, an inhibitor of creatine phosphokinase. Biochim Biophys Res Comm 3:884–889, 1983

96. Ingwall JS, Weiner CD, Morales, MF, et al: Specificity of creatine in the control of muscle protein synthesis. J Cell Biol 63:145–151, 1974

97. Meyer RA, Brown TR, Krilowicz BL, Kushmerick MJ: Phosphagen and intracellular pH changes during contraction of creatine-depleted rat muscle. Am J Physiol 250:C264–C274, 1986

98. Steegers K, Benders A, Oerlamans F, et al: Altered Ca^{2+} responses in muscles with combined mitochondrial and cytosolic creatine kinase deficiences. Cell 89:93–103, 1997

99. Carmelli E, Hochberg Z, Livne E, et al: Effect of growth hormone on gastrocnemius muscle of aged rate after immobilization: biochemistry and morphology. J Appl Physiol 75:1529–1535, 1993

100. Stockler S, Holzbach U, Hanefeld F, et al: Creatine deficiency in the brain: a new, treatable inborn error of metabolism. Pediatr Res 36:409–413, 1994

101. Guthmiller P, Van Pilsum JF, Boen JR, McGuire DM: Cloning and sequencing of rat kidney L-arginine : glycine amidinotransferase. J Biol Chem 269:17556–17560, 1994

102. Delanghe J, De Slypere JP, Buyzere M, et al: Normal reference values for creatine, creatinine, and carnitine are lower in vegetarians. Clin Chem 35:1802–1803, 1989

103. Harris RC, Soderlund K, Hultman E: Elevation of creatine in resting and exercised muscle of normal subjects by creatine supplementation. Clin Sci 83:367–374, 1992

104. Guimbal C, Killimann MW: A Na^+-dependent creatine transporter in rabbit brain, muscle heart and kidney. J Biol Chem 268:8418–8421, 1993

105. Soro I, Richman J, Santoro G, et al: The cloning and expression of a human creatine transporter. Biochim Biophys Res Comm 204:419–426, 1994

106. Loike JD, Zalutsky DL, Kaback E, et al: Extracellular creatine regulates creatine transport in rat and human muscle cells. Proc Natl Acad Sci USA 85:807–811, 1988

107. Green AL, Simpson EJ, Littlewood JJ, et al: Carbohydrate ingestion augments creatine retention during creatine feeding in humans. Acta Physiol Scand 158:195–202, 1996

108. Forsberg AM, Nilsson E, Werneman J: Muscle composition in relation to age and sex. Clin Sci 81:249–256, 1991

109. Matthews PM, Allaire C, Shoubridge EA, et al: In vivo muscle magnetic resonance spectroscopy in the clinical investigation of mitochondrial disease. Neurology 41:114–120, 1991

110. Arnold DL, Taylor DJ, Radda GK: Investigation of human mitochondrial myopathies by phosphorus magnetic resonance spectroscopy. Ann Neurol 18:189–196, 1985

111. Eleff SM, Barker PB, Blackband SJ, et al: Phosphorus magnetic resonance spectroscopy of patients with mitochondrial cytopathies demonstrates decreased levels of brain phosphocreatine. Ann Neurol 27:626–630, 1990

112. Gamrin L, Essen P, Forsberg AM, et al: A descriptive study of skeletal muscle metabolism in critically ill patients: free amino acids, energy-rich phosphates, protein, nucleic acids, fat, water, and electrolytes. Crit Care Med 24:575–583, 1996

113. MacDougall JD, Ward GR, Sale DG, Sutton JR: Biochemical adaptation of human skeletal muscle to heavy resistance training and immobilization. J Appl Physiol 43:700–703, 1977

114. Odland LM, MacDougall JD, Tarnopolsky MA: The effect of oral Cr supplementation on muscle [PCr] and short-term maximum power output. Med Sci Sports Exerc 2(2):216–219, 1997

115. Gordon A, Hultman E, Kaijser L, et al: Creatine supplementation in chronic heart failure increases skeletal muscle creatine phosphate and muscle performance. Cardiovasc Res 30:413–418, 1995

116. Hultman E, Soderlund K, Timmons JA, et al: Muscle creatine loading in men. J Appl Physiol 81:232–237, 1996

117. Ingwall JS, Morales MF, Stockdale FM: Creatine and the control of myosin synthesis in differentiating skeletal muscle. Proc Natl Acad Sci USA 69:2250–2253, 1972

118. Adams GR, Haddad F, Baldwin KM: Interaction of chronic creatine depletion and muscle unloading: effects on postural and locomotor muscles. J Appl Physiol 77:1198–1205, 1994

119. Adams GR, Baldwin KM: Age dependency of myosin heavy chain transitions induced by creatine depletion in rat skeletal muscle. J Appl Physiol 78:368–371, 1995

120. Laskowski MB, Chevli R, Fitch CD: Biochemical and ultrastructural changes in skeletal muscle induced by a creatine antagonist. Metabolism 30:1080–1085, 1981

121. Crim MC, Calloway DH, Margen S: Creatine metabolism in men: urinary creatine and creatinine excretions with creatine feeding. J Nutr 105:428–438, 1975

122. Vannas-Sulonen K, Sipila I, Vannas A, et al: Gyrate atrophy of the choroid and retina: a 5-year follow-up of creatine supplementation. Ophthalmology 92:1719–1727, 1985

123. Earnest CP, Snell PG, Rodriquez R, et al: The effect of creatine monohydrate ingestion on anaerobic power indices, muscular strength, and body composition. Acta Physiol Scand 153:207–209, 1995

124. Hallbrucker C, Ritter M, Lang F, et al: Hydroperoxide metabolism in rat liver, K^+ channel activation, cell volume changes and eicosanoid formation. Eur J Biochem 211:449–458, 1993

125. Gerber GB, Gerber G, Koszalka TR, Emmel VM: Creatine metabolism in vitamin E deficiency in the rat. Am J Physiol 202:453–460, 1962

126. Hoberman HD, Sims EAH, Engstrom WW: The effect of methyltesterone on the rate of synthesis of creatine. J Biol Chem 173:111–116, 1948

127. Matthews RT, Yang L, Jenkins BG, et al: Neuroprotective effects of creatine and cyclocreatine in animal models of Huntington's disease. J Neurosci 18:156–163, 1998

128. Tarnopolsky MA, Roy BD, MacDonald JR: A randomized, controlled trial of creatine monohydrate in patients with mitochondrial cytopathies. Muscle Nerve 20:1502–1509, 1997

129. Satolli F, Marchesi G: Creatine phosphate in the rehabilitation of patients with muscle hypotonotrophy of the lower extremity. Curr Ther Res 46:67–73, 1989

130. Poortmans JR, Auquier H, Renaut V, et al: Effect of short-term creatine supplementation on renal responses in men. Eur J Appl Physiol 76:566–567, 1997

131. Pritchard NR, Kalra PA: Renal dysfunction accompanying oral creatine supplements. Lancet 351:1252–1253, 1998

4

Exercise and Core Temperature

C. BRUCE WENGER

Temperature changes affect biologic processes through configurational changes that alter the function of protein molecules such as enzymes, receptors, and membrane channels, and through a general effect on chemical reactions rates as described by the law of Arrhenius. Within the physiologic range of temperatures, most chemical reaction rates vary approximately as an exponential function of temperature, and raising temperature by 10°C increases the reaction rate two- to threefold. A familiar clinical consequence of this effect is described by the rule that each 1°C of fever increases fluid and calorie needs 13%.[1] The thermoregulatory responses of homeotherms keep internal or body core temperature within a narrow range, thereby providing a more stable physicochemical environment for their biologic processes.

Normal human body temperature is conventionally said to be 37°C (98.6°F), a figure that may be misleadingly precise. Core temperature at rest undergoes a daily or circadian rhythm with an amplitude of about 1°C, and is lowest in the early morning and highest in the late afternoon.[2-4] In women of childbearing age, this circadian rhythm is superimposed on another rhythm, with a somewhat smaller amplitude, associated with the menstrual cycle.[5-7] These rhythms are produced by underlying rhythms in the control of the thermoregulatory responses, in what we may think of as the setting

of the body's "thermostat." These rhythms, plus other factors such as individual variation and acclimatization to heat, account for a range of core temperatures of healthy subjects at rest (Fig. 4–1). In addition, heavy exercise or fever may raise core temperature several degrees, and more extreme disturbances of core temperatures may result from neurologic disease or from heat or cold stress that overwhelms the capacity of the thermoregulatory system.

Adverse effects of heat stress include impairment of physical and mental performance,[8,9] heat-related illnesses and syndromes,[10-12] aggravation of preexisting illnesses,[13-15] and direct injury caused by high tissue temperature. Apart from burns, direct thermal injury may include some of the tissue injury associated with heat stroke. In healthy individuals, the physiologic defenses against heat are ordinarily so powerful and effective that tissue temperature rarely reaches harmful levels during heat stress, and most adverse effects of heat stress owe much more to secondary consequences of thermoregulatory and other homeostatic responses than to direct thermal injury to tissue. With the exception of local tissue injury, adverse effects of cold are chiefly those associated with hypothermia, ie, clinically significant lowering of core temperature, which include depression of central nervous system function, cardiac output, and respiration, and electrical disturbances of the heart. Because of the high rates of metabolic heat production associated with exercise, heat stress is a much more frequent threat than cold stress during exercise. Nevertheless, hypothermia may be a significant problem during marathons and other prolonged exercise performed in cold or

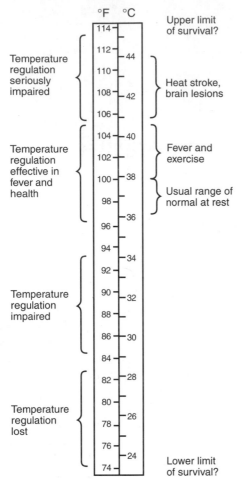

°F   °C

114 —— Upper limit of survival?

112 — — 44

Temperature regulation seriously impaired
110 —
108 — — 42   Heat stroke, brain lesions
106 —

104 — — 40   Fever and exercise
Temperature regulation effective in fever and health
102 —
100 — — 38
98 —   Usual range of normal at rest
— 36
96 —

94 —
— 34
92 —

Temperature regulation impaired
90 — — 32
88 —
86 — — 30
84 —

82 — — 28
80 —
Temperature regulation lost
78 — — 26
76 —
74 — — 24   Lower limit of survival?

FIGURE 4–1. Ranges of rectal temperature in healthy persons, patients with fever, and persons with impairment or failure of thermoregulation. (Modified from Du Bois EF: Fever and the Regulation of Body Temperature. Charles C. Thomas, Springfield, IL, 1948.)

wet weather.[16–18] This chapter discusses normal physiologic responses to heat and cold, especially in combination with exercise; events that lead to deterioration of performance or frank illness during heat or cold stress; and factors that affect tolerance to heat and cold. In addition, clinical aspects of heat and cold stress are briefly summarized.

BODY TEMPERATURE AND HEAT TRANSFER IN THE BODY

Thermal physiologists divide the body into a warm internal core and a cooler outer shell. The regulated internal body temperature is the temperature of the vital organs inside the head and trunk. The core includes these organs, along with a variable amount of other more superficial and peripheral tissue. The amount of the body included in the core is greater in a warm environment and when metabolic heat production is high. Within the core, temperature is relatively uniform and close to the temperature of the central blood.

Shell temperature is strongly influenced by the environment and thus is not regulated within narrow limits, as core temperature is, even though thermoregulatory responses strongly affect the temperature of the shell and especially its outermost layer, the skin. The thickness of the shell depends on the environment and the body's need to conserve heat. In a warm environment, the shell may be less than 1 cm thick, but in a subject conserving heat in a cold environment, it may extend several centimeters below the skin.

Heat is lost to the environment only from tissues in contact with the environment, chiefly from skin but to a lesser extent from the respiratory passages also. Therefore, body heat balance depends on the flow of heat from the sites of heat production to the skin. Heat is transported within the body by two means: conduction through the tissues and convection by the blood, a process in which flowing blood carries heat from warmer tissues to cooler tissues. Heat flow through tissue by conduction depends on the thermal conductivity of the tissue, whereas heat flow by convection depends on the rate of blood flow through the tissues. Changes in skin blood flow in a cool environment change the thickness of the shell. When skin blood flow is reduced in the cold, the affected skin becomes cooler, and the underlying tissues, which may include the more superficial muscles of the neck and trunk and most of the volume of nonexercising limbs, become cooler as they lose heat by conduction to cool overlying skin and ultimately to the environment. In this way, these underlying tissues, which in a warm environment were part of the body core, now become part of the shell. Since the shell lies between the core and the environment, all heat leaving the body core via the skin passes through the shell before being given up to the environment, and thus the shell insulates the core from the environment. In a cool subject, skin blood flow is low, and core-to-skin heat transfer is dominated by conduction, and since the shell is thicker under these conditions, it provides more insulation to the core. Thus changes in skin blood flow, which directly affect core-to-skin heat transfer by convection, also indirectly affect core-to-skin heat transfer by conduction, by changing the thickness of the shell.

REGULATION OF BODY TEMPERATURE

Physiologic and Behavioral Temperature Regulation

Two distinct control systems, physiologic and behavioral, operate in parallel to regulate body temperature. Physiologic thermoregulation utilizes involuntary responses. In humans the most important responses involved in physiologic thermoregulation are changes in skin blood flow, which controls flow of heat from the interior of the body to the skin; sweating, which increases heat loss by evaporation, in the heat and during exercise; and shivering, which increases metabolic heat production, in the cold. The physiologic control system is capable of fine adjustments to these responses, and enables homeotherms to achieve fairly precise regulation of their core temperature. Behavioral thermoregulation involves the conscious use of any means available and operates primarily to reduce the level of thermal discomfort. Since thermal discomfort is closely related to the underlying physiologic strain,[19] behavioral thermoregulation reduces the demand on the physiologic thermoregulatory responses. Familiar behavioral responses include adding or removing clothing, seeking a more comfortable environment, and drinking hot or cold liquids, and reducing physical activity in hot environments. Behavioral thermoregulation is strongly influenced by learned responses, and may be compromised or overridden when there is enough motivation to persist in a situation that produces a high degree of thermal stress, as during intense physical training or athletic competition or in the performance of certain jobs. In healthy young persons, harmful effects of heat and cold are most often the result of failure to make the appropriate behavioral responses, owing to excessive motivation, improper supervision, or lack of foresight.

Balance Between Heat Production and Heat Loss

Although the body exchanges some energy with the environment in the form of mechanical work, most is exchanged as heat, by conduction, convection, and radiation, and as latent heat through evaporation or, rarely, condensation of water (Fig. 4–2). If the sum of energy production and energy gain from the environment does not equal energy loss, the extra heat is "stored" in or lost from the body. This is summarized in the following heat balance equation:

$$M = E + R + C + K + W + S \qquad \text{Eq 1}$$

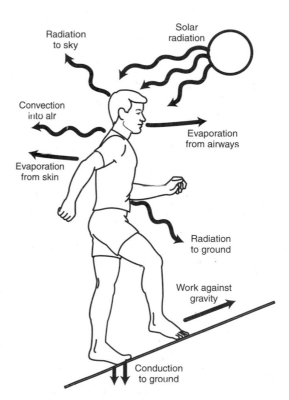

FIGURE 4–2. Exchange of energy with the environment. This hiker gains heat from the sun by radiation, and loses heat by conduction to the ground through the soles of his feet, by convection into the air, by radiation to the ground and sky, and by evaporation of water from his skin and respiratory passages. In addition, some of the energy released by his metabolic processes is converted into mechanical work, rather than heat, since he is walking uphill. (Redrawn from Wenger CB: The regulation of body temperature. In: Rhodes RA, Tanner GA [eds]: Medical Physiology. Little, Brown & Co, Boston, 1995, pp. 587–613. Used with permission.)

where M is metabolic rate, E is rate of heat loss by evaporation, R and C are rate of heat loss by radiation and convection, respectively, K is the rate of heat loss by conduction (only to solid objects, in practice, as explained later), W is rate of energy loss as mechanical work, and S is rate of heat storage in the body,[20,21] which is positive when mean body temperature is increasing.

Metabolic Rate and Sites of Heat Production

At thermal steady state, the rate of heat production in the body is equal to the rate of heat loss to the environment and can be measured precisely by direct calorimetry, a cumbersome technique in which all heat and water vapor leaving the body are captured and measured with special apparatus. More usually, metabolic rate is estimated by indirect calorimetry[22] from measurements of oxygen consumption, since virtually all energy available to the body depends on oxygen-consuming chemical reactions. The heat production associated with consumption of 1 L of oxygen varies somewhat according to the proportions of carbohydrate, fat, and protein that are oxidized. An average value of 20.2 kJ (4.83 kcal) per liter of oxygen is often used for metabolism of a mixed diet. Since the ratio of carbon dioxide produced to oxygen consumed varies according to the fuel, indirect calorimetry can be made more accurate by also measuring carbon dioxide production and calculating the amount of protein oxidized from urinary nitrogen excretion.

Metabolic rate for a fasting young man at rest is about 45 W/m² of body surface area, or 81 W (70 kcal/h) for a surface area of 1.8 m². At rest, the trunk viscera and the brain account for about 70% of energy production, even though they comprise only about 36% of the body mass (Table 4–1). During exercise, however, the muscles are the chief site of energy production and may account for 90% during heavy exercise (Table 4–1). A healthy but sedentary young man performing moderate exercise may reach a metabolic rate of 600 W, and a trained athlete performing intense exercise, 1,400 W or more. The overall mechanical efficiency of exercise varies enormously, depending on the activity; but, at best, no more than one fourth of the metabolic energy is converted into mechanical work outside the body, and the remaining three fourths

TABLE 4–1. Relative Mass and Rate of Metabolic Heat Production of Various Body Compartments During Rest and Strenuous Exercise

	BODY MASS (%)	HEAT PRODUCTION (%)	
		REST	EXERCISE
Brain	2	16	1
Trunk viscera	34	56	8
Muscle and skin	56	18	90
Other	8	10	1

Modified from Wenger CB, Hardy JD: Temperature regulation and exposure to heat and cold. In: Lehmann JF (ed): Therapeutic Heat and Cold. Williams & Wilkins, Baltimore, MD, 1990, pp. 150–178.

or more is converted into heat within the body.[23] Since exercising muscles produce so much heat, they may be nearly 1°C warmer than the core. They warm the blood that perfuses them, and this blood, returning to the core, warms the rest of the body.

Biophysics of Heat Exchange with the Environment

Radiation, convection, and evaporation are the dominant means of heat exchange with the environment. In humans, respiration usually accounts for a minor part of total heat exchange and is not predominantly under thermoregulatory control, although hyperthermic subjects may hyperventilate. Humans, therefore, exchange most heat with the environment through the skin, and the rate of heat exchange between the body and the environment depends on the surface area of the skin.

Every surface emits energy as electromagnetic radiation with a power output that depends on its area, reflectivity, and temperature, and every surface absorbs electromagnetic radiation from its environment at a rate that depends on its area and reflectivity and on the radiant temperature of the environment (T_r). Radiative heat exchange (R) between the skin and the environment is proportional to the difference between the fourth powers of the respective absolute temperature of the surfaces; but if the difference between skin temperature (T_{sk}) and T_r is much smaller than the absolute temperature of the skin, R is approximately proportional to $(T_{sk} - T_r)$. At ordinary tissue and environmental temperatures, virtually all radiant energy is in the far infrared range, where nearly all surfaces except polished metals have low reflectivity. However, bodies such as the sun that are hot enough to glow emit large amounts of radiation in the near infrared and visible range, in which light-colored surfaces have higher reflectivity than dark surfaces do. The practical importance of this is that skin and clothing color have little effect on heat exchange except in sunlight or intense artificial light.

Convection is transfer of heat via moving fluid, either liquid or gas. In thermal physiology the fluid is usually air or water in the environment or blood inside the body. Fluids conduct heat in the same way as solids do, and a perfectly still fluid transfers heat only by conduction. Since air and water are not good conductors of heat, perfectly still air or water is not effective in heat transfer. However, it is rare that a fluid is perfectly still, and slight movement produces enough convection to have a large effect on heat transfer. Thus, although conduction contributes to heat transfer by moving fluids, convection so dominates the overall heat transfer that we refer to the entire process as convection. The conduction term (K) in equation 1 is therefore, in practice, restricted to heat flow between the body and other solid objects, and usually represents only a small part of the total heat exchange with the environment. Convective heat exchange between the skin and the ambient air is proportional to the skin surface area and the difference between skin and air temperature. Convective heat exchange depends also on geometric factors that affect heat exchange with moving air and on the degree of air movement. It is approximately proportional to the square root of air speed, except at very low air speeds.

A gram of water that is converted into vapor at 30°C absorbs 2,425 J (0.58 kcal) in the process. In subjects who are not sweating, evaporative water loss is typically about 13 to 15 g/$(m^2 \cdot h)$, corresponding to a heat loss of 16 to 18 W for a surface area of 1.8 m^2. About half of this amount is lost through breathing, and half as insensible perspiration[24,25] (ie, evaporation of water that diffuses through the skin). Insensible perspiration is independent of the sweat glands and is not under thermoregulatory control.

These modes of water loss, however, are quite small compared with what is possible during sweating. Evaporation of sweat is proportional to the skin surface area that is wet with sweat, and depends also on air movement, since water vapor is carried away by moving air, and on the temperature of the skin and the moisture content of the air. The most familiar way of representing the moisture content of air is as relative humidity, the ratio between the actual moisture content of the air and the maximum moisture content that is possible at the temperature of the air. However relative humidity is not the most useful measure of the evaporative cooling power of the environment for thermal physiology, and may be misleading. A more useful index is the wet bulb temperature, which is the temperature of a completely wet ventilated surface that is not artificially heated or cooled. Wet bulb temperature is measured with a psychrometer, a device that includes a thermometer, a water source with a wick to keep the thermometer bulb wet, and some means of blowing ambient air across the wick. The temperature inside a closed vehicle or poorly ventilated building in direct sunlight may easily reach 50°C (122°F), and if there are sources of moisture inside, the relative humidity may reach 37%, which may not sound particularly high; however, the wet bulb temperature in such an environment is 35°C (95°F), the same as in a 35°C environment at 100% relative humidity.

Tissue Blood Flow and Heat Transport in the Body

Heat travels within the body by two parallel means: conduction through the tissues and convection by the blood, the process by which flowing blood carries heat from warmer to cooler tissues. Heat flow by conduction is proportional to the change of temperature with distance in the direction of heat flow and to the thermal conductivity of the tissues. Heat flow by convection depends on the rate of blood flow through the tissue and the temperature difference between the tissue and the blood supplying it. The power of the body to transport heat through a layer of tissue by conduction and convection combined is expressed as conductance, C, defined as $C = HF/(\Delta T)$, where HF is the rate of heat flow through the tissue layer, and ΔT is the temperature difference across the tissue layer.

The most important conductance for thermal physiology is that involved in heat transfer from body core to skin. The skin and other superficial and peripheral tissues are, in general, cooler than the core. These cooler tissues, lying between the core and the skin surface, compose the shell. The shell is defined functionally, rather than anatomically, and is thinnest when the body is warm and skin blood flow is high. Since all heat leaving the body via the skin passes through the shell, the shell insulates the core from the environment. In a cold subject, vasoconstriction reduces skin blood flow so much that the conductance of the shell, and thus core-to-skin heat transfer, is dominated by conduction. A representative value for shell conductance of a lean man under these conditions is $8.9 \text{ W}/(\text{m}^2 \cdot {}^\circ\text{C})$, or about $16 \text{ W}/{}^\circ\text{C}$ for a whole body with a typical surface area of 1.8 m^2. The subcutaneous fat layer adds to the insulation value of the shell of a vasoconstricted subject, because it increases the thickness of the shell and because its thermal conductivity is only about 0.4 times that of dermis or muscle; thus it is a more effective insulator. In a warm subject, however, the shell is relatively thin and provides little insulation. Furthermore, a warm subject's skin blood flow is high, so heat flow from the core to the skin is dominated by convection. In these circumstances the subcutaneous fat layer, which affects conduction but not convection, has little effect on heat flow. Obese persons do tend to be less heat-tolerant than thinner persons, for two main reasons. First, the obese are at a relative disadvantage for dissipating heat because they have less skin surface area in proportion to their weight than do their thinner counterparts. Second, obese individuals tend to be less physically fit and therefore to have less well-developed heat-dissipating responses, as discussed later.

Let us return to our vasoconstricted man with a shell conductance of $16 \text{ W}/{}^\circ\text{C}$. Under these conditions, a temperature difference between core and skin of 5°C allows a typical resting metabolic heat production of 80 W to be conducted to the skin surface. In a cool environment, T_{sk} may be low enough for this to occur easily; however, in a warm environment or especially during exercise, shell conductance must increase substantially to allow all the heat produced to be conducted to the skin without at the same time causing core temperature to rise to dangerous or lethal levels. For example, without an increase in shell conductance, T_c would have to be 30°C higher than T_{sk} to allow heat production of 480 W during moderate exercise to be carried to the skin. Fortunately, under such circumstances, increases in skin blood flow occur that can raise shell conductance 10-fold or more. Thus a crucial thermoregulatory function of skin blood flow is to control the conductance of the shell and the ease with which heat travels from core to skin. A closely related function is to control T_{sk}. In a person who is not sweating, an increase in skin blood flow tends to bring T_{sk} toward T_c, and a decrease allows T_{sk} to approach ambient temperature. Since convective and radiative heat exchange (R + C) depend directly on skin temperature, the body can control heat exchange with the environment by adjusting skin blood flow. If the heat stress is so great that increasing R + C through increasing skin blood flow is not enough to maintain heat balance, the body secretes sweat to increase evaporative heat loss. Once sweating begins, skin blood flow continues to increase as the person becomes warmer, but now the tendency of an increase in skin blood flow to warm the skin is approximately balanced by the tendency of an increase in sweating to cool the skin. Therefore, after sweating begins, further increases in skin blood flow usually cause little change in skin temperature or R + C. The increases in skin blood flow that accompany sweating are important to thermoregulation, nevertheless, since they deliver to the skin the heat that is being removed by evaporation of sweat and facilitate evaporation by keeping the skin warm. Skin blood flow and sweating thus work in tandem to dissipate heat that is produced in the body.

Physiologic Heat-Dissipating Responses

Humans have two physiologic responses for dissipating heat, dilation of the cutaneous vasculature and sweating. Each of these may affect cardiovascular homeostasis.

Responses of Skin Vascular Beds, and Pooling of Blood. Blood vessels in human skin are under dual vasomotor control, involving separate nervous signals for vasoconstriction and for vasodilation.[26-28] Reflex vasoconstriction, occurring in response to cold and also as part of certain nonthermal reflexes such as baroreflexes, is mediated primarily through adrenergic sympathetic fibers distributed widely over most of the skin.[29] Reducing the flow of impulses in these nerve fibers allows the blood vessels to dilate. In the so-called acral regions ie, lips, ears, nose, palms of the hands, and soles of the feet,[27,29] and in the superficial veins,[27] vasoconstrictor fibers are the predominant vasomotor innervation, and the vasodilation occurring during heat exposure is largely a result of withdrawal of vasoconstrictor activity.[30] Reflex control of skin blood flow in these regions, unlike that in the rest of the skin,[30] is sensitive to small temperature changes in the thermoneutral range, ie, the range of thermal conditions in which the body is neither chilled nor sweating, and may "fine tune" heat loss to maintain heat balance in this range.

In most of the skin, the vasodilation occurring during heat exposure depends on sympathetic nervous signals that cause the blood vessels to dilate, and is prevented or reversed by regional nerve block.[31] Since it depends on the action of nervous signals, such vasodilation is sometimes referred to as active vasodilation. Active vasodilation occurs in almost all the skin outside the acral regions.[30] In skin areas where active vasodilation occurs, vasoconstrictor activity is minimal in the thermoneutral range, and as the body is warmed, active vasodilation begins near the point of onset of sweating.[27,32] The neurotransmitter or other vasoactive substances responsible for active vasodilation in human skin is not known.[29] However, since sweating and vasodilation operate in tandem in the heat, there has been considerable interest in the notion that the mechanism for active vasodilation is somehow linked to the action of sweat glands.[27,33] Active vasodilation is impaired or absent in the skin of patients with anhidrotic ectodermal dysplasia,[34] even though their vasoconstrictor responses are intact, implying that active vasodilation either is linked to an action of sweat glands or is mediated through nerves that have not developed or are nonfunctional in these patients.

The superficial venous beds receive blood from the skin. Dilation of these beds, which is complete at mild levels of heat stress, enhances transfer of heat from blood to skin. However, in regions below the level of the heart, these veins readily become engorged with blood, especially when skin blood flow is high, and the resulting peripheral pooling of blood impairs venous return, reduces central blood volume and compromises diastolic filling of the heart, and limits cardiac output, especially during exercise. Compensatory responses that maintain cardiac function in the face of peripheral pooling are discussed later in the chapter.

Sweating and Loss of Fluid and Electrolytes. Humans can dissipate large amounts of heat by secretion and evaporation of sweat. When the environment is warmer than the skin, usually when the environment is warmer than about 35°C, evaporation is the only way to lose heat. Human sweat glands are controlled through postganglionic sympathetic nerves that release acetylcholine,[35] rather than norepinephrine like most other sympathetic nerves. Human skin contains 2 million to 3 million functional eccrine sweat glands,[35] the histologic type most important in thermoregulation. Their secretory capacity can be increased by aerobic exercise training and heat acclimatization. A fit man well acclimatized to heat can achieve a peak sweating rate greater than 2.5 L/h.[36,37] Such rates cannot long be maintained, however, and the maximum daily sweat output is probably about 15 L.[38]

Eccrine sweat is formed from a precursor fluid in the secretory coil of the gland. This fluid is initially isotonic with plasma; but as it moves along the duct, Na^+ is reabsorbed from the fluid by active transport. When it emerges from the duct as sweat, it is the most dilute body fluid, with $[Na^+]$ ranging from less than 5 to 60 mEq/L.[39] As the rate of sweat secretion increases, the precursor fluid moves through the duct more quickly, and a smaller fraction of its initial sodium content is reabsorbed, and $[Na^+]$ in the resulting sweat is higher. Thus salt losses through sweating increase disproportionately as sweat production rises.

Large amounts of water and salt can be lost in a few hours of profuse sweating, and the consequent reduction in plasma volume may compromise cardiovascular homeostasis and cardiac output. In addition, since sweat is hypotonic to plasma, loss of sweat progressively increases the osmolality of the bodily fluids if the water is not replaced. Both the reduction in plasma volume and the increase in osmolality will compromise thermoregulation by shifting the thresholds for sweating and vasodilation in the skin toward higher core temperature. If large amounts of salt are lost, and only the water but not the salt is replaced, plasma volume will not return to normal because the loss of salt reduces the total number of osmoles in the extracellular fluid, and a disproportionate amount of the water that is replaced goes into the intracellular space.

During prolonged (several hours) heat exposure with high sweat output, sweat rates often gradually diminish, and the response of the sweat glands to locally applied cholinergic drugs is reduced also. The reduction of sweat gland responsiveness is sometimes called sweat gland "fatigue." One mechanism involved is hydration of the stratum corneum, which swells and mechanically obstructs the sweat duct, causing a reduction in sweat secretion, an effect called hidromeiosis.[40] The glands' responsiveness can be at least partly restored if the skin is allowed to dry, eg, by increasing air movement,[41] but prolonged sweating also causes histologic changes in the sweat glands.[42]

Compensatory Cardiovascular Responses

During heat stress, peripheral pooling of blood and decreased plasma volume due to unreplaced fluid losses combine to impair venous return and diastolic filling of the heart. Several compensatory mechanisms help to defend cardiac filling, cardiac output, and arterial blood pressure under such circumstances. The most important compensatory reflexes are constriction of the renal and splanchnic vascular beds. Reduction of blood flow through these beds increases the fraction of cardiac output that is available to perfuse exercising muscle. In addition, the splanchnic vascular bed is very compliant; thus, reduction in splanchnic blood flow reduces the volume of blood contained in the splanchnic vascular bed, allowing a partial restoration of central blood volume and cardiac diastolic filling. The effect of pooling of blood in the skin on central blood volume and the compensatory effect of splanchnic vasoconstriction are shown schematically in Figure 4–3. The degree of splanchnic vasoconstriction is graded according to the levels of heat stress and exercise

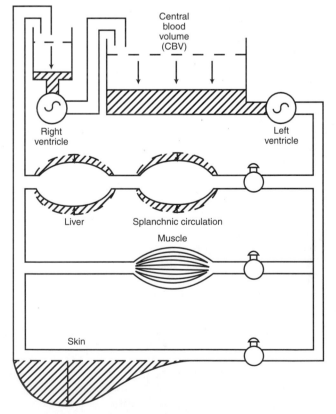

FIGURE 4–3. Schema of the effects of skin vasodilation on peripheral pooling of blood and the thoracic reservoirs from which the ventricles are filled, and the effects of compensatory vasomotor adjustments in the splanchnic circulation. The valves drawn at the right sides of liver–splanchnic circulation, muscle, and skin vascular beds represent the resistance vessels that control blood flow through those beds. *Arrows* show the direction of the changes during heat stress. (Redrawn from Rowell LB: Cardiovascular adjustments to thermal stress. In: Shepherd JT, Abboud FM [eds]: Handbook of Physiology, Section 2: The Cardiovascular System, Vol 3: Peripheral Circulation and Organ Blood Flow. American Physiological Society, Bethesda, MD, 1983, pp. 967–1023; and Rowell LB: Cardiovascular aspects of human thermoregulation. Circ Res 52:367–379, 1983.)

intensity. During strenuous exercise in the heat, renal and splanchnic blood flow may decrease to 20% of their values in a cool resting subject.[27,43] Splanchnic vasoconstriction may help to explain nausea and vomiting accompanying heat exhaustion, and gastrointestinal symptoms that some athletes experience after endurance events.[44]

In addition, the superficial veins, which drain the skin, constrict during exercise and thus reduce the volume of blood pooled in them. Because of the essential thermoregulatory function of skin blood flow during exercise and heat stress, the body preferentially compromises splanchnic and renal flow to maintain cardiovascular homeostasis[45]; but above a certain level of cardiovascular strain, skin blood flow too is compromised to maintain cardiac filling. Another important mechanism that opposes pooling of blood in dependent veins during leg exercise is the so-called muscle pump. Since the valves in the veins of the limbs permit blood flow only toward the heart, rhythmic contraction of skeletal muscle assists the movement of venous blood toward the heart. Exhausted runners often collapse only after finishing a race, partly because they lose most of the effect of the muscle pump.

Despite these compensatory responses, heat stress markedly increases the thermal and cardiovascular strain that exercise produces in subjects unacclimatized to heat. In Figure 4–6, a comparison of responses on the first day of exercise in the heat with those on cool days shows some effects of unaccustomed environmental heat stress on the responses to exercise. On the first day in the heat, heart rate during exercise reached a level about 40 beats/min higher than in the cool environment, to help compensate for the effects of impaired cardiac filling and to maintain cardiac output, and rectal temperature during exercise rose 1°C higher than in the cool environment.

Responses to Cold

The body maintains core temperature in the cold by minimizing heat loss and, when this is not sufficient, by increasing heat production. In humans, constriction of peripheral blood vessels to reduce core-to-skin thermal conductance is the chief physiologic means of conserving heat in the cold. Skin blood flow is the principal determinant of conductance, and constriction of cutaneous arterioles reduces conductance by reducing skin blood flow. In addition, constriction of the superficial limb veins further improves heat conservation by diverting venous blood to the deep limb veins, which lie close to the major arteries of the limbs and do not constrict in cold. (Since many penetrating veins connect the superficial veins to the deep veins, venous blood from anywhere in the limb potentially can return to the heart via either superficial or deep veins.) In the deep veins, cool venous blood returning to the core can take up heat from the warm blood in the adjacent deep limb arteries. Thus some of the heat contained in the arterial blood as it enters the limbs takes a "short circuit" back to the core, and when the arterial blood reaches the skin, it is already cooler than the core and so loses less heat to the skin than it otherwise would. (When the superficial veins dilate in heat, most venous blood returns via superficial veins to maximize core-to-skin heat flow.) The transfer of heat from arteries to veins by this short circuit is called countercurrent heat exchange, and it can cool the blood in the radial artery of a cool but comfortable subject to as low as 25°C by the time it reaches the wrist.[46]

Once skin blood flow is near minimal, metabolic heat production increases. In human adults, nearly all of this increase occurs in skeletal muscles, as a result first of increased tone and later of frank shivering. Shivering may increase metabolic rate at rest by more than fourfold, eg, to 350 to 400 W, comparable to mild-to-moderate exercise. It is frequently stated that the shivering response diminishes substantially after several hours and is impaired following exhaustive exercise, but these effects have not been studied systematically and are not well understood. In a reasonably fit athlete exercising in cold air, exercise rather than shivering would ordinarily be expected to account for most of the metabolic heat production. Since warm clothing tends to restrict movement, an athlete will improve his or her competitive advantage by wearing the lightest clothing that will maintain heat balance with the expected rate of heat production. Thus an athlete who cannot maintain the expected pace due to exhaustion or musculoskeletal injury may be at increased risk of hypothermia during competition in a cold environment.

The shell's insulating properties increase in the cold, as its blood vessels constrict and its thickness increases. In the cold the shell includes a substantial amount of skeletal muscle, whose blood flow is reduced by direct cooling. The resulting reduction of blood flow through muscle in the shell of a cool subject increases the shell's insulating properties.[47] This effect limits the ability of skeletal muscle activity to warm the core, since peripheral or superficial exercising muscles will be warmed by their own heat production and by the blood flow required by aerobic exercise and thus may lose large amounts of heat to the environment through the overlying skin, especially when the overlying skin is very cold,[48] as during immersion in cold water.

Control of Thermoregulatory Responses

Integration of Thermal Information. Temperature receptors in the body core and the skin transmit information about their temperatures through afferent nerves to the brain stem, and especially the hypothalamus, where much of the integration of temperature information takes place. Core temperature receptors involved in thermoregulation have been found in several sites, including the spinal cord and medulla,[49] but they are concentrated especially in the hypothalamus,[49] and in experimental mammals temperature changes of only a few tenths of 1°C in the anterior preoptic area of the hypothalamus elicit changes in the thermoregulatory effector responses.

Most physiologic control systems produce a response that is graded according to the disturbance in the regulated variable. In many such systems, changes in the effector responses are proportional to displacement of the regulated variable from some threshold value.[24] Such control systems are called proportional control systems. Changes in the heat-dissipating responses are proportional to displacement of core temperature from some threshold value (Fig. 4–4). Each response has a core temperature threshold, a temperature at which the response starts to increase. These thresholds depend on mean skin temperature; thus, at any given skin temperature, the change in each response is proportional to the change in core temperature, and increasing the skin temperature lowers the threshold level of core temperature and increases the re-

sponse at any given core temperature. Control of the heat-dissipating responses is more complicated than the most simple proportional control systems, since the heat-dissipating responses are controlled according to both core and skin temperature. The sensitivity of the thermoregulatory system to core temperature enables it to adjust heat loss so as to resist disturbances in core temperature, and the system's sensitivity to skin temperature enables it to respond appropriately to moderate changes in the environment with little or no change in body core temperature. For example, the skin temperature of someone who enters a hot environment rises and may elicit sweating even if there is no change in core temperature. On the other hand, an increase in heat production due to exercise elicits the appropriate heat-dissipating responses through an increase in core temperature.

Both sweating and skin blood flow participate in reflexes other than thermoregulatory responses. For the purposes of this chapter, the most important nonthermoregulatory reflexes are those that involve the blood vessels of the skin in responses that help to maintain cardiac output, blood pressure, and tissue oxygen delivery. During heat stress, thermoregulatory requirements usually dominate the control of these responses, but in conditions of high cardiovascular strain, thermoregulatory requirements for skin blood flow may be overridden to support circulatory function. An important and dramatic example is the reduction in skin blood flow that accounts for the cool, ashen skin characteristic of heat exhaustion.

Thermoregulatory Responses During Exercise. At the start of exercise, metabolic heat production increases rapidly, but there is little change in heat loss initially, so heat is stored in the body and core temperature rises. The increase in core temperature, in turn, elicits heat-loss responses, but core temperature continues to rise until heat loss has increased enough to match heat production; thus heat balance is restored and core temperature and the heat-loss responses reach new steady-state levels. The rise in core temperature that elicits heat-dissipating responses sufficient to reestablish thermal balance during exercise is an example of a load error,[24] which occurs when any proportional control system resists the effect of some imposed

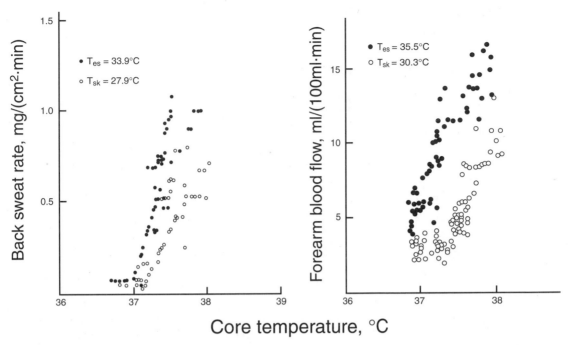

FIGURE 4–4. The relations of back sweat rate (*left panel*) and forearm blood flow (*right panel*) to esophageal (T_{es}) and mean skin temperatures ($\overline{T}_{sk}$). Sweating data are from four subjects performing cycle exercise at an oxygen consumption rate of 1.6 L/min; blood flow data are from one subject. During measurements of blood flow, forearm temperature was kept at 36.8°C to eliminate a difference in local temperature between experiments. Local temperature was not controlled independently during measurements of sweating; thus the difference between conditions includes a small effect of local skin temperature, appearing as a difference in slope. (*Left panel* drawn from data of Sawka MN, Gonzalez RR, Drolet LL, Pandolf KB: Heat exchange during upper- and lower-body exercise. J Appl Physiol 57:1050–1054, 1984; *right panel* modified from Wenger CB, Roberts MF, Stolwijk JAJ, Nadel ER: Forearm blood flow during body temperature transients produced by leg exercise. J Appl Physiol 38:58–63, 1975.)

disturbance or "load." In a proportional control system, the load error is proportional to the load, and indeed the magnitude of core temperature elevation at steady state during exercise is proportional to the metabolic rate[50] and thus to the rate of heat production. Although the elevated core temperature during exercise superficially resembles that during fever due to resetting of the body's thermostat, there are some crucial differences. First, although heat production may increase substantially (through shivering) at the beginning of a fever, it does not need to stay high to maintain the fever but returns nearly to prefebrile levels once the fever is established; during exercise, however, an increase in heat production not only causes the elevation in core temperature but also is necessary to sustain it. Second, the rate of heat loss while core temperature is rising during a fever, is, if anything, lower than before the fever began; but the rate of heat loss during exercise starts to increase as soon as core temperature starts to rise and continues to increase as long as core temperature is rising. Because of the role of skin temperature in thermoregulatory control, the steady-state core temperature during exercise is largely independent of ambient temperature and humidity[51] over a range of environmental conditions called the "prescriptive zone," whose limits depend on exercise intensity.[52] Figure 4–5 shows steady-state rectal temperatures during exercise at three intensities in a broad range of environmental conditions. The higher the metabolic rate during exercise, the lower the upper limit of the prescriptive zone.

During prolonged exercise there is a gradual "drift" in several cardiovascular and thermoregulatory responses. This may include a continuous rise in heart rate, accompanied by a fall in stroke volume and reductions in aortic, pulmo-

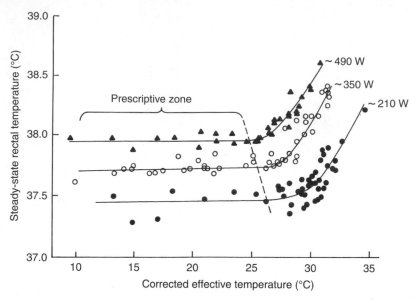

FIGURE 4–5. Relation between environmental conditions and steady-state rectal temperature during exercise at three metabolic rates. The abscissa is "corrected effective temperature," a function of globe temperature (which combines air temperature and radiant temperature), wet-bulb temperature, and air speed, chosen to be an index of environmental stress. (Redrawn from Lind AR: A physiological criterion for setting thermal environmental limits for everyday work. J Appl Physiol 18:51–56, 1963.)

nary arterial, and right ventricular end-diastolic pressures.[43] Rowell[43] named these changes "cardiovascular drift," and thought of them as appearing as early as after 15 minutes of exercise. He[43] and Johnson and Rowell[53] emphasized the role of thermoregulatory increases in skin blood flow in producing cardiovascular drift. However, later authors[54–56] described, as part of the picture of cardiovascular drift, an upward creep in core temperature, which may begin only after a period of apparent thermal steady state (eg, after 30–60 minutes of exercise). In some of these studies, most but not all of the changes in cardiovascular and thermoregulatory responses could be prevented by replacing fluid lost in sweat, suggesting that these changes were mostly secondary to changes in plasma volume and osmolality due to sweating. Other factors that may affect cardiovascular and thermoregulatory function during prolonged exercise include changes in myocardial function,[57] changes in baroreceptor sensitivity or peripheral α-adrenergic receptor responsiveness,[58] or an upward adjustment of the thermoregulatory set point,[59] presumably due to some sort of inflammatory response and perhaps elicited by products of muscle injury.[59] These effects have

not been investigated extensively, and little is known about the underlying physiologic or pathologic mechanisms. Some of these effects have been reported only after several hours of exercise or near exhaustion, and little is known about the conditions of exercise duration and intensity required to produce them, or their persistence after the end of exercise. Although their functional significance is, as yet, only poorly understood, these changes may be important in limiting performance during prolonged strenuous activity, such as forced marches, marathons, and other endurance athletic events.

ADVERSE EFFECTS OF HEAT AND COLD STRESS

Heat Disorders

Exercise is often an important factor in heat disorders because of both the metabolic heat produced during exercise, and the combined effects of thermoregulation and exercise on several physiologic systems, particularly the circulatory system. Although hyperthermia is often associated with heat disorders and may be involved in their pathogenesis, the relation between body temperature and clinical manifestations is complex,[60] and levels of core temperature that are typically associated with heat stroke have been observed in athletes who apparently suffered no ill effects.[61,62] For convenience, the heat disorders may be divided into two groups: those with primarily local manifestations and those with more general manifestations. This division is not absolute, however; for example, extensive miliaria rubra, a skin disorder, may impair thermoregulation. For more detailed discussion of pathogenesis and clinical management, the reader is referred elsewhere.[10,11] The heat disorders are discussed in brief.

Disorders with Primarily Local Manifestations

Heat edema, a dependent edema of the hands, legs, and feet, typically occurs within the first week of adaptation to tropical heat, and is worsened by prolonged standing. Heat edema is probably due to the retention of salt and water, which is a normal part of acclimatization to heat, and peripheral vasodilation probably has a contributory role. Heat edema is benign and self-limiting. Treatment with diuretics is not indicated and will impair development of acclimatization by interfering with retention of salt and water.

Miliaria rubra, commonly called heat rash or prickly heat, is characterized by blockage of the sweat ducts with plugs of keratin debris, and typically occurs following repeated or prolonged exposure to heat. The resulting rash is irritating, but the most serious effect is marked impairment of sweating in the affected skin, which may precede the appearance of the rash by up to a week and may persist for some time after the rash clears.[63] Some patients may be unable to sweat below the neck. The impairment of sweating, if extensive, substantially limits the ability to tolerate exercise in heat.

Heat Syncope

Heat syncope is a temporary circulatory failure due to pooling of blood in the peripheral veins and a consequent decrease in diastolic filling of the heart. The primary cause of the peripheral pooling is the large increase in skin blood flow that is part of the thermoregulatory response to heat exposure, but an inadequate baroreflex response may be an important contributing factor. Heat syncope usually occurs in individuals who are standing with little activity. Symptoms may range from lightheadedness to loss of consciousness. Core temperature typically is no more than slightly elevated, except when an attack follows exercise, and the skin is wet and cool. Recovery is rapid once the patient sits or lies down, though complete recovery of blood pressure and heart rate often take an hour or two. Heat syncope affects mostly those who are not acclimatized to heat, presumably because the expansion of plasma volume that occurs with acclimatization compensates for the peripheral pooling of blood. Patients being treated for hypertension with diuretics or medications that impair the baroreflexes are at particular risk and should exercise care when standing in crowds or lines in hot surroundings.

Continuum of Heat Cramps, Heat Exhaustion, and Heat Stroke

Traditionally, heat cramps, heat exhaustion, and heat stroke were considered three distinct clinical entities. However, these disorders have overlapping features, and the concept that they are syndromes representing different parts of a continuum[64,65] has gained favor. In keeping with this concept, some recent literature describes a syndrome called exertional heat injury, intermediate in severity between heat exhaustion and heat stroke. However, there does not seem to be a consensus on diagnostic criteria for distinguishing exertional heat injury from heat exhaustion, on one hand, or from heat stroke, on the other; compare, for example, Petersdorf[66] and Kark and Ward.[67]

Water loss from the sweat glands can exceed 1 L/h during exercise in the heat. The amount of salt lost in the sweat is quite variable, and persons who are well acclimatized to heat can often secrete very dilute sweat. However, those who are less well acclimatized may lose large amounts of salt in their sweat and become substantially salt depleted. Consider the following conditions.

Heat Cramps. Heat cramps is an acute disorder consisting of brief, recurrent, and often agonizing cramps in skeletal muscle of the limbs and trunk. The cramp produces a hard lump in the affected muscle, which typically has recently been used in intense exercise. Although the cramps are brief, generally lasting only a few minutes, they may recur for many hours in severe, untreated cases. Patients are characteristically physically fit men, well acclimatized to heat, who have been drinking adequate amounts of water but not replacing salt lost in the sweat. They usually have hyponatremia, which is thought to be involved in the pathogenesis of heat cramps, though the mechanism is obscure. Hyponatremia is common, however, whereas heat cramps are an unusual accompaniment. Intravenous infusion of 0.5 to 1 L of normal saline solution or, alternatively, somewhat smaller amounts of hypertonic saline solution is the treatment of choice in severe cases. However, oral administration of 0.1% salt in water is also effective,[11] somewhat unexpectedly, given the usual association of heat cramps with hyponatremia. The immediate goal of treatment is relief of the cramps, not restoration of salt balance, which takes longer and is best achieved by giving salted food or fluids by mouth.

Heat Exhaustion. Heat exhaustion is characterized by circulatory collapse occurring after prolonged or repeated exercise-heat stress. Most patients have lost both salt and water, but heat exhaustion may be associated predominantly with either salt depletion or water depletion. Salt-depleted patients have hypovolemia out of proportion to the degree of dehydration and are hypovolemic even if not greatly dehydrated, since their body water is distributed preferentially to the intracellular space to maintain osmotic balance between the intracellular and extracellular spaces. Salt-depleted persons tend either to be unacclimatized to heat or to be consuming small amounts of salt in their diet, and they have replaced at least some of their water loss. Heat exhaustion due primarily to water depletion tends to develop more rapidly than that due to salt depletion, and is characterized by greater thirst. In addition, hypovolemia occurring during water-depletion heat exhaustion is associated with less hemoconcentration, since water is lost from both the red blood cells and the plasma.

Heat exhaustion spans a clinical spectrum, from fairly mild disorders that respond well to rest in a cool environment and fluid replacement by mouth, to severe forms with collapse, confusion, and hyperpyrexia. Loss of consciousness is uncommon, but there may be vertigo, ataxia, headache, weakness, nausea and vomiting, pallor, tachycardia, and orthostatic hypotension. The patient usually is sweating profusely. Muscle cramps indistinguishable from heat cramps may occur, especially if salt depletion is part of the pathogenesis. Treatment consists primarily of laying the patient down away from the heat, and replacing fluid and salt, as needed. In severe cases, intravenous administration of normal saline solution may be required. Active cooling measures may be called for if the patient's core temperature is 40.6°C (105°F) or higher, since water-depletion heat exhaustion may lead to heat stroke.

Restoration of Fluid Loss. As $[Na^+]$ in the extracellular fluid is reduced, water moves from the extracellular fluid into the intracellular fluid to maintain osmotic balance, causing the cells to swell. Since the brain occupies most of the space within a rigid case, even a modest degree of cerebral edema can increase intracranial pressure, leading to encephalopathy and brain stem herniation in extreme cases. By removal of interstitial fluid and by loss of solutes from within the cells, the brain can protect itself from osmotic swelling if plasma $[Na^+]$ changes slowly enough.[68] Although osmotic swelling of the brain is usually associated with hyponatremia, its occurrence is related to the rate of change of plasma $[Na^+]$ rather than the level of $[Na^+]$. For this reason, care should be taken to prevent reducing plasma $[Na^+]$ too rapidly when replacing water in water-depleted patients.[11] In addition, a few individuals who are drinking large amounts of fluid during sustained exercise in the heat may become hyponatremic if they lose excessive amounts of salt in their sweat or drink and retain more fluid than is required to replace their losses.[69–71] Although hyponatremia is far less common than water-depletion heat exhaustion, it may be difficult to differentiate the two conditions in the early stages without laboratory tests. Patients with water-depletion heat exhaustion respond quickly to fluid replacement, whereas hyponatremia is aggravated by administering hypotonic fluids, and may progress to life-threatening cerebral edema. Therefore, in a patient presumed to have heat exhaustion but who does not improve quickly in response to administration of hypotonic fluids, such treatment should not be continued without further medical evaluation. A rule suggested for field use is that a patient with presumed heat exhaustion should be given 2 quarts of water to drink over the course of an hour and needs medical evaluation if noticeable improvement has not occurred by the end of the hour.

Heat Stroke

Heat stroke is the most severe heat disorder and as such deserves special attention.

Heat stroke is characterized by hyperthermia, which often develops rapidly, and severe neurologic disturbances, frequently including convulsions. Although these disturbances typically are characteristic of a nonfocal encephalopathy, some patients may show abnormalities of cerebellar function, which may be transient or may persist. Heat stroke may be divided into two forms depending on the pathogenesis. In the classic form, the primary pathogenic factor is environmental heat stress that overwhelms an impaired thermoregulatory system, whereas in exertional heat stroke the primary factor is metabolic heat production (see Knochel and Reed[11] for a more extensive discussion). Consequently, victims of exertional heat stroke tend to be younger and more physically fit (typically, soldiers, athletes, and laborers) than victims of the classic form. Heat stroke may be complicated by liver damage, electrolyte abnormalities, and, especially in the exertional form, by rhabdomyolysis, disseminated intravascular coagulation, or renal failure.

Loss of consciousness may occur suddenly or may be preceded by up to an hour of prodromal symptoms including headache, dizziness, drowsiness, restlessness, ataxia, confusion, and irrational or aggressive behavior. The physiologic pathology is not well understood, and there is evidence that factors other than hyperthermia contribute to the development of heat stroke. The traditional diagnostic criteria of heat stroke—coma, hot dry skin, and temperature above 41.1°C (106°F)—reflect experience primarily with the classic form. Rigid adherence to these criteria will lead to underdiagnosis, since cessation of sweating may be a late event, especially in exertional heat stroke. Moreover, patients may come to medical attention either in the prodromal phase or after they have had a

chance to cool somewhat and regain consciousness, especially if they still are sweating.

Measurement of rectal temperature or other deep body temperature is essential for clinical evaluation of hyperthermia and for observing response to treatment. A diagnosis of heat stroke must not be excluded on the basis of either oral temperature or temperature measured at the external auditory meatus or tympanic membrane. Because of hyperventilation, oral temperature may be 2° to 3°C lower than rectal temperature in heat stroke, and the temperature of the external auditory meatus or tympanum may be as much as 5°C lower than rectal temperature in collapsed hyperthermic athletes.[72] Low temperature of the tympanum may be due in part to cooling of its blood supply, which comes mostly from branches of the external carotid artery and thus follows a superficial course. It is sometimes asserted that since the tympanum is so close to the cranium, tympanic temperature represents intracranial temperature, and thus the temperature of the brain, more accurately than any other noninvasive temperature measurement. Thus tympanic temperature measurements that are appreciably lower than measurements of trunk core (eg, rectal or esophageal) temperature in hyperthermic human subjects are sometimes adduced to argue for the existence of physiologic heat exchange mechanisms that protect the human brain during hyperthermia by cooling it below the temperature of the central blood. However, there is little empirical support either for the claims made for tympanic temperature or for the existence of special mechanisms to cool the human brain (see Sawka et al[33] and Brengelmann[73] for further discussion).

Heat stroke is an extreme medical emergency, and prompt appropriate treatment is critical in reducing morbidity and mortality. Cooling the patient to lower the core temperature is the cornerstone of early treatment and should begin as soon as possible. The patient should be removed from hot surroundings without delay, excess clothing and any equipment that obstructs free flow of air should be removed, the patient's skin should be wetted if water is available, and the patient should be fanned to promote evaporative cooling. Although helpful, these measures are no substitute for more vigorous cooling once appropriate means are available, and cooling is accomplished most effectively by immersion in cold water. Costrini et al[74] lowered the rectal temperature of patients with heat stroke at a mean rate of 0.18°C/min by immersing them in ice water. There is some disagreement as to the optimal water temperature, since lowering the temperature not only increases the core-to-skin thermal gradient for heat flow but also reduces skin blood flow. Observations in dogs with heat stroke suggest that while water at 15° to 16°C (59°–61°F) is more effective than warmer water, little further advantage is gained with lower water temperature.[75]

However, there is no empirical support for the superiority of cooling methods, such as tepid baths or evaporation of sprayed water, that achieve only modest skin cooling. Some arguments in favor of such cooling methods are based on studies that compared different cooling methods in healthy persons with mild hyperthermia, whose peripheral vascular and other thermal responses may, however, be substantially different from those of patients with heat stroke. The pitfalls in relying on such studies may be seen by comparing the following two reports: In tests in hot but normal young subjects, an evaporative cooling method was reported to be more effective than other cooling methods, causing tympanic temperature to fall at a rate of 0.31°C/min.[76] However, in a series of patients with heat stroke the same authors found that the same cooling method lowered rectal temperature at a rate of only 0.06°C/min,[77] one fifth the rate they had reported in healthy subjects[76] and one third the rate that Costrini et al[74] achieved.

There is evidence for a systemic inflammatory component in heat stroke,[64] and elevated levels of several inflammatory cytokines have been reported in patients with heat stroke.[78–80] Leakage of gram-negative endotoxin from the gut, perhaps facilitated by splanchnic ischemia, may be a trigger for secretion of these cytokines, since treatments aimed at preventing leakage of endotoxin[81,82] or neutralizing endotoxin[83] partially protect experimental animals against heat stroke during subsequent heating. Gaffin and Hubbard[84] discussed the implications of these concepts for prevention and treatment of heat stroke, but their proposed measures are not supported by clinical data sufficient to allow their recommendation.

Aggravation of Other Diseases by Heat Stress

Besides causing more or less characteristic disorders, heat stress can worsen the clinical state of patients with a number of other diseases. For example, patients with congestive heart failure have substantially impaired sweating and circulatory responses to environmental heat stress, and exposure to moderately hot environments worsens the signs and symptoms of congestive heart failure.[14] Conversely, air conditioning improves the clinical progress of patients hospitalized in the summer with a variety of cardiorespiratory and other chronic diseases.[14] The harmful effects of heat stress on patients with other diseases are also shown by analysis of the effects of unusually hot weather on total mortality and causes of death. Ellis[15] examined monthly mortality statistics for the years 1952 to 1967 and identified 5 years in each of which more than 500 deaths were reported as due to "excessive heat and insolation." In June and July of these "heat wave" years there was excess mortality, ie, above that expected for the month, from diabetes; cerebrovascular accident; arteriosclerotic, degenerative, and hypertensive heart disease; and diseases of the blood-forming organs. Ellis estimated the total number of excess deaths was more than 10 times greater than the number of deaths actually reported as due to heat. The greatest increase in mortality during heat wave years was in infants and persons 65 or older.[15]

Hypothermia

Hypothermia occurs when the body's defenses against cold are disabled or overwhelmed. The direct effect of hypothermia is to slow the body's metabolic processes and thus to reduce the metabolic rate, via the law of Arrhenius. In this way, hypothermia prolongs the time that tissues can safely tolerate loss of blood flow and oxygen delivery. Controlled hypothermia is often used to protect the brain, which is especially vulnerable to anoxia, during surgical procedures in which its circulation is interrupted. Much of what we know about the physiologic effects of hypothermia comes from observations in surgical patients.

During the initial phases of cooling, stimulation of shivering through thermoregulatory reflexes far outweighs the direct effect of the law of Arrhenius, so that metabolic rate increases, reaching a peak at a core temperature of 30° to 33°C. At lower core temperatures, however, metabolic rate is dominated by the law of Arrhenius, and thermoregulation is lost. A vicious circle develops, wherein a fall in core temperature depresses metabolism and allows core temperature to fall further, so that at 17°C, oxygen consumption is about 15% and cardiac output 10% of precooling values.

Hypothermia that is not induced for therapeutic purposes is called accidental hypothermia. Accidental hypothermia occurs in individuals whose defenses are impaired by drugs (especially ethanol, in the United States) or by disease or other physical condition, and in healthy individuals who are immersed in cold water or become exhausted during exposure to cold. Hypothermia is classified according to the patient's core temperature as mild (32°–35°C), moderate (28°–32°C), or severe (<28°C). Shivering is usually prominent in mild hypothermia, but diminishes in moderate hypothermia, and is absent in severe hypothermia.

The pathophysiology is characterized chiefly by the depressant effect of cold (via the law of Arrhenius) on multiple physiologic processes and differences in the degree of depression of each process. Apart from shivering, the most prominent features of mild and moderate hypothermia are due to depression of the central nervous system. These begin with mood changes (commonly apathy, withdrawal, and irritability) progressing, as hypothermia deepens, to confusion and lethargy, ataxia, and speech and gait disturbances, which may mimic a cerebrovascular accident ("stroke"). In severe hypothermia, voluntary movement, reflexes, and consciousness are lost, and muscular rigidity appears. Cardiac output and respiration decrease as core temperature falls.

Myocardial irritability increases in severe hypothermia, causing substantial danger of ventricular fibrillation, with the risk increasing as cardiac temperature falls. The primary mechanism presumably is that cold depresses conduction velocity in Purkinje fibers more than in ventricular muscle, favoring the development of circus-movement propagation of action potentials, but myocardial hypoxia also contributes. In more profound hypothermia, cardiac sounds become inaudible, and pulse and blood pressure cannot be measured because of circulatory depression; the electrical activity of the heart and brain becomes unmeasurable, and extensive muscular rigidity may mimic rigor mortis. The patient may appear clinically dead, but patients have been revived with core temperatures as low as 17°C; thus, "no one is dead until warm and dead." The usual causes of death during hypothermia are cessation of respiration and failure of cardiac pumping, because of either ventricular fibrillation or direct depression of cardiac contraction.

Depression of renal tubular metabolism by cold impairs reabsorption of sodium, causing diuresis and leading to dehydration and hypovolemia. Acid-base disturbances in hypothermia are complex. Respiration and cardiac output typically are depressed more than metabolic rate, and mixed respiratory and metabolic acidosis results, due to carbon dioxide retention and lactic acid accumulation and also to the cold-induced shift of the hemoglobin-oxygen dissociation curve to the left. Acidosis aggravates the susceptibility to ventricular fibrillation.

Treatment consists of preventing further cooling, and restoring fluid, acid-base, and electrolyte balance. Patients with mild to moderate hypothermia may be warmed solely by providing abundant insulation to promote retention of metabolically produced heat, but those who are more severely affected require active rewarming. The most serious complication associated with treating hypothermia is development of ventricular fibrillation. Vigorous handling of the patient may trigger ventricular fibrillation, but an increase in the patient's circulation (eg, associated with warming or skeletal muscle activity) may itself increase susceptibility to such an occurrence. This may happen as follows: peripheral tissues of a hypothermic patient are, in general, even cooler than the core, including the heart, and acid products of anaerobic metabolism will have accumulated in underperfused tissues while the circulation was most depressed. As the circulation increases, a large increase in blood flow through cold, acidotic peripheral tissue may return enough cold, acidotic blood to the heart to cause a transient drop in the temperature and pH of the heart and increase its susceptibility to ventricular fibrillation.

The diagnosis of hypothermia is usually straightforward in a patient rescued from cold, but may be far less clear in a patient in whom hypothermia results from serious impairment of the defenses against cold. A typical example is the elderly person, living alone, who is discovered at home, cool and obtunded or unconscious. The setting may not particularly suggest hypothermia, and when the patient comes to medical attention, the diagnosis may easily be missed, since standard clinical thermometers are not graduated low enough (usually only to 34.4°C) to detect hypothermia, and in any case do not register temperature below the level to which the mercury has been shaken. Since hypothermia depresses the brain, the patient's condition may be misdiagnosed as a cerebrovascular accident or other primary neurologic disease. Thus, recognition of hypothermia in such a setting depends on the physician's considering it when he or she is examining a cool, obtunded patient and on obtaining a true core temperature with a thermometer that registers low temperatures.

FACTORS AFFECTING TOLERANCE TO HEAT AND COLD

Many factors, including heat acclimatization, physical fitness, gender, body fat, age, drugs, and a number of diseases, affect thermoregulatory responses and tolerance to heat and cold.

Acclimatization and Physical Fitness

Prolonged or repeated heat stress, especially when combined with exercise sufficient to elicit profuse sweating, produces acclimatization to heat,[85] a set of physiologic changes that reduces the physiologic strain associated with exercise-heat stress. The classic signs of heat acclimatization are reductions in core and skin temperatures and heart rate and increases in sweat production during a given level of exercise in heat. These changes begin to appear during the first few days, and approach full development within a week. Figure 4–6 illustrates some of these effects in three young men who were acclimatized by daily treadmill walks in dry heat for 10 days.[86] On the first day in the heat, heart rate

and rectal temperature during exercise reached much higher levels than in cool control (25°C) conditions, but on the tenth day in the heat, final heart rate and rectal temperature during exercise were 40 beats/min and 1°C, respectively, lower than on the first day. In addition, sweat production increased 10%, skin temperature was about 1.5°C lower, and the metabolic cost of treadmill walking decreased 4%.

The mechanisms that produce these changes are not fully understood, but include a modest (~0.4°C) reduction in the setting of the body's "thermostat," thus reducing the thresholds for sweating and cutaneous vasodilation; increased sensitivity of the sweat glands to cholinergic stimulation[87,88] and a decrease in sweat gland susceptibility to hidromeiosis and fatigue; and retention of salt and water and expansion of plasma volume to compensate for peripheral pooling of blood in dilated blood vessels in the skin. Heat acclimatization produces other changes[85] also, including improved ability to sustain high rates of sweat production; an aldosterone-mediated reduction in sweat sodium concentration, to levels as low as 5 mEq/L at low sweat rates, which minimizes salt depletion; an increase in the fraction of sweat secreted on the limbs; and perhaps other changes that help protect against heat illness.

The effect of heat acclimatization on performance can be quite dramatic, and acclimatized subjects can easily complete exercise in the heat that previously was difficult or impossible.[89] The benefits of acclimatization are lessened or reversed by sleep loss, infection, alcohol abuse, dehydration, and salt depletion.[85] These factors impair thermoregulation in the heat in the unacclimatized also. Heat acclimatization disappears in a few weeks if not maintained by repeated heat exposure.

Some of the changes that occur with heat acclimatization are mediated by "training" the heat-dissipating responses, particularly sweating, through repeated use.[85] Repeated exercise that is intense enough and lasts long enough to improve maximal oxygen consumption also expands plasma volume and, by elevating core temperature, trains the heat-dissipating responses and produces an improvement in heat tolerance similar to that associated with heat acclimatization.[85] This effect probably explains the association of physical fitness with heat tol-

FIGURE 4–6. Change in the responses of heart rate, rectal temperature, and mean skin temperature during exercise in a 10-day program of acclimatization to dry heat (50.5°C, 15% relative humidity), together with responses during exercise in a cool environment before and after acclimatization. (The "cool control" condition was 25.5°C, 39% relative humidity.) Each day's exercise consisted of five 10-minute treadmill walks at 2.5 mph (1.12 m/s) up a 2.5% grade. Successive walks were separated by 2-minute rest periods. *Large circles* show values before the start of the first exercise period each day; *small circles* show values at the end of successive exercise periods; and the *dashed* line connects final values each day. (Redrawn from Eichna, LW, Park CR, Nelson N, et al: Thermal regulation during acclimatization in a hot, dry [desert type] environment. Am J Physiol 163:585–597, 1950.)

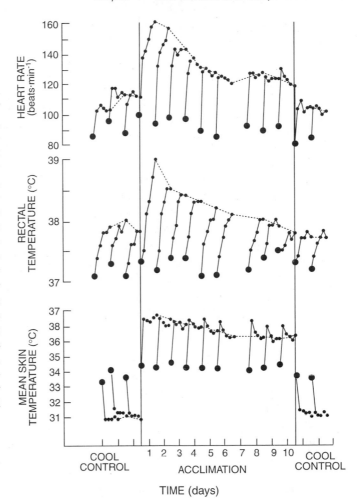

erance. In marked contrast to acclimatization to heat, the responses that comprise human cold acclimatization are inconsistent and appear to confer no more than a modest advantage.[90]

Gender

Although women as a group are less tolerant to exercise-heat stress than men are, the difference appears to be explained by differences in size, acclimatization, and maximal oxygen consumption, and when subjects are matched according to these variables, gender differences largely disappear.[91] The exertional form of heat stroke is said to be rare in women.[10] Its apparent rarity probably does not indicate that women are not susceptible to exertional heat stroke, since in active-duty soldiers, a population in which most heat stroke is of the exertional type, annual incidence of heat stroke in women is at least half that in men (unpublished data, Defense Medical Surveillance System, 1997-1998). The effect of the menstrual cycle has not been well studied. However, Pivarnik et al,[92] studying women's responses during cycle exercise at 22°C, found that after 60 minutes of exercise, heart rate was 10 beats/min higher in the luteal than in the follicular phase, and rectal temperature increased 1.2°C in the luteal phase and was still rising, whereas it increased 0.9°C in the follicular phase and was near steady state. Although they examined only one set of experimental conditions, using a temperate rather than a warm environment, their data suggest a decline in tolerance to exercise-heat stress during the luteal phase.

Age, Obesity, Drugs, and Physical Disorders

Heat tolerance and the effectiveness of the thermoregulatory system are reduced with increasing age, and in healthy 65-year-old men the sensitivity of the sweating response is half that in 25-year-old men. This effect is opposite to the effect of physical fitness, and it is not clear how much of the decrease is a direct effect of aging itself and how much owes to changes that tend to accompany increased age, such as reduced physical fitness.[91] In addition, newborn infants and many healthy elderly persons are less able than older children and younger adults to maintain body temperature in the cold. This appears to be due to a reduced ability both to conserve body heat by reducing heat loss and to increase metabolic heat production in the cold.

Obesity also is associated with reduced heat tolerance; Kenney[91] reviews mechanisms that may explain this association. However, obesity enhances cold tolerance, apparently because of the thermal insulation provided by the subcutaneous layer of fat.

Thermoregulation in the heat is impaired by diuretics, which cause loss of fluid and electrolytes, and by drugs that suppress sweating, most obviously those used for their anticholinergic effects, such as atropine and scopolamine. However, many drugs used for other purposes, such as glutethimide (a sleep medicine), tricyclic antidepressants, phenothiazines (tranquilizers and antipsychotic drugs), and antihistamines also have some anticholinergic action, and have been associated with heat stroke.[11] Furthermore, some drugs, including tricyclic antidepressants, butyrophenones, and amphetamines, increase the risk of heat-associated illness through other mechanisms.[11] In addition, certain drugs, such as barbiturates, alcohol, and phenothiazines, impair the defenses against cold.

Several congenital and acquired skin disorders—including ichthyosis, anhidrotic ectodermal dysplasia, and miliaria rubra—impair sweating and may seriously reduce heat tolerance. Anhidrotic ectodermal dysplasia is especially interesting in this regard, since not only sweating but also active vasodilation in the skin is impaired or absent. Thus artificially wetting the skin only partially corrects the thermoregulatory deficit during exercise, when large amounts of body heat need to be carried to the skin. Artificial wetting is probably most effective in a dry environment, in which evaporation can produce a cool skin.

Neurologic diseases that involve the thermoregulatory structures in the brain stem can impair thermoregulation. Although such disorders can produce hypothermia, hyperthermia is more usual and typically is characterized by loss of sweating and disruption of the circadian rhythm.

Certain diseases, such as hypothyroidism, hypopituitarism, congestive heart failure, and septicemia, impair the defenses against cold. This impairment may explain why septicemia, especially in debilitated patients, is often accompanied by hypothermia instead of the usual febrile response to infection.

Prevention of Heat and Cold Illnesses

Careful attention to risk factors is the key to prevention of heat and cold illnesses. Candidates for occupations or other activities that subject them to prolonged or severe cold stress or exercise-heat stress should be screened for individual risk factors, including use of therapeutic or recreational drugs that would increase their risk of illness. Unacclimatized personnel, especially those who are physically unfit, should be allowed to acclimatize to heat gradually. Consideration should be given to excusing personnel with mild infections from activities that involve prolonged or severe exercise-heat stress. Provision should be made for adequate sleep, and alcohol abuse should be guarded against.

Perhaps the most important measure for preventing heat illness is provision of ample cool palatable water or other beverages and frequent opportunities to drink. Although acclimatization reduces loss of salt, it does not reduce water requirements; indeed, the biophysics of heat exchange largely preclude any such effect during sustained exercise-heat stress. The persistent myth that withholding water during exercise-heat stress produces toughening is unsupported by evidence.

Persons undergoing prolonged exercise-heat stress should drink frequently and not wait until they feel thirsty, since thirst is not a reliable guide to water requirements under such conditions. Soldiers on a long march, for example, gradually become progressively dehydrated if they drink only according to their feelings of thirst.[93] Provision of flavored beverages may enhance consumption, but carbonated or caffeinated beverages should not be drunk, since carbonation may give a sense of fullness and caffeine promotes fluid loss by diuresis. Beverages containing electrolytes may be beneficial during intense sustained exercise-heat stress or when food intake is reduced.

REFERENCES

1. Du Bois EF: Fever and the Regulation of Body Temperature. Charles C Thomas, Springfield, IL, 1948

2. Aschoff J: Circadian rhythm of activity and of body temperature. In: Hardy JD, Gagge AP, Stolwijk JAJ (eds): Physiological and Behavioral Temperature Regulation. Charles C Thomas, Springfield, IL, 1970, pp. 905–919

3. Gisolfi CV, Wenger CB: Temperature regulation during exercise: old concepts, new ideas. Exerc Sports Sci Rev 12:339–372, 1984

4. Mackowiak PA, Wasserman SS, Levine MM: A critical appraisal of 98.6°F, the upper limit of the normal body temperature, and other legacies of Carl Reinhold August Wunderlich. JAMA 268:1578–1580, 1992

5. Hessemer V, Brück K: Influence of menstrual cycle on shivering, skin blood flow, and sweating responses measured at night. J Appl Physiol 59:1902–1910, 1985

6. Kolka MA: Temperature regulation in women. Med Exerc Nutr Health 1:201–207, 1992

7. Stephenson LA, Kolka MA: Menstrual cycle phase and time of day alter reference signal controlling arm blood flow and sweating. Am J Physiol 249:R186–R191, 1985

8. Johnson RF, Kobrick JL: Psychological aspects of military performance in hot environments. In: Burr RE, Pandolf KB (eds): Textbook of Military Medicine. Medical Aspects of Harsh Environments, Vol 1. Borden Institute, Office of the Surgeon General, Department of the Army, Washington, DC, (in press)

9. Sawka MN, Pandolf KB: Physical exercise in hot climates: physiology, performance and biomedical issues. In: Burr RE, Pandolf KB (eds): Textbook of Military Medicine. Medical Aspects of Harsh Environments, Vol 1. Borden Institute, Office of the Surgeon General, Department of the Army, Washington, DC, (in press)

10. Knochel JP: Heat stroke and related heat stress disorders. Dis Month 35:301–377, 1989

11. Knochel JP, Reed G: Disorders of heat regulation. In: Maxwell MH, Kleeman CR, Narins RG (eds): Clinical Disorders of Fluid and Electrolyte Metabolism, McGraw-Hill, New York, 1987, pp. 1197–1232

12. Leithead CS, Lind AR: Heat Stress and Heat Disorders. F.A. Davis, Philadelphia, 1964

13. Bridger CA, Helfand LA: Mortality from heat during July in Illinois. Int J Biometeorol 12:51–70, 1968

14. Burch GE, DePasquale NP: Hot Climates, Man and His Heart. Charles C Thomas, Springfield, IL, 1962

15. Ellis FP: Mortality from heat illness and heat-aggravated illness in the United States. Environ Res 5:1–58, 1972

16. Armstrong LE, Epstein Y, Greenleaf JE, et al: American College of Sports Medicine position stand: heat and cold illnesses during distance running. Med Sci Sports Exerc 28(12):i–x, 1996

17. Jones BH, Roberts WO: Medical management of endurance events: incidence, prevention, and care of casualties. In: Cantu RC, Micheli LJ (eds): ACSM's Guidelines for the Team Physician. Lea & Febiger, Philadelphia, 1991, pp. 266–286

18. Thompson RL, Hayward JS: Wet-cold exposure and hypothermia: thermal and metabolic responses to prolonged exercise in rain. J Appl Physiol 81:1128–1137, 1996

19. Cabanac M: Physiological role of pleasure. Science 173:1103–1107, 1971

20. Bligh J, Johnson KG: Glossary of terms for thermal physiology. J Appl Physiol 35:941–961, 1973

21. Gagge AP, Hardy JD, Rapp GM: Proposed standard system of symbols for thermal physiology. J Appl Physiol 27:439–446, 1969

22. Ferrannini E: Equations and assumptions of indirect calorimetry: some special problems. In: Kinney JM, Tucker HN (eds): Energy Metabolism: Tissue Determinants and Cellular Corollaries. Raven Press, New York, 1992, pp. 1–17

23. Åstrand P-O, Rodahl K: Temperature regulation. In: Textbook of Work Physiology: Physiological Bases of Exercise. McGraw-Hill, New York, 1977, pp. 523–576

24. Hardy JD: Physiology of temperature regulation. Physiol Rev 41:521–606, 1961

25. Kuno Y: Insensible perspiration. In: Human Perspiration. Charles C Thomas, Springfield, IL, 1956, pp. 3–41

26. Fox RH, Edholm OG: Nervous control of the cutaneous circulation. Br Med Bull 19:110–114, 1963

27. Rowell LB: Cardiovascular adjustments to thermal stress. In: Shepherd JT, Abboud FM (eds): Handbook of Physiology, section 2: The Cardiovascular System, Vol 3: Peripheral Circulation and Organ Blood Flow. American Physiological Society, Bethesda, MD, 1983, pp. 967–1023

28. Sawka MN, Wenger CB: Physiological responses to acute exercise-heat stress. In: Pandolf KB, Sawka MN, Gonzalez RR (eds): Human Performance Physiology and Environmental Medicine at Terrestrial Extremes. Benchmark Press, Indianapolis, IN, 1988, pp. 97–151

29. Johnson JM, Proppe DW: Cardiovascular adjustments to heat stress. In: Fregly MJ, Blatteis CM (eds): Handbook of Physiology, Section 4: Environmental Physiology. Oxford University Press, for the American Physiological Society, New York, 1996, pp. 215–243

30. Roddie IC: Circulation to skin and adipose tissue. In: Shepherd JT, Abboud FM (eds): Handbook of Physiology, Section 2: The Cardiovascular System, Vol 3: Peripheral Circulation and Organ Blood Flow. Bethesda, MD, 1983, pp. 285–317

31. Rowell LB: Active neurogenic vasodilatation in man. In: Vanhoutte PM, Leusen I (eds): Vasodilatation, Raven Press, New York, 1981, pp. 1–17

32. Love AHG, Shanks RG: The relationship between the onset of sweating and vasodilatation in the forearm during body heating. J Physiol (Lond) 162:121–128, 1962

33. Sawka MN, Wenger CB, Pandolf KB: Thermoregulatory responses to acute exercise-heat stress and heat acclimation. In: Fregly MJ, Blatteis CM (eds): Handbook of Physiology, Section 4: Environmental Physiology. Oxford University Press, for the American Physiological Society, New York, 1996, pp. 157–185

34. Brengelmann GL, Freund PR, Rowell LB, et al: Absence of active cutaneous vasodilation associated with congenital absence of sweat glands in humans. Am J Physiol 240:H571–H575, 1981

35. Kuno Y: The sweat apparatus. In: Human Perspiration. Charles C Thomas, Springfield, IL, 1956, pp. 42–97

36. Eichna LW, Ashe WF, Bean WB, Shelley WB: The upper limits of environmental heat and humidity tolerated by acclimatized men working in hot environments. J Indust Hyg Toxicol 27:59–84, 1945

37. Ladell WSS: Thermal sweating. Br Med Bull 3:175–179, 1945

38. Kuno Y: The loss of water and salt by sweating, their replenishment and changes in the blood. In: Human Perspiration. Charles C Thomas, Springfield, IL, 1956, pp. 251–276

39. Robinson S, Robinson AH: Chemical composition of sweat. Physiol Rev 34:202–220, 1954

40. Brown WK, Sargent F II: Hidromeiosis. Arch Environ Health 11:442–453, 1965

41. Nadel ER, Stolwijk JAJ: Effect of skin wettedness on sweat gland response. J Appl Physiol 35:689–694, 1973

42. Dobson RL, Formisano V, Lobitz WC, Jr, Brophy D: Some histochemical observations on the human eccrine sweat glands. III: The effect of profuse sweating. J Invest Dermatol 31:147–159, 1958

43. Rowell LB: Human cardiovascular adjustments to exercise and thermal stress. Physiol Rev 54:75–159, 1974

44. Fogoros RN: 'Runner's trots' gastrointestinal disturbances in runners. JAMA 243:1743–1744, 1980

45. Wenger CB: Non-thermal factors are important in the control of skin blood flow during exercise only under high physiological strain. Yale J Biol Med 59:307–319, 1986

46. Bazett HC, Love L, Newton M, et al: Temperature changes in blood flowing in arteries and veins in man. J Appl Physiol 1:3–19, 1948

47. Toner MM, McArdle WD: Human thermoregulatory responses to acute cold stress with special reference to water immersion. In: Fregly MJ, Blatteis CM (eds): Handbook of Physiology, Section 4: Environmental Physiology. Oxford University Press, for the American Physiological Society, New York, 1996, pp. 379–397

48. Shephard RJ: Metabolic adaptations to exercise in the cold: an update. Sports Med 16:266–289, 1993

49. Jessen C: Interaction of body temperatures in control of thermoregulatory effector mechanisms. In: Fregly MJ, Blatteis CM (eds): Handbook of Physiology, Section 4: Environmental Physiology. Oxford University Press, for the American Physiological Society, New York, 1996, pp. 127–138

50. Nielsen M: Die Regulation der Körpertemperatur bei Muskelarbeit. Skand Arch Physiol 79:193–230, 1938

51. Stolwijk JAJ, Saltin B, Gagge AP: Physiological factors associated with sweating during exercise. Aerospace Med 39:1101–1105, 1968

52. Lind AR: A physiological criterion for setting thermal environmental limits for everyday work. J Appl Physiol 18:51–56, 1963

53. Johnson JM, Rowell LB: Forearm skin and muscle vascular responses to prolonged leg exercise in man. J Appl Physiol 39:920–924, 1975

54. Hamilton MT, Gonzalez-Alonso J, Montain SJ, Coyle EF: Fluid replacement and glucose infusion during exercise prevent cardiovascular drift. J Appl Physiol 71:871–877, 1991

55. Montain SJ, Coyle EF: Influence of graded dehydration on hyperthermia and cardiovascular drift during exercise. J Appl Physiol 73:1340–1350, 1992

56. Shaffrath JD, Adams WC: Effects of airflow and work load on cardiovascular drift and skin blood flow. J Appl Physiol 56:1411–1417, 1984

57. Tibbits GF: Regulation of myocardial contractility in exhaustive exercise. Med Sci Sports Exerc 17:529–537, 1985

58. Raven PB, Stevens GHJ: Cardiovascular function and prolonged exercise. In: Lamb DR, Murray R (eds): Prolonged Exercise. Benchmark Press, Indianapolis, IN, 1988, pp. 43–74

59. Haight JSJ, Keatinge WR: Elevation in set point for body temperature regulation after prolonged exercise. J Physiol (Lond) 229:77–85, 1973

60. Kark JA, Gardner JW, Hetzel DP, et al: Fever in classification of exertional heat injury. Clin Res 39:143A, 1991

61. Maron MB, Wagner JA, Horvath SM: Thermoregulatory responses during competitive marathon running. J Appl Physiol 42:909–914, 1977

62. Pugh LGCE, Corbett JL, Johnson RH: Rectal temperatures, weight losses, and sweat rates in marathon running. J Appl Physiol 23:347–352, 1967

63. Pandolf KB, Griffin TB, Munro EH, Goldman RF: Persistence of impaired heat tolerance from artificially induced miliaria rubra. Am J Physiol 239:R226–R232, 1980

64. Hales JRS, Hubbard RW, Gaffin SL: Limitation of heat tolerance. In: Fregly MJ, Blatteis CM (eds): Handbook of Physiology, Section 4: Environmental Physiology. Oxford University Press, for the American Physiological Society, New York, 1996, pp. 285–355

65. Lind AR: Pathophysiology of heat exhaustion and heat stroke. In: Khogali M, Hales JRS (eds): Heat Stroke and Temperature Regulation. Academic Press, New York, 1983, pp. 179–188

66. Petersdorf RG: Hypothermia and hyperthermia. In: Wilson JD, Braunwald E, Isselbacher KJ, et al (eds): Harrison's Principles of Internal Medicine. McGraw-Hill, New York, 1991, pp. 2194–2220

67. Kark JA, Ward FT: Exercise and hemoglobin S. Semin Hematol 31:181–225, 1994

68. Berl T: Treating hyponatremia: damned if we do and damned if we don't. Kidney Int 37:1006–1018, 1990

69. Armstrong LE, Curtis WC, Hubbard RW, et al: Symptomatic hyponatremia during prolonged exercise in heat. Med Sci Sports Exerc 25:543–549, 1993

70. Frizzell RT, Lang GH, Lowance DC, Lathan SR: Hyponatremia and ultramarathon running. JAMA 255:772–774, 1986

71. Noakes TD, Goodwin N, Rayner BL, et al: Water intoxication: a possible complication during endurance exercise. Med Sci Sports Exerc 17:370–375, 1985

72. Roberts WO: Assessing core temperature in collapsed athletes: what's the best method? Phys Sports Med 22:49–55, 1994

73. Brengelmann GL: Dilemma of body temperature measurement. In: Shiraki K, Yousef MK (eds): Man in Stressful Environments: Thermal and Work Physiology. Charles C Thomas, Springfield, IL, 1987, pp. 5–22

74. Costrini AM, Pitt HA, Gustafson AB, Uddin DE: Cardiovascular and metabolic manifestations of heat stroke and severe heat exhaustion. Am J Med 66:296–302, 1979

75. Magazanik A, Epstein Y, Udassin R, et al: Tap water, an efficient method for cooling heatstroke victims—a model in dogs. Aviat Space Environ Med 51:864–867, 1980

76. Weiner JS, Khogali M: A physiological body-cooling unit for treatment of heat stroke. Lancet 1:507–509, 1980.

77. Khogali M, Weiner JS: Heat stroke: report on 18 cases. Lancet 2:276–278, 1980

78. Bouchama A, Al-Sedairy S, Siddiqui S, et al: Elevated pyrogenic cytokines in heatstroke. Chest 104:1498–1502, 1993

79. Bouchama A, Parhar RS, El-Yazigi A, et al: Endotoxemia and release of tumor necrosis factor and interleukin 1α in acute heatstroke. J Appl Physiol 70:2640–2644, 1991

80. Chang DM: The role of cytokines in heat stroke. Immunol Invest 22:553–561, 1993

81. Butkow N, Mitchell D, Laburn H, Kenedi E: Heat stroke and endotoxaemia in rabbits. In: Hales JRS (ed): Thermal Physiology. Raven Press, New York, 1984, pp. 511–514

82. Bynum G, Brown J, DuBose D, et al: Increased survival in experimental dog heatstroke after reduction of gut flora. Aviat Space Environ Med 50:816–819, 1978

83. Gathiram P, Wells MT, Brock-Utne JG, Gaffin SL: Antilipopolysaccharide improves survival in primates subjected to heat stroke. Circ Shock 23:157–164, 1987

84. Gaffin SL, Hubbard RW: Experimental approaches to therapy and prophylaxis for heat stress and heatstroke. Wilderness Environ Med 4:312–334, 1996

85. Wenger CB: Human heat acclimatization. In: Pandolf KB, Sawka MN, Gonzalez RR (eds): Human Performance Physiology and Environmental Medicine at Terrestrial Extremes. Benchmark Press, Indianapolis, IN, 1988, pp. 153–197

86. Eichna LW, Park CR, Nelson N, et al: Thermal regulation during acclimatization in a hot, dry (desert type) environment. Am J Physiol 163:585–597, 1950

87. Collins KJ, Crockford GW, Weiner JS: The local training effect of secretory activity on the response of eccrine sweat glands. J Physiol (Lond) 184:203–214, 1966

88. Kraning KK, Lehman PA, Gano RG, Weller TS: A non-invasive dose-response assay of sweat gland function and its application in studies of gender comparison, heat acclimation and anticholinergic potency. In: Mercer JB (ed): Thermal Physiology 1989. Elsevier, Amsterdam, 1989, pp. 301–307.

89. Pandolf KB, Young AJ: Environmental extremes and endurance performance. In: Shephard RJ, Åstrand PO (eds): Endurance in Sport. Blackwell Scientific Publications, New York, 1992, pp. 270–282.

90. Young AJ: Homeostatic responses to prolonged cold exposure: human cold acclimatization. In: Fregly MJ, Blatteis C (eds): Handbook of Physiology, Section 4: Environmental Physiology. Oxford University Press, for the American Physiological Society, New York, 1996, pp. 419–438

91. Kenney WL: Physiological correlates of heat intolerance. Sports Med 2:279–286, 1985

92. Pivarnik JM, Marichal CJ, Spillman T, Morrow JR Jr: Menstrual cycle phase affects temperature regulation during endurance exercise. J Appl Physiol 72:543–548, 1992

93. Rothstein A, Adolph EF, Wills JH: Voluntary dehydration. In: Visscher MB, Bronk DW, Landis EM, Ivy AC (eds): Physiology of Man in the Desert. Interscience, New York, 1947, pp. 254–270.

5

Inflammation: Its Influence and Consequences in Athletes

W. WATSON BUCHANAN

Sport has its origins in training for the hunt and battle. It is therefore appropriate that the Father of Sports Medicine, Galen (130–200 AD) (Fig. 5–1) of Pergamum (Gr., *Pergamon*), was team physician to the gladiators of Rome as well as court physician to Marcus Aurelius Antonius (121–180 AD), emperor of Rome 161–180 AD.[1-4] Although Galen may be considered the father of such modern-day gladiatorial sports as American football and Canadian ice hockey, a case can be made for the Italian Bernardino Ramazzini (1633–1714) (Fig. 5–2) as being the father of less violent sports such as running and rowing.[5] In his *De Morbis Artificum* (*Diseases of Workers*) (Fig. 5–3), Ramazzini discusses not only afflictions associated with certain occupations (he is recognized as Father of Occupational Medicine) but also diseases that may occur in runners ("De Cursonum Morbis") and athletes ("De Athletarium Morbis").[6] Ramazzini noted that "runners suffer from hernia and asthma" and that "sometimes they burst a small vein in the kidneys and pass bloody urine." He considered exercise beneficial to the knees of runners and may also have been aware that sudden death could occur during strenuous exercise, citing Hippocrates, "It is more dangerous to change from idleness to work than from work to idleness."

DEFINITION AND NATURE OF SPORTS INJURIES

Noyes et al[7] proposed that "sports-related injury or illness prevents the player from practicing or competing on the day after the injury and requires medical or dental care beyond icing or wrapping. All concussions, nerve injuries and eye injuries, no matter how transient are included." This definition is purely clinical, without any pathologic basis.

Although some sports are more frequently associated with certain types of injuries, such as Achilles tendinitis in runners and meniscal injuries of the knee in soccer players, it is meaningless to talk of "football" or "tennis" injuries, since no such sport-related, as opposed to mechanism-related, injuries exist. Some of the injuries in contact or collision sports such as boxing and wrestling, American football and rugby, ice hockey and lacrosse, and horseback riding and downhill skiing, to mention but a few, are more than "lumps, bumps, and bruises." Indeed, such injuries can be devastating, resulting in permanent brain damage, blindness, cervical spinal fractures, brachial plexus tears, and even sudden death from ruptured aortic aneurysm (in Marfan syndrome) and myocardial infarction.[8] Nevertheless, many of the effects of exercise and sports are beneficial, including improved cardiovascular function, lowering of blood pressure, greater muscle strength and endurance, and a general sense of well-being.

EPIDEMIOLOGY

It has been estimated that some 7 million schoolchildren participate regularly in sports in the United States.[9] The incidence of sports injuries in these children has been estimated at 3% to 11%.[9,10] A survey in Ireland of 6,799 schoolchildren between 10 and 18 years of age who

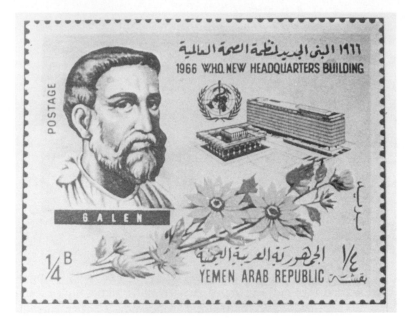

FIGURE 5–1. Postage stamp from the Arab Yemen Republic commemorates Galen (130–200 AD).

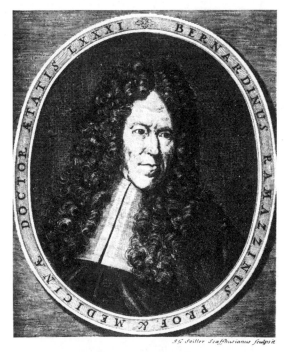

BERNARDINO RAMAZZINI

From the *Opera Omnia*, Geneva, 1717

FIGURE 5–2. Portrait of the Italian Bernardino Ramazzini (1633–1714) by an unknown artist, in the Municipal Museum of Carpi, Modena, Italy.

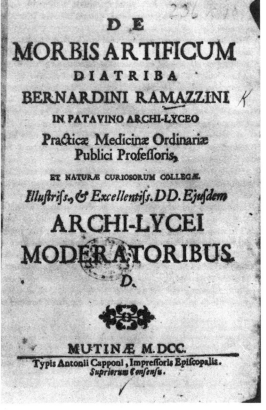

Title-page of the Editio Princeps, 1700

FIGURE 5–3. Title page of the original Latin edition of *De Morbis Artificum*, published in 1700.

were active in sports revealed an overall incidence of 2.94 injuries per 100 children per year, mostly sprains, strains, and contusions.[11] Most injuries in US high school football players were also of soft tissue: contusions (26.6%), sprains (21.6%), strains (8.6%), and suspected fractures (8.6%). Many more injuries were recorded among adult and professional soccer players than among young players, some 15 to 30 times, probably reflecting a greater intensity of the game.[12] Injuries in female athletes tend to be less frequent and less severe but take longer to heal.[13]

The sites of injuries depend on the sport. Most sports injuries involve the lower extremities,[14] although shoulder injuries are more common in swimmers and baseball players.[15] In a review of 1,280 urban sports persons with an average age of 30, the most frequently injured joints were the knee (45.5%), ankle (9.8%), and shoulder (7.7%).[16] More than half of these injuries involved the soft tissues about the knee,[16] especially the ligaments.[17] Soft tissue inflammatory lesions are also the most common sports injuries in the elderly.[15]

INFLAMMATION

Since the majority of sports injuries are inflammatory, involving soft tissues, it is important that those treating such injuries understand what is now known about inflammation. Many definitions of inflammation have been proposed, but essentially, inflammation is a reaction of irritated or damaged tissues that still retain their vitality. It is to be seen as a process, not a state. John Hunter (1729–1793) (Fig. 5–4), in his famous *A Treatise on the Blood, Inflammation, and Gun-shot Wounds,*[18] concluded that "Inflammation is itself not to be considered as a disease, but as a salutary operation consequent either to some violence or some disease." Hunter also appreciated that the inflammatory response is usually beneficial and ends in healing: "But if inflammation develops, regardless of its cause, still it is an effect whose purpose is to restore the parts to their natural functions." It is often forgotten that wound healing requires an inflammatory response.

Historically, inflammation has been considered either acute or chronic, depending on the persistence and nature of the inflammatory re-

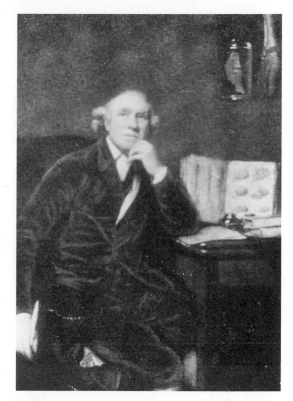

FIGURE 5–4. Portrait of the Scottish surgeon-anatomist John Hunter (1729–1793), by the English portrait painter Sir Joshua Reynolds (1723–1792).

sponse. Tendinitis has been defined clinically as acute (symptoms present for less than 2 weeks), subacute (symptoms present for 2 to 6 weeks), or chronic (symptoms present for 6 weeks or longer).[19] This, it will be appreciated, is entirely arbitrary in the absence of histologic examination. Pathologists, although clear in defining acute and chronic on the basis of the cellular infiltrate, are equally vague about their duration; one standard undergraduate text states that "acute inflammation lasts for days or a few weeks; chronic inflammation persists for weeks, months or even years."[20] In the discussion that follows, the two categories of inflammation, acute and chronic, are considered from a pathologic point of view.

Acute Inflammation

Vascular Events

The initial events in acute inflammation include transient vasoconstriction of arterioles, followed by vasodilation of precapillary arterioles and an increase in the permeability of the endothelial cell barrier. The capillaries become suffused with blood, additional channels open, and there is increased flow through the postcapillary venules. In 30 to 60 minutes the blood flow in the capillary bed slows or even stops, for reasons as yet unknown. This hemoconcentration leads to reduced blood flow velocity (sludging), with resulting increase in interstitial fluid pressure. Separation of endothelial cells occurs, leaving gaps 800 nm in diameter, which facilitates exudation of plasma and diapedesis of cells. Inflammation, in its early stages, is a vascular phenomenon and therefore cannot occur in avascular tissues such as cornea or cartilage. Likewise, repair is also a vascular phenomenon.

These vascular changes are brought about by vasoactive mediators, originating from both plasma and cellular sources at the site of injury. These vasoactive mediators include histamine, serotonin (5-hydroxytryptamine), bradykinin, anaphylatoxins, prostaglandins and leukotrienes, and platelet-activating factors. These mediators bind to specific receptors on vascular endothelial and smooth muscle cells, especially in the postcapillary venule, causing both vasoconstriction and vasodilation. Histamine is released from mast cells, and is responsible for an increase in vascular permeability by inducing H_1 receptor activations.[21,22] Serotonin is derived from the dense granules of platelets and, like histamine, induces changes in vascular permeability. Kinins are derived from plasma precursors, enhance vascular permeability of postcapillary venules, increase blood flow, and produce pain.[23,24] It is uncertain, however, how important they are in vivo, because they are rapidly inactivated (<15 seconds) by a group of enzymes called kininases.[24] Captopril, an inhibitor of one of the two degradative kininases, kininase II, can, however, give rise to inflammatory skin eruptions.[25]

The anaphylatoxins (C3a and C5a) are products of complement activation (Fig. 5–5). These molecules have potent effects on smooth muscle contraction and increase vascular permeability. C3a and C5a also can induce degranulation of mast cells and basophils, with consequent release of histamine, and C5a is a highly potent chemotactic factor for neutrophils.[26]

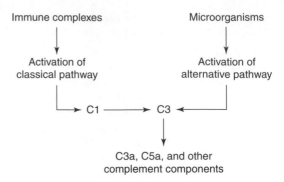

FIGURE 5–5. Simple diagram of the classical and alternative complement pathways. Note how the alternative pathway can activate C3 without prior activation of C1. Activation of C3 is the central event leading to opsonization of bacteria and viruses, target cell killing, and macrophage activation. The anaphylatoxins, C3a and C5a are important in chemotaxis, increased vascular permeability, and adhesion of leukocytes to endothelium.

Arachidonic acid products include prostaglandins, thromboxanes, and leukotrienes (known collectively as eicosanoids [Fig. 5–6]). Their precursors are polyunsaturated fatty acids, including dihomo-γ-linolenic acid, arachidonic acid, and eicosapentaneoic acid, found in cell membrane phospholipids. The most abundant of these precursors is arachidonic acid, which is formed from membrane phospholipids by phospholipase A_2, which can be inhibited by glucocorticoid-induced proteins known as lipocortins (lipomodulin and macrocortin). Nonsteroidal anti-inflammatory drugs (NSAIDs), such as aspirin, inhibit the enzyme cyclooxygenase.[27] Prostaglandins, especially E_2 and I_2 (prostacyclin), enhance blood flow at sites of inflammation[28,29] but have no effect on permeability.[30,31] It is uncertain, however, whether prostaglandins have a direct effect on the microvasculature or whether their effect is mediated by the release of vasoactive substances such as bradykinin and histamine.[32,33] Prostaglandins I_2 and E_2 contribute to pain, not directly but by sensitizing pain receptors to other substances (eg, bradykinin and histamine).[34] Thromboxane A_2 is a potent vasoconstrictor. The second pathway by which arachidonic acid is metabolized is lipoxygenation, with formation of the leukotrienes. Leukotrienes C_4, D_4, and E_4, known collectively as the slow-reacting substances of anaphylaxis, stimulate smooth muscles to contract and increase

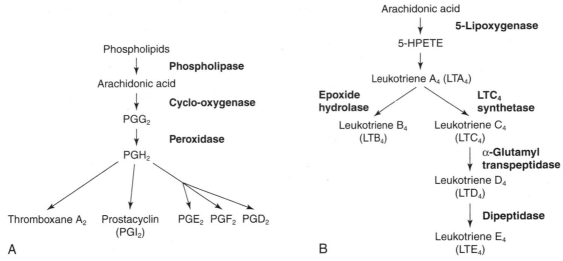

FIGURE 5–6. **A,** Synthesis of thromboxane and prostaglandins. The compounds produced have similar structure but markedly different actions. Thus, thromboxane A_2 is a powerful vasoconstrictor and producer of platelet aggregation, whereas prostacyclin (prostaglandin I_2) has the opposite effect. Prostaglandins E_2 and I_2 play an important role in the vascular events in inflammation, causing vasodilation and, in collaboration with histamine and kinins, increased capillary permeability (see text). They also promote osteoclastic activity and probably play a predominant role in causing articular erosions in inflammatory joint disease. *PG,* prostaglandin. **B,** Synthesis of leukotrienes (LT) from arachidonic acid. The enzyme 5-lipoxygenase leads to the formation of leukotrienes through 5-hydroperoxyeicosatetraenoic acid (5-HPETE) and cyclic 5,6-epoxide (LTA_4). Four different leukotrienes are then formed: LTB_4, by the enzyme epoxide hydrolase, and LTC_4, LTD_4, and LTE_4 by the enzymes α-glutamyl transpeptidase and dipeptidase. The latter three leukotrienes were previously known as the slow-reacting substance of anaphylaxis. LTB_4 is a powerful chemoattractant for polymorphonuclear leukocytes and causes adherence of these cells to endothelial cells.

vascular permeability. Leukotriene B_4 is derived from leukotriene A_4 present in macrophages, and has potent chemotactic activity for leukocytes.[35] Phospholipid metabolism and the activity of the various arachidonic acid derivatives is extremely complex. Suffice it to say, prostaglandin E_2 can inhibit macrophages and T lymphocytes, perhaps by inhibiting the cytokines interleukin-1 and tumor necrosis factor.[36]

Platelets also contribute significantly to the inflammatory process with the release of serotonin and the production of thromboxane A_2. Low molecular weight fibrin degradation products increase vascular permeability.[37]

Cellular Accumulation

Adherence of polymorphonuclear leukocytes to vascular endothelium is the second key event in acute inflammation. Adherence of polymorphonuclear leukocytes to the endothelial cells comes about by cell adhesion molecules, present both on the polymorphonuclear leukocyte (eg,

integrins)[38,39] and endothelial cells (eg, selectins).[40] The initial recruitment of polymorphonuclear leukocytes to sites of tissue injury is believed to be largely due to the chemotactic action of C5a. After 6 to 48 hours, other chemotactic low-molecular-weight cell-derived factors known as cytokines (eg, leukotriene B_4 and interleukin-8) become active in recruitment of polymorphonuclear leukocytes. Interleukin-1 and tumor necrosis factor-α stimulate chemotactic cytokine production.[41–43] Hypoxia can also cause endothelial cells to produce a chemoattractant for polymorphonuclear leukocytes[44] and facilitate adhesion.[45]

Polymorphonuclear leukocytes have an important role in inflammation, despite their short half-life of approximately 7 hours. They have the ability to phagocytose and digest foreign material and bacteria by virtue of their phagolysosomes.[46] They undergo apoptosis, or programmed death, and are phagocytosed by mononuclear cells (in synovial fluid, described formerly as Reiter's cells).[47] Polymorphonuclear leukocytes secrete metalloproteases (eg, collagenase and gelatinase), which break down collagen, normally resistant to most proteolytic enzymes because of its unusual amino acid sequence and triple-helical structure.[48,49] Polymorphonuclear leukocytes also secrete neutral proteases (eg, cathepsin G and elastase), but their role in inflammation is still uncertain.[50]

Polymorphonuclear leukocytes and other cells and processes (eg, arachidonic acid cascade[51]) involved in inflammation produce oxygen-derived free radicals: superoxide (O_2^-), hydroxyl (OH^-), and hydrogen peroxide (H_2O_2).[52] The chemistry of these free radicals is complex and as yet poorly understood. Ferric iron (Fe^{++}) is believed to play a role in producing OH^- radicals from H_2O_2, which may explain why there is a correlation between free iron and severity of inflammation,[53] why iron chelators have a protective role in inflammation (at least in animals),[54] and why intravenously administered iron causes joint inflammation flare-ups in patients with rheumatoid arthritis.[55] Oxygen free radicals degrade hyaluronic acid[56,57] and enhance the destructive effects of lysosomal proteases.[58] They also can generate a chemoattractant for polymorphonuclear leukocytes from extracellular fluid.[59,60] It appears that the body has scavengers, such as superoxide dismutase and catalase, which "mop up" these oxygen free radicals.[61,62]

Accumulation of polymorphonuclear leukocytes in extravascular sites results in pus formation. Certain bacteria, such as *Staphylococcus aureus,* produce coagulase, which walls off pus, producing what is often referred to as "good and laudable pus" (L., *pus bonum et laudabile*).[63] Organisms such as β-hemolytic streptococci are highly adapted to spread through tissues, being not only able to resist destruction by polymorphonuclear leukocytes because of their antiphagocytic M protein, but also because they make a number of extracellular enzymes, such as streptokinase, hyaluronidase, and deoxyribonuclease, which liquefy tissue components and allow it to escape the confines of the area of inflammation. This results in thin, watery, and often blood-stained pus.

Those physicians who treat sports injuries seldom see suppuration supervening on acute inflammation. However, if such suppuration persists, the presence of foreign material within the inflamed area must be considered. A piece of dead bone (sequestrum), for instance, in osteomyelitis is an example of an endogenous foreign body.

Chronic Inflammation

Chronic inflammation initially is characterized by a pleomorphic cellular reaction including lymphocytes, macrophages, and plasma cells. The transition from acute to chronic inflammation is difficult to pinpoint without examination of serial biopsy specimens. Chronic inflammation may begin insidiously and not necessarily follow the classic acute inflammatory state. The histologic hallmark is infiltration by monocytes, principally, lymphocytes, macrophages, and plasma cells, proliferation of fibroblasts and small blood vessel formation (angiogenesis), and fibrosis. When monocytes reach the extravascular tissue, they are "activated" to become macrophages. A number of chemotactic factors have been identified in the recruitment of monocytes, including C5a and transforming growth factor-β. Macrophages produce a great number of biologically active products (eg, interleukin-1), which causes fibroblast proliferation and release of free oxygen radicals and proteases, which are toxic to tissues. Plasma cells produce antibody, eg, rheumatoid factor in rheumatoid arthritis. Lymphocytes produce lymphokines, which stimulate monocytes and macrophages, which in turn influence both T- and B-cell functions.

The complexity of inflammation is nothing short of daunting; the phenomenon can be visualized as a series of waterfalls tumbling into a pool. The kallikrein-kinin, complement, coagulation, and fibrolytic systems, which are all activated by Hageman factor (factor XII) are all interlinked (Fig. 5–7). In addition, there are both vascular and cellular reactions. The following comment by Mark Twain[63] appears apt:

> The researches of many commentators have already thrown much darkness on the subject, and it is probable that, if they continue, we shall soon know nothing about it.

Systemic Effects

Fever is one of the most prominent systemic manifestations of inflammation but usually is not a feature of common soft tissue sports inju-

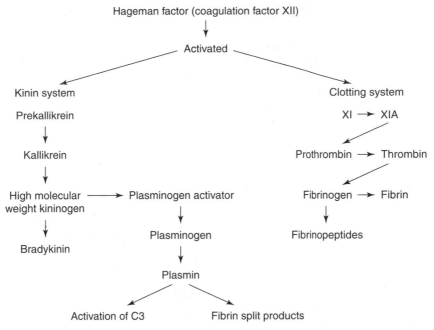

FIGURE 5–7. The three mediator systems triggered by activated Hageman factor (coagulation factor XII). Bradykinin is not chemotactic but causes contraction of smooth muscle, blood vessel dilation, and pain. The final step in the clotting system cascade is the conversion of fibrinogen to fibrin by the action of thrombin. Fibrinopeptides are produced during this conversion and are chemotactic for leukocytes and increase vascular permeability. High-molecular-weight kininogen activates plasminogen to produce plasmin. This multifunctional protease not only lyses fibrin clots but also cleaves C3, and forms fibrin split products.

ries. Bacteria, viruses, and damaged cells cause the production of endogenous pyrogens, including interleukin-1 and tumor necrosis factor-α. Interleukin-1 stimulates the synthesis of prostaglandin in the hypothalamus, which causes stimulation of the vasomotor center, resulting in sympathetic nerve stimulation, vasoconstriction of dermal vessels, decrease in heat dissipation, and fever.[64] The antipyretic effects of acetaminophen and aspirin-like drugs can be explained by their ability to suppress prostaglandin synthesis.[65] Acetaminophen, it should be noted, suppresses prostaglandin formation in brain tissue.[27]

Interleukin-1 and tumor necrosis factor-α also accelerate release and increase production of polymorphonuclear leukocytes from the bone marrow. The presence of immature neutrophils in the blood is referred to as a "shift to the left." Prolonged inflammation leads to production of colony-stimulating factors, which cause proliferation of leukocytes in the bone marrow, the stimulation being made by interleukin-1 and tumor necrosis factor-α.

In addition to causing fever and leukocytosis, interleukin-1 and tumor necrosis factor-α, as well as interleukin-6, promote the synthesis by hepatocytes of a series of proteins known as acute-phase proteins.[66,67] These include C-reactive protein, haptoglobin, α₁-antitrypsin, fibrinogen, ceruloplasmin, α₁-acid glycoprotein (orosomucoid), complement components, plasminogen, fibrinogen, serum amyloid A, and kinin polypeptides. These acute-phase proteins help cope with the consequences of inflammation, especially by activation of the complement pathway, proteinase inhibition, and antioxidant activity, but may be injurious as well as beneficial.[68]

The erythrocyte sedimentation rate is not an acute-phase protein, but can be considered to reflect the acute-phase response. Fibrinogen has the greatest effect on the erythrocyte sedimentation rate. Elevated immunoglobulin concentrations, as occur in multiple myeloma and Waldenström's macroglobulinemia, may increase the erythrocyte sedimentation rate in the absence of inflammation. Anemia and polycythemia also affect the erythrocyte sedimentation rate. Treatment of rheumatic disease with NSAIDs has little or no effect on the erythrocyte sedimentation rate.[69] On the other hand, treatment of rheumatoid arthritis with gold, penicillamine, sulphasalazine, methotrexate,[70] and cyclosporin A has, however, no effect.[71] If measurement of the erythrocyte sedimentation rate is to be done in clinical trials of sports injuries, the method preferred is that of Westergren.[72] A case has been made for measurement of plasma viscosity rather than the erythrocyte sedimentation rate in clinical therapeutic trials in rheumatoid arthritis,[73,74] but there are no data to indicate whether this might be useful in sports medicine clinical trials.

HEALING

It would be surprising if the body were not endowed with a number of mechanisms to combat inflammation and promote the healing process. If there are, for example, a large number of plasma proteases (elastase, collagenase, plasmin, trypsin, chymotrypsin, Hageman factor, kallikrein, and thrombin), then there are at least half a dozen inhibitors (α_1-antitrypsin, α_2-macroglobulin, antithrombin III, C1-inactivator, α_1-antichymotrypsin, inter-α-trypsin inhibitor). Inflammation may undergo resolution or may heal with fibrosis and scar formation. Angiogenesis is required and is initiated by hypoxia and by products of inflammation such as prostaglandins E_2 and I_2[75] and fibroblast growth factor[76] released by lymphocytes and macrophages. The collagen that is first laid down is type III (embryonal). Myofibroblasts, which have the morphologic and synthetic characteristics of fibroblasts and the contractile properties of smooth muscle cells, cause contracture of scar tissue.[77] This specialized type of tissue, composed of fibroblasts and new blood vessels, is known as granulation tissue. There may be an excess of this soft red (because of neovascularization) tissue, which is often termed "proud flesh." Occasionally, this granulation tissue may produce excessive fibrous tissue known as keloid.

Infection and the presence of foreign bodies are the two most likely causes of delay in the inflammatory-reparative process. Age does not appear to be a major factor, and nutrition has

an effect only with prolonged severe protein deprivation and vitamin C deficiency, neither of which are likely in sports persons. Wound healing is also delayed in patients with zinc deficiency, again unlikely in those who participate in sports. Absence of neutrophils, as in hematologic disease, also influences wound healing, as in diabetes mellitus. Glucocorticoids have been shown experimentally to have the potential to delay wound healing, but there is no strong evidence that short-term administration of even large doses of corticosteroids has any appreciable effect. Long-term corticosteroid therapy, especially in large doses, does have an effect on skin collagen, leading to spontaneous bruising and thin skin.

PAIN

Pain is the cardinal feature of sports-induced soft tissue injuries. Research by neuroscientists has shed much light on the pathophysiology of pain, the understanding of which is important for today's sports medicine physician. What follows is a brief and simplified account of the evolution of knowledge about pain, from Descartes (1596–1650), who considered nerves to be tubes that contain fine threads connecting nerve endings in the skin and other tissues to the brain.[78] He believed pain and other sensations were transmitted to the brain by means of these threads, as illustrated in the famous picture from his book, *L'Homme* (Fig. 5–8). Data acquired over the last half century, especially the gate control theory of Melzack and Wall,[79] finally put to rest Descartes' concept of a fixed, direct-line communication between nerve ending and brain. The transmission of nerve impulses is now known to be modulated by a spinal gating mechanism at the dorsal root ganglion and dorsal horn, and probably also at other levels in the spinal cord and midbrain.[80–82]

The complex nature of the neural and biochemical substrates that process nociceptive information can be considered in three parts.

Peripheral Nervous System

Nociceptors are neural sensors that signal potentially harmful stimuli to the central nervous system (CNS). The nociceptors of joint, muscle, bone, periosteum, and fascia are conducted by

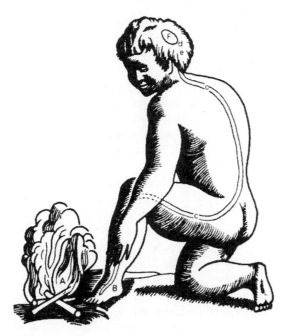

FIGURE 5–8. René Descartes (1596–1650), a contemporary of William Harvey (1578–1657), believed that the brain was the seat of both sensation and motor function. His concept of the pain pathway is illustrated in this drawing from his book *L'Homme.* Descartes believed that pain was conducted by threads contained in nerves, which he considered to be tubes.

thinly myelinated A delta (group III) and unmyelinated C (type IV) afferent fibers. Large sensory fibers (A alpha, A beta, and groups I and II) have mechanosensitive functions involved in proprioception and motor control.[83–85] Synovium, which is relatively insensitive to pain formerly was considered to have no pain receptors,[86] and any nerve endings present are mainly of autonomic origin.[87] However, Grönblad et al[88] confirmed the presence of neurofilaments and neuropeptides in synovium. No nervous elements have been detected in cartilage.[89]

Tissue damage causes release of a large number of algesiogenic substances, including H^+, K^+, serotonin, histamine, prostaglandins (especially E_2), leukotrienes, bradykinin, substance P, and calcitonin gene–related peptides, among many others. Some of these algesiogenic chemicals (H^+, K^+, prostaglandins, leukotrienes) are derived from tissue; others are derived from plasma (bradykinin) or as in the case of substance P and calcitonin gene–related peptide from C fiber nerve endings.[90–92] The release of substance P

and calcitonin gene–related peptide increases local microcirculation and plasma extravasation[93–95] and stimulates mast cells and other factors of the immune system, resulting, in turn, in release of histamine and serotonin.[93] Topical application of capsaicin, derived from *Capsicum,* the common red pepper plant,[96] was effective in double-blind controlled trials in osteoarthritis[97,98] by virtue of its ability to block release of substance P.[99] When capsaicin is applied locally, some of the endogenous chemicals (eg, bradykinin) produce pain, but if the capsaicin application is preceded by the application of serotonin or prostaglandin E_2, the response is much enhanced.[100]

The two types of nerve fibers carrying information about pain account for the double pain response.[101] Unmyelinated C fibers conduct pain slowly (<1–2 m/s), whereas fine myelinated A delta fibers conduct pain rapidly (4–>20 m/s). The latter fibers transmit "sharp" pain, eg, finger prick; the former conduct pain of a dull, aching nature, which is often diffuse and poorly localized and often felt some distance from the point stimulated, ie, "referred" pain.[102] This dull type of pain arises from deep structures such as muscles and gives rise to pain with segmental distribution, different from the dermatomes of spinal nerves and often referred to as sclerotomes.[103–105] Muscle spasm accompanies all types of severe pain[106] and is an important secondary source of pain[107]; muscle tenderness can be quantified by pressure measurements.[108]

Dorsal Root Ganglion and Horn

An incredible number of chemical neurotransmitters have been identified in the dorsal root ganglia, trigeminal or medullary root horn, and dorsal horn.[81,82] These include enkephalins, such as dynorphin, gamma-aminobutyric acid (GABA), substance P, somatostatin, angiotensin II, cholecystokinin, gastrin-releasing peptide, avian pancreatic peptide, and norepinephrine.[81] These various neuropeptides function to modulate the transmission of pain, not only at the sites mentioned but also, as is now believed, at many levels of the nervous system. The modulation can be enhanced or facilitated, impaired or inhibited, as described by Melzack and Wall[79] in their gate control theory. Thus, counterirritants, of whatever nature, probably act by changing the chemistry, thus shutting the "gate," with resulting relief from pain. Pain may do the opposite, ie, open the gate, which may not shut after the source of pain is removed, as in phantom limb pain after amputation. Extreme excitement, as in battle, may change the chemistry, thus shutting the gate, so the soldier feels no pain when his foot is blown off by a landmine. Athletes do not suffer, as a rule, from postpain syndromes, such as occur in whiplash injuries from automobile accidents. The reason may be that in the athlete the gate is shut when the injury occurs, whereas the opposite is the case in persons involved in car accidents.

Spinal Cord, Thalamus, and Cortex

Transmission of pain impulses continues in two ascending pathways, the spinothalamic and spinoreticulothalamic. These pathways end in the lateral and medial thalamic nuclei and the medullary reticular system, from which they are relayed to the sensory cortex of the brain. Considerable research has concluded that there must also be descending pain-modulating pathways, for which there is now anatomic evidence. These descending pain-modulating pathways can be activated by stress and by "thought," as well as by morphine and other opioids. Naloxone, a morphine antagonist, consistently worsens clinical pain, especially when severe,[109] but not experimental pain.[110]

Analgesics

Despite the vigorous and enormously expensive research into new drugs to relieve pain, the "magic bullet" remains to be discovered. Medicines such as NSAIDs and corticosteroid drugs reduce inflammation at the periphery but do not abolish pain. Drugs directed at blocking the many algesiogenic agents in inflamed tissue, eg, capsaicin, which blocks substance P and calcitonin gene–related peptide, may be successful in reducing, but not abolishing, pain. The best hope is to find a centrally acting drug like morphine but without addictive properties and without the rapid enzyme degradation associated with the enkephalins. Pain, however, has a biologic function in preventing injury and tissue damage. The rare syndrome of congenital ab-

sence of pain, for example, can be associated with severe neuropathic joint destruction.[111]

Acetaminophen

Acetaminophen is a weak cyclooxygenase inhibitor and has no demonstrable anti-inflammatory effect. It does, however, inhibit brain cyclooxygenase, which presumably accounts for its antipyretic and analgesic effects. Although acetaminophen relieves pain of osteoarthritis,[112,113] controversy exists as to its efficacy in rheumatoid arthritis.[114–121] No increase in pain relief was noted in patients with rheumatoid arthritis treated with pentazocine, compared with placebo.[122] There are, to my knowledge, no properly controlled therapeutic trials of acetaminophen in sports injuries, although its use is frequently recommended.[123–126] The combination of dextropropoxyphene and acetaminophen has, however, been useful in soft tissue injuries.[127]

DRUGS FOR TREATMENT OF PAIN

Mode of Action

Nonsteroidal Anti-Inflammatory Drugs

NSAIDs inhibit cyclooxygenase, thus reducing the production of prostaglandins.[27] Although there is some correlation between cyclooxygenase inhibition and anti-inflammatory effect, this only partly explains their therapeutic action.[128] Nonacetylated salicylates are 50 times less effective than acetylsalicylic acid in inhibiting cyclooxygenase but are no less effective.[129–131] On the other hand, full therapeutic doses, ie, 3 g/d, of nonacetylated salicylate reduces the urinary output of cyclooxygenase to the same extent (85%–95%) as aspirin.[132] Weissmann[133] has suggested that in rheumatoid arthritis only 25% to 30% of the inflammatory response is mediated by arachidonic acid–derived products. Certainly, NSAIDs have multiple effects on cellular functions other than cyclooxygenase inhibition, including antagonizing generation and activity of kinin polypeptides, altering lymphocyte responses, decreasing granulocyte and monocyte migration and phagocytosis, coupling oxidative phosphorylation, inhibiting lysosomal enzyme release, activating the complement system, and displacing an endogenous anti-inflammatory peptide from plasma proteins.[128,134,135] Abramson and Weissmann[136] have put forward the intriguing suggestion that NSAIDs may interfere with a cell receptor that triggers immobilization of intracellular calcium and activation of the cell. Aspirin is the only NSAID that permanently inhibits cyclooxygenase, hence its value in prevention of blood clotting.

Unlike cyclooxygenase which is present in all tissues of the body, lipoxygenase is found only in neutrophils, eosinophils, monocytes and macrophages, basophils, and certain mast cells.[137] Apart from benoxaprofen (now withdrawn) and to a lesser extent diclofenac and ketoprofen, none of the NSAIDs affect lipoxygenases product formation.[138]

All NSAIDs, with the exception of nabumetone, which is a pro-drug administered as a base, are weak organic acids with low pKa, which is believed to facilitate their concentration in inflamed tissue.[139] Ninety to ninety-five percent of NSAIDs is bound to plasma proteins; in some (eg, salicylates), the free or unbound fraction increases proportionately with the dose.[140] Dose-response relationships have been demonstrated with only a few NSAIDs, including naproxen, fenclofenac, and carprofen, and although therapeutic concentrations of salicylates and phenylbutazone have been suggested, there is no clear correlation between plasma concentration of salicylate or any other NSAID and clinical outcome in therapeutic doses.[141] Boardman and Hart[142] showed that anti-inflammatory effect of aspirin could be demonstrated only with daily doses of 3 g. However, the method used to demonstrate anti-inflammatory effects was relatively insensitive, ie, measurement of digital joint circumference in patients with rheumatoid arthritis. Smaller doses of salicylate may have had an anti-inflammatory effect, but not capable of detection. Likewise, small doses of indomethacin have only analgesic effect.[143] Ketorolac, a pyrrolo-pyrole derivative, is marketed as an analgesic but is an NSAID that at analgesic doses has virtually no anti-inflammatory effect.

The NSAIDs are lipid-soluble, which enables them to pass easily through cell membranes and, perhaps, is why they can give rise to headaches and confusion, especially in the elderly.[144] NSAIDs vary in their rate of biotransformation or metabolism, and elimination. They can be conveniently divided into those with a relatively short plasma half-life (t½ less than 6 hours) and those with a long plasma half life (t½ more than 12 hours). It takes five times the plasma half-life to reach steady state; thus, if rapid action is desired, a drug with a short half-life is preferred. Drugs with a short half-life need not be given any more frequently than twice a day, probably because of their persistence in synovial fluid.[145]

Recently, two isoenzymes of cyclooxygenase have been identified. One, COX-1, as it is generally called, is present in the stomach, platelets, endothelium of blood vessels, and kidney, and the other, COX-2, is induced only in inflammation. Efforts to find an NSAID that will inhibit only COX-2, thus avoiding many of the side effects associated with inhibition of COX-1, have finally been successful.[146]

Corticosteroid Drugs

The mechanism of action of corticosteroids is still not fully understood. They inhibit both prostaglandin and leukotriene synthesis by blocking the action of phospholipase enzyme, which converts phospholipids in cell membranes to arachidonic acid. Corticosteroids couple to a specific cytoplasmic receptor and then transfer to the nucleus, where the complex binds to chromatin, thus modulating protein synthesis.[147] As a result of their multiple effects on cellular function, corticosteroids have a long list of adverse effects, most of which are type A, or dose related.[148]

Narcotic Analgesics

Administration of narcotic analgesics may be necessary in serious sports injuries when an athlete is in severe pain. Morphine, the prototype of this class of drug, acts on the periaqueductal gray matter of the midbrain.[149,150]

Evaluation of Effects
Pain Relief

One of the problems in analyzing analgesic and anti-inflammatory drug therapy in sports injuries is the inadequacy of study designs. A review of the literature, albeit not exhaustive, reveals only 18 placebo-controlled double-blind trials of NSAIDs in acute sports injuries.[151–168] A large number of studies have been published in which one NSAID has been compared with another but without a placebo or no-treatment group. Most sports injuries improve over time, and even when large numbers of patients are studied,[164,169–171] it is difficult to avoid the conclusion that drug A = drug B = drug C . . . = 0. This is particularly true since none of the NSAIDs studied in placebo-controlled trials performed much better than placebo, and, indeed, in seven studies,[151,152,154,158,159,163,164] performed no differently.

This poor or no response compared with placebo may be due to the fact that, as suggested in one of the first trials to be published,[151] inflammation may not be of great importance in most soft tissue sports injuries. On the other hand, six controlled clinical trials[166,172–175] demonstrated superiority of NSAID gels compared with placebo. It has been well established that the response to analgesic medication depends on the severity of pain when it is prescribed[131,176–178] (Fig. 5–9), and it is interesting that in one study,[163] "advantage appeared to be evident in patients in whom injury was judged to be severe." Patients with sports soft-tissue injury may have insufficient severe pain to allow a clear distinction between active drug and placebo. This is supported by the findings in at least one study, in which 68 soccer players were treated for 14 days with either naproxen or dextropropoxyphene napsylate.[179] Patients receiving naproxen returned to normal activities 1 day sooner than did those receiving the analgesic![179]

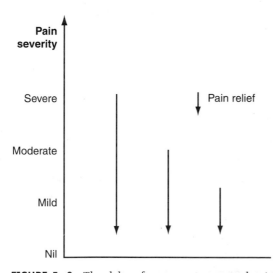

FIGURE 5–9. The delta of response to an analgesic is determined by the severity of pain when medication is given. Note that pain is never eradicated.

There is only one placebo-controlled trial of a nonopiate centrally acting analgesic in sports injuries.[180] It is thus not possible to know how much of the benefit of NSAIDs is the result of their analgesic effect as opposed to their anti-inflammatory effect. Despite the large number of local corticosteroid injections that have been administered to injured athletes, not a single peer-reviewed placebo-controlled study could be found in the literature. This also applied to administration of oral corticosteroids.[181]

Sports injuries take many forms, and several of the trials of NSAIDs can be criticized for selecting patients with different types of injury, thereby adding an uncontrolled variable.[151,153,155,157,161,164,165] The methods used in sports medicine trials have largely been subjective, with only occasional use of objective criteria such as volumetric estimation of swelling[182] or thermography.[156,166,167,172]

Perhaps the major problem in sports medicine injuries is the absence of biochemical and histologic information regarding injuries, which has been commented upon in several reviews.[181–186] Is there an acute-phase protein response, and, if so, for how long? What cells are present in the inflamed tissues? When do mononuclear cells appear? These questions need answering.

Pain is measured in terms of its relief,[187] and an argument can be made that pain relief is what should be measured in clinical therapeutic trials. In practice, however, it has seldom been done. More debatable is whether patients should have access to their previous scores. With the passage of time, patients tend to overestimate pain severity but quickly correct this when shown their previous scores.[188–190] Bird and Dixon[191] argued against showing patients their previous scores, but overall it seems to make little difference.[192,193] In clinical trials in sports injuries, this is probably not a serious consideration, since few studies exceed 14 days.

Joint Tenderness

In sports injuries, usually only one joint is involved; thus the articular indices of joint tenderness, which have proved useful in trials of rheumatic disease, are not relevant. The method used to assess joint or soft tissue tenderness should be consistent to ensure reliability. It is important, therefore, to standardize the procedure. Various pressure algometers[194,195] and do-lorimeters[196,197] are available that have acceptable reproducibility. In addition, Atkins et al[198] described an electronic method for measuring joint tenderness, which may also prove useful in clinical therapeutic trials of sports injuries. These instruments could be profitably investigated for use in determining tenderness in sports injuries.

Joint Movement

When sports injuries involve joints, either directly or indirectly, it may be useful to estimate the range of movement as an outcome measure. This does not appear to have been done, despite the fact that measurement of joint movement is highly reproducible.[199] In trials in rheumatoid arthritis, no difference in joint movement has been recorded between NSAID therapy and placebo.[200]

Swelling

The amount of tissue swelling in a limb can be determined by measurement of the circumference. A volumetric method, such as described in the hand by Scott,[201] can be used but only for hand and wrist and foot and ankle injuries.

Heat and Redness

Thermographic evaluation of increased temperature has occasionally been used in therapeutic trials in sports injuries[156,166,167,172] but has largely been abandoned in rheumatic disease trials because of the initial high cost of the equipment and the strict attention required to ambient temperature.[69] However, thermography is a noninvasive, reproducible, sensitive, and quantifiable method for assessing improvement in joint inflammation.[202,203] The more simple infrared thermographic instrument is not sufficiently sensitive.[204]

Ultrasonography is relatively simple and inexpensive and may be of value in sports injuries. It is, for example, capable of detecting even relatively small amounts of effusion in hip joints.[205,206] Radionuclide scans may also provide useful information, although the method is no longer used in clinical trials in rheumatic disease because of its insensitivity.[129,207,208] It should be noted that in rheumatoid arthritis the time courses of clinical indices, radionuclide uptake studies, and thermography show differences, which probably also would occur in sports inju-

ries. Whether magnetic resonance imaging (MRI) may be of value in assessment of swelling remains to be determined. Difficulties have been encountered with MRI in volumetric assessments.[209]

Redness occurs in only a few joint diseases, eg, gout and pseudogout, septic arthritis, and occasionally reactive arthritis. To my knowledge it is not a prominent feature of the majority of sports injuries.

Functional Impairment

Many functional indices have been introduced since their origin in 1937,[210] but all have been for arthritic disorders and are not appropriate to sports injuries. For injuries of the lower limbs the time to walk a certain distance, eg, 50 feet (15 m), might prove useful, although this has not proven sensitive to change in rheumatoid arthritis.[211] A version of the functional index described by Lee et al[212] might be of value, since it gives scores for both upper and lower limbs. There are three categories of impairment: 0, able to perform; +1, able to perform, but with difficulty; and +2, unable to perform. The index has not been of value in clinical trials of antirheumatic drugs in rheumatoid arthritis, although it will change after reconstructive surgery. A walking capacity scale, which gives numerical scores for the distance covered, might be considered for sports injury trials.[213]

Global Assessment

Patient and physician global assessments are frequently incorporated in clinical trials, but it is uncertain how they are compiled, and to date there is no study to determine their reliability.[214,215]

Compliance

Compliance can be estimated by patient reporting, either verbal or by diary, counting of pills, and plasma drug monitoring. In patients with arthritis, compliance is good when the patient has pain,[216] and it is presumed the same is true in patients with sports injuries. There is, however, no estimate of the level of compliance below which a therapeutic response is significantly impaired. Although therapeutic ranges have been suggested for some NSAIDs, eg, salicylates and phenylbutazone, there is scant evidence that estimation of blood concentrations is of any clinical value, although indomethacin levels correlate with headache.[217] Pill counting has generally been found adequate.[218,219] In general, compliance of 80% or greater is considered adequate.

Countervention

Countervention, the administration of an efficacious treatment other than the one being studied, is probably the most serious threat to the validity of any therapeutic trial.[220]

Double Blindedness

The controlled therapeutic trial is double blinded or, if necessary, triple blinded. However, many patients are able to break the code, especially if they have been told which side effects may develop and whether these side effects are dramatic, as in the case of cyclosporin A.[221] The question arises, How double blind is double blind, and does it matter?[222] It is also worth pointing out that both mild and serious side effects augment pain relief.[223] Insofar as possible, every effort should be made to ensure double blindedness and a record made of how many patients were able to break the code.

Drug Dosage

Most drug trials are of fixed doses, but it can be argued that patients be allowed to increase dosage (including placebo medication) if adequate pain relief is not achieved. In clinical therapeutic trials in sports injuries, this may be of considerable importance, since the recommended therapeutic dose of an analgesic may be suboptimal in a large person with a football injury. Increased dosing would require careful recording of the number of pills used. The use of acetaminophen as an escape drug is probably less desirable than a titration strategy.

Analysis

The two approaches to statistical analysis are explicative, or per protocol, and management, or intention to treat. In explicative analysis, patients who do not complete a trial are excluded; in the management approach they are included. The latter is now the preferred approach.[224]

Codification

There is a need for codification of clinical therapeutic trials in sports injuries. This could be done along the lines of the codification proposed for rheumatic disease.[225] Codification enables the reader to know immediately the trial design, how patients were selected, whether the study is placebo controlled, and whether compliance was determined, among other factors.

Treatment

Drugs used in the treatment of sports injuries generally are NSAIDs. For minor pain, acetaminophen may suffice, and 4 g/d can safely be taken. In severe injury, narcotic analgesics may be required to relieve pain.

There is some evidence of individual variation in response to NSAIDs,[226-230] but this could not be confirmed by Preston et al,[178] who prescribed flurbiprofen on two separate occasions in patients with rheumatoid arthritis. The apparent variability in response may be due to variation in clinical severity of disease (Fig. 5–10). Thus a patient with active disease who is prescribed an NSAID and in whom the disease activity decreases (patient improves) is considered a responder, whereas if the disease activity increases (worsens), the patient is considered a nonresponder (Fig. 5–10). If there is variation in response with NSAIDs, it is surprising it has not been observed in acute situations, such as acute rheumatic fever or acute gouty arthritis.[231]

Like acetaminophen and aspirin, ibuprofen and naproxen are available over-the-counter and may be used to treat pain from sports injuries. In Third World countries, such as Brazil, various other medications are available, including corticosteroids.[232] Athletes, especially those involved in contact sports such as boxing, should be

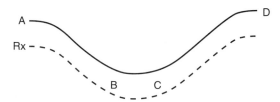

FIGURE 5–10. Treatment with a nonsteroidal antiinflammatory analgesic reduces pain and other indices of inflammation. Rheumatoid arthritis varies in severity over time, whether treatment is given or not. If the patient receives treatment between *A* and *B,* the patient is considered a responder, whereas the patient who receives treatment between *C* and *D* is a nonresponder (see text).

warned against taking aspirin because it increases the risk for hemorrhage into injured tissues.[233] NSAIDs have been reported to affect cognitive functions, especially in the elderly,[234–236] and conceivably could affect reaction time in sprinters. It may also be dangerous for athletes to take salicylates or other NSAIDs during physical exertion in the heat.[237] Further, dehydration with exercise may increase the risk of renal dysfunction.[238]

Acute gastrointestinal hemorrhage, although rare, may result from use of any of the currently available NSAIDs. Nonacetylated salicylates are less likely to cause hemorrhage than is aspirin.[239] Ketorolac is an NSAID that acts principally as an analgesic at therapeutic doses but can cause gastrointestinal bleeding.[240] It is probably reasonable to administer misoprostol with NSAIDs, because it can reduce the likelihood of serious gastrointestinal complications by approximately 50%.[241] Patients with a past history of peptic ulcer probably should not take NSAIDs.[242] It is generally not recognized that the likelihood of acute gastrointestinal hemorrhage is as likely with a short course of treatment as at any time during chronic administration.[243,244] Acetaminophen increases the likelihood of gastrointestinal hemorrhage in rats[245] but not in humans.[246] There is evidence that administration of acetaminophen prior to NSAID administration may have a cytoprotective effect.[247] The risk of acute gastrointestinal hemorrhage with oral corticosteroid administration is small but increases with coadministration of NSAIDs.[242,248,249]

Current information on the effects of smoking and drinking on NSAID-induced gastrointestinal lesions is conflicting.[250–252] Nevertheless, it might be wise to suggest that athletes not drink alcoholic beverages if they are taking an NSAID. Certainly athletes who are receiving NSAIDs, even one as mild as ibuprofen, should be warned of the hazards of binge drinking, which can lead to acute renal failure.[253,254] NSAIDs also can induce asthma,[255] which may be of importance in athletes who experience cold-induced bronchospasm. Cutaneous reactions to NSAIDs are not uncommon[256] and may be precipitated in athletes participating in sports in which there is prolonged exposure to ultraviolet light.

It must be appreciated that side effects of NSAIDs are relatively uncommon.[257] This is particularly true of those obtained over-the-counter,[258,259] although both gastrointestinal hemorrhage[260] and elevation of blood pressure[261] have been noted. No deaths have been reported with even massive overdoses of ibuprofen.[262,263]

Data regarding the efficacy of corticosteroid injections are based primarily on experience in rheumatic diseases, and even in these diseases, most of the evidence is anecdotal. The few good studies that have been performed[264] have given conflicting results.[265] There are no properly controlled randomized clinical trials dealing with sports-related tendon injuries,[266,267] and there is no evidence that corticosteroid injections increase the rate of return to function, either in acute or repetitive tendon injuries.

The most common adverse reaction to injection of corticosteroid drugs is crystal-induced inflammation. This may be painful but usually is short-lived, 4 to 12 hours.[268] Atrophy of overlying skin may occur if corticosteroid leaks into the subcutaneous tissues. This is especially likely with fluorinated compounds. Infection following corticosteroid injection is rare, provided the injection is not made through infected or psoriatic skin. Septic arthritis following intra-articular corticosteroid injections in rheumatoid arthritis usually occurs in severely debilitated patients and those receiving immunosuppressive therapy.[269] It is important that corticosteroid not be injected into a tendon, since it might cause the tendon to rupture. It is also worth keeping in mind that hypersensitivity reactions, including anaphylactoid shock, have been reported after intra-articular injection of methylprednisolone acetate.[270]

Rest

An argument can be made for letting Father Time and Mother Nature heal sports injuries. It is important to keep in mind that physical rest is the most potent anti-inflammatory agent we have. This has been amply testified by the sparing effect of paralysis, from whatever cause, on the development of osteoarthritis,[271–274] rheumatoid arthritis,[275–279] psoriatic arthritis,[280] gout[281] and pseudogout or chondrocalcinosis.[282] Controlled trials of hospital bed rest and immobilization have clearly demonstrated amelioration in joint inflammation in rheumatoid arthritis.[283,284]

In an excellent review of anti-inflammatory therapy in sports medicine, Leadbetter[285] makes the comment that inflammation is not the primary problem in sports injuries, but performance recovery. The advocacy of anti-inflammatory treatment, he maintains, deemphasizes the role of physical rehabilitation and even well-timed surgical repair.

Diet

Fish oils and evening primrose oil have been shown to reduce formation of leukotriene B_4 in both healthy subjects and patients with rheumatoid arthritis[286,287]; however, in double-blind trials, fish oils and evening primrose oil produced only modest pain reduction in patients with rheumatoid arthritis.[288,289]

An interesting study was recently reported from Japan on the metabolic effects of 10 g of hot red pepper ingested by long-distance runners. The results indicated stimulation of carbohydrate oxidation both at rest and during exercise.[290] Whether this leads to any difference in performance remains to be determined.

SUMMARY

In its many forms, inflammation plays a major role in both sports and recreational activities at all ages. This survey chapter of its medical history, etiologies, and therapies and their efficacies prepares readers for all subsequent chapters.

REFERENCES

1. Garrison FH: An Introduction to the History of Medicine, with Medical Chronology, Suggestions for Study and Bibliographic Data, 4th Ed. W.B. Saunders, Philadelphia, 1963, p. 225
2. Lyons AS, Petrucell RJ: Medicine: An Illustrated History. Harry N. Abrams, New York, 1978, pp. 251–261
3. Snook GA: The father of sports medicine (Galen). Am J Sports Med 6:126–131, 1978
4. Snook GA: The history of sports medicine, Part 1. Am J Sports Med 12:252, 1984
5. Buchanan WW: Bernardino Ramazzini (1633–1714): Physician and tradesman and possibly one of the "fathers" of sports medicine. Clin Rheumatol 10:136, 1991
6. Ramazzini B: Diseases of Workers (Latin text of 1713. Wright WC, trans, 1940). The Classics of Medicine Library, Birmingham, Ala, 1983
7. Noyes ER, Lindenfeld TN, Marshall MT: What determines an athletic injury (definition)? Who determines an injury (occurrence)? Am J Sports Med 16(suppl 1):65, 1988
8. Mellion MB: Sports Medicine Secrets. Hanley and Belfus, Philadelphia, 1993
9. Goldberg B: Injury patterns in youth sports. Phys Sports Med 17:175, 1989
10. Hoffman MD, Lyman KA: Medical needs at high school football games in Milwaukee. J Orthop Sports Phys Ther 1:67, 1988
11. Watson AW: Sports injuries during one academic year in 6799 Irish school children. Am J Sports Med 12:65, 1984
12. Keller CS, Noyes FR, Buncher CR: The medical aspects of soccer injury epidemiology. Am J Sports Med 15:230, 1987
13. Chandry DA, Grana WA: Secondary school athletic injury in boys and girls: a three year comparison. Phys Sports Med 13:106, 1985
14. Witman PA, Melvin M, Nicholas JA: Common problems seen in a metropolitan sports injury clinic. Phys Sports Med 9:105, 1981
15. De Haven KE, Lintner DM: Athletic injuries: comparison by age, sport, and gender. Am J Sports Med 14:218, 1986
16. Witman PA, Melvin M, Nicholas JA: Common problems seen in a metropolitan sports injury clinic. Phys Sports Med 9:105, 1981
17. Woo SL-Y, Buckwalter JA (eds): Injury and Repair of the Musculoskeletal Soft Tissues. American Academy of Orthopaedic Surgeons, Park Ridge, Ill, 1988
18. Hunter J: A Treatise on the Blood, Inflammation, and Gun-shot Wounds. Printed by John Richardson, London, England, 1794. Reprinted by The Classics of Medicine Library, Birmingham, Ala, 1982
19. Leadbetter WB, Buckwalter JA, Gordon SL (eds): Sports-Induced Inflammation: Clinical and Basic Science Concepts. American Academy of Orthopaedic Surgeons, Park Ridge, Ill, 6:14, 1990
20. Hurley JV: Inflammation. In: Anderson JR (ed): Muir's Textbook of Pathology, 12th Ed. Edward Arnold, London, 4:1, 1985
21. Beaven MA: Histamine. N Engl J Med 294:30–36, 320, 1976
22. Asako H, Kurose I, Wolf R, et al: Role of H1 receptors and P-selectin in histamine-induced leukocyte rolling and adhesion in postcapillary venules. J Clin Invest 93:1508, 1994
23. Armstrong D, Jepson J, Keel CA, Stewart JS: Pain-producing substances in human inflammatory exudates and plasma. J Physiol 135:350, 1957
24. Sharma JN, Buchanan WW: Pathogenic responses to bradykinin system in chronic inflammatory rheumatoid disease. Exp Toxic Pathol 46:421, 1994

25. Luderer JR, Lookingbill DP, Schneck DW, et al: Captopril-induced skin eruptions. J Clin Pharmacol 22:151, 1982

26. Hugli FA, Morgan EL: Mechanisms of leukocyte regulation by complement-derived factors. Contemp Topics Immunol 14:109, 1984

27. Vane JR: Inhibition of prostaglandin synthesis as a mechanism for aspirin-like drugs. Nature New Biol 231:232, 1971

28. Lewis GP, Westwick J, Williams TJ: Microvascular responses produced by the prostaglandin endoperoxide PGG_2 in vivo. Br J Pharmacol 59:442P, 1977

29. Williams KI, Higgs GE: Eicosanoids and inflammation. J Pathol 156:101, 1988

30. Crunkhorn P, Willis AL: Interaction between prostaglandins E and F given intradermally in the rat. Br J Pharmacol 41:507, 1971

31. Williams TJ, Morley J: Prostaglandins as potentiators of increased vascular permeability in inflammation. Nature 246:215, 1973

32. Kuehl FA, Humes JL, Egan RW, et al: Role of prostaglandin endoperoxide in inflammatory processes. Nature 265:170, 1977

33. Williams TJ, Peck MJ: Role of prostaglandin mediated vasodilatation in inflammation. Nature 270:530, 1977

34. Ferreira SH, Nakamura M, Castro MSA: The hyperalgesic effects of prostacyclin and prostaglandin E_2. Prostaglandins 16:31, 1978

35. Soter WA, Lewis RA, Corey EJ, Austen KF: Local effects of synthetic leukotrienes (LTC4, LTD4, LTE4, and LTB4) in human skin. J Invest Dermatol 80:115, 1983

36. Pettifer ER, Higgs GA, Salmon JA: Eicosanoids (prostaglandins and leukotrienes). In: Wicher J, Evans S (eds): Biochemistry of Inflammation. Kluwer Academic Publishers, Dordrecht, The Netherlands, p. 91, 1992

37. Belew M, Gardin B, Lindberg G, et al: Structure-activity relationships of vasoactive peptides derived from fibrin and fibrinogen degraded by plasmin. Biochim Biophys Acta 621:169, 1980

38. Pober JS, Cotran RS: The role of endothelial cells in inflammation. Transplantation 50:537, 1990

39. Etzioni A, Frydman M, Pollack S, et al: Recurrent severe infections caused by a novel leukocyte adhesion deficiency. N Engl J Med 327:1789, 1992

40. Bevilacqua MP, Stengelin S, Gimbrone MA Jr, Seed B: Endothelial leukocyte adhesion molecule 1: an inducible receptor for neutrophils related to complement regulatory proteins and lectins. Science 243:1160, 1989

41. Martin M, Resch K: Interleukin-1: more than a mediator between leukocytes. Trends Pharmacol Sci 9:171, 1988

42. Dinarello CA: Interleukin-1. Rev Infect Dis 6:51, 1984

43. Symons JA, Eastgate JA, Duff GW: Interleukin-1 as an inflammatory mediator. In: Wicher J, Evans S (eds): Biochemistry of Inflammation. Kluwer Academic Publishers, Dordrecht, The Netherlands, p. 183, 1992

44. Farber HW, Center DM, Rounds S: Effect of ambient oxygen on cultured endothelial cells from different vascular beds. Am J Physiol 253:H875, 1987

45. Mullane FM, Pinto A: Endothelium, arachidonic acid on coronary vascular tone. Fed Proc 46:54, 1987

46. Weiss SJ: Mechanisms of disease: tissue destruction by neutrophils. N Engl J Med 320:365, 1989

47. Savill JS, Wyllie AH, Henson JE, et al: Macrophage phagocytosis of aging neutrophils in inflammation: programmed cell death in the neutrophil leads to recognition by macrophages. J Clin Invest 83:865, 1989

48. Weiss SJ, Peppin GJ: Collagenolytic metallo enzymes of the human neutrophil. Biochem Pharmacol 35:3189, 1986

49. Docherty AJP, Murphy G: The tissue metalloproteinase family and the inhibitor TIMP: a study using DNAs and recombinant proteins. Ann Rheum Dis 49:469, 1990

50. Pettipher R, Edwards J, Cruwys S, et al: Pathogenesis of antigen-induced arthritis in mice deficient in neutrophil elastase and cathepsin G. Am J Pathol 137:1077, 1990

51. Egan RW, Paxton J, Kuehl FA: Mechanisms for the irreversible self deactivation of prostaglandin synthetase. J Biol Chem 251:7329, 1976

52. Dormandy TL: Free-radical pathology and medicine. J R Coll Phys Lond 23:221, 1989

53. Blake DR, Gallagher PJ, Potter AR, et al: The effect of synovial iron on the progression of rheumatoid disease. Arthritis Rheum 27:495, 1984

54. Andrews FJ, Morris CJ, Kondratowicz G, Blake DR: Effect of iron chelation on inflammatory joint disease. Ann Rheum Dis 46:327, 1987

55. Winyard PG, Blake DR, Chirico S, et al: Mechanism of exacerbation of rheumatoid synovitis by total-dose iron-dextran infusion: in vivo demonstration of iron-promoted oxidant stress. Lancet 1:69, 1987

56. McCord JM: Free radicals and inflammation: protection of synovial fluid by superoxide dismutase. Science 185:529, 1974

57. Greenwald RA, Moy WW: Effect of oxygen-derived free radicals on hyaluronic acid. Arthritis Rheum 23:455, 1980

58. Gutteridge JMC, Stocks J: Caeruloplasmin: physiological and pathological perspectives. CRC Crit Rev Clin Lab Sci 13:257, 1981

59. Perez HD, Weksler BB, Goldstein JM: Generation of a chemotactic lipid from arachidonic acid by exposure to a superoxide-generating system. Inflammation 4:313, 1980

60. Petrone WF, English DK, Wong K, McCord JM: Free radicals and inflammation: superoxide-dependent activation of a neutrophil chemotactic factor in plasma. Proc Natl Acad Sci U S A 77:1159, 1980

61. Merry P, Winyard PG, Morris CJ, et al: Oxygen free radicals, inflammation and synovitis: the current status. Ann Rheum Dis 48:864, 1989

62. Greenwald RA: Oxygen radicals, inflammation, and arthritis: pathophysiological considerations and implications of treatment. Semin Arthritis Rheum 20:219, 1991

63. Majno G: The Healing Hand: Man and Wound in the Ancient World. Harvard University Press, Cambridge, Mass, 1975, p. 4

64. Dinarello CA: Tumor necrosis factor (cachectin) is an endogenous pyrogen and induces IL-1. J Clin Invest 77:1734, 1986

65. Feldberg W, Melton AS: Prostaglandins and body temperature. In: Vane JR, Ferreira SH (eds): Inflammation. Springer-Verlag, New York, 1978, p. 617

66. Ballou SP, Kushner J: C-reactive protein and the acute phase response. Adv Intern Med 37:313, 1992

67. Kushner J: Regulation of the acute phase response to cytokines. Perspect Biol Med 36:611, 1993

68. Colton HR: Airway inflammation in cystic fibrosis. N Engl J Med 332:886, 1995

69. Bellamy N, Buchanan WW: Clinical evaluation in rheumatic diseases. In: McCarty DJ (ed): Arthritis and Allied Diseases: A Textbook of Rheumatology, 11th ed. Lea & Febiger, Philadelphia, 1989, pp. 158–185

70. Anderson JJ, Felson DT, Meenan RF, Williams HJ: Which traditional measures should be used in rheumatoid clinical trials? Arthritis Rheum 32:1093, 1989

71. Khawar K, Al-Jarallah K, Buchanan WW: Cyclosporin A in rheumatoid arthritis: a critical review. Inflammopharmacol 2:141, 1993

72. International Council for Standardization in Haematology (Expert Panel in Blood Rheology): ICSH recommendations for measurement of erythrocyte sedimentation rate. J Clin Pathol 46:198, 1993

73. Dixon JS: Relationship between plasma viscosity or ESR and the Ritchie Articular Index. Br J Rheumatol 23:233, 1984

74. Dixon JS, Hayes S, Constable PDL, Bird HA: What are the "best" measurements for monitoring patients during short-term second-line therapy. Br J Rheumatol 27:37, 1988

75. Williams TJ: Prostaglandin E_2, prostaglandin I_2 and the vascular changes in inflammation. Br J Pharmacol 65:517, 1979

76. Fibroblast growth factors: time to take note [editorial]. Lancet 336:777, 1990

77. Roche WR: Myofibroblasts. J Pathol 161:281, 1990

78. Descartes R: *L'Homme*. E Angot, Paris, 1664

79. Melzack R, Wall PD: Pain mechanisms: a new theory. Science 150:971, 1965

80. Melzack R, Wall PD: The Challenge of Pain. Penguin Books, New York, 1982

81. Iversen LL: The possible role of neuropeptides in the pathophysiology of rheumatoid arthritis [editorial]. J Rheumatol 12:399, 1985

82. Bonica JJ, Yaksh T, Liebeskind JC, et al: Biochemistry and modulation of nociception and pain. In: Bonica JJ, Loesev JD, Chapman CR, et al (eds): Management of Pain, 2nd ed. Lea & Febiger, Philadelphia, 1990, pp. 95–121

83. Wyke B: The neurology of joints: a review of general principles. Clin Rheum Dis 7:223, 1981

84. Kennedy JC, Alexander IJ, Hayes KC: Nerve supply of the human knee and its functional importance. Am J Sports Med 10:329, 1982

85. Lawson, SN: Morphological and biochemical cell types of sensory neurones. In: Scott SA (ed): Sensory Neurones: Diversity, Development and Plasticity. Oxford University Press, New York, p. 27, 1992

86. Harvey AR: Neurophysiology of rheumatic pain. Clin Rheumatol 1:1, 1987

87. Kellgren JH, Samuel EP: The sensitivity and innovation of the articular capsule. J Bone Joint Surg 32B:84, 1950

88. Grönblad M, Konttinen YT, Korkala O, et al: Neuropeptides in synovium of patients with rheumatoid arthritis and osteoarthritis. J Rheumatol 15:1807, 1988

89. Kellgren JH: Pain in osteoarthritis. J Rheumatol 10(suppl 9):108, 1983

90. Merighi A, Polak JM, Gibson SJ, et al: Ultrastructure studies on calcitonin gene-related peptide-, tachy kinins-, and somatostatin-immunoreactive nerves in rat dorsal root ganglia: evidence for the colocalisation of different peptides in single secretary granules. Cell Tissue Res 254:101, 1987

91. Mapp PI, Stevens CR, Blake DR: The physiology of the joint and its disturbance in inflammation. In: Maddison PJ, Isenberg DA, Woo P, Glass DN (eds): Oxford Textbook of Rheumatology. Oxford University Press, Oxford, England, 1993, pp. 256–268

92. Konttinen YT, Sorsa T, Santravirtha S, Russell A: Via dolorosa: from the first to second station [editorial]. J Rheumatol 21:783, 1994

93. Lembeck F, Gamse R: Substance P in peripheral sensory processes. In: Porter R, O'Connor R (eds): Substance P in the Nervous System. CIBA Foundation Symposium '91. Pitman, London, 1982, pp. 35–49

94. Brain SD, Williams TJ, Tippins JP, et al: Calcitonin gene-related peptide is a potent vasodilator. Nature 313:54, 1985

95. O'Halloran J, Bloom SR: Calcitonin gene related peptide. Br Med J 302:739, 1991

96. Virus RM, Gebhart GF: Pharmacologic actions of capsaicin: apparent involvement of substance P and serotonin. Life Sci 25:1273, 1979

97. Deal CL, Schnitzer TJ, Lipstein E, et al: Treatment of arthritis with topical capsaicin: a double-blind trial. Clin Ther 13:383, 1991

98. McCarthy GM, McCarthy DJ: Effect of topical capsaicin in the therapy of painful osteoarthritis of the hands. J Rheumatol 19:604, 1992

99. Zimmerman M: Pain mechanisms and mediators in osteoarthritis. Semin Arthritis Rheum 18(suppl 2):22, 1989

100. Mense S: Sensitization of group IV muscle receptors to bradykinin by 5-hydroxytryptamine and prostaglandin E_2. Brain Res 225:95, 1981

101. Lewis T, Pochin EE: The double pain response of the human skin to a single stimulus. Clin Sci 3:67, 1937

102. Kellgren JH: Observations on referred pain arising from muscle. Clin Sci 3:175, 1938

103. Kellgren JH: On the distribution of pain arising from deep somatic structures with charts of segmental pain areas. Clin Sci 4:35, 1939

104. Kellgren JH: Somatic simulating visceral pain. Clin Sci 44:303, 1939

105. Inman VT, Saunders JBM: Referred pain from skeletal structures. J Nerv Mental Dis 99:660, 1944

106. Lewis T, Kellgren J: Observations relating to referred pain, viscero-motor reflexes and other associated phenomena. Clin Sci 4:47, 1939

107. Simons DJ, May E, Goodell H, Wolff HG: Experimental studies on headache: muscles of the scalp and neck as sources of pain. Proc Assoc Res Nerv Mental Dis 23:228, 1943

108. Newham DJ: The consequences of eccentric contractions and their relation to delayed onset muscle pain. Eur J Appl Physiol 57:353, 1988

109. Levene JD, Gordon NC, Fields HL: Naloxone dose dependently produces analgesia and hyperalgesia in post operative pain. Nature 278, 1979

110. Grevert P, Goldstein A: Endorphins: naloxone fails to alter experimental pain on mood in humans. Science 199:1093, 1978

111. Dearborn GVN: A case of congenital general pure analgesia. J Nerv Med Dis 75:612, 1932

112. Brooks PM, Dougan MA, Mugford A, Meffin E: Comparative effectiveness of five analgesics in patients with rheumatoid arthritis and osteoarthritis. J Rheumatol 9:732, 1982

113. Bradley JD, Brandt KD, Katz BP, et al: Comparison of an anti-inflammatory dose of ibuprofen, an analgesic dose of ibuprofen, and acetaminophen in the treatment of patients with osteoarthritis of the knee. N Engl J Med 325:87, 1991

114. Huskisson EC: Simple analgesics for arthritis. Br Med J 4:196, 1974

115. Lee P, Watson M, Webb J, et al: Therapeutic effectiveness of paracetamol in rheumatoid arthritis. Int J Clin Pharmacol Biopharm 11:68, 1975

116. Lee P, Anderson JA, Miller J, et al: Evaluation of analgesic action and efficacy of anti-rheumatic drugs: study of 10 drugs in 684 patients with rheumatoid arthritis. J Rheumatol 3:283, 1976

117. Hardin JG, Kirk KA: Comparative effectiveness of five analgesics for the pain of rheumatoid arthritis. J Rheumatol 6:405, 1979

118. Kantor TG: Analgesics for arthritis. Clin Rheum Dis 6:525, 1980

119. Nuki G: Non-steroidal analgesics and anti-inflammatory agents. Br Med J 287:39, 1983

120. Hart FD: Rational use of analgesics in the treatment of rheumatic disorders. Drugs 33:85, 1987

121. Brooks PM, Buchanan WW: Prediction of the clinical efficacy of an intolerance to anti-rheumatic drug therapy. Prog Rheum Dis 17:347, 1991

122. Nuki G, Downie WW, Dick WC, et al: Clinical trial of pentazocine in rheumatoid arthritis: observations in the values of potent analgesics and placebos. Ann Rheum Dis 32:436, 1973

123. Martin J (ed): Handbook of Pharmacy Health Education. Pharmaceutical Press, London, 1991, p. 161

124. Nykamp D: Sports injuries. US Pharm 17:34, 1992

125. Edward C, Stillman P: Musculoskeletal disorders. Pharm J 251:733, 1993

126. Lum L: Tackling sports injuries: helping patients prevent and treat injuries from sports and exercise. Pharm Pract 13:58, 1997

127. Sleet RA, Khan MA: Comparative study of mefenamic acid and dextropropoxyphene plus paracetamol in the accident and emergency department. Curr Med Res Opin 7:77, 1980

128. Clements PJ, Paulus HE: Nonsteroidal anti-rheumatic drugs In: Kelley WN, Harris ED, Ruddy S, Sledge CB (eds): Textbook of Rheumatology, 5th Ed. W.B. Saunders, Philadelphia, 1997, p. 707

129. Deodhar SD, Dick WC, Hodgkinson R, Buchanan WW: Measurement of clinical response to anti-inflammatory drug therapy in rheumatoid arthritis. Q J Med 42:387, 1973

130. The Multicentre Salicylate/Aspirin Comparison Study Group: Does the acetyl group of aspirin contribute to the anti-inflammatory efficacy of salicylic acid in the treatment of rheumatoid arthritis? J Rheumatol 16:321, 1989

131. Preston SJ, Arnold MH, Beller EM, et al: Comparative analgesic and anti-inflammatory properties of sodium salicylate and acetylsalicylic acid (aspirin) in rheumatoid arthritis. Br J Clin Pharmacol 27:607, 1989

132. Vane J: The evolution of non-steroidal anti-inflammatory drugs and their mechanisms of action. Drugs 33(suppl 1):18, 1987

133. Weissmann G: Discussion 1987. Drugs 33(suppl 1), 8, 1987

134. Schlegel SI: General characteristics of non-steroidal anti-inflammatory drugs. In: Paulus HE, Furst DE, Dromgoole S (eds): Drugs for Rheumatic Disease. Churchill Livingstone, New York, 1987, p. 203

135. Forrest MJ, Brooks PM: Mechanism of action of non-steroidal anti-rheumatic drugs. Baillières Clin Rheumatol 2:275, 1988

136. Abramson SB, Weissmann G: The mechanisms of action of nonsteroidal anti-inflammatory drugs. Arthritis Rheum 32:1, 1989

137. Lewis RA, Austin KF, Soberman RJ: Leukotrienes and other products of the 5-lipoxygenase pathway. N Engl J Med 323:645, 1990

138. Dawson W, Boot JR, Harvey J, Walker JR: The pharmacology of benoxaprofen with particular reference to effects on lipoxygenase product formation. Eur J Rheumatol Inflam 5:61, 1982

139. Brune K, Glatt M, Graf P: Mechanisms of action of anti-inflammatory drugs. Gen Pharmacol 2:27, 1976

140. Furst DE, Tozer RN, Melmon KL: Salicylate clearance, the resultant of protein binding and metabolism. Clin Pharmacol Ther 26:380, 1979

141. Bellamy N, Buchanan WW, Kean WF: Variations in responses to NSAIDs. In: Famaey JP, Paulus HE (eds): Therapeutic Applications of NSAIDs: Subpopulations and New Formulations. Marcel Dekker, New York, 1992, p. 3

142. Boardman PL, Hart FD: Clinical measurement of the anti-inflammatory effects of salicylates in rheumatoid arthritis. Br Med J 2:264, 1967

143. Sunshine A, Laska E, Meisner M, Morgan S: Analgesic studies of indomethacin analyzed by computer techniques. Clin Pharmacol Ther 5:699, 1964

144. O'Brien WM, Bagby GF: Rare adverse reactions to nonsteroidal anti-inflammatory drugs. J Rheumatol 12:13, 347, 562, 785, 1985

145. Day RO, Graham GG, Williams KM: Pharmacokinetics of non-steroidal anti-inflammatory drugs. Baillières Clin Rheumatol 2:363, 1988

146. Vane JR: Toward a better aspirin. Nature 367:215, 1994

147. Chan L, O'Malley BW: Steroid hormone action: recent advances. Ann Intern Med 89:694, 1978

148. Stein CM, Pincus T: Glucocorticoids. In: Kelley WN, Harris ED, Ruddy S, Sledge CB (eds): Textbook of Rheumatology, 5th Ed. W.B. Saunders, Philadelphia, 1997, p. 787

149. Snyder SH: Opiate receptors and internal opiates. Sci Am 236:44, 1977

150. Yaksh TL: Spiral opiate analgesia: characteristics and principles of action. Pain 11:293, 1981

151. Huskisson EC, Berry H, Street FG, Madhurst HE: Indomethacin for soft tissue injuries. Rheumatol Rehab 12:159, 1973

152. Van Marion WF: Indomethacin in the treatment of soft tissue injuries: a double-blind trial against placebo. J Int Med Res 1:151, 1973

153. Fitch KD, Gray SD: Indomethacin in soft tissue sports injuries. Med J Aust 1:260, 1974

154. Goldie JF, Gunterberg B, Jacobson C: Foot volumetry as an objective test of the effect of antiphogistic drugs in ankle sprains. Rheumatol Rehab 13:204, 1974

155. Krishnan G: A placebo controlled, double-blind trial of benoxylate tablets in the treatment of bursitis and synovitis. Rheumatol Rehab 16:180, 1977

156. VanHeerden JJ: Diclophenac sodium, oxyphenbutazone and placebo in sports injuries of the knee. S Afr Med J 52:396, 1977

157. Santilli G, Tuccimei U, Cannistra FM: Comparative study with piroxicam and ibuprofen versus placebo in supportive treatment of minor sports injuries. J Int Med Res 8:265, 1980

158. Anderson S, Fredin H, Lindbory H, et al: Ibuprofen versus compression bandage in the treatment of ankle sprain. Acta Orthop Scand 54:322, 1983

159. Viijakko T, Rokkanen P: The treatment of ankle sprain by bandaging and antiphlogistic drugs. Ann Chir Gynaecol 72:66, 1983

160. McLatchie GR, Allister G, MacEwan C, et al: Variable schedules of ibuprofen for ankle sprains. Br J Sports Med 19:203, 1985

161. Duranceau JA, Lacoste F, Bourgouin J, Philips R: Double-blind comparison of ketoprofen and placebo in the treatment of sprains and strains. Clin Ther 8:187, 1986

162. Hutson MA: A double-blind study comparing ibuprofen 1800 mg or 2400 mg daily and placebo in sports injuries. J Int Res 14:142, 1986

163. Dupont M, Beliveau P, Theriault G: The efficacy of anti-inflammatory medication in the treat-

ment of the acutely sprained ankle. Am J Sports Med 15:41, 1987

164. Jenner PN: Nabumetone in the treatment of skin and soft tissue injury. Am J Med 83(suppl 4B):101, 1987

165. Lereim P, Gabor I: Piroxicam and naproxen in acute sports injuries. Am J Med 84(suppl 5A):45, 1988

166. Garagiola U: Comparison of diclofenac sodium and aspirin in the treatment of acute sports injuries [letter]. Am J Sports Med 17:589, 1989

167. Giani E: Telethermographic evaluation of NSAIDs in the treatment of sports injuries. Med Sci Sports Exerc 21:1, 1989

168. Bakshi R, Rotman H, Shaw M, Sussman H: Double-blind, multi-center evaluation of the efficacy and tolerability of diclofenac dispersible in the treatment of acute soft-tissue injuries. Clin Ther 17:30, 1995

169. Heere LP: Piroxicam in acute musculoskeletal disorders and sports injuries. Am J Med 84(suppl 5A):50, 1988

170. Calligaris A, Scaricabarozzi I, Vecchiet L: A multi-center double-blind investigation comparing nimesulide and naproxen in the treatment of minor sports injuries. Drugs 46(suppl 1):187, 1993

171. Gepner P: Volarene Emulgel et tendinites d'origine sportive: resultats sur 2046 observations. Cinesiologie 36:39, 1995

172. Commandre F-A: Traitement percutane par le diclofenac en emulsion gel de la petite traumatologie et pathologic locomotrice du sport (control blethermographique). Lyon Mediterr Med 24:11699, 1988

173. Almekinders LC: The efficacy of nonsteroidal anti-inflammatory drugs in the treatment of ligament injuries. Sports Med 9:137, 1990

174. Campbell J, Dunn J: Evaluation of topical ibuprofen cream in the treatment of acute ankle sprains [abstract]. J Accident Emerg Med 11:178, 1994

175. Hosie G, Bird H: The topical NSAID felbinac versus oral NSAIDs: a critical review. Eur J Rheumatol Inflamm 14:21, 1994

176. Maclagan TJ: The treatment of acute rheumatism by salicin. Lancet 1:342, 1876

177. Lee P, Watson TL, Webb J, et al: Method for assessing therapeutic potential of anti-inflammatory anti-rheumatic drugs in rheumatoid arthritis. Br Med J 2:685, 1973

178. Preston SJ, Arnold MH, Beller EM, et al: Variabililty in response to non-steroidal anti-inflammatory analgesics: evidence from controlled clinical therapeutic trials of flurbiprofen in rheumatoid arthritis. Br J Clin Pharmacol 26:759, 1988

179. Beveridge K: Treatment of sports injuries with naproxen sodium and dextropropoxyphene napylate. Pharmatherapeutica 3:393, 1985

180. Friedel HA, Fitton A: Flupirtine: a review of its pharmacological properties and therapeutic efficacy in pain states. Drugs 45:548, 1993

181. Fredberg U: Local corticosteroid injection in sport: review of literature and guidelines for treatment. Scand J Med Sci Sports 7:131, 1997

182. Almekinders LC: The efficacy of nonsteroidal anti-inflammatory drugs in the treatment of ligament injuries. Sports Med 137:143, 1990

183. Micheli LJ: Common painful sports injuries: assessment and treatment. Clin J Pain 5(suppl 2):51, 1989

184. Weiler JM, Albright JP, Buckwalter JA: Nonsteroidal anti-inflammatory drugs. In: Lewis AJ, Furst DE (eds): Anti-Inflammatory Agents in Sports Medicine. Marcel Dekker, New York, 1987, pp. 71–78

185. Price KO, Goldwine MA: Treatment of athletic injuries. US Pharm 19(suppl 7):15, 1994

186. Leadbetter WB: Anti-inflammatory therapy in sports injury: the role of nonsteroidal drugs and corticosteroid injection. Clin Sports Med 14:353, 1995

187. Beecher HK: Measurement of subjective responses. Oxford University Press, New York, 1959

188. Scott J, Huskisson EC: Accuracy of subjective measurements made with or without previous scores: an important source of error in serial measurement of subjective states. Ann Rheum Dis 38:558, 1979

189. Carlsson AM: Assessment of chronic pain: aspects of the reliability and validity of the visual analogue scale. Pain 16:87, 1983

190. Jacobsen M: The use of rating scales in clinical research. Br J Psychol 111:545, 1965

191. Bird HA, Dixon JS: Measurement of pain. In: Wright V (ed): Clinical Rheumatology: Pain. Bailliere Tindall, London, 1987, p. 71

192. Bellamy N, Goldsmith H, Buchanan WW, et al: Prior score availability: observations using the WOMAC Osteoarthritis Index. Br J Rheumatol 30:150, 1991

193. Van den Burg MJ, Young KA, Wojtulewski J, et al: Does it matter how visual analogue scales are used in clinical studies? Pharm Med 1:47, 1984

194. Buchanan HM, Midgley JA: Evaluation of pain threshold using a simple pressure algometer. Clin Rheumatol 6:510, 1987

195. Gerecz-Simon EM, Tunks ER, Heale J-A, et al: Measurement of pain threshold in patients with rheumatoid arthritis, osteoarthritis, ankylosing spondylitis and healthy controls. Clin Rheumatol 8:467, 1989

196. McCarty DJ, Gatter RA, Phelps P: A dolorimeter for quantification of articular tenderness. Arthritis Rheum 8:551, 1965

197. McCarty DJ: A twenty-pound dolorimeter for quantification of articular tenderness. Arthritis Rheum 11:696, 1968

198. Atkins CJ, Zielinski A, Klinkhoff AA, et al: An electronic method for measuring joint tenderness in rheumatoid arthritis. Arthritis Rheum 34:407, 1992

199. Mitchell WS, Miller J, Sturrock R: An evaluation of goniometry as an objective parameter for measuring joint motion. Scott Med J 20:57,1975

200. Thune S: A comparative study of azapropazone and indomethacin in the treatment of rheumatoid arthritis. Curr Med Res Opin 4:70, 1976

201. Scott JT: Morning stiffness in rheumatoid arthritis. Ann Rheum Dis 19:361, 1960

202. Ingpen ML: The quantitative measurement of joint changes in rheumatoid arthritis. Ann Phys Med 9:322, 1968

203. Bacon PA, Collins A-J, Ring EFJ, Cosh JA: Thermography in the assessment of inflammatory arthritis. Clin Rheum Dis 2:51, 1976

204. Arnold MH, Preston SJL, Beller EM, Buchanan WW: Infra-red surface thermography: evaluation of a new radiometry instrument for measuring skin temperature over joints. Clin Rheumatol 8:225, 1989

205. Foldes K, Gaal M, Balint P, et al: Ultrasonography after hip arthroplasty. Skeletal Radiol 21:297, 1992

206. Foldes K, Konrad K, Balint G, et al: Non-invasive imaging methods in painful hip arthroplasties: correlation of pain with radionuclide uptake and ultrasonography in conservatively managed patients. J Orthop Rheumatol 8:199, 1995

207. Dick WC: The use of radioisotopes in normal and diseased joints. Semin Arthritis Rheum 1:301, 1972

208. Lee P: Isotopes in the measurement of joint inflammation. J Rheumatol 9:767, 1982

209. Pilch L, Stewart C, Gordon D, et al: Assessment of cartilage volume in the femorotibial joint with magnetic resonance imaging and 3D computer reconstruction. J Rheumatol 21:2307, 1994

210. Bellamy N, Buchanan WW: Dr Douglas Taylor and half a century of musculoskeletal kelvinism. Clin Rheumatol 7:272, 1988

211. Grace EM, Gerecz EM, Kassam YB, et al: 50-foot walking time: a critical assessment of an outcome measure in clinical trials of antirheumatic drugs. Br J Rheumatol 27:372, 1988

212. Lee P, Jasani MK, Dick WC, Buchanan WW: Evaluation of a functional index in rheumatoid arthritis. Scand J Rheumatol 2:71, 1973

213. Guttman L: The basis of scalogram analysis. In: Stouffer SA (ed): Measurement and Prediction. Princeton University Press, New York, 1950

214. Bellamy N, Buchanan WW: Clinical evaluation in the rheumatic diseases. In: Koopman WJ (ed): Arthritis and Allied Conditions: A Textbook of Rheumatology, 13th Ed. Williams & Wilkins, Baltimore, Md, vol 2, 1997, p. 47

215. Buchanan WW, Bellamy N: NSAIDs: clinical efficacy and toxicity. Inflammopharmacology 1: 115, 1991

216. Lee P, Tan LJP: Drug compliance in outpatients with rheumatoid arthritis. Aust NZ J Med 9:274, 1979

217. Helleberg L: Clinical pharmacokinetics of indomethacin. Clin Pharmacokinet 6:245, 1981

218. Deyo RA, Inuit TS, Sullivan B: Non-compliance with arthritis drugs: magnitude correlates and clinical implications. J Rheumatol 8:931, 1981

219. Constant F, Guillemin F, Herbeth B, et al: Measurement methods of drug consumption as a secondary judgment criterion for clinical trials in chronic rheumatic diseases. Am J Epidemiol 145:826, 1997

220. Feinstein AR: Clinical biostatistics III: the architecture of clinical research. Clin Pharmacol Ther 11:432, 1970

221. Tugwell P, Bombardier C, Gent M, et al: Low dose cyclosporin versus placebo in patients with rheumatoid arthritis. Lancet 355:1051, 1990

222. Huskisson EC, Scott J: How blind is double-blind and does it matter? Br J Clin Pharmacol 3:331, 1976

223. Max MB, Schafer SC, Culnane M, et al: Association of pain relief with drug side effects in post herpetic neuralgia: a single-dose study of clonidine, codeine, ibuprofen and placebo. Clin Pharm Ther 43:363, 1988

224. Sackett DL, Gent M: Controversy in counting and attributing events in clinical trials. N Engl J Med 301:1410, 1979

225. Bellamy N, Buchanan WW: The codification of clinical trial methodology. Eular Bull 13:61, 1984

226. Scott DL, Roden S, Marshall T, Kendall MJ: Variations in response to non-steroidal anti-inflammatory drugs. Br J Clin Pharmacol 14:691, 1982

227. Day RO, Brooks PM: Variations in responses to non-steroidal anti-inflammatory drugs. Br J Clin Pharmacol 23:655, 1987

228. Brooks PM, Day RO: Non-steroidal anti-inflammatory drugs: differences and similarities. N Engl J Med 324:1716, 1991

229. Furst DE: Are there differences among non-steroidal anti-inflammatory drugs? Arthritis Rheum 57:1, 1994

230. Robbins D, Taylor MAH, Brown MD, McIlwain H: Ketoprofen versus ibuprofen for acute sports injuries: are there differences between nonsteroidal anti-inflammatory drugs? Curr Ther Res Clin Exp 48:780, 1990

231. Bellamy N, Buchanan WW, Kean WF: Variations in responses to NSAIDs. In: Famaey JP, Paulus HE (eds): Therapeutic Applications of NSAIDs Subpopulations and New Formulations. Marcel Dekker, New York, 1992, pp. 3–26

232. Ferraz MB, Pereira RB, Paiva JG, et al: Availability of over-the-counter drugs for arthritis in Sao Paulo, Brazil. Soc Sci Med 42:1129, 1996

233. Beall S, Gardner J, Coxley D: Anterolateral compartment syndrome related to drug-induced bleeding: a case report. Am J Sports Med 11:454, 1983

234. Anderson RJ, Potts DE, Gabow PA, et al: Unrecognized adult salicylate intoxication. Ann Intern Med 85:745, 1976

235. Bowen JD, Larson EB: Drug-induced cognitive impairment: defining the problems and finding solutions. Drugs Aging 3:349, 1993

236. Goodwin JS, Regan M: Cognitive dysfunction associated with naproxen and ibuprofen in the elderly. Arthritis Rheum 25:1013, 1982

237. Fred HL: Reflections on a 100 mile run: effects of aspirin therapy. Med Sci Sports Exerc 12:212, 1980

238. Buchanan WW, Rainsford KD: Aspirin and non-acetylated salicylates: use in inflammatory injuries incurred during sporting activities. In: Leadbetter WB, Buckwalter JA, Gordon SL (eds): Sports-Induced Inflammation: Clinical and Basic Science Concepts. American Academy of Orthopaedic Surgeons, Park Ridge, Ill, 1990, p. 431

239. Scheiman JM, Behler EM, Berardi RR, Elta GH: Salicylic acid causes less gastro-duodenal mucosal damage than enteric-coated aspirin: an endoscopic comparison. Dig Dis Sci 34:229, 1989

240. Strom BL, Berlin JA, Kinman JL, et al: Parenteral ketorolac and risk of gastrointestinal and operative site bleeding: a postmarketing surveillance study. JAMA 275:376, 1996

241. Silverstein RE, Graham DY, Senior JR, et al: Misoprostil reduces serious gastrointestinal complications in patients with rheumatoid arthritis receiving nonsteroidal anti-inflammatory drugs. Ann Intern Med 123:241, 1995

242. Fries JF: NSAID gastropathy: the second most deadly rheumatic disease? Epidemiology and risk appraisal. J Rheumatol 18(suppl 28):6, 1991

243. MacDonald TM: Side-effects of non-steroidal anti-inflammatory drugs: studies from the Tayside Medicines Monitoring Unit. In: Rainsford KD (ed): Side Effects of Anti-Inflammatory Drugs IV. Kluwer Academic Publishers, London, 1997, pp. 25–33

244. Gabriel SE, Jaaiskimaimen I, Bombardier C: Risk for serious gastrointestinal complications related to use of nonsteroidal anti-inflammatory drugs: a meta-analysis. Ann Intern Med 115:787, 1991

245. Bhattacharya SK, Tandon R: Potentiation of gastric toxicity of ibuprofen by paracetamol in the rat. J Pharm Pharmacol 43:520, 1991

246. Lanza FL, Royer GL, Nelson RS, et al: Effect of acetaminophen on human gastric mucosal injury caused by ibuprofen. Gut 27:440, 1986

247. Stern RS, Hogan AI, Kahm LH, Isenberg JJ: Protective effect of acetaminophen against aspirin and ethanol induced damage to the human gastric mucosa. Gastroenterology 86:728, 1984

248. Piper JM, Ray WA, Daugherty JR, et al: Corticosteroid use and peptic ulcer disease: role of nonsteroidal anti-inflammatory drugs. Ann Intern Med 114:735, 1991

249. Pecora PG, Kaplan B: Corticosteroids and ulcers: is there an association? Ann Pharmacother 30:870, 1996

250. Savage RL, Moller PW, Ballantyne CL, Wells JE: Variation in the risk of peptic ulcer complications with nonsteroidal anti-inflammatory drug therapy. Arthritis Rheum 36:84, 1993

251. Griffin MR, Piper JM, Daugherty JR, et al: Nonsteroidal anti-inflammatory drug use and increased risk of peptic ulcer disease in elderly persons. Ann Intern Med 114:257, 1991

252. Holvoet J, Terriere L, Van Hee V, et al: Relation of upper gastrointestinal bleeding to nonsteroidal anti-inflammatory drugs and aspirin: a case-control study. Gut 32:730, 1991

253. Elsasser GN, Lopez L, Evans E, et al: Reversible acute renal failure associated with ibuprofen ingestion and binge drinking. J Fam Pract 27:221, 1988

254. Wen SF, Parthasarathy R, Liiopoulos O, Oberley TD: Acute renal failure following binge drinking and nonsteroidal anti-inflammatory drugs. Am J Kidney Dis 20:381, 1992

255. Szczeklik A: Antipyretic analgesics and the allergic patient. Am J Med 75:82, 1983

256. Simon IS: Actions and toxic effects of the nonsteroidal anti-inflammatory drugs. Curr Opin Rheumatol 6:238, 1994

257. Buchanan WW, Brooks PM: Prediction of organ system toxicity with anti-rheumatic drug therapy. In: Bellamy N (ed): Prognosis in the Rheumatic Diseases. Kluwer Academic Publishers, Dordrecht, The Netherlands, 18:403, 1991

258. Furey SA, Waksman JA, Dash BH: Nonprescription ibuprofen: side effect profile. Pharmacotherapy 12:403, 1992

259. De Armond B, Francisco CA, Lin JS, et al: Safety profile of over-the-counter naproxen sodium. Clin Ther 17:587, 1995

260. Liang NM, Fortin P: Management of osteo-arthritis of the hip and knee. N Engl J Med 325:125, 1991

261. Bradley JG: Nonprescription drugs and hypertension: which one affects blood pressure? Postgrad Med 89:195, 1991

262. Linden CH, Townsend PL: Metabolic acidosis after acute ibuprofen overdosage. J Pediatr 111:922, 1987

263. Veltri JC, Rollins DE: A comparison of the frequency and severity of poisoning cases for ingestion of acetaminophen, aspirin and ibuprofen. Am J Emerg Med 6:104, 1988

264. Fitzgerald RF Jr: Intrasynovial injections of steroids. Mayo Clin Proc 51:655, 1976

265. Owen DS Jr: Aspiration and injection of joints and soft tissues. In: Kelley WN, Harris ED, Ruddy S, Sledge CB (eds): Textbook of Rheumatology, 5th Ed. W.B. Saunders, Philadelphia, 1997, vol 1, p. 591

266. Scott WA: Injection techniques and use in the treatment of sports injuries. Sports Med 22:406, 1966

267. Sandmeier R, Renström PAFH: Diagnosis and treatment of chronic tendon disorders in sports. Scand J Med Sci Sports 7:96, 1997

268. Gatter RA: Arthrocentesis technique and intra-synovial therapy. In: Koopman WJ (ed): Arthritis and Allied Conditions: A Textbook of Rheumatology, 13th Ed. Williams & Wilkins, Baltimore, Md, 1997, p. 751

269. Ostensson A, Geborek P: Septic arthritis as a non-surgical complication in rheumatoid arthritis: relation to disease severity and therapy. Br J Rheumatol 22:211, 1991

270. Mace S, Vadas P, Prozanski W: Anaphylactic shock induced by intra articular injection of methyl prednisolone acetate. J Rheumatol 24:1191, 1997

271. Coste F, Forestier J: Hémiplégie et nodosités d'Heberden controlatérales. Bull Soc Med Hôp Paris 51:772, 1935

272. Hench PS: Heberden's nodes: hereditary in hypertrophic arthritis of the finger joints (a discussion). JAMA 115:2025, 1940

273. Glynn JH, Sutherland I, Walker GF, et al: Low incidence of osteoarthritis in hip and knee after anterior polymyelitis! a late review. Br Med J 2:739, 1966

274. Földes K, Marietta B, Piroska E, Balint G: Hemiplégia protektiu sizerepe nodáles generalizált kéy arthrosisban. Mugyar Rheumatol 34:407, 1993

275. Bland JH, Eddy WM: Hemiplegia and rheumatoid hemiarthritis. Arthritis Rheum 11:72, 1968

276. Kamerman JS: Protective effect of traumatic lesions in rheumatoid arthritis following hemiplegia. Ann Rheum Dis 21:370, 1962

277. Glick EN: Assymetrical rheumatoid arthritis after poliomyelitis. Br J Med 3:26, 1967

278. Thompson M, Bywaters EGL: Unilateral rheumatoid arthritis following hemiplegia. Ann Rheum Dis 21:370, 1962

279. Yoghmai I, Rooholamini SM, Faunce HF: Unilateral rheumatic arthritis: protective effects of neurological defects. Am J Roentgenol 128:299, 1977

280. Veale D, Farrel M, Fitzgerald O: Mechanism of joint sparing in a patient with unilateral psoriatic arthritis and a longstanding hemiplegia. Br J Rheumatol 32:413, 1993

281. Glynn JL, Clayton ML: Sparing effect of hemiplegia on tophaceous gout. Ann Rheum Dis 35:534, 1976

282. Fontanet A, Menkes CJ: Hemiplegie et polyarthropathie controlaterale de la chondrocalcinose. Rev Rhum 56:789, 1989

283. Partridge REH, Duthie JJR: Controlled trial of immobilisation of the joints in rheumatoid arthritis. Ann Rheum Dis 22:91, 1963

284. Lee P, Kennedy AC, Anderson J, Buchanan WW: Benefits of hospitalisation in rheumatoid arthritis. Q J Med 63:205, 1974

285. Leadbetter WB: Anti-inflammatory therapy in sports injury: the role of nonsteroidal drugs and corticosteroid injection. Clin Sports Med 14:353, 1995

286. Payan DG, Wong MYS, Chernov-Rogan T, et al: Alterations in human leucocyte function induced by ingestion of eicosapentanoic acid. J Clin Immunol 6:402, 1986

287. Prescott SM: The effect of eicosapentanoic acid on leukotriene production by human neutrophils. J Biol Chem 259:7615, 1984

288. Belch JJF, Ansell D, Madhok R, et al: Effects of altering dietary essential fatty acids on requirements for nonsteroidal anti-inflammatory drugs in patients with rheumatoid arthritis: a double-blind placebo controlled study. Ann Rheum Dis 47:96, 1988

289. Buchanan HM, Preston SJ, Brooks PM, Buchanan WW: Is diet important in rheumatoid arthritis? Br J Rheumatol 30:125, 1991

290. Lim K, Yoshioka M, Kikuzato S, et al: Dietary red pepper ingestion increases carbohydrate oxidation at rest and during exercise in runners. Med Sci Sports Exerc 29:355, 1997

6

Arthritis and Exercise

LAWRENCE E. HART

Physical activity is widely recognized as an essential component of a healthy lifestyle. There is a growing consensus that adequate and regular exercise reduces the risk of cardiovascular disease, facilitates weight reduction, prevents osteoporosis, improves quality of life, and may postpone death.[1-3] However, to dogmatically accept that exercise is a health-promoting practice already infers that we have prejudged its benefits without fully accounting for its risks.[4]

With regard to musculoskeletal conditions in general, there is an emerging literature that identifies various forms of physical activity as risk factors for a spectrum of tendon, ligament, and muscle injuries.[5] What is much less definitive is the relationship between physical activity and the onset or acceleration of joint disorders. A further important aspect of the exercise and arthritis conundrum relates to the role of exercise as a therapeutic intervention in patients with diagnosed arthropathies. This chapter focuses on these two issues.

For purposes of this overview a methodologic approach is used that assesses the quality of evidence of published research according to predetermined critical appraisal criteria. The evidence-based approach described in Chapter 1 provides the basis for this model. To retrieve the relevant studies on exercise and arthritis, a Medline search of the available English-language literature for 1976 to 1998 was conducted. Additional contributions were identified through reference lists in some of the searched reports and in textbooks of sports medicine, rehabilitation, and rheumatology.

DOES EXERCISE CAUSE ARTHRITIS?

Osteoarthritis (OA), or degenerative joint disease, is the commonest form of arthritis and is the condition referred to when the relation of physical activity to joint disease is considered. The American Academy of Orthopedic Surgeons and the National Institutes of Health have proposed the following definition of OA[6]:

Osteoarthritis (OA) is the result of both mechanical and biologic events that destabilize the normal coupling of degradation and synthesis of articular cartilage and subchondral bone. Although it may be initiated by multiple factors including genetic, developmental, metabolic and traumatic, OA involves all of the tissues of the diarthroidal joint. Ultimately, OA is manifested by morphologic, biochemical, molecular and biomechanical changes of both cells and matrix which lead to a softening, fibrillation, ulceration and loss of articular cartilage, sclerosis, and eburnation of subchondral bone, osteophytes, and subchondral cysts. When clinically evident, OA is characterized by joint pain, tenderness, limitation of movement, crepitus, occasional effusions, and variable degrees of local inflammation.

Mechanical stresses of differing types are thought to damage articular cartilage. Such factors include joint dysplasia or malalignment, a single major impact, repeated minor impact loading, minute mechanical derangement, joint hypermobility, and protracted overuse.[7] Comprehensive descriptions of the effects of mechanical insults on articular cartilage are provided by Radin et al[8] and Mankin.[9] Intuitively, there is little debate on the likely evolution of OA changes that result from joint malalignment or dysplasia, hypermobility, or a single major impact. It has been plausibly demonstrated, for example, that surgical removal of a meniscus following knee injury represents a significant risk factor for radiologically corroborated tibiofemoral OA.[10] Earlier studies have also found this association. In addition, there is evidence to suggest that cruciate or collateral injuries of the knee increase the risk of premature OA.[11–21]

When and how repeated minor impact loading or protracted overuse precipitates or aggravates joint degeneration is somewhat less clearcut. The oft-cited example in support of such an association is the purportedly increased incidence of OA in the shoulders and elbows of pneumatic drill operators, in the hips of farm workers, and in the elbows and knees of miners.[22] However, critical appraisal of the literature reveals that such relationships have been supported by less than optimal methodology that really does not make the case for unequivocal associations between the onset of OA and the identified causal stressors.[23] Moreover, such uncertainty makes it impossible to establish whether normal joints might be affected by exercise or whether, instead, there needs to be some incongruity of the joint surface, provoked by exercise-induced trauma, or other factors, before OA becomes evident.[24]

Confounding Factors

The association between exercise and arthritis is further confounded by various other factors that might influence the development or acceleration of arthritic change.

Age. The incidence of severe OA increases exponentially with age. In older athletes, therefore, it is difficult to determine whether aging or exercise is the predominant element in worsening joint symptoms.[25] At the other end of the age spectrum, it has been suggested, but never proved, that frequent involvement in sports at an early age and at an intense level might predispose to arthritis in later life.[26,27]

Gender. While it is recognized that OA likely affects men and women in similar numbers, symptoms tend to occur in women earlier in life. Once symptoms develop, arthritis tends to have a different anatomic distribution in men and women. Quite what effect these gender dif-

ferences might have in possible sports-related OA needs to be explored.[28]

Ethnicity. The incidence of OA differs across ethnic groups. Chinese populations, for example, have a lower prevalence of hip OA than Caucasian comparison groups have.[29]

Geography. Some populations, especially those in colder climates such as Finland and Alaska, are thought to have a lower prevalence of OA than people who live in warmer environments.[30,31]

Body Habitus. Obesity is a risk factor for OA of the knee, the great toe, and the hand.[32]

Six of the most popular forms of exercise—running, walking, swimming, aerobics, cycling, and racquet sports—meet the US Public Health Service definition of appropriate physical activity; ie, they involve large muscle groups in dynamic movement for periods of 20 minutes or longer, 3 or more days of the week, requiring 60% or more of an individual's cardiorespiratory capacity.[4,5] The incidence of radiographically demonstrated OA of the hips and knees of former elite tennis players has been explored,[33] but because of a small sample size and the combination of these data with a broader cohort, of runners, the findings for the tennis players need to be viewed with caution, and only a larger, preferably prospective, cohort study would provide the appropriate information on whether playing tennis is itself a factor in the subsequent onset of OA. In a study[34] that compared runners and swimmers, no increase in OA prevalence was detected in either group. No studies, to date, have looked prospectively at cycling, walking, or aerobics as possible determinants of lower extremity joint disorders. By comparison, much more has been done to explore the development of OA in distance runners, and it is, therefore, this population that provides the model for further discussion.

Running and Arthritis

Various musculoskeletal conditions are thought to be directly or indirectly related to running.[5,35–39] While most studies have examined associations with soft tissue injuries, some reports have focused specifically on joint problems.

When scrutinizing any literature, it is important to examine strength of association according to accepted paradigms. While it is well recognized that conducting an experiment, or *randomized controlled trial* (RCT), is the most powerful way to determine whether exposure to a potential risk factor results in an increased incidence of disease, it is nonetheless accepted that the effects of most risk factors for humans cannot be explored with this study design.[40] Though less robust than RCTs, observational study designs, either *cohort studies* or *case-control studies,* have been used to determine risk. Of the two, the prospective cohort is considered the stronger study design. A review by Walter and Hart[41] provides further information on the relative strengths and weaknesses of various study designs, particularly with reference to the sports medicine literature. For purposes of determining a relationship between running and OA, only satisfactorily designed cohort and case-control studies have been selected.

Research Showing No Association Between Running and Osteoarthritis

In a study by Panush et al,[12] the clinical and radiographic profiles of 17 male distance runners were compared with those of 18 nonrunners matched for height and weight. The identified group of runners had run a mean of 28 miles per week for 12 years. There were no significant difference between the two groups for all of the variables assessed. These observations suggested that runners who train over relatively long distances for extended periods are not at increased risk for premature development of OA of the lower extremities.[43,44]

In January 1984, investigators at the Stanford Arthritis Center began a prospective 5-year longitudinal study that examined the effect of running on bone density and the later development of OA. Distance runners, who had exercised for an average of 224 minutes per week over a mean of 8.5 years, and matched controls, aged 50 to 72 years, participated in the study.[45–47] Radiographs of 41 runners and nonrunners assessed at baseline demonstrated that female runners, but not their male counterparts, had somewhat more sclerosis and spur formation on their spine and weight-bearing knee films but not on hand

films. There were no differences between the groups in joint space narrowing, crepitation, joint stability, or symptomatic OA.[45]

When 34 of these matched pairs were reevaluated 2 years later, almost all the runners and control subjects were found to have statistically significant within-group progression of radiographic scores. The largest average increase was in spur progression in the female matched control group.[46] Thirty-three runners and their matched controls were assessed at the 5-year termination of this study. There was radiologic progression of OA of the knees, hands, and lumbar spine in all subjects but no demonstrable difference in the extent of OA changes in the two groups. With aging, OA of the hands developed in 13% of all subjects and OA of the knees in 12%.[47]

In studies by Puranen et al,[48] radiographic data for the hips demonstrated no appreciable differences between runners and controls. Sohn and Micheli[34] compared the incidence of OA in runners and swimmers and were unable to detect any added risk for OA in the runners. Also, Konradsen et al[49] reported no association between running and lower extremity OA in a group of Danish runners who had continued to run over a period of 40 years.

In addition to these studies, there is some literature that suggests that running should *not* be dismissed as a possible precipitant of accelerated OA in later life.

Research Showing a Positive Association Between Running and Osteoarthritis

In a study by Marti et al[50] the hip radiographs of 27 former elite distance runners were compared with radiographs of nine former bobsledders and 23 control subjects. All participants had been assessed in 1973 as part of a study on athletic training practices, and all were reevaluated in 1988. Results of this investigation showed that an additive radiologic index of hip disease, based on grades of subchondral sclerosis, osteophyte formation, and joint space narrowing, was significantly increased among runners compared with the bobsledders and untrained controls. In multivariate analyses, age and mileage run emerged as independent, significant, and positive predictors of radiologic signs of hip OA. Among runners alone, running pace in 1973 rather than mileage run, was considered the stronger predictor of subsequent joint degeneration.

In a study by Kujala et al,[51] hospital admissions with OA of the hips, knees, or ankles were recorded for male athletes who had represented Finland in selected sports between 1920 and 1965. When compared with healthy, nonathletic controls, the athletes were at a slightly higher risk of requiring hospitalization because of demonstrated lower extremity OA. Compared with participants in mixed sports and power sports, eg, boxing, wrestling, weight lifting, and throwing, endurance athletes, eg, distance runners and cross-country skiers, required hospital-based care at an older age.

Spector et al[33] explored the risk of OA of the hips and knees in female distance runners who had competed at a national or international level between 1950 and 1979. Compared with age-matched controls, the former athletes had greater rates of radiologically demonstrated OA at all sites.

Conclusions

Given the inherent differences in the populations studied, the varying strengths of the study designs, the relatively small numbers of some of the individual study samples, inconsistencies in the measurement of the radiologic and clinical outcome measures, and a host of confounding variables that may have been incompletely accounted for in some of the studies, it is difficult, based on the literature, to determine with any conclusiveness whether running is or is not a significant risk factor for lower extremity OA. However, the balance of available evidence does support the contention that running is likely **not** a significant factor in promoting the development of OA in later life.

When seeking consensus in studies on running, certain other important issues also need to be recognized. For example, while there is an assumption that running may affect normal joints, it still remains unclear whether joint incongruities might be precipitated by repetitive foot strikes on hard surfaces, thereby traumatizing the joints and predisposing them to degenerative changes.

A further potential bias that needs to be considered relates to the selection of those who choose to run. It has been conjectured that a sizeable number of runners quit after a short

time because of joint pain. This may indicate early arthritis or a propensity for it, and, if so, those who are able to continue may already represent a population that is less prone to joint problems.

Other Sports and Arthritis

In addition to the studies on running, several published reports have explored the possible association between other sports activities and subsequent development of OA. However, because this literature is, in general, smaller and less methodologically rigorous than that available to explore the relation between running and arthritis, criteria for study selection have been pragmatically loosened to permit the inclusion of case series designs.

In two separate studies that compared radiologic changes of the knee[52] and hip[53] in elite and recreational soccer players and a group of age-matched controls, a higher rate of OA was found in the elite players, with no demonstrable differences between the nonelite and control groups. In contrast, Adams[54] found only a low incidence (3%) of clinically and radiologically demonstrated OA of the knees in a group of former professional soccer players. Degenerative changes of the hips, knees, ankles, and cervical spine have also been reported in soccer players.[55,56]

An increased incidence of OA affecting the ankle, knee, feet, and spine has been reported in football players.[57–62] Vincellete et al[58] suggest that linemen, possibly because of their weight, are at greatest risk for joint damage and subsequent arthritis. Rugby players may also be at increased risk for knee changes.[63]

Ballet dancers may have an increased incidence of OA involving the cervical spine, the hips, knees, talar joints, and metatarsophalangeal articulations of the feet.[57,64–67]

In baseball, OA of the elbow and shoulder may occur with greater frequency[68–70]; in cricket, changes in the fingers have been observed[71]; and in gymnastics, elbow, shoulder, and wrist lesions have been demonstrated.[72] Downhill skiers may be at increased risk for OA of the finger joints.[73]

One study has suggested that Lacrosse players may have an increased incidence of degenerative changes in their ankles and knees,[74] and parachutists are possibly at increased risk for ankle, knee, and spine lesions.[75]

In a critical appraisal of the literature that purports to examine the linkage between OA and each of these sports activities, some important methodologic pitfalls need to be recognized:

1. These studies span a lengthy time frame, from 1941 to 1994, with the majority reported before 1980. In many of the earlier studies, criteria for the clinical and radiologic definition of OA are not clearly stated, and terms such as "osteoarthrosis" or even "joint abnormality" are used to describe underlying degenerative changes. Comparisons both within and between studies were, therefore, much less robust than might be acceptable in current practice, where standard criteria have been recommended, particularly for OA of the hands, hips, and knees.[76]

2. One of the key issues in determining risk factors for OA relates to the question of whether changes have occurred with or without joint trauma. However, in many of the studies reported, this important issue has been incompletely addressed. Nonetheless, it would seem to be intuitively obvious that in contact or collision sports, eg, football, rugby, and martial arts, or "single-impact loading" activities, eg, parachuting, joint trauma is likely a precursor to OA in later life. Also, "repetitive loading" of specific joints, eg, in soccer, weight lifting, and ballet, is likely a precipitant for joint damage that may predispose to OA over time.

3. In several reports, conclusions were based on relatively weak study designs such as case series.[41] Moreover, in many instances in which control populations were included, insufficient information was provided to determine whether the respective study and control groups were satisfactorily identified and matched, thus raising the possibility of selection biases. Also, denominator-based data, when available, were often incompletely presented.

4. Factors such as intensity and duration of exercise, length of follow-up, and identification of confounding variables were often incompletely reported in the published studies.

DOES EXERCISE HAVE A ROLE IN MANAGEMENT OF ARTHRITIS?

The role of exercise in the comprehensive management of arthritis has evoked considerable debate. Some have advised against physical activity on the grounds that vigorous motion to an arthritic joint may damage delicate periarticular tissue.[77] For such practitioners, rest was prescribed as the preferred alternative. What has become increasingly evident, however, is that prolonged inactivity tends to add measurably to the problems of pain, stiffness, loss of motion, weakness, functional limitation, and disability.[77]

To explore the effects of therapeutic exercise in the management of arthritis, a selection of the literature that again meets the methodologic criteria outlined in Chapter 1 is used. However, as a further stage in the process, the *quality* of the accumulated evidence is graded according to a recognized framework (Table 6–1). Within this framework, grade I evidence reflects the conclusions of at least one properly designed RCT, and grade II and III ratings indicate descending strengths of study design. Isolated case reports are not included in the overview. Although exercise has been recommended for a spectrum of rheumatic diseases, this discussion focuses only on OA and inflammatory (rheumatoid) arthritis (RA). For a further scientific overview that includes the role of exercise in arthritis, readers are referred to Puett and Giffin.[78]

TABLE 6–1. Categories for Quality of Evidence on Which Treatment Recommendations Are Made

GRADE	DEFINITION
I	Evidence from at least one properly randomized, controlled trial
II	Evidence from at least one well-designed clinical trial without randomization, from cohort or case-controlled analytic studies, preferably from more than one center, from multiple time series, or from dramatic results in uncontrolled experiments
III	Evidence from opinions of respected authorities on the basis of clinical experience, descriptive studies, or reports of expert committees

From Hart LE: Arthritis. In Basmajian JV, Banerjee SN (eds): Clinical Decision Making in Rehabilitation: Efficacy and Outcomes. Churchill Livingstone, New York, 1996, p. 203

The goals of an integrated exercise program are to increase muscle strength and joint range of motion, improve stamina and general fitness, and provide patients with a sense of well-being and enhanced psychosocial function.[79–81] In general, exercise routines can be categorized as passive, active, or active-assisted. Active exercise is further classified as isotonic, isometric, or isokinetic. A usual regimen is customized to a patient's needs and includes combinations of different types of exercises, performed either on land or in an aquatic medium (hydrotherapy). Stretching routines and recreational activity are also emphasized in such programs.[82]

Ytterberg et al[83] alluded to some of the potential pitfalls in the methodology and interpretation of the existing literature on exercise for arthritis. Despite their concerns, however, an emerging body of knowledge, based on credible grade I evidence, attests to the efficacy of therapeutic exercise in both RA and OA.

A low-intensity aerobic exercise protocol (three times a week for 12 weeks) was effective in patients with RA.[84] Subjects enrolled in the exercise arm demonstrated improvements in activities of daily living and reduced joint pain and fatigue, compared with those in the nonexercising control group. Improvements in activities of daily living were also shown in a long-term follow-up of 23 patients with RA who were enrolled in a home-based aerobic exercise program.[85] Although this Scandinavian study met the requirements of an RCT and reported a positive outcome, results may not be generalizable to a North American population because of some apparent differences in management style and patient assessment. Minor et al[86] demonstrated the efficacy of physical conditioning exercises in patients with either RA or OA compared with controls. Both aquatic and walking exercise improved aerobic capacity, 50-foot walking time, depression, anxiety, and physical activity (following a 12-week protocol). In patients with OA, a supervised walking program for 8 weeks was effective.[87]

Rogind et al[88] have demonstrated that a physical training program improves walking speed and quadriceps muscle strength in patients with OA.

Two RCTs have provided grade I recommendations for the use of exercise programs in improving the grip strength of patients with RA of the hands.[89,90]

Grade II and III evidence exists to support the use of the following:

- Dynamic rather than static training techniques in RA affecting lower extremity joints[91]
- Physical training in an elderly population of patients with RA receiving corticosteroid treatment[92]
- Isokinetic knee extension training in RA[93]
- Evening exercise to reduce morning stiffness in patients with RA[94]
- Muscle strengthening to improve the exercise capacity and aerobic fitness in patients with OA[95]
- Passive muscle stretching to increase abduction in OA of the hip[96]
- A quantitative progressive rehabilitative program to increase muscle strength and endurance in patients with knee OA[97]
- A customized range of motion dance program to increase joint range in patients with RA[98]
- A structured exercise program to improve quadriceps strength, and thereby reduce sensorimotor dysfunction, in patients with OA of the knee[99]
- An aerobic or resistance exercise program to improve physical performance, reduce pain, and improve measures of disability in older disabled persons with OA of the knee[100]
- Exercise therapy to reduce pain and disability in patients with OA of the hip or knee[101]

In addition to land-based exercise programs, exercise routines in water are widely advocated for management of rheumatic conditions. It is generally acknowledged that hydrotherapy provides the patient with an opportunity to perform movements in a medium that not only provides buoyancy but also allows movement with much less effort so that seriously weakened limbs may be moved and exercised in a manner not possible without support.[82,102,103]

Several studies have provided grade II and III evidence that support hydrotherapy protocols of various sorts in the overall management of RA.[104–107] However, these need to be appraised together with at least two other reports that shed some doubt on the effectiveness of this intervention. Green et al[108] demonstrated that a home exercise program is as effective as hydrotherapy for OA of the hips, and a study by Hart et al[109] did not detect any significant differences in outcome between patients with RA who were enrolled in a structured pool exercise program and an age-matched control group that did not receive hydrotherapy. These studies provided grade I and II evidence, respectively.

Conclusions

Based on the strength of evidence in the available literature, there is an emerging consensus that land-based exercise not only is a useful adjunct but also should be considered an essential component in the management of OA and RA. In particular, aerobic conditioning exercises have been endorsed by the American College of Rheumatology as important components in the nonpharmacologic treatment of OA of the hips[110] and knees.[111]

Relatively few studies, using variable methods, have explored the use of hydrotherapy in the routine management of OA and RA. Their conclusions differ, and, therefore, until further evidence is forthcoming, it is not possible to make any definitive recommendations on the value of this intervention.

SUMMARY

Physical activity is recognized as an integral component of a healthy lifestyle. However, while the benefits of regular exercise have been well accepted, there is a growing realization that the potential advantages of exercise often need to be weighed against possible adverse effects, particularly on the musculoskeletal system.

This chapter has explored the possible association between sustained physical activities of various sorts and the subsequent onset or acceleration of OA. For most of the sports that have been scrutinized to date, evidence is quantitatively and methodologically insufficient to arrive at definitive conclusions. Running is the notable exception, and the balance of available evidence tends to indicate that this activity does not trigger OA in apparently normal joints. Nonetheless, even the running literature includes studies that plausibly challenge this view.

A clearer picture emerges with regard to the use of exercise as a therapeutic intervention in the management of arthritis. Although the results of hydrotherapy have been mixed, a sizeable literature demonstrates the effectiveness of land-based exercises for patients with both RA and OA.

REFERENCES

1. Lane NE, Buckwalter JA: Exercise: a cause of osteoarthritis? Rheum Dis Clin North Am 19: 617, 1993
2. Paffenbarger RS Jr, Hyde RT, Wing AL, et al: Some interrelations of physical activity, physiological fitness, health, and longevity. In: Bouchard C, Shephard RJ, Stephens T (eds): Physical Activity, Fitness, and Health. Human Kinetics, Champaign, Ill, 1994, p. 119
3. Pate RR, Pratt M, Blair SN, et al: Physical activity and public health: a recommendation from the Centers for Disease Control and Prevention and the American College of Sports Medicine. JAMA 273:402, 1995
4. Koplan JP, Siscovick DS, Goldbaum GM: The risks of exercise: a public health view of injuries and hazards. Pub Health Rep 100:189, 1985
5. Hart LE: Exercise and soft tissue injury. Bailliere Clin Rheumatol 8:137, 1994
6. Hochberg MC: Clinical features and treatment. In: Klippel JH (ed): Primer on the Rheumatic Diseases, 11th Ed. Arthritis Foundation, Atlanta, 1997, p. 218
7. Peyron JG: Epidemiologic and etiologic approach of osteoarthritis. Semin Arthritis Rheum 8:288, 1979
8. Radin EL, Burr DB, Caterson DF, et al: Mechanical determinants of osteoarthritis. Semin Arthritis Rheum 21(suppl 2):12, 1991
9. Mankin HJ: The reaction of articular cartilage to injury and osteoarthritis. N Engl J Med 291:1285, 1335, 1974
10. Roos H, Lauren M, Adalberth T, et al: Knee osteoarthritis after meniscectomy. Arthritis Rheum 41:687, 1998
11. Appel H: Late results after meniscectomy in the knee joint. Acta Orthop Scand Suppl 133:1, 1970
12. Brown AR, Rose BS: Familiar precocious polyarticular osteoarthritis of chondroplastic type. N Z Med J 65:449, 1966
13. Charnely RK: Late joint changes as a result of internal derangement of the knee. Am J Surg 76:496, 1948
14. Dandy DJ, Jackson RW: The diagnosis of problems after meniscectomy. J Bone Joint Surg (Br) 57:349, 1975

15. Fairbank TJ: Knee joint changes after meniscectomy. J Bone Joint Surg (Br) 30:644, 1948
16. Gear MWL: The late results of meniscectomy. Br J Surg 54:270, 1967
17. Jackson JP: Degenerative changes in the knee after meniscectomy. BMJ 2:525, 1968
18. Jones RE, Smith EC, Reisch JS: Effects of medical meniscectomy in patients older than forty years. J Bone Joint Surg (Am) 50:73, 1978
19. Kirk JA, Ansel BM, Bywater EGL: The hypermobility syndrome. Ann Rheum Dis 26:419, 1967
20. O'Donohue DH, Frank GH, Jeter GL, et al: Repair and reconstruction of the anterior cruciate ligament in dogs: factors influencing long-term results. J Bone Joint Surg (Am) 53:710, 1971
21. Tapper EM, Hoover NW: Late results after meniscectomy. J Bone Joint Surg (Am) 51:517, 1969
22. Smith EL, Smith KA, Gilligan C: Exercise, fitness, osteoarthritis, and osteoporosis. In: Bouchard C, Shephard RJ, Stephens T, et al (eds): Exercise, Fitness, and Health: A Consensus of Current Knowledge. Human Kinetics, Champaign, Ill, 1990, p. 517
23. Hadler NM: Industrial rheumatology. Arthritis Rheum 20:1019, 1977
24. Dorr LD: Arthritis and athletics. Clin Sports Med 10:343, 1991
25. Ettinger WH Jr: Physical activity, arthritis, and disability in older people. Clin Ger Med 14: 633, 1998
26. McKeag DB: The relationship of osteoarthritis and exercise. Clin Sports Med 11:471, 1992
27. Murray RO, Duncan C: Athletic activity in adolescence as an etiological factor in degenerative hip disease. J Bone Joint Surg (Br) 53:406, 1971
28. Scott JC, Hochberg MC: Osteoarthritis. I: Epidemiology. MD State Med J 33:712, 1984
29. Hoaglund FT, Yau AC, Wong WL: Osteoarthritis of the hip and other joints in southern Chinese in Hong Kong. J Bone Joint Surg (Am) 55:545, 1973
30. Blumberg BS: A study of the prevalence of arthritis in Alaskan Eskimos. Arthritis Rheum 4:325, 1961
31. Lawrence JS, Degraaf R, Laine VAI: Degenerative joint disease in random samples and occupational groups. In: Keligren JH, Jeffrey MR, Ball J (eds): The Epidemiology of Chronic Rheumatism. Blackwell, Oxford, 1963, p. 212
32. Kellgren JH: Osteoarthrosis in patients and populations. BMJ 2:1, 1961
33. Spector TD, Harris PA, Hart DJ, et al: Risk of osteoarthritis associated with long-term weight-bearing sports. Arthritis Rheum 39:988, 1996
34. Sohn RS, Micheli LJ: The effect of running on the pathogenesis of osteoarthritis of the hips and knees. Clin Orthop Rel Res 198:106, 1985
35. Walter SD, Hart LE, Sutton JR, et al: Training habits and injury experiences in distance runners: age- and sex-related factors. Physician Sports Med 16:101, 1988
36. Walter SD, Hart LE, McIntosh JM, et al: The Ontario cohort study of running-related injuries. Arch Intern Med 149:2561, 1989
37. Marti B, Vader JP, Minder CE, Abelin T: On the epidemiology of running injuries: the 1984 Bern Grand-Prix study. Am J Sports Med 16:285, 1988
38. Koplan JP, Powell KE, Sikes RK, et al: An epidemiologic study of the benefits and risks of running. JAMA 248:3118, 1982
39. Macera CA, Pate RR, Powell KE, et al: Predicting lower extremity injuries among habitual runners. Arch Intern Med 149:2565, 1989
40. Fletcher RH, Fletcher SW, Wagner EH (eds): Clinical Epidemiology: The Essentials, 3rd Ed. Williams & Wilkins, Baltimore, Md, 1996
41. Walter SD, Hart LE: Application of epidemiological methodology to sports and exercise science research. Exerc Sport Sci Rev 18:417, 1990
42. Panush RS, Schmidt C, Caldwell JR, et al: Is running associated with degenerative joint disease? JAMA 255:1152, 1986
43. Panush RS, Lane NE: Exercise and the musculoskeletal system. Bailliere Clin Rheumatol 8:79, 1994
44. Panush RS: Does exercise cause arthritis? Long-term consequences of exercise on the musculoskeletal system. Rheum Dis Clin North Am 16:827, 1990
45. Lane NE, Bloch DA, Jones HH, et al: Long-distance running, bone density, and osteoarthritis. JAMA 255:1147, 1986
46. Lane NE, Bloch DA, Hubert HB, et al: Running, osteoarthritis and bone density: initial 2-year longitudinal study. Am J Med 88:452, 1990
47. Lane NE, Michel B, Bjorkengren A, et al: The risk of osteoarthritis with running and aging: a 5-year longitudinal study. J Rheumatol 20: 461, 1993
48. Puranen J, Ala-Ketola L, Peltokalleo P, Saarela J: Running and primary osteoarthritis of the hip. BMJ 1:424, 1975
49. Konradsen L, Hansen EB, Sondergaard L: Long distance running and osteoarthrosis. Am J Sports Med 18:379, 1990
50. Marti B, Knobloch M, Tschopp A, et al: Is excessive running predictive of degenerative hip disease? controlled study of former elite athletes. BMJ 299:91, 1989
51. Kujala UM, Kaprio J, Sarna S: Osteoarthritis of weight bearing joints of lower limbs in former elite male athletes. BMJ 308:231, 1994

52. Roos H, Lindberg H, Gardsell P, et al: The prevalence of gonarthrosis and its relation to meniscectomy in former soccer players. Am J Sports Med 22:219, 1994

53. Lindberg H, Roos H, Gardsell P: Prevalence of coxarthrosis in former soccer players: 286 players compared with matched controls. Acta Orthop Scand 64:165, 1993

54. Adams ID: Osteoarthrosis and sport. Clin Rheum Dis 2:523, 1976

55. Sortland O, Tysvaer AT, Storli OV: Changes in the cervical spine in association football players. Br J Sport Med 16:80, 1982

56. Klunder KB, Rud B, Hansen J: Osteoarthritis of the hip and knee joints in retired football players. Acta Orthop Scand 51:925, 1980

57. Brodelius A: Osteoarthritis of the talar joints in footballers and ballet dancers. Acta Orthop Scand 30:309, 1961

58. Vincelette P, Laurin CA, Levesque HP: The footballer's ankle and foot. Can Med Assoc J 107:872, 1972

59. Rall KL, McElroy GL, Keats TE: A study of the long term effects of football injury to the knee. Missouri Med 61:435, 1964

60. Ferguson RJ, McMaster JH, Stanitski CL: Low back pain in college football linemen. J Sports Med 2:63, 1975

61. Albright JP, Moses JM, Feldick HG, et al: Nonfatal cervical spine injuries in interscholastic football. JAMA 13:1243, 1976

62. Moretz JA, Harlan SD, Goodrich J, Walters R: Long-term follow-up of knee injuries in high school football players. Am J Sport Med 12:298, 1984

63. Slocum DB: Overuse syndrome of the lower leg and foot in athletes. Instructor's Lecture at American Academy of Orthopedic Surgery. 17:359, 1960

64. Ambre T, Nilsson BE: Degenerative changes in the first metatarso-phalangeal joint of ballet dancers. Acta Orthop Scand 49:317, 1978

65. Miller EH, Schneider HJ, Bronson JL, McLain D: A new consideration in athletic injuries: the classical ballet dancer. Clin Orthop Rel Res 3:181, 1975

66. Ende LS, Wickstrom J: Ballet injuries. Physician Sport Med 10:101, 1982

67. Washington EL: Musculoskeletal injuries in theatrical dancers: site, frequency and severity. Am J Sport Med 2:75, 1978

68. Adams JE. Injury to the throwing arm: a study of traumatic changes in the elbow joints of boy baseball players. California Med 102:127, 1965

69. Hansen NM: Epiphyseal changes in the proximal humerus of an adolescent baseball pitcher. Am J Sport Med 10:380, 1982

70. Bennett GE: Shoulder and elbow lesions of the professional baseball pitcher. JAMA 117:510, 1941

71. Vere Hodge N: Chronic injury: cricket. In: Larson LA (ed): Encyclopedia of Sports Sciences and Medicine. Macmillan, New York, 1971, p. 605

72. Bozdech A: Chronic injury: gymnastics. In: Larson LA (ed): Encyclopedia of Sports Sciences and Medicine. Macmillan, New York, 1971, p. 616

73. Gerber C, Senn E, Matter P: Skier's thumb: surgical treatment of recent injuries to the ulnar collateral ligament of the thumb's metacarpophalangeal joint. Am J Sport Med 9:171, 1981

74. Thomas RB: Chronic injury: lacrosse. In: Larson LA (ed): Encyclopedia of Sports Sciences and Medicine. Macmillan, New York, 1971, p. 621

75. Murray-Leslie CF, Lintott DJ, Wright V: The knees, ankles, and spine in sport and veteran military parachutists. Ann Rheum Dis 36:327, 1977

76. Klippel JH (ed): Primer on the Rheumatic Diseases, 11th Ed. Arthritis Foundation, Atlanta, Ga, 1997, p. 464

77. Minor MA, Lane NE: Recreational exercise in arthritis. Rheum Dis Clin North Am 22:563, 1996

78. Puett DW, Griffin MR: Published trials of nonmedical and noninvasive therapies for hip and knee osteoarthritis. Ann Intern Med 121:133, 1994

79. Schnitzer TJ: Management of osteoarthritis. In: McCarty DJ, Koopman WJ (eds): Arthritis and Allied Conditions, 12th Ed. Lea & Febiger, Philadelphia, 1993, p. 1761

80. Basmajian JV: Therapeutic exercise in the management of rheumatic diseases. J Rheumatol 14(suppl 15):22, 1987

81. Hicks JE, Nicholas JJ, Swezey RL (eds): Handbook of Rehabilitative Rheumatology. American Rheumatism Association, Atlanta, Ga, 1988

82. Hart LE: Arthritis. In: Basmajian JV, Banerjee SN (eds): Clinical Decision Making in Rehabilitation: Efficacy and Outcomes. Churchill Livingstone, New York, 1996, p. 203

83. Ytterberg SR, Mahowald ML, Krug HE: Exercise for arthritis. Bailliere Clin Rheumatol 8:161, 1994

84. Harkcom TM, Lampman RM, Banwell BF, Castor CW: Therapeutic value of graded aerobic exercise training in rheumatoid arthritis. Arthritis Rheum 28:32, 1985

85. Nordemar R: Physical training in rheumatoid arthritis: a controlled long-term study. Scand J Rheumatol 10:25, 1981

86. Minor MA, Hewett JE, Webel RR, et al: Efficacy of physical conditioning exercise in patients with rheumatoid arthritis. Arthritis Rheum 32:1396, 1989

87. Kovar PA, Allegrante JP, MacKenzie CR, et al: Supervised fitness walking in patients with osteoarthritis of the knee: a randomized, controlled trial. Ann Intern Med 116:529, 1992

88. Rogind H, Bibow-Nielsen B, Jensen B, et al: The effects of a physical training program on patients with osteoarthritis of the knees. Arch Phys Med Rehabil 79:1421, 1998

89. Brighton SW, Lubbe JE, van der Merwe CA: The effect of long-term exercise programme on the rheumatoid hand. Br J Rheumatol 32:392, 1993

90. Hoenig H, Groff G, Pratt K, et al: A randomized controlled trial of home exercise on the rheumatoid hand. J Rheumatol 20:785, 1993

91. Ekdahl C, Andersson SI, Moritz U, et al: Dynamic versus static training in patients with rheumatoid arthritis. Scand J Rheumatol 19:17, 1990

92. Lyngberg KK, Harreby M, Bentzen H, et al: Elderly rheumatoid arthritis patients on steroid treatment tolerate physical training without an increase in disease activity. Arch Phys Med Rehabil 75:1189, 1994

93. Lyngberg KK, Ramsing BU, Nawrocki A, et al: Safe and effective isokinetic knee extension training in rheumatoid arthritis. Arthritis Rheum 37:623, 1994

94. Byers PH: Effect of exercise on morning stiffness and mobility in patients with rheumatoid arthritis. Res Nurs Health 8:275, 1985

95. Fisher NM, Pendergast DR: Effects of a muscle exercise program on exercise capacity in subjects with osteoarthritis. Arch Phys Med Rehabil 75:792, 1994

96. Leivseth G, Torstensson J, Reikeras O: Effect of passive muscle stretching in osteoarthritis of the hip. Clin Sci 76:113, 1989

97. Fisher NM, Gresham G, Pendergast DR: Effects of quantitative progressive rehabilitation program applied unilaterally to the osteoarthritic knee. Arch Phys Med Rehabil 74:1319, 1993

98. Van Deusen J, Harlowe D: The efficacy of the ROM dance program for adults with rheumatoid arthritis. Am J Occup Ther 41:90, 1987

99. Hurley MV, Scott DL: Improvements in quadriceps sensorimotor function and disability of patients with knee osteoarthritis following a clinically practicable exercise regime. Br J Rheumatol 37:1181, 1998

100. Ettinger WH Jr, Burns R, Messier SP, et al: A randomized trial comparing aerobic exercise and resistance exercise with a health education program in older adults with knee osteoarthritis: the fitness arthritis and seniors trial (FAST). JAMA 277:25, 1997

101. Van Baar JE, Dekker J, Oostendorp RAB, et al: The effectiveness of exercise therapy in patients with osteoarthritis of the hip or knee: a randomized clinical trial. J Rheumatol 25:2432, 1998

102. Banwell BF: Physical therapy in arthritis management. In: Ehrlich GE (ed): Rehabilitation Management of Rheumatic Conditions. Williams & Wilkins, Baltimore, Md, 1986, p. 264

103. Duffield MH: Exercise in Water. Balliere Tindall, Cassell, London, 1969

104. Goldby LJ, Scott DL: The way forward for hydrotherapy. Br J Rheumatol 32:771, 1993

105. Damneskiold-Samsoe B, Lyngberg K, Risum T, et al: The effect of water exercise therapy given to patients with rheumatoid arthritis. Scand J Rehabil Med 19:31,1987

106. Dial C, Windsor RA: A formative evaluation of a health education–water exercise program for class II and class III adult rheumatoid arthritis patients. Patient Educ Couns 7:33, 1985

107. Langridge JC, Phillips D: Group hydrotherapy exercises for chronic back pain sufferers: introduction and monitoring. Physiotherapy 74:269, 1988

108. Green J, McKenna F, Redfern EF, Chamberlain MA: Home exercises are as effective as outpatient hydrotherapy for osteoarthritis of the hip. Br J Rheumatol 32:812, 1993

109. Hart LE, Goldsmith CH, Churchill ER, et al: A randomized controlled trial to assess hydrotherapy in the management of patients with rheumatoid arthritis. Arthritis Rheum 37(suppl):416, 1994

110. Hochberg MC, Altman RD, Brandt KD, et al: Guidelines for the medical management of osteoarthritis, Part I: Osteoarthritis of the hip. Arthritis Rheum 38:1535, 1995

111. Hochberg MC, Altman RD, Brandt KD, et al: Guidelines for the medical management of osteoarthritis, Part II: Osteoarthritis of the knee. Arthritis Rheum 38:1541, 1995

CHAPTER

7

Psychological and Sociologic Factors in Sport

LARRY M. LEITH

Few observers would argue that athletic performance is becoming increasingly more skilled, complex, and physical. Athletes are faster, stronger, and more technically advanced, and in many cases they are even more tempermental. In response, sports physicians and other allied health professionals who assess and treat sports injuries are being forced to meet new challenges and adapt to the ever-changing nature of sports.

Success at elite levels of sport may be 10% to 20% physiologic and 80% to 90% psychological.[1] This observation places a tremendous onus on athletes and coaches to completely master mental training techniques. It also suggests that practitioners of sports medicine would be well-advised to consider the psychological and sociologic aspects of sports injuries along with the obvious clinical trauma. For example, research within the general population[2] and the athletic population[3-8] reveals that certain specific psychological factors may predispose some individuals to injury and reinjury. In addition, certain situational aspects are likely to play a major role.

This chapter considers some of the psychological and sociologic factors that have the potential to affect sports medicine rehabilitation. Because of its planned eclectic nature, it is not practical to categorize the studies in terms of "level of research" for each subsection. For this reason, only research that can be categorized as level I and level II is cited. Exceptions are identified and classified within the text.

Some of the problematic psychological and sociologic factors that interact with the more traditional causes of sports injuries are examined, specifically, pregame anxiety and nonpharmacologic methods of management; self-perception and personality development; motivation and performance promotion; violence and aggression and their consequences; and leadership in the sport environment.

PREGAME ANXIETY AND NONPHARMACOLOGIC MANAGEMENT

One of the factors that has repeatedly been found to significantly influence the quality of the athletic experience is the level of state anxiety during the time leading up to the competition. This concept is referred to as *precompetitive anxiety*. Several researchers have studied the temporal changes in state anxiety as the time-to-event approaches. One well-controlled study measured precompetition anxiety in collegiate wrestlers 1 week, 48 hours, 24 hours, 2 hours, and 20 minutes before actual competition.[9] Similar time-to-event research has been conducted by other researchers in a variety of sports.[10-13] While some of their results differed in specifics, general findings are consistent.

First, these studies pointed out the importance of differentiating between *cognitive state anxiety* and *somatic state anxiety*. Cognitive state anxiety can be viewed as the mental component of state anxiety and is caused by fear of negative evaluation and threat to self-esteem. Somatic state anxiety, on the other hand, is the physiologic and affective aspects of anxiety and is directly related to physiologic arousal.[12,14]

Second, research indicates that precompetitive cognitive anxiety is relatively high and remains high and stable as the time-to-event approaches. Conversely, somatic state anxiety is relatively low and remains low until approximately 24 hours before the event and then increases rapidly as game time approaches. Once the performance begins, somatic anxiety dissipates rapidly,[12,15] whereas cognitive state anxiety fluctuates throughout the contest as the probability of success or failure changes.[16] Therefore, high cognitive state anxiety is believed to be a major psychological contributor to performance error. Of special interest to the practitioner is a study I made[17] which found that simply talking about "choking" has the effect of hindering actual performance, probably by increasing cognitive state anxiety. Conversely, somatic anxiety can be viewed as an indicator of readiness in the athlete. Since it dissipates rapidly, it is not believed to have a negative effect on athletic performance. For this reason, the sports practitioner should be concerned with techniques of managing cognitive state anxiety. Some of the more popular management techniques that have evolved from level I and level II research are discussed.

Decision-Making Recommendations

The following recommendations include only grade A (supported by at least one, and preferably more, level I randomized trials) and grade B (supported by at least one level II randomized trial) classifications.

The *Competitive State Anxiety Inventory*—2[18] appears to be the best psychological instrument for assessing multidimensional anxiety in the sports setting. It is sport specific and adequately measures cognitive and state anxiety.[19,20]

In terms of pregame anxiety management, the practitioner has the option of considering several workable strategies, including *active coping strategies, progressive relaxation, meditation,* and *stress management training*. A brief overview of each follows. In deciding which technique is best, it is advisable to find the one the athlete is most comfortable with.

Active Coping Strategies

In conducting research with athletes from a variety of sports and competition levels, sport scientists[21–23] have identified the strategies used by athletes to manage anxiety. One of the commonest techniques used was active coping strategies. Rathus and Nevid[24] state that active coping strategies are preferred because they reflect attempts to alter or remove the stressor, thereby reducing or eliminating its effect. Self-statements such as "I knew what I had to do, so I doubled my efforts to make things work" reflect an active coping approach to anxiety management. In contrast, passive coping strategies, such as wishful thinking and daydreaming, are least effective.[20]

Progressive Relaxation

Progressive relaxation, a technique originally developed by Jacobsen,[25,26] involves the systematic tension and relaxation of muscle groups in an attempt to reduce anxiety. In this procedure, athletes are asked to lie or sit in a comfortable position. The environment is kept quiet and free of distractions while the athlete inhales and tenses a specific muscle group for approximately 5 seconds, then exhales and releases the tension while concentrating on the "feeling" of relaxation. This procedure is repeated for several different muscle groups. Using progressive relaxation for the entire body can be a lengthy process, lasting up to an hour. After a few weeks of practice, however, the athlete is usually able to tense and relax several muscle groups simultaneously, thereby shortening the time needed to complete the procedure. Several studies have documented the performance benefits of progressive relaxation.[27–29]

Meditation

Meditation, a relaxation training technique that has been used for thousands of years, involves the use of mental focus to calm the body.[30] Although there are many different forms of meditation,[31] most share several features. When meditating, individuals usually sit in a comfortable position in a quiet and dark environment, breathing slowly and deeply. The athlete then concentrates on a single stimulus, such as a candle flame or specific mental picture. Some individuals prefer to repeat a certain repetitive sound or word, called a *mantra* (eg, the sound "ohm"). By concentrating on the single stimulus, the athlete attempts to eliminate all thoughts from consciousness, thereby excluding negative thoughts and relaxing the body.

Research has documented the beneficial effects of meditation on athletic performance.[30,32] As a caveat to the practitioner, however, the positive effect of meditation on performance may be limited to activities involving gross motor movements, such as running and weight lifting.[33,34]

Stress Management Training

Stress management training is a comprehensive stress management program that teaches relaxation and control of anxiety. Individuals learn not only about stress in general but also about personal tendencies and reactions to stressors. They learn to recognize situations or events that typically lead to anxiety and learn new coping strategies to handle stress better.

Smith[35] developed a stress management training program for use in sports. The program consists of five phases:

1. **Pretreatment phase.** The pretreatment or assessment phase attempts to identify events that lead to high anxiety and typical ways of handling this anxiety.
2. **Treatment rationale phase.** This is the educational section of the program, in which the athlete learns about anxiety in general, and the most effective ways of handling anxiety.
3. **Skill acquisition phase.** The athlete is trained to cope with stress and anxiety in a positive manner with the help of strategies such as positive self-talk.
4. **Skill rehearsal.** The athlete practices muscle relaxation and cognitive restructuring skills learned in phase three. To be most effective, these skills should be practiced under conditions that approximate the "real life" situations in which they will be used.
5. **Posttreatment evaluation.** This last phase involves analyzing the effectiveness of stress management training on the athlete.

Stress management programs have been successful in lowering anxiety and improving athetic performance.[36,37]

SELF-PERCEPTION AND PERSONALITY DEVELOPMENT

Personality is best defined as "that pattern of characteristic thoughts, feelings, and behaviors that distinguishes one person from another and that persists over time and situations."[38] Currently, most sport psychologists view personality from an *interactional approach*,[39–42] which reflects the fact that athletes bring their own particular personality with them to the athletic environment. For this reason, to fully understand the athlete's behavior, the practitioner must consider the individual's personality, the situation, and the interaction between the two.

Self-Confidence

Almost every practitioner of sport will quickly agree that self-confidence is important to successful athletic performance. As an aid to understanding this important psychological construct, sport psychologists have targeted Bandura's[43,44] *self-efficacy theory*. Self-efficacy is the belief that one can succeed at a particular task.

Unlike other stable personality traits, self-efficacy is situation specific. Bandura[44] believes that feelings of self-efficacy evolve from four sources:

1. **Successful performance.** The first and most important source of self-efficacy is successful performance. As one experiences success, one integrates information about the accomplishment, resulting in the belief that future success is possible or even probable. Conversely, failure has the opposite effect, leading to the expectation of future failure.
2. **Social comparison.** Athletes receive efficacy information vicariously through social comparison. Bandura[44] suggests that when individuals see others succeed at a task, they persuade themselves that if others can do it, they should also be able to achieve at least some improvement in performance.
3. **Comparison.** Another source of self-efficacy is persuasion, as when a coach or parent attempts to convince an athlete that he or she has the ability to succeed at a task.
4. **Emotional arousal.** Athletes also receive efficacy information through emotional arousal. If one experiences a heightened level of arousal prior to an important contest, one may believe the arousal is due to lack of ability, thus lowering expectancy for success.

Proven methods of increasing self-efficacy are examined in the Decision-Making Recommendations discussion.

Personality Profile

Another common sport personality research theme concerns the extent to which the personality profiles of athletes and nonathletes differ. Morgan's[45] literature review concluded that athletes are more stable and extroverted than nonathletes are. An earlier review by Cooper[46] reported that athletes are more competitive, dominant, self-confident, and achievement oriented. Similar findings were reported by Butt and Cox.[47] In addition, athletes have been found to be more psychologically well adjusted[46,48,49] and often display higher levels of self-esteem than nonathletes do.[50–53] Research has also revealed that, compared with nonathletes, athletes hold more conservative political views,[54] are more authoritarian, and demonstrate higher levels of persistence.[55] It is important for the practitioner to note, however, that although differences have been documented with levels I and II research, a clear pattern will not emerge until more research is performed.

Risk of Injury

Recently, sport psychologists have attempted to identify personality traits associated with athletic injury. If successful, this approach would make it possible to predict when an athlete is most susceptible to injury. So far, the personality traits of *vigor,* an inverse relationship,[56] and *tendermindedness*[57] have been found to correlate with the occurrence of injuries. However, the strongest relationship with injury prevalence involves *stress,* especially in contact sports.[58–62] These findings indicate that athletes who experience high levels of stress are most likely to report injuries. These findings once again point to the need for stress management programs.

Decision-Making Recommendations

In addition to the incorporation of stress management programs, completed research offers the following grade A and B recommendations.

The best psychometric instrument for measuring personality is the Cattell 16 PF.[63] This viewpoint is shared by several experts.[19,20,64]

Imagery

In terms of enhancing self-efficacy, research suggests that the use of *positive imagery* has ex-

cellent potential. It is important for the practitioner to remember, however, that some athletes prefer *internal imagery* while others rely more exclusively on *external imagery.*

In internal imagery, athletes imagine their surroundings and behaviors from their own vantage point (ie, through their own eyes). In external imagery, athletes imagine the situation from the perspective of someone watching the performance.

Regardless of the method preferred, numerous research studies have documented the beneficial effects of positive imagery on athletic performance.[65–69] Such consistent findings recommend that practitioners solicit the help of a sport psychologist to ensure that athletes are using imagery in the most effective manner.

MOTIVATION AND PERFORMANCE PROMOTION

Motivation can best be defined as a process of arousal within an organism that helps direct and sustain behavior. Most theorists agree that motivation can be *intrinsic* or *extrinsic.* Intrinsic motivation lies within an individual and involves interest in and enjoyment of a task. Extrinsic motivation lies outside the individual and involves the rewards and benefits of performing a task. Trophies, praise, money, and ribbons are extrinsic motivators. Often overlooked by practitioners is the finding that using extrinsic motives to enhance performance is not always a good idea. Indeed, when an athlete is performing a task for solely intrinsic motives, presenting extrinsic rewards often lowers intrinsic motivation.[70]

To date, a wide variety of motivational theories has been advanced, including instinctual models,[71] drive models,[72] and expectancy theories.[73] Each of these has its own strengths and weaknesses. Little, if any, research has been performed on these models in the sport setting. One model that has received a fair amount of attention in athletics is the achievement motivation concept, as originated by McClelland et al.[74] The results of these studies are so inconsistent that they will not be reported here. Instead, attention is focused solely on the relationship between goal setting as a motivational technique and performance enhancement.

Goal Setting

Only recently have researchers become interested in the effect and importance of goal setting. As a general overview, it has been found that to be effective, goals must be established in the correct manner; otherwise they actually may inhibit motivation, effort, and ultimately performance.[75]

Research reveals that *specific goals* lead to better performance than "do your best" goals.[76,77] An accumulating body of literature also finds that goal specificity alone may not be enough to enhance performance. To be effective, specific goals should be paired with *difficult but attainable goals.*[78] Burton[79] reported that fewer than 20 empirical studies on the relationship between goal setting and sport performance have been conducted but also discovered that two of every three studies (67%) documented positive benefits of goal setting on athletic performance.

Decision-Making Recommendations

The previous discussion provided some guidelines for enhancing self-efficacy. It should be noted that increasing efficacy can also be viewed as a motivational technique.[19,20] In addition, the following grade A and B recommendations are offered.

Research suggests that the best psychometric instrument for measuring intrinsic and extrinsic motivation in sport is the *Sport Motivation Scale* (SMS).[20,80] Research also suggests that coaches and practitioners should not simply ask athletes to perform to their best ability but should be specific and precise in terms of what they want the individual to accomplish. And finally, coaches should assign specific goals that will force the athlete to exert a fairly large amount of effort. Both of these goal-setting techniques will help to enhance performance.

VIOLENCE AND AGGRESSION AND THEIR CONSEQUENCES

One of the most popular definitions of aggression is provided by Baron and Richardson,[81] who suggest that "aggression is any form of behavior directed toward the goal of harming or injuring another living being who is motivated to avoid such treatment." While very good, this definition does not account for aggressive acts directed against an object, such as an athlete throwing a tennis racket or kicking a volleyball in frustration. Acts of this nature are by no means uncommon.

Types of Aggression

In a discussion of aggression in sport, it is necessary to distinguish between two types of behavior. *Hostile aggression* is an aggressive act motivated by anger that has as its main intent or goal to harm another individual or object. *Instrumental aggression,* on the other hand, is an aggressive act that also has the intent of harming another individual, but that does not have as its main goal the other person's suffering. Aggression of this nature is not motivated by anger but is performed as a means to an end, such as victory in a sporting event.

In addition to these two categories of aggression, it is also necessary to consider another type of behavior, assertiveness. *Assertiveness* is the use of legitimate force and strategy to achieve a goal. Unlike actions defined as aggressive, assertiveness does not involve intent to harm. Generally speaking, when coaches encourage their athletes to play more aggressively, they really mean to play more assertively. This involves utilizing a higher energy level to make their presence felt. Although assertiveness is not a form of aggression, it is included in this discussion because of the tendency of many practitioners to mislabel appropriate forms of behavior as "aggressive."

Situational Factors

Research has consistently found that situational factors can increase the tendency toward aggressive behavior.[82,83] It is therefore appropriate to provide a brief overview of situational factors that have the potential to increase the likelihood of aggressive behavior in the sports environment.

It is thought that some situational factors in sport facilitate aggressive behavior because they increase physiologic arousal, ie, increased heart rate, respiration, and blood pressure. Empirical research has reported that increased arousal can intensify already existing negative emotional responses, thereby increasing the likelihood of aggressive behavior.[81]

The concept of *excitation transfer*[84] has been used to account for this effect. This viewpoint maintains that residual arousal from one setting can be misattributed to another emotional setting, thereby intensifying the emotional response, and that any factor that increases player arousal can increase the potential for overt aggressive behavior. Two factors that have been consistently reported in the literature are environmental temperature[85] and noise.[86]

Intent is another situational factor that has been linked in two studies to increased aggressiveness.[87,88] The results indicated that the best predictor of player aggression was prior intentional aggression from an opponent. In other words, athletes are most likely to respond aggressively when they themselves have been the initial target of aggression from an opponent.

Losing outcomes have been associated with aggressive behavior.[89] In addition, three research studies suggest that *point differential* of the score may be an important instigator of aggressive behavior[90–92]; ie, athlete aggression increases as the point spread between the competitors increases.

There appears to be a relationship between *league standing* and the incidence of aggressive behavior. Research indicates that teams not in first place exhibit higher levels of aggressive behavior.[93,94] The general opinion is that such teams are frustrated by their league standing and, as a result, respond more aggressively in league play.

Use of *anabolic steroids* is a situational factor that can increase player aggressiveness.[95–97] Steroids are said to allow athletes to train for longer periods to increase their muscle mass. The research[95–97] indicates that aggression is a major negative side effect of these drugs.

Decision-Making Recommendations

The following grade A and B recommendations are offered as suggestions for reducing aggression in sport. Each strategy has been developed from the research and critical reviews.[98–103]

The *Bredemeier Aggression Inventory* (BAAGI)[104] is an excellent sport-specific instrument for measuring aggression. It adequately differentiates instrumental from hostile aggression.

Young athletes must be provided with nonaggressive role models. Coaches who act aggressively themselves or who allow older athletes to behave aggressively teach young athletes that aggression is acceptable.

Coaches must make every effort not to reward aggressive behavior. Although assertive behavior is acceptable and should be encouraged, athletes who display aggression should be removed from the contest and counselled about the unacceptable nature of aggression in sport.

Coaches who encourage or even allow athletes to behave aggressively should be fined, censured, or even suspended from coaching duties. This will send a strong message to athletes predisposed to aggressive behavior.

Coaches and officials should receive formal training in dealing with and curbing aggressive behavior in their sports. This could be done in workshops, as well as in formal training in the National Coaching Certification Program (NCCP). Only certified coaches and officials should be allowed to work with athletes.

As well as being punished for acts of aggression, athletes should receive positive reinforcement for controlling their temper in highly volatile situations. They should be taught strategies and coping skills designed to curtail acts of aggression.

LEADERSHIP IN THE SPORTING ENVIRONMENT

Like most organizations, sports teams require qualified leaders to be successful. In its simplest terms, leadership is a behavioral process in which one group member influences other members to attain the group's goals.

Theories and Models

Over the years various leadership theories have been advanced, including *trait theories*,[105] *behavior theories*,[106] *contingency theory*,[107] *path-goal theory*,[108] and *life cycle theory*.[109] Although all of these theories have some merit, there does not appear to be a consensus, from a research perspective, on their acceptability in the sporting environment. For this reason, attention is focused on a relatively new model that appears to have direct relevance in the sporting environment.

Multidimensional Theory

The multidimensional theory of leadership[110] is a sport-specific model that focuses on the congruence among three leadership behavioral states: required, actual, and preferred. This theory predicts that as the congruence among these states increases, the group performance and satisfaction also increase. The antecedents of these leadership behaviors are situational, leader, and member characteristics.

Required leader behaviors are witnessed in the demands and constraints placed on the leader by the situation and characteristics of the members. A professional coach, for example, has to exhibit different leader behaviors than does a coach of youth sport. *Actual leader behaviors* are actions displayed by the leader regardless of the situation and member characteristics. These behaviors often reflect the leader's personal disposition and leadership style. *Preferred leader behaviors* are those behaviors desired by athletes, for a variety of personal reasons. It is important to note, however, that preferred leader behaviors are subject to change with changes in the situation.

To date, research on the multidimensional model of leadership in the sports environment has been encouraging. In research involving college basketball, Chelladurai[111] found that as a player's perception of the coach's behavior becomes more incongruent with the player's preferences, overall satisfaction decreases. Similarly, in a study involving intercollegiate coach-athlete dyads, Horne and Carron[112] reported that discrepancies between an athlete's preferred leadership behaviors and perceived leadership behaviors were related to athlete satisfaction and performance. Other studies[113–115] also support the multidimensional model.

Research to date indicates that the multidimensional model of leadership is valid and useful for understanding the leadership process in the sports environment. Of the various theories, it appears to hold the most promise for sports-specific applications.

Decision-Making Recommendations

The following grade A and B recommendations deal with leadership in the sports environment.

It appears that the best psychometric instrument for assessing leadership in the sports setting is the *Leadership Scale for Sports* (LSS),[116,117] which consists of 40 items measuring five dimensions of leader behavior.

It appears important that the coach "tune in" to the preferences of the athletes. Because player satisfaction and performance are related to the degree to which their preferences match the leader's behavior, it is important to open up the lines of communication with the athletes. One of the best places for this is in a group goal-setting environment.

Similarly, it is important for athletes to know that their ultimate goals, especially in terms of performance, will to some extent dictate the type of leadership required. For example, athletes must be made aware of the fact that if their primary goal is performance based, it will not always be possible to have a friendly and carefree practice environment. Again, this necessitates open communication between the coach and athlete.

When goals are arrived at jointly, discrepancies between the preferred and the required or actual leadership behaviors can be largely eliminated, resulting in greater athlete satisfaction and improved performance.

REFERENCES

1. Kozar B, Lord R: Psychological considerations for training the elite athlete. In: Hall ER, McIntyre M (eds): Olympism: a movement of the people. Proceedings of the United States Olympic Academy VII. Texas Tech University, Lubbock, 1983, pp. 78–96
2. Levenson H, Hirschfeld L, Hirschfeld A, Dzubay B: Recent life events and accidents: the role of sex differences. J Human Stress 10:4–11, 1983
3. Bramwell ST, Masuda M, Wagner NN, Holmes TH: Psychosocial factors in athletic injuries. J Human Stress 2:6–20, 1975
4. Coddington RD, Troxell JR: The effects of emotional factors on football injury rates: a pilot study. J Human Stress 7:3–5, 1980
5. Cryan PD, Alles WF: The relationship between stress and college football injuries. J Sports Med 23:52–58, 1983
6. Guttman MC, Knapp DM, Foster C, et al: Age, experience, and gender as predictors of psychological response to training in Olympic speedskaters. Presented at the 1984 Olympic Scientific Congress, Eugene, Oregon, 1984

7. Passer MW, Seese MD: Life stress and athletic injury: examination of positive versus negative events and three moderator variables. J Human Stress 10:11–16, 1983

8. Smith RE, Smoll FL, Ptacek JT: Conjunctive moderator variables in vulnerability and resiliency life research: life stress, social support, and coping skills, and adolescent sport injuries. J Personality Social Psychol 58:360–369, 1990

9. Gould D, Petlichkoff L, Weinberg RS: Antecedents of temporal changes in, and relationships between CSAI-2 subcomponents. J Sport Psychol 6:289–304, 1984

10. Jones JG, Cale A: Precompetition temporal patterning of anxiety and self-confidence in males and females. J Sport Behav 12:183–195, 1989

11. Jones JG, Swain A, Cale A: Gender differences in precompetition temporal patterning and antecedents of anxiety and self-confidence. J Sport Exerc Psychol 13:1–15, 1991

12. Martens R, Vealey RS, Burton D: Competitive Anxiety in Sport. Human Kinetics Books, Champaign, Ill, 1990

13. Swain A, Jones G: Relationship between sport achievement orientation and competitive state anxiety. Sport Psychol 6:42–54, 1992

14. Endler NS: The interaction model of anxiety: some possible implications. In: Landers DM, Christina RW (eds): Psychology of Motor Behavior and Sport—1977. Human Kinetics, Champaign, Ill, 1978, pp. 332–351

15. Fenz WD: Learning to anticipate stressful events. J Sport Exerc Psychol 10:223–238, 1988

16. Hardy L, Parfitt G: A catastrophe model of anxiety and performance. Br J Psychol 82:163–178, 1991

17. Leith LM: Choking in sports: are we our own worst enemies? Int J Sport Psychol 19:59–64, 1988

18. Martens R, Burton D, Vealey RS, et al: Development and validation of the Competitive State Anxiety Inventory—2. In: Martens R, Vealey RS, Burton D (eds): Competitive Anxiety in Sport. Human Kinetics Books, Champaign, Ill, 1990, pp. 117–190

19. Cox RH: Sport Psychology: Concepts and Applications. Brown & Benchmark, Dubuque, Ia, 1994

20. Wann DL: Sport Psychology. Prentice-Hall, Upper Saddle River, NJ, 1997

21. Crocker P: Managing stress by competitive athletes: ways of coping. Int J Sport Psychol 23:161–175, 1992

22. Crocker P, Graham T: Coping by competitive athletes with performance stress: gender differences and relationships with affect. Sport Psychol 9:325–338, 1995

23. Madden CC, Summers JJ, Brown DF: The influence of perceived stress on coping with competitive basketball. Int J Sport Psychol 21:21–35, 1990

24. Rathus SA, Nevid JS: Psychology and the Challenges of Life: Adjustment and Growth, 4th Ed. Holt, Rinehart & Winston, New York, 1989

25. Jacobson E: Progressive Relaxation. University of Chicago Press, Chicago, 1929

26. Jacobson E: You Must Relax. McGraw-Hill, New York, 1976

27. Carlson CR, Howe RH: Efficacy of abbreviated progressive muscle relaxation training: a quantitative review of behavioral medicine research. J Consult Clin Psychol 61:1059–1067, 1993

28. Maynard IW, Hemmings B, Warwick-Evans L: The effects of a somatic intervention strategy on competitive state anxiety and performance in semiprofessional soccer players. Sport Psychol 9:51–64, 1995

29. Onestak DM: The effects of progressive relaxation, mental practice, and hypnosis on athletic performance: a review. J Sport Behav 14:247–274, 1991

30. Schafer W: Stress Management for Wellness, 2nd Ed. Harcourt Brace Jovanovich, New York, 1992

31. Zaichkowsky LD, Takenaka K: Optimizing arousal levels. In: Singer RN, Murphey M, Tennant LK (eds): Handbook of Research on Sport Psychology. Macmillan, New York, 1993, pp. 511–527

32. Layman EM: Meditation and sport performance. In: Straub W (ed): Sport Psychology: An Analysis of Athlete Behavior, 2nd Ed. Mouvement Publications, Ithaca, NY, pp. 266–273

33. Hall EG, Hardy CJ: Ready, aim, fire: relaxation strategies for enhancing pistol marksmanship. Percept Motor Skills 72:775–786, 1991

34. Williams LRT: Transcendental meditation and mirror-tracing skill. Percept Motor Skills 46:371–378, 1978

35. Smith RE: A cognitive-affective approach to stress management training for athletes. In: Neadeau CH, Halliwell WR, Newell KM, Roberts GC (eds): Psychology of Motor Behavior and Sport—1979. Human Kinetics, Champaign, Ill, 1980, pp. 54–72

36. Crocker PR: Evaluating stress management training under competition conditions. Int J Sport Psychol 20:191–204, 1989

37. Ziegler S, Klinzing J, Williamson K: The effects of two stress management training programs on cardiorespiratory efficiency. J Sport Psychol 4:280–289, 1982

38. Phares EJ: Introduction to Personality, 3rd Ed. Harper Collins, New York, 1991

39. Carron AV: Personality and athletics: a review. In: Rushall B (ed): The Status of Psycho-Motor Learning and Sport Psychology Research. Sport Science, Dartmouth, Nova Scotia, 1975, pp. 5.1–5.12

40. Cox RH, Qui Y, Liu Z: Overview of sport psychology. In: Singer RN, Murphey M, Tennant LK (eds): Handbook of Research on Sport Psychology. Macmillan, New York, 1993, pp. 3–31

41. Cratty BJ: Psychology in Contemporary Sport, 3rd Ed. Prentice Hall, Englewood Cliffs, NJ, 1989

42. Vanden Auweele Y, De Cuyper B, Van Mele B, Rzewnicki R: Elite performance and personality: from description and prediction to diagnosis and intervention. In Singer RN, Murphey M, Tennant LK (eds): Handbook of Research on Sport Psychology. Macmillan, New York, 1993, pp. 257–289

43. Bandura A: Self-efficacy: toward a unifying theory of behavior change. Psychol Rev 84:191–215, 1977

44. Bandura A: Social Foundations of Thought and Action: A Social-Cognitive Theory. Prentice-Hall, Englewood Cliffs, NJ, 1986

45. Morgan WP: The trait psychology controversy. Res Q Exerc Sport 51:50–76, 1980

46. Cooper L: Athletics, activity, and personality: a review of the literature. Res Q 40:17–22, 1969

47. Butt DS, Cox DN: Motivational patterns in Davis Cup, university and recreational tennis players. Int J Sport Psychol 23:1–13, 1992

48. LeUnes AD, Nation JR: Saturday's heroes: a psychological portrait of college football players. J Sport Behav 5:139–149, 1982

49. Snyder EE, Kivlin JE: Women athletes and aspects of psychological well-being and body image. Res Q 46:191–199, 1975

50. Kamal AF, Blais C, Kelly P, Ekstrand K: Self-esteem attributional components of athletes versus nonathletes. Int J Sport Psychol 26:189–195, 1995

51. Mahoney MJ: Psychological predictors of elite and non-elite performance in Olympic weightlifting. Int J Sport Psychol 20:1–12, 1989

52. Marsh HW, Perry C, Horsely C, Roche L: Multidimensional self-concepts of elite athletes: how do they differ from the general population? J Sport Exerc Psychol 17:70–83, 1995

53. Trujillo CM: The effect of weight training and running exercise intervention programs on the self-esteem of college women. Int J Sport Psychol 14:162–173, 1983

54. Rehberg RA, Schafer WE: Participation in interscholastic athletics and college expectations. Am J Sociol 73:732–740, 1968

55. Lufi D, Tenenbaum G: Persistence among young male gymnasts. Percept Motor Skills 72:479–482

56. Meyers MC, LeUnes AD, Elledge JR, et al: Injury incidence and psychological mood state patterns in collegiate rodeo athletes. J Sport Behav 15:297–305, 1992

57. Jackson DW, Jarrett H, Bailey D, et al: Injury prediction in the young athlete: a preliminary report. Am J Sport Med 6:6–14, 1978

58. Andersen MB, Williams JM: A model of stress and athletic injury: prediction and prevention. J Sport Exerc Psychol 10:294–306, 1988

59. Hanson SJ, McCullagh P, Tonymon P: The relationship of personality characteristics, life stress, and coping resources to athletic injury. J Sport Exerc Psychol 14:262–272, 1992

60. Nidefer RM: Psychological aspects of sports injuries: issues in prevention and treatment. Int J Sport Psychol 20:241–255, 1989

61. Rotella RJ, Heyman SR: Stress, injury, and the psychological rehabilitation of athletes. In: Willams JM (ed): Applied Sport Psychology: Personal Growth to Peak Performance, 2nd Ed. Mayfield, Mountain View, Calif, 1993, pp. 338–355

62. Williams JM, Roepke N: Psychology of injury and injury rehabilitation. In Singer RN, Murphey M, Tennant LK (eds): Handbook of Research on Sport Psychology. MacMillan, New York, 1993, pp. 815–839

63. Cattell RB: Personality pinned down. Psychol Today July 1973, 40–46

64. Williams JM: Applied Sport Psychology: Personal Growth to Peak Performance. Mayfield, Mountain View, Calif, 1993

65. Grouios G: The effect of mental practice on diving performance. Int J Sport Psychol 23:60–69, 1992

66. Lee C: Psyching up for a muscular endurance task: effects of image content on performance and mood state. J Sport Exerc Psychol 12:66–73, 1990

67. Predebon J, Docker SB: Free-throw shooting performance as a function of preshot routines. Percept Motor Skills 75:167–171, 1992

68. Templin DP, Vernacchia RA: The effect of highlight music videotapes upon the game performance of intercollegiate basketball players. Sport Psychol 9:41–50, 1995

69. Underleider S, Golding JM: Mental practice among Olympic athletes. Percept Motor Skills 72:1007–1017, 1991

70. Deci EL, Ryan RM: Intrinsic Motivation and Self-Determination in Human Behavior. Plenum Press, New York, 1985

71. McDougall M: An Introduction to Social Psychology. Methuen, London, 1908

72. Hull CL: Principles of Behavior. Appleton, New York, 1943

73. Vroom VH: Work and Motivation. John Wiley & Sons, New York, 1964

74. McClelland DC, Atkinson JW, Clark RA, Lowell EL: The Achievement Motive. Appleton-Century-Crofts, New York, 1953

75. Burton D: The Jekyl/Hyde nature of goals: reconceptualizing goal setting in sport. In: Horn TS (ed): Advances in Sport Psychology. Human Kinetics, Champaign, Ill, 1992, pp. 267–297

76. Baron RA, Greenberg J: Behavior in Organizations: Understanding and Managing the Human Side of Work, 3rd Ed. Allyn & Bacon, Needham Heights, Mass, 1990

77. Weinberg RS: Goal setting and performance in sport and exercise settings: a synthesis and critique. Med Sci Sports Exerc 26:469–477, 1994

78. Locke EA, Latham GP: Goal setting theory. In: O'Neil HF, Jr, Drillings M (eds): Motivation: Theory and Research. Erlbaum, Hillsdale, NJ, pp. 13–29

79. Burton D: Goal setting in sport. In: Singer RN, Murphey M, Tennant LK (eds): Handbook of Research on Sport Psychology. Macmillan, New York, 1993, pp. 467–491

80. Pelletier LG, Fortier MS, Vallerand RJ, et al: Toward a new measure of intrinsic motivation, extrinsic motivation, and amotivation in sports: the Sport Motivation Scale (SMS). J Sport Exerc Psychol 17:35–53, 1995

81. Baron RA, Richardson DR: Human Aggression, 2nd Ed. Plenum Press, New York, 1994

82. Berkowitz L: Aggression: Its Causes, Consequences, and Control. McGraw-Hill, New York, 1993

83. Geen RG: Human Aggression. Brooks/Cole, Pacific Grove, Calif, 1990

84. Zillman D: Cognition-excitation interdependencies in aggressive behavior. Aggress Behav 14:51–64, 1988

85. Reifman AS, Larrick RP, Fein S: Temper and temperature on the diamond: the heat-aggression relationship in major league baseball. Personality Social Psychol Bull 17:580–585, 1991

86. Geen RG: Effects of attack and uncontrollable noise on aggression. J Res Personality 12:15–29, 1978

87. Betancourt H, Blair I: A cognitive (attribution)–emotion model of violence in conflict situations. Personality Social Psychol Bull 18:343–350, 1992

88. Harrel WA: Aggression by high school basketball players: an observational study of the effects of opponents' aggression and frustration-inducing factors. Int J Sport Psychol 11:290–298, 1980

89. Leith LM: The effect of various physical activities, outcome, and emotional arousal on subject aggression scores. Int J Sport Psychol 20:57–66, 1989

90. Rainey DW, Cherilla K: Conflict with baseball umpires: an observational study. J Sport Behav 16:49–59, 1993

91. Russell GW: Psychological issues in sports aggression. In: Goldstein JH (ed): Sports Violence. Springer-Verlag, New York, 1983, pp. 157–181

92. Wankel LM: An examination of illegal aggression in intercollegiate hockey. In: Williams ID, Wankel LM (eds): Proceedings of the Fourth Canadian Psycho-Motor Learning and Sport Psychology Symposium. Fitness and Amateur Sport Directorate, Ottawa, Ont, Canada, 1973, pp. 531–544

93. Russell GW, Drewry BR: Crowd size and competitive aspects of aggression in ice hockey: an archival study. Human Relations 29:723–735, 1976

94. Volkamer N: Investigations into the aggressiveness in competitive social systems. Sportwissenschaft 1:33–64, 1971

95. Gregg E, Rejeski WJ: Social psychobiologic dysfunction associated with anabolic steroid abuse: a review. Sport Psychol 4:275–284, 1990

96. Lubell A: Does steroid abuse cause—or excuse—violence? Physician Sports Med 17:176–180, 185, 1989

97. Yates WR, Perry P, Murray S: Aggression and hostility in anabolic steroid users. Biol Psychiatry 31:1232–1234, 1992

98. DeBenedette V: Spectator violence at sports events: what keeps enthusiastic fans in bounds? Physician Sports Med 16:203–211, 1988

99. Lefebvre LL, Leith LM, Bredemeier BB: Modes for aggression assessment and control. Int J Sport Psychol 11:11–21, 1980

100. Leith LM: Reinforcers and aggression control in sport. Coach Sci Update 1:20–23, 1983

101. Leith LM: Do coaches encourage aggressive behavior in sport? Can J Sport Sci 16:85–86, 1991

102. Leith LM: Aggression in sport. In: Bull S (ed): Sport Psychology for the Practitioner. Crowood Publishers, London, 1991, pp. 52–69

103. Luxbacher J: Violence in sport: an examination of the theories of aggression, and how the coach can influence the degree of violence in sport. Coach Rev 9:14–17, 1986

104. Bredemeier BJ: The assessment of reactive and instrumental athletic aggression. Proceedings of the International Symposium on Psychological

Assessment in Sport. Wingate Institute for Physical Education and Sport, Netanya, Israel, 1978, pp. 136–149

105. Stogdill RM: Personal factors associated with leadership: survey of literature. J Psychol 25:35–71, 1948

106. Hemphill JK, Coons AE: Development of the leader behavior description questionnaire. In: Stogdill RM, Coons AE (eds): Leader Behavior: Its Description and Measurement. Ohio State University Press, Columbus, 1957

107. Fiedler FE: A Theory of Leadership Effectiveness. McGraw-Hill, New York, 1967

108. House RJ: A path-goal theory of leader effectiveness. Adm Sci Q 16:321–338, 1971

109. Hersey P, Blanchard KH: Management of Organizational Behavior. Prentice-Hall, Englewood Cliffs, NJ, 1977

110. Chelladurai P: Leadership in sports: a review. Int J Sport Psychol 21:328–354, 1990

111. Chelladurai P: Discrepancy between preferences and perceptions of leadership behavior and satisfaction of athletes in varying sports. J Sport Behav 6:27–41, 1984

112. Horne T, Carron AV: Compatibility in coach-athlete relationships. J Sport Psychol 7:137–149, 1985

113. Chelladurai P, Imaumura H, Yamaguchi Y, et al: Sport leadership in a cross-national setting: the case of Japanese and Canadian university athletes. J Sport Exerc Psychol 10:374–389, 1985

114. Laughlin N, Laughlin S: The relationship between the similarity in perceptions of teacher/coach leader behavior and evaluations of their effectiveness. Int J Sport Psychol 22:396–410, 1994

115. Riemer HA, Chelladurai P: Leadership and satisfaction in athletics. J Sport Exerc Psychol 17:276–293, 1995

116. Chelladurai P, Saleh SD: Preferred leadership in sports. Can J Appl Sport Sci 3:85–92, 1978

117. Chelladurai P, Saleh SD: Dimensions of leader behavior in sports: development of a leadership scale. J Sport Psychol 2:34–45, 1980

Caffeine and Carbohydrate Loading in Endurance Exercise

MARK A. TARNOPOLSKY

Striving for an edge in competition, athletes have used various training strategies and dietary supplements. Many of the supplements taken by athletes have shown no ergogenic benefit in properly designed, randomized, controlled trials; thus, an exhaustive review of the plethora of nutraceuticals and other compounds on the commercial market (eg, coenzyme Q_{10}, various vitamins and minerals, branched-chain amino acids, glycerol) is not included here. This chapter explores the scientific basis and applied studies of the potential ergogenic benefits of carbohydrate loading and caffeine administration. These were chosen because of the extensive numbers of studies of both basic and applied aspects of their use. Thus, sound conclusions as to their efficacy and safety can be drawn.

One of the first strategies to be used by endurance athletes was the manipulation of dietary carbohydrate to maximize performance. An understanding of the mechanisms behind such strategies and their development and refinement mushroomed in the 1960s with the advent of the Bergström muscle biopsy technique.[1] Many thousands of studies have since been published, and some general conclusions are elucidated in this chapter. Manipulation of nutritional carbohydrate is not considered "illegal" under international sporting rules, and there are, at most, minimal side effects from their use.

A second strategy that became of great interest in the 1970s was caffeine administration. The original idea behind the putative role for caffeine in endurance exercise came from its potential to increase free fatty acid oxidation and to "spare" muscle glycogen use. This role has come into question, yet the ergogenic effects are well documented. Therefore, other effects of caffeine may be ergogenic, and these are discussed.

Unlike carbohydrates, which form the largest component of our macronutrient intake, caffeine is found in only a few foods and drinks and would meet many of the criteria for labeling it a drug. As such, and given the potential ergogenic effects, caffeine is considered a restricted drug by the International Olympic Committee (IOC; urine concentration >12 mg/L). Although the modest intake of caffeine on a habitual basis appears to be without side effects,[2,3] there may be acute effects that would be deleterious to an athlete. For example, caffeine-induced insomnia could be ergolytic if caffeine is consumed on the evening prior to a competition. Caffeine, particularly in nonhabitual consumers, can result in anxiety, restlessness, and tremor that may be ergolytic in sports requiring accuracy, eg, shooting, biathlon. Another common side effect is diuresis and increased gastric motility, both of which could be ergolytic during an endurance event. These potential side effects, and ethical concerns about doping, are significant factors for the individual athlete to consider when contemplating caffeine consumption for ergogenic purposes.[4]

This chapter reviews the essential details of the basic biologic principles and the applied applications of carbohydrate nutrition and caffeine supplementation during endurance athletics.

BRIEF REVIEW OF METABOLISM DURING ENDURANCE EXERCISE

The transition from rest to endurance exercise results in massive cardiovascular and metabolic adjustment. For example, heart rate, stroke volume, and ventilation may increase even in the anticipatory phase prior to exercise and increase significantly at exercise onset. The changes can be highlighted by considering that in the average male athlete, oxygen consumption (V_{O_2}) is about 3 to 5 ml/kg/min at rest and increases to more than 60 ml/kg/min during a marathon run. This represents a 15- to 20-fold increase in V_{O_2}. In addition to oxygen delivery and uptake, there is a large need for carbon energy sources to support electron transport and oxidative phosphorylation. Oxidative phosphorylation is ultimately responsible for the vast majority of the adenosine triphosphate (ATP) required to support actin-myosin cross-bridge action (muscle contraction) in endurance activity.

Oxygen consumption and energy or substrate delivery are tightly coupled processes. Approximately 5 kcal is used for each 1 L of oxygen consumed during aerobic activities. This changes slightly, depending on the proportion of the macronutrients being oxidized; however, it is a close estimate, for the majority of the energy for endurance exercise (between 55% to 80% of maximal oxygen consumption [V_{O_2max}]) comes from carbohydrate sources (Table 8-1). This range of endurance exercise intensity is important because it covers the average intensity of a training workout (55%–70% V_{O_2max}) and

the average 10 to 42 km race (65%–80%). Unless otherwise stated, endurance exercise refers to activities performed within these ranges.

At the onset of exercise there is rapid ATP hydrolysis, with a resultant increase in ADP. Adenosine triphosphate is not "stored," and biochemical pathways must buffer the alteration in energy charge. Initially, phosphocreatine (PCr) hydrolysis rephosphorylates adenosine diphosphate (ADP) to ATP via the creatine kinase (CK) reaction (PCr + ADP <CK> ATP + creatine). This "temporal" buffering capacity by PCr can last only about 10 seconds, and within seconds there is contribution from the anaerobic breakdown of glycogen through the glycolytic pathway (anaerobic glycogenolysis). Cardiovascular adaptation to endurance exercise may commence even before the onset of exercise; however, the central and peripheral mechanisms are not sufficient to deliver all of the required oxygen to the mitochondria during this transition period. Thus, even in so-called aerobic activities, there is an initial increase in lactate production owing to a mismatch between glycogenolysis and oxidative phosphorylation. Rapidly, however, oxidative phosphorylation is activated, and intramuscular glycogen, glucose, free fatty acids (FFA), and proteins can be oxidized to provide ATP equivalents.

Most of the energy for endurance activities at 55% to 80% V_{O_2max} comes from intramuscular glycogen stores. This had been observed directly in muscle biopsy specimens in the late 1960s.[1,5] In addition to these observations, Bergström et al[1] and Ahlborg et al[5] also showed good correlation between the depletion of muscle glycogen and fatigue during endurance exercise. It is estimated that the total available glycogen within the muscles is about 300 to 500 g (~1,200–2,000 kcal), with a further 50 to 75 g in the liver. Once the intramuscular glycogen stores are depleted, an athlete can maintain an exercise intensity of only about 50% to 55% V_{O_2max} because lipid, although energetically dense, can only support an energy delivery *rate* at about this intensity. For the athlete, this results in an increased perception of effort and an obligatory requirement to reduce exercise intensity. The lay term for this is "hitting the wall." From a practical standpoint, this implies that even with normal glycogen stores, there is only

TABLE 8-1. Fuel Utilization During 60 Minutes of Endurance Exercise

FUEL	65% V_{O_2peak} (% TOTAL)	80% V_{O_2peak} (% TOTAL)
Intramuscular glycogen	30–45	65–80
Intramuscular triglycerides	15–20	5–10
Plasma free fatty acids	25–40	10–20
Plasma glucose	5–10	5–15
Protein	1–4	2–8

See Tarnopolsky MA, Atkinson SA, Phillips SM, MacDougall JD: J Appl Physiol 78:1360–1368, 1995; Ivy JL, Katz AL, Cutler CL, et al: J Appl Physiol 64:1480–1485, 1988; Tarnopolsky MA, Dyson K, Atkinson SA, et al: Int J Sport Nutr 6:323–336, 1996 enough energy to support 90 to 120 minutes of exercise at 75% VO_{2max}.

On the basis of the observations of the importance of carbohydrates to the provision of energy and the correlation of glycogen depletion with fatigue, strategies were devised to prevent this depletion. One strategy was to increase the dietary intake of carbohydrates to "load" the muscles with more glycogen. The theory was that this would prolong the time to fatigue during exercise by starting with a higher basal glycogen concentration. Many studies have now shown the efficacy of this strategy, which has been termed glycogen loading or carbohydrate loading.[6–8]

Another strategy centers around the concept that slowing the rate of carbohydrate utilization during exercise will result in a longer time until depletion and resultant fatigue. A few studies had shown that the provision of increased FFA to muscle attenuated the rate of glycogen depletion.[9] The impracticality of the methods used to elevate FFA levels in these studies (synthetic triglyceride intravenous infusion plus heparin injection) led to alternate strategies. It was known that caffeine could elevate plasma FFA concentration, and studies conducted in the late 1970s showed an ergogenic effect of caffeine that was partially attributed to increased FFA delivery and glycogen sparing.[10,11] Over the past 20 years, many studies have yielded interesting insights into the mechanisms of action of carbohydrate supplementation and caffeine administration. Further examination of these concepts forms the bulk of this chapter.

CAFFEINE

Pharmacokinetics

Caffeine (1,3,7-trimethylxanthine) is an alkaloid derivative found in many plant species throughout the world. Caffeine is primarily consumed in beverages such as coffee and tea, but is also present in a number of other sources (Table 8–2). It is important to note that most of the ergogenic benefits reported for caffeine are at doses of 4 to 6 mg/kg (ie, 280–420 mg for a 70 kg man).

Caffeine is rapidly absorbed following an oral dose, and peak plasma levels are achieved within about 60 minutes (range, 15–120 minutes).[12]

TABLE 8–2. Caffeine Content of Some Common Foods

SUBSTANCE	CAFFEINE (mg)
Coffee (instant)	50–80
Coffee (drip)	75–125
Coffee (percolated)	90–175
Coffee (decaffeinated)	3–15
Tea (strong)	60–85
Tea (weak)	20–35
Cola	25–35
Chocolate (50 g)	10–15

See also Tarnopolsky MA: Caffeine and endurance performance. Sports Med 18:109–125, 1994; Bunker ML, McWilliams M: Caffeine content of some common beverages. J Am Diet Assoc 74:28–32, 1989

The plasma half-life of caffeine varies considerably, from 3 to 10 hours,[4] and is prolonged following oral contraceptive use.[13] Caffeine metabolism is accelerated in habitual caffeine consumers yet is not affected significantly by acute exercise.[4] Caffeine is metabolized in the liver via mixed-function oxidases (p450 system) to yield mono- and dimethylxanthines and urates; however, 0.5% to 3% is excreted unchanged in the urine.[4,14] In spite of the variability in fractional urinary excretion rate, the IOC uses urinary caffeine concentrations to determine doping infractions. This means that the same oral dose of caffeine cannot be used to reliably predict the urinary excretion concentration.

In one study of nine male endurance athletes[14] the postexercise urine caffeine concentrations were 10.4 mg/L following an oral dose of 450 mg (~6.5 mg/kg). Another study[15] used a higher dose of caffeine (9 mg/kg) and found that the IOC limit was just marginally exceeded in only 20% of subjects. Similarly, only 33% of the subjects in still another study[16] exceeded the IOC limit with a very high dose (13.5 mg/kg). On average, the usual ergogenic dose of 4 to 6 mg/kg will result in a urine concentration that, although varied (4–8 mg/L), is still below the IOC guidelines.

Mechanisms of Action That May Be Ergogenic

Many of the cellular effects of caffeine (CNS stimulant effects, diuresis, increased gastric secretion, increased adipocyte lipolysis) are due to adenosine receptor antagonism.[4] Adenosine is structurally similar to caffeine, and functions to inhibit (A_1 receptor) or stimulate (A_2 receptor) adenylate cyclase within the cell. Adenylate cyclase activation increases the intracellular second messenger, cyclic adenosine monophosphate (cAMP), and induces a cellular response.

The A_1 receptor antagonism on adipocytes first intrigued physiologists because it predicted an increase in cAMP and an increase in lipolysis (?increased FFA utilization by muscle with resultant glycogen sparing). This hypothesis was based upon the observation that physiologic caffeine concentrations increase adipocyte lipolysis in vitro[17] and that artificially increased [FFA](Intralipid and heparin) "spares" muscle glycogen utilization during exercise.[9] It was proposed that increased FFA oxidation increases citrate, which inhibits glycogenolysis.[18] The existence of this so-called glucose–fatty acid cycle has been debated in the literature over the years.[18,19]

Several studies have shown that caffeine increases plasma [FFA],[10,11,20–24] whereas others have not.[25–27] It is interesting that in most of the studies that show an increase in plasma [FFA], it usually occurs in the early stages of exercise.[20,23,24,28] It is also of interest that levels of the putative mediators of the glucose–fatty acid cycle (citrate and acetyl coenzyme A/reduced coenzyme A [CoA/CoA-SH]) were elevated only immediately before exercise after caffeine supplementation.[29] This may suggest that caffeine-increased plasma [FFA] and muscle FFA utilization occurs only in the early rest-exercise transition phase. Nevertheless, caffeine has been shown to spare glycogen utilization in every study in which it was directly measured.[20,24,27] Of interest, Spriet et al[24] showed that caffeine-induced glycogen sparing occurred within the first 15 minutes of exercise and that thereafter utilization was similar to that with placebo. Another group[20] also showed an increase in intramuscular triglycerides prior to exercise after caffeine ingestion. These observations support the theory that the glucose–fatty acid cycle, or some other mechanism, may function to spare glycogen utilization in the rest-exercise transition phase.

Even the original proponents of the FFA-glycogen-sparing theory suggested that either central nervous system (CNS) stimulation or enhanced neuromuscular function could be partly responsible for the ergogenic effects of caffeine ingestion.[10,11] The degree of CNS stimulation is difficult to assess, particularly as it may relate to an ergogenic effect in exercise performance. Studies have shown that the rating of perceived exertion was lower during exercise following caffeine ingestion, and speculated that this may represent CNS arousal.[10,30] However, others have not found this,[23,31] and the relationship to the central perception of fatigue is unclear.

Another attractive mechanism of action that may contribute to an ergogenic effect is the potentiation of calcium (Ca^{++}) release from the sarcoplasmic reticulum calcium release channel (ryanodine receptor).[32] Fatigue at low frequencies of electrical stimulation is due to failure of Ca^{++} release from the sarcoplasmic reticulum.[33,34] The methylxanthines are well known to potentiate Ca^{++} release from the sarcoplasmic reticulum of skeletal muscle in both pharmacologic[34,35] and physiologic[36,37] concentrations.

Studies in humans support a role for methylxanthines enhancing muscle contractile function, presumably via enhanced sarcoplasmic reticulum Ca^{++} release. At least three studies have shown that methylxanthines potentiated diaphragmatic contractility-force in humans.[38–40] Lopes et al[41] showed that caffeine (500 mg) potentiated the force of submaximal, electrically stimulated contractions in humans.[41] We[42] showed that caffeine (6 mg/kg) increased low-frequency force in electrically stimulated dorsiflexor muscles of both habitual and nonhabitual caffeine consumers. In another study[23] we found no effect of caffeine (5 mg/kg) on the maximal voluntary contraction strength nor single twitch strength of the quadriceps muscle group either before or after endurance exercise in young men.[23]

It appears that some of the potential ergogenic effects of caffeine may come from a direct effect on the skeletal muscle ryanodine receptor (potentiation of Ca^{++} release). This is likely to be of most benefit to submaximal efforts based upon the experimental evidence, and it is also inherently logical that at submaximal contractions there is more potential Ca^{++} to be released.

One final mechanism of action that has been suggested to be of potential ergogenic benefit is an attenuation of the exercise-induced K^+ accumulation.[43] Accumulation of K^+ in the transverse tubule may lead to conduction block and be important in the genesis of muscular fatigue. Lindinger et al[43] found that caffeine (9 mg/kg) attenuated the increase in plasma K^+ during exercise at approximately 80% VO_{2max} and attributed this to a stimulation of Na^+ and K^+ pumps in noncontracting muscle.[44]

It is probable that there are interactive effects of caffeine that may be of ergogenic potential to athletic performance. Which, if any, of the effects will predominate depends on the task specificity and its resultant mechanism of fatigue. I shall now review several of the studies that have investigated the potential ergogenic effects of caffeine in sports performance. Also of interest, though not well studied, is the potential for caffeine to be of benefit in selected patient populations. For example, I have found profound low-frequency fatigue in patients with mitochondrial cytopathies (Tarnopolsky M, unpublished observations, 1998), and there is the potential for caffeine to be an adjunctive ergogenic agent in these and other patient populations.

Studies in High-Intensity Exercise

In theory, caffeine could enhance high-intensity exercise performance through one of several mechanisms. First, it could enhance CNS drive and perhaps increase effort in uncomfortable high-intensity tasks. Furthermore, K^+ accumulation could be attenuated and lessen its potential to induce T tubule conduction block. It is also possible that there could be a potentiation of Ca^{++} release from the sarcoplasmic reticulum; however, impaired Ca^{++} release is more significant in the genesis of fatigue at lower intensities. Finally, it is extremely unlikely that any FFA-carbohydrate effects would be of any use in this type of activity, in which muscle glycogen is not limiting to exercise performance.

In progressive cycle and running exercise tasks leading to fatigue in 12 to 25 minutes (ie, VO_{2max} test), the vast majority of studies show no ergogenic effect of caffeine.[45–48] Furthermore, in exercise tasks at 90%[49] and 100%[22] VO_{2max}, there was no improvement after caffeine ingestion, even at the extremely high dose (12.9 mg/kg) used in the latter study.

In higher intensity tasks there is some variability in the results. For example, the same investigators used maximal anaerobic tests and reported both positive[50] and no[51] ergogenic effects following 3.7 and 5 mg/kg caffeine ingestion, respectively. These same investigators later demonstrated a statistically significant improvement in sprint swimming performance following 4.3 mg/kg caffeine ingestion.[52] A 1998 study[53] did not find any ergogenic benefit from caffeine administration (6 mg/kg) on performance in four repeated maximal 30-second cycle ergometer trials in nine men.

Studies in Endurance Exercise

Much of the interest in the potential ergogenic effects of caffeine arises from the potential benefits derived from the cellular processes. For example, most of the energy for a marathon race comes from muscle glycogen,[54] and these stores are insufficient to support a race duration of much more than 2 hours (the current world record is 2 h, 6 min, 22 s). Therefore, if caffeine can spare muscle glycogen or potentiate the force of submaximal contractions (less effort per stride), it may be ergogenic. In addition, the CNS effects could partially ameliorate the negative effects of central fatigue.

A review of the many studies over the years that have examined the potential ergogenic potential of caffeine in endurance exercise performance would be tedious and relatively uninformative. For this reason, I have chosen to review only the studies that have actually used open-ended performance tasks or some other measure of performance (eg, total force output over 2 h). Several studies have used closed-ended methods, with no true performance indicators. These studies help in understanding mechanisms but do not address performance per se and are not considered here. Only studies published in peer-reviewed journals that used randomized double-blind designs are included, with the exception of the two reports[10,11] from Costill's laboratory, where a single-blind (subject only) design was used. However, because of the pioneering nature of this work and the careful controls and important outcome variables that were measured, these were included.

The pioneering studies by Costill's laboratory in the late 1970s were instrumental in popularizing caffeine use among athletes during the big explosion of marathon running at that time. In the first study,[10] nine subjects were randomized to caffeinated ($\sim$5 mg/kg) or decaffeinated coffee and cycled at 80% VO_{2max} until exhaustion. They found a 20% improvement in the time to fatigue when the subjects consumed caffeine. In a similar study reported the next year,[11] these same authors reported a 7.4% improvement in total force output over a 2-hour cycle after ingestion of about 7 mg/kg caffeine in nine subjects. A study by Graham and Spriet[15] showed a 44% increase in cycling time to fatigue at 85% VO_{2max} in seven elite athletes for caffeine (9 mg/kg) compared with placebo. This same group[55] later showed a 27% increase in fatigue time in eight subjects during cycle ergometry at 80% VO_{2max}[29] and similar results in habitual caffeine-consuming athletes after 0, 2, and 4 days of caffeine withdrawal.

In treadmill running, four studies[15,22,56,57] have demonstrated even more impressive increases in performance. Two of the studies[22,56] used treadmill running at 80% VO_{2max}, and found improvements in performance time of 37% and 33% with caffeine doses of 4.4 and 6.6 mg/kg, respectively. In addition to the cycling trial above, Graham and Spriet[15] also incorporated a running trial at approximately 85% VO_{2max} and found a 51% increase in running time. A subsequent study by the same group[57] showed that 3 and 6 mg/kg caffeine improved running performance at 85% VO_{2max} in eight male subjects by 22%.

In spite of the difficulties in completing "field" studies, a randomized, double-blind study of elite nordic skiers[58] showed performance improvements of 1.7% and 3.2% at sea level and 2,900 m after caffeine administration (6 mg/kg). It should be noted that the difficulties in controlling extraneous factors make field studies prone to type II errors (failure to detect a difference when in reality one exists).

Taken together, the above studies show that caffeine is ergogenic to endurance activities at 75% to 85% VO_{2max} and that it may be ergogenic in high-intensity anaerobic activities. However, the data are much more convincing for the long-term endurance activities. An interesting recent study[12] showed that equivalent doses of caffeine consumed in coffee or as caffeine citrate in a liquid vehicle increased performance at 85% VO_{2max} only in the caffeine citrate trial. This may indicate that the consumption of large amounts of caffeine as coffee may not be ergogenic and still could result in a doping infraction! It is critical to note that all of the aforementioned performance studies used caffeine doses that would not likely be considered a doping infraction under current IOC guidelines. This calls into question the rationale for the current IOC guidelines and suggests that consideration should be given to lowering it. Even halving the current urine level of 12 mg/L to 6 mg/L would go a long way toward curtailing its ergogenic use yet allow moderate use by those who enjoy a cup of coffee in the morning before a race! A summary of the effects of caffeine during endurance exercise and the potential ergogenic effects is presented in Table 8–3.

CARBOHYDRATES

Structure and Metabolism

The macronutrient carbohydrates important in athletics are glucose, fructose, sucrose, and glucose polymers or starch. Glucose and fructose are monosaccharides (each a 6-carbon sugar); sucrose is a disaccharide (2 monosaccharides, glucose and fructose); glucose polymers are synthetic polysaccharides of 8 to 24 glucose moieties; and starch is a natural polysaccharide of many glucose moieties. The monosaccharides and disaccharides are also referred to as simple sugars, and starch and glucose polymers are considered complex carbohydrates. This distinction has physiologic relevance because the polysaccharides are absorbed more slowly than the simple sugars and induce a lesser peak insulin plasma concentration. All of these carbohydrates are compounds containing carbon (C), hydrogen (H), and oxygen (O) at a ratio of about

TABLE 8–3. Potential Ergogenic Effects of Caffeine in Endurance Exercise

EFFECT	REFERENCE
Increased free fatty acid oxidation	10,11,20–24
Glycogen sparing	20,24,27
Increase in low-frequency forcep	41,42
Central facilitation	10,11

$1C:2H:1O$, which is partially responsible for their increased metabolic efficiency (energy/mol O_2) as compared with fats, which are more reduced (ie, less O).

A detailed discussion of carbohydrate digestion and absorption is beyond the scope of this chapter, and thus the focus here is on the intestinal transport of glucose and fructose. Glucose is absorbed in the jejeunum via a Na^+-dependent facilitated process that is linked to an ATP-dependent process. The glucose is transported via a glucose transporter called GLUT–2 along with Na^+; the glucose then enters the blood via the basolateral intestinal membrane via a GLUT–5 transporter, and Na^+ is actively (ATP dependent) transported via a basolateral membrane Na^+/K^+ ATPase pump. Thus the facilitated glucose transport is linked to an active process. Fructose transport is independent of glucose transport, and occurs via a distinct facilitated transport process. This has relevance to sports, because it has been shown[59] that the oxidation of 50 g of fructose + 50 g of glucose during exercise was greater than 100 g of glucose, and this was partially attributed to the distinct transport pathways described. Caution must be used with fructose ingestion because the intestinal transport capacity may be as low as 30 g in some individuals, and intake higher than this can lead to diarrhea.[60]

Another practical aspect of intestinal transport is that high concentrations of simple sugars in the intestine inhibit gastric emptying owing to high osmolality.[61,62] This was the impetus for companies to manufacture glucose polymers (several glucose molecules joined together) because the osmolality of a solution is a function of the number of particles and not the total gram molecular weight. In theory one should be able to deliver a greater total sugar load to the intestine with glucose polymers than with monomers, particularly during exercise, when splanchnic perfusion is already reduced. An additional benefit from the lower osmolality of glucose polymers comes from the lesser requirements for water secretion into the intestinal lumen to dilute the sugar, leading to a net loss of fluid from the bloodstream.[63]

Once in the bloodstream, glucose is transported into the muscle via GLUT–4 and GLUT–1 transporters. GLUT–1 is considered a basal transporter, and GLUT–4 migration to the sarcolemma is sensitive to both muscle contraction and insulin.[64,65] Both of these transporters increase in total numbers in response to endurance exercise training, which may explain the enhanced ability of trained athletes to carbohydrate load.[65,66]

In the resting state, much of the glucose that enters the muscle is converted to glycogen via the glycogen synthase pathway. Glycogen is a form of stored polysaccharide that consists of a protein backbone (glycogenin) and linear and branched glucose moieties. Glycogen is found as a dynamic and smaller molecular weight species termed proglycogen, and at higher glycogen concentrations a larger and less metabolically labile form termed macroglycogen is formed. The exact role of these two forms of glycogen during exercise is currently being explored.[67]

During exercise, glycogen is broken down by the enzyme phosphorylase and enters the glycolytic pathway. Fructose is predominantly taken up by the liver for glycogen storage and oxidation, yet it can enter the glycolytic pathway as well; however, during endurance exercise the vast majority of carbon comes from intramuscular glycogenolysis.

Pyruvate is the 3-C molecule "at the end" of glycolysis and under aerobic conditions enters the tricarboxylic acid (TCA) after a decarboxylation step catalyzed by pyruvate dehydrogenase. The TCA cycle produces reducing equivalents that enter oxidative phosphorylation at complex I (NADH) and complex II ($FADH_2$) and form ATP via ATP synthase (complex V).

A summary of glucose metabolism is presented in Figure 8–1.

Habitual Diet/Carbohydrate Loading

It was known in the 1930s that a high-carbohydrate diet increased endurance exercise performance, compared with a high-fat diet.[68] It was not until the late 1960s that this was shown to be due to a higher intramuscular glycogen concentration. The "classic" studies of glycogen loading were reported in 1967, and showed that exhaustive exercise, followed by 3 days of high fat and protein intake, followed by 3 days of high carbohydrate intake (>75% CHO), resulted in higher muscle glycogen than did a high-carbohydrate diet alone.[1,69] For more than a de-

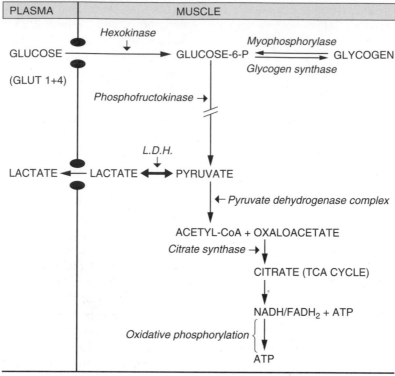

Italicized words indicate important enzymes (except oxidative phosphorylation where 5 enzyme complexes [I–V] are required). *LDH* = lactate dehydrogenase.

FIGURE 8–1. Summary of glucose metabolism in skeletal muscle. Italicized words represent important enzymes, except oxidative phosphorylation, in which five enzyme complexes (I–V) are required.

cade, this classic form of glycogen loading was utilized by long-distance runners.

In 1981, Sherman et al[70] showed that similar increases in intramuscular glycogen were observed with a "modified" glycogen-loading strategy consisting of exhaustive exercise followed by tapering of training volume and a carbohydrate intake of more than 70% (~8 g/kg/d) for 4 days. This method averts the unpleasant high fat and protein phase of the classic method, and with similar improvements in performance, it has become the favored method. Another consideration is that there are gender differences in glycogen loading. In 1995, Tarnopolsky et al[8] reported that male athletes increased muscle glycogen and endurance exercise performance time by just over 40%, whereas females neither increased muscle glycogen nor performance in response to a modified glycogen-loading protocol. This may be partially due to the lower overall energy intake by the female athletes even when expressed relative to lean body mass; however, there may be other intrinsic differences, which

we are now investigating (GLUT–4, glycogen synthase, hexokinase activity).

Anecdotally, some athletes have complained of a feeling of stiffness in the muscles after loading and weight gain. These are both due to the net water retention that is obligatory with the increased glycogen intake. It should be noted that glycogen loading is likely to benefit only athletes competing in events that require intensity of 65% to 85% $V_{O_{2max}}$ and that last longer than 60 minutes, ie, when glycogen stores may become limiting.

Experts commonly recommend that carbohydrates represent at least 65% of daily energy intake based upon the early work in dietary-glycogen relationships. In addition, a 1971 study by Costill et al[71] showed that runners who ran j10 miles per day on a treadmill could not complete their workout on the third day while consuming a diet that contained 45% carbohydrate but could do so on a diet supplying 70% carbohydrate. Another study[72] showed that after 7 days of adaptation there were no performance impairments when subjects consumed 42% as opposed to 84% dietary carbohydrate. Humans can adapt to a prolonged high-fat diet during endurance exercise training and show no performance decrement.[73] However, these low-carbohydrate diets do not conform to American Heart Association and Canadian Recommended Nutrient Intake guidelines, which suggest that at least 60% of energy intake be carbohydrate. Furthermore, the popular 40:30:30 diet has not been shown to confer any advantage to the traditional recommendations, and there is no scientific basis in recommending that 30% of energy intake be in the form of protein.[74] A summary of glycogen loading strategies is found in Table 8–4.

Supplementation Before and During Competition

The prerace period depends upon the time of the event. Most sporting events take place in the morning; thus there are usually only a few hours before a race. To my knowledge, no specific studies have indicated whether a particular early morning snack is of ergogenic benefit. However, some general suggestions are prudent, based upon physiologic principles. These include high carbohydrate content, to optimize liver glycogen stores to be used in maintenance of plasma glucose; low fiber, to prevent gas and fecal bulk; and an energy content of no more than 4 to 5 kcal/kg to prevent the presence of undigested food in the gut at the onset of vigorous exercise. There was initial concern about carbohydrate consumption in the hour before exercise, based upon a single study[75] that showed that glucose consumed 1 hour prior to exercise

resulted in a large increase in insulin, which at the onset of exercise inhibited FFA use and promoted hypoglycemia (impaired exercise performance).

Subsequent studies have shown that consumption of carbohydrate 1 to 2 g/kg in the hour prior to exercise increases glucose availability and oxidation,[76,77] and others have shown improved endurance exercise performance.[78,79] There is no general consensus as to the type of carbohydrate supplement to be taken during this time. In theory, however, a combination of fructose and glucose polymers (the latter representing the largest proportion) would be ideal. This would take advantage of the different sugar transporters at a time when splanchnic blood-flow is adequate, the fructose would optimize liver glycogen stores, and the lower osmolality of the polymers would facilitate gastric emptying and attenuate lumenal water flux.

Dozens of studies have examined carbohydrate supplementation during exercise. These supplements have been shown to increase carbohydrate oxidation,[27,59,80–83] reduce intramuscular glycogen utilization,[27] and enhance endurance exercise performance.[22,81,84,85] There is no consensus as to the type of carbohydrate supplement because these effects have been seen with glucose, glucose polymers, and fructose (the latter only as a mixture with glucose). As a rule the concentration of carbohydrate is typically 6% to 8%, and the rate of provision must be at least 1 g/kg/h.

In most studies, the carbohydrate was provided in divided doses, usually every 10 to 15 minutes or as wanted. In every case there was sodium in the drinks (to promote glucose uptake via the Na^+-dependent transporter), and the concentration was 20 to 60 mmol/L. For some reason, most commercially available drinks also contain K^+ between 2 to 8 mmol/L. I do not see the logic behind this *during* exercise because plasma $[K^+]$ increases with exercise, and its accumulation in the T tubule can cause conduction block and may be involved in the genesis of fatigue.[86] Nevertheless, it is difficult to avoid K^+ because it is in the commercial products and is also found in most juices. It would seem to make sense to design a commercial drink that does not contain K^+ for use *during* exercise (before and after exercise, some K^+ may be of benefit to maintain or replace intracellular stores).

TABLE 8–4. Glycogen Loading Strategies

STRATEGY	REFERENCE
Classic method	1,7,69
Exhaustive exercise for 3 days at ~10% CHO, then 3 days at ~90% CHO	
Modified method	7,70
Taper exercise over 6 days at ~50% CHO for 3 days, then 70% CHO for 3 days	

CHO, carbohydrate.

A summary of before and during exercise carbohydrate supplementation is presented in Table 8–5.

Supplementation After Exercise

There was a burst of interest in the timing of postexercise nutritional supplementation in the late 1980s with a clever study by Ivy et al,[87] who showed that the provision of carbohydrate immediately after exercise resulted in a more rapid rate of glycogen synthesis over the ensuing 2 hours as compared with the same supplement provided 2 hours after exercise. Subsequent work by the same group[88] showed that the form of carbohydrate (ie, liquid, solid, IV) did not influence the rate of glycogen resynthesis. Further research by the same group[89] showed that the addition of protein to the carbohydrate sup-

---

TABLE 8–5. Carbohydrate Supplementation Before and During Exercise

Preexercise Supplementation

4 Hours before*
　~200–400 kcal
　Low fiber
　High carbohydrate (complex/starch)
1 Hour before
　Liquid supplement (function of heat and
　　humidity)†
　6%–8% carbohydrate
　Glucose or glucose polymers + fructose
　　(maximum, 30 g of fructose)
　Warm up during this time
　Sodium (20–60 mmol/L) and potassium
　　(2–8 mmol/L)

During Exercise Supplementation

　Liquid supplement (function of heat and
　　humidity)
　6%–8% glucose or glucose polymers
　Sodium (20–60 mmol/L) and potassium (as low
　　as possible)
　Drink frequently

---

*Only if the competition is in the late morning.

†The amount of fluid is hard to determine and is a function of temperature and humidity. At 20°C, with low humidity, consume at least 125–150 mlq 15 min, and this can be increased substantially with increased humidity and temperature. As a rule of thumb, try to keep the urine clear before a race and start drinking fluids early. Also, practice any suggestion in training to determine individual tolerance.

---

plement resulted in an even greater rate of resynthesis. However, the additional protein also added 43% more energy, so it was unclear whether it was the macronutrient ratio or the total energy that was responsible for this observation.

We[90] showed that the rate of glycogen repletion is similar for *isoenergetic* carbohydrate and carbohydrate protein postexercise supplements, which suggests that protein per se does not increase the rate of resynthesis. We also extended these observations by showing that female athletes demonstrate a postexercise resynthesis response similar to that in male athletes.[90] This is important because it demonstrates that an athlete can consume a more "balanced" supplement in the post-exercise period and derive the same benefits. This is important when one considers that a 50-kg female consuming 2,000 kcal/d could consume 600 to 700 kcal of simple sugar replacement drinks if carbohydrate-only drinks are taken during and after exercise.

A subsequent study showed that the timing of the postexercise supplements did not affect glycogen concentrations after 24 hours, provided carbohydrate intake was high during this period.[90] Therefore, the timing and rapidity of postexercise supplementation may not be so important to subsequent performance, provided a high carbohydrate intake is consumed and that adequate time is taken between bouts of exercise (?24 h). However, if an athlete is performing more than one bout of exercise in a day (training or competition), the timing may take on greater importance. The issue of postexercise supplementation in resistance exercise is discussed in Chapter 3.

I am aware of only one study in which the effects of postexercise, preexercise, and during-exercise carbohydrate supplementation were compared with those of placebo and two different preexercise and during-exercise supplements. We[90] compared a placebo drink during a simulated duathalon (running for 1 h at 76% VO_{2max} plus cycling at 85%–90% VO_{2max} to exhaustion) in elite male athletes with three other conditions:

- Trial A consisted of 3 days of postexercise carbohydrate-protein supplementation + 600 ml over the hour before exercise (8% solution of 75% glucose polymers + 25%

fructose) + 600 ml over the hour of running (8% solution of 37% glucose + 63% glucose polymers [no potassium]).

- Trial B was the same as trial A but with no postexercise supplement for 3 days before exercise.
- Trial C was the same as trial B, but the drink was 100% glucose and contained 3.7 mmol/L potassium.

We found a 24% increase in endurance time for trial A ($P <.05$), 21% for trial B (NS), and 7% for trial C (NS), as compared with placebo. The improvements in exercise capacity in trial A were cotemporal with lower plasma $[K^+]$, higher total carbohydrate oxidation, and higher plasma glucose concentrations.[91] Essentially, this experiment was a practical trial designed to test the performance efficacy of a combination of the aforementioned suggestions contained in this review of the literature.

CONCLUSIONS

Caffeine

Caffeine consumption (4–6 mg/kg) 1 hour before exercise appears to enhance endurance exercise performance at intensities of 65% to 85% $V_{O_{2max}}$. There does not appear to be any benefit to maximal strength, nor to graded exercise to exhaustion tests (ie, $V_{O_{2max}}$ tests), although in high-intensity exercise, predominantly anaerobic bouts, there may be some performance improvement. Intake of 4 to 6 mg/kg caffeine likely would not exceed the current IOC "legal" limit. Consideration should be given to lowering the IOC limit because as it currently stands, many athletes could obtain an ergogenic effect. Any athlete considering caffeine ingestion should consider the pharmacokinetics, ethical considerations related to doping per se, and potential short-term side effects (anxiety, diuresis, increased intestinal motility).

Carbohydrate Supplementation

The current evidence still supports that most individuals should habitually derive more than 60% of daily energy intake from carbohydrates, despite some reports showing that persons can adapt to a higher fat or protein diet. For endurance events in which intramuscular glycogen may limit performance (ie, exercise at 70%–85% $V_{O_{2max}}$ for >75 min), the modified glycogen loading protocol outlined above should improve performance in male athletes. Further work is required to determine whether modifications (ie, increased absolute carbohydrate or energy) may allow carbohydrate loading by female athletes.

Four hours before a race, depending on the start time of the race, an athlete should consume a high-carbohydrate snack with low fiber content. In the hour before a race, the consumption of 600 to 1,000 ml of a liquid CHO supplement will likely improve performance at the above-mentioned intensities and duration. During exercise, consumption of a liquid carbohydrate supplement (6%–8% carbohydrate) at 150 to 250 ml every 15 minutes will likely improve performance. Carbohydrate intake before exercise may contain fructose; however, during exercise the fructose intake should be low to none, and potassium concentration should be as low as possible.

After exercise, it is important to consume a carbohydrate supplement (1–2 g/kg) within the first 30 minutes if one is going to exercise later in the day. Supplements with 10 to 15 g of protein and even small amounts of fat in addition to the carbohydrate do not affect the rate of glycogen resynthesis, and they allow for a more "balanced" supplement. If an athlete is not training or competing until the next day, it is not critical to consume carbohydrate within the first 30 minutes after exercise; however, overall carbohydrate intake over the ensuring 24 hours should be high (>6 g/kg).

REFERENCES

1. Bergström J, Hermansen L, Hultman E, Saltin B: Diet, muscle glycogen and physical performance. Acta Physiol Scand 71:140–150, 1967
2. Grobbee DE, Rimm EB, Giovannucci E, et al: Coffee, caffeine, and cardiovascular disease in men. N Engl J Med 323:1026–1032, 1990
3. Pozniak PC: The carcinogenicity of caffeine and coffee: a review. J Am Diet Assoc 85:1127–1132, 1985
4. Tarnopolsky MA: Caffeine and endurance performance. Sports Med 18:109–125, 1994
5. Ahlborg B, Bergström J, Ekelund L-G, Hultman E: Muscle glycogen and muscle electrolytes during

prolonged physical exercise. Acta Physiol Scand 70:129–142, 1967

6. Karlsson J, Saltin B: Diet, muscle glycogen, and endurance performance. J Appl Physiol 31:203–206, 1971

7. Burke LM, Read RSD: A study of carbohydrate loading techniques used by marathon runners. Can J Sport Sci 12:6–10, 1987

8. Tarnopolsky MA, Atkinson SA, Phillips SM, MacDougall JD: Carbohydrate loading and metabolism during exercise in males and females. J Appl Physiol 78:1360–1368, 1995

9. Costill DL, Coyle E, Dalsky G, et al: Effects of elevated plasma FFA and insulin on muscle glycogen usage during exercise. J Appl Physiol 43:695–699, 1977

10. Costill DL, Dalsky G, Fink W: Effects of caffeine ingestion on metabolism and exercise performance. Med Sci Sports Exerc 10:155–158, 1978

11. Ivy JL, Costill DL, Fink WJ, Lower RW: Influence of caffeine and carbohydrate feedings on endurance performance. Med Sci Sports Exerc 11:6–11, 1979

12. Graham TE, Hibbert E, Sathasivam P: Metabolic and exercise endurance effects of coffee and caffeine ingestion. J Appl Physiol 85:883–889, 1998

13. Patwardhan RV, Desmond PV, Johnson RF, et al: Impaired elimination of caffeine by oral contraceptive steroids. J Lab Clin Med 95:603–608, 1980

14. van der Merwe PJ, Luus HG, Barnard JG: Caffeine in sports: influence of endurance exercise on the urinary caffeine concentration. Int J Sports Med 13:74–76, 1992

15. Graham TE, Spriet LL: Performance and metabolic responses to a high caffeine dose during prolonged exercise. J Appl Physiol 71:2292–2298, 1991

16. Wagner JC: How much caffeine is too much in athletes? [letter]. Am J Hosp Pharm 47:303, 1990

17. Zhang Y, Wells J: The effects of chronic caffeine administration on peripheral adenosine receptors. J Pharmacol Exp Ther 254:757–763, 1990

18. Rennie MJ, Holloszy JO: Inhibition of glucose uptake and glycogenolysis by availability of oleate in well-oxygenated perfused skeletal muscle. Biochem J 168:161–170, 1977

19. Hargreaves M, Kiens B, Richter EA: Effect of increased plasma free fatty acid concentrations on muscle metabolism in exercising men. J Appl Physiol 70:194–201, 1991

20. Essig D, Costill DL, vanHandel PJ: Effects of caffeine ingestion on utilization of muscle glycogen and lipid during leg ergometer cycling. Int J Sports Med 1:86–90, 1980

21. Fisher SM, McMurray RG, Berry M, et al: Influence of caffeine on exercise performance in habitual caffeine users. Int J Sports Med 7:276–280, 1986

22. Sasaki H, Takaoka I, Ishiko T: Effects of sucrose or caffeine ingestion on running performance and biochemical responses to endurance running. Int J Sports Med 8:203–207, 1987

23. Tarnopolsky MA, Atkinson SA, MacDougall JD, et al: Physiological responses to caffeine during endurance exercise in habitual caffeine users. Med Sci Sports Exerc 21:418–424, 1989

24. Spriet LL, MacLean DA, Dyck DJ, et al: Caffeine ingestion and muscle metabolism during prolonged exercise in humans. Am J Physiol 262: E891–E898, 1990

25. Knapik JJ, Jones BH, Toner MM, et al: Influence of caffeine on serum substrate changes during running in trained and untrained individuals. In: Knuttgen HG, Vogel JA, Poortmans J (eds): Biochemistry of Exercise. Human Kinetics Publishers, Champaign, Ill, 1983, pp. 514–519.

26. Weir J, Noakes TD, Myburgh K, Adams B: A high carbohydrate diet negates the metabolic effects of caffeine during exercise. Med Sci Sports Exerc 19:100–105, 1987

27. Erickson MA, Schwarzkopf RJ, McKenzie RD: Effects of caffein, fructose, and glucose ingestion on muscle glycogen utilization during exercise. Med Sci Sports Exerc 19:579–583, 1987

28. Bangsbo J, Jacobsen K, Nordberg N, et al: Acute and habitual caffeine ingestion and metabolic responses to steady-state exercise. J Appl Physiol 72:1297–1303, 1992

29. Spriet LL, MacLean DA, Dyck DJ, et al: Caffeine ingestion and muscle metabolism during prolonged exercise in humans. Am J Physiol 262(Endocrinol Metab 25):E891–E898, 1992

30. Giles D, MacLaren D: Effects of caffeine and glucose ingestion on metabolic and respiratory functions during prolonged exercise. J Sport Sci 2:35–46, 1984

31. Casal DC, Leon AS: Failure of caffeine to affect substrate utilization during prolonged running. Med Sci Sports Exerc 17:174–179, 1985

32. Penner R, Neher E, Takeshima H, et al: Functional expression of the calcium release channel from skeletal muscle ryanodine receptor cDNA. FEBS Lett 259:217–220, 1989

33. Edwards RHT, Hill DK, Jones DA, et al: Fatigue of long duration in human skeletal muscle after exercise. J Physiol 272:769–778, 1977

34. Westerblad H, Duty S, Allen DG: Intracellular calcium concentration during low-frequency fatigue in isolated single fibers of mouse skeletal muscle. J Appl Physiol 75:382–388, 1993

35. Weber A, Herz R: The relationship between caffeine contracture of intact skeletal muscle and

the effect of caffeine on reticulum. J Gen Physiol 52:750–759, 1968

36. Connett RJ, Ugol LM, Hammack MJ, et al: Twitch potentiation and caffeine contractures in isolated rat soleus muscle. Comp Biochem Physiol 74C: 349–354, 1983

37. Block BM, Barry SR, Falukner JA: Aminophyline increases submaximal power but not intrinsic velocity of shortening of frog muscle. J Appl Physiol 73:30–35, 1992

38. Aubier M, DeTroyer A, Sampson M, et al: Aminophyline improves diaphragmatic contractility. N Engl J Med 305:249–252, 1981

39. Supinski GS, Deal EC Jr, Kelsen SG: The effects of caffeine and theophylline on diaphragm contractility. Am Rev Respir Dis 130:429–433, 1984

40. Supinski GS, Levin S, Kelsen SG: Caffeine effect on respiratory muscle endurance and sense of effort during loading breathing. J Appl Physiol 60:2040–2047, 1986

41. Lopes JM, Jardim AJ, Aranda JV, Macklem PT: Effect of caffeine on skeletal muscle function before and after fatigue. J Appl Physiol 54:1303–1305, 1983

42. Tarnopolsky M, Hicks A, Cupido C, McComas AJ: Caffeine and neuromuscular function in humans: no effects of tolerance. Physiologist 35:A 30.15, 201, 1992

43. Lindinger MI, Graham TE, Spriet LL: Caffeine attenuates the exercise-induced increase in plasma $[K^+]$ in humans. J Appl Physiol 74:1149–1155, 1993

44. Clausen T, Flatman JA: The effect of catecholamines on Na-K transport and membrane potential in rat soleus muscle. J Physiol 270:383–414, 1977

45. Perkins R, Williams MH: Effect of caffeine upon maximal muscular endurance of females. Med Sci Sports 7:221–224, 1975

46. Powers SK, Byrd RJ, Tulley R, Callender T: Effects of caffeine ingestion on metabolism and performance during graded exercise. Eur J Appl Physiol Occup Physiol 50:301–307, 1983

47. Gaesser GA, Rich RG: Influence of caffeine on blood lactate responses during incremental exercise. Int J Sports Med 6:207–211, 1985

48. Dodd SL, Brooks E, Powers SK, et al: The effects of caffeine on graded exercise performance in caffeine naïve versus habituated subjects. Eur J Physiol 62:424–429, 1991

49. Falk B, Burstein R, Rosenblum J, et al: Effects of caffeine ingestion on body fluid balance and thermoregulation during exercise. Can J Physiol Pharmacol 68:889–892, 1990

50. Anselme F, Collomp K, Mercier B, et al: Caffeine increases maximal anaerobic power and blood lactate concentration. Eur J Appl Physiol 65: 188–193, 1992.

51. Collomp K, Ahmaidi S, Audran M, et al: Effects of caffeine ingestion on performance and anaerobic metabolism during the Wingate test. Int J Sports Med 12:439–443, 1991

52. Collomp K, Ahmidi S, Chatard JC, et al: Benefits of caffeine ingestion on sprint performance in trained and untrained swimmers. Eur J Appl Physiol 64:377–380, 1992

53. Greer F, McLean C, Graham TE: Caffeine, performance, and metabolism during repeated Wingate exercise tests. J Appl Physiol 85:1502–1508, 1998

54. O'Brien MJ, Viguie CA, Mazzeo RS, et al: Carbohydrate dependence during marathon running. Med Sci Sports Exerc 25:1009–1017, 1993

55. Van Soeren MH, Graham TE: Effect of caffeine on metabolism, exercise endurance, and catecholamine responses after withdrawal. J Appl Physiol 85:1493–1501, 1998

56. Cadarette BS, Levine L, Berube CL, et al: Effects of varied dosages of caffeine on endurance exercise to fatigue. Biochem Exerc 13:871–877, 1983

57. Graham TE, Spriet LL: Metabolic, catecholamine, and exercise performance responses to various doses of caffeine. J Appl Physiol 78:867–874, 1995

58. Berglund B, Hemmingsson P: Effects of caffeine ingestion on exercise performance at low and high altitudes in cross-country skiers. Int J Sports Med 3:234–236, 1982

59. Adopo E, Peronnet F, Massicote D, et al: Respective oxidation of exogenous glucose and fructose given in the same drink during exercise. J Appl Physiol 76:1014–1019, 1994

60. Ravich WJ, Bayless TM, Thomas M: Fructose: incomplete intestinal absorption in humans. Gastroenterology 84:26–29, 1983

61. Mitchell JB, Costill DL, Houmard JA, et al: Gastric emptying: influence of prolonged exercise and carbohydrate concentration. Med Sci Sports Exerc 21:269–274, 1989

62. Rehrer NJ, Wagenmakers AJM, Beckers EJ, et al: Gastric emptying, absorption, and carbohydrate oxidation during prolonged exercise. J Appl Physiol 72:468–475, 1992

63. Massiocotte D, Péronnet F, Brisson G, et al: Oxidation of a glucose polymer during exercise: comparison with glucose and fructose. J Appl Physiol 66:179–183, 1989

64. Roberts CK, Barnard RJ, Scheck SH, Balon TW: Exercise-stimulated glucose transport in skeletal muscle is nitric oxide dependent. Am J Physiol 273(Endocrinol Metab 36):E220–E225, 1997

65. Hickner RC, Fisher JS, Hansen PA, et al: Muscle glycogen accumulation after endurance exercise in trained and untrained individuals. J Appl Physiol 83:897–903, 1997

66. Vukovich MD, Arciero PJ, Kohrt WM, et al: Changes in insulin action and GLUT-4 with 6 days of inactivity in endurance runners. J Appl Physiol 80:240–244, 1996

67. Adamo KB, Tarnopolsky MA, Graham TE: Dietary carbohydrate and the post-exercise synthesis of proglycogen and macroglycogen in human skeletal muscle. Am J Physiol (Endocrinol Metab) 38:E229–E234, 1998

68. Christensen EH, Hansen O: Arbeitsfähigkeit und Ernährung. Skand Arch Physiol 81:160–171, 1939

69. Hultman E, Bergström J: Muscle glycogen synthesis in relation to diet studied in normal subjects. Acta Med Scand 182:109–116, 1967

70. Sherman WM, Costill D, Fink WJ, Miller JM: The effect of exercise and diet manipulation on muscle glycogen and its subsequent utilization during performance. Int J Sports Med 2:114–118, 1981

71. Costill DL, Bowers R, Branan G, Sparks K: Muscle glycogen utilization during prolonged exercise on successive days. J Appl Physiol 31:834–838, 1971

72. Sherman WM, Doyle JA, Lamb DR, Strauss RH: Dietary carbohydrate, muscle glycogen, and exercise performance during 7 d of training. Am J Clin Nutr 57:27–31, 1993

73. Helge JW, Wulff B, Kiens B: Impact of a fat-rich diet on endurance in man: role of the dietary period. Med Sci Sports Exerc 30:456–461, 1998

74. Tarnopolsky MA, MacDougall JD, Atkinson SA: Influence of protein intake and training status on nitrogen balance and lean body mass. J Appl Physiol 64:187–193, 1988

75. Foster C, Costill DL, Fink WJ: Effects of pre-exercise feedings on endurance performance. Med Sci Sports Exerc 11:1–5, 1979

76. Brouns F, Rehrer NJ, Saris WHM, et al: Effect of carbohydrate intake during warming-up on the regulation of blood glucose during exercise. Int J Sports Med 10(suppl 1):S68–S75, 1989

77. Febbraio MA, Stewart KL: CHO feeding before prolonged exercise: effect of glycemic index on muscle glycogenolysis and exercise performance. J Appl Physiol 81:1115–1120, 1996

78. Sherman WM, Peden MC, Wright DA: Carbohydrate feedings 1 h before exercise improves cycling performance. Am J Clin Nutr 54:866–870, 1991

79. Coggan AR, Swanson SC: Nutritional manipulations before and during endurance exercise: effects on performance. Med Sci Sports Exerc 24:S331–S335, 1992

80. Sasaki H, Maeda J, Usui S, Ishiko T: Effect of sucrose and caffeine ingestion on performance of prolonged strenuous running. Int J Sports Med 8:261–265, 1987

81. Davis JM, Lamb DR, Pate RR, et al: Carbohydrate-electrolyte drinks: effects on endurance cycling in the heat. Am J Clin Nutr 48:1023–1030, 1988

82. Brouns F, Saris WHM, Beckers E, et al: Metabolic changes induced by sustained exhaustive cycling and diet manipulation. Int J Sports Med 10(suppl 1):S49–S62, 1989

83. Tarnopolsky MA, Bosman M, MacDonald JR, et al: Postexercise protein-carbohydrate and carbohydrate supplements increase muscle glycogen in men and women. J Appl Physiol 83:1877–1883, 1997

84. Brouns F, Saris WHM, Stroecken J, et al: Eating, drinking, and cycling: a controlled Tour de France simulation study. Part II: Effect of diet manipulation. Int J Sports Med 10 (suppl 1):S41–S48, 1989

85. Murray R, Seifert DE, Eddy DE: Carbohydrate feeding and exercise: effect of beverage carbohydrate content. Eur J Apply Physiol 59:152–158, 1989

86. Sjögaard G: Exercise-induced muscle fatigue: the significance of potassium. Acta Physiol Scand 593(suppl):1–63, 1990

87. Ivy JL, Katz AL, Cutler CL, et al: Muscle glycogen synthesis after exercise: effect of time of carbohydrate ingestion. J Appl Physiol 64:1480–1485, 1988

88. Reed MJ, Brozinick JT Jr, Lee MC, Ivy JL: Muscle glycogen storage postexercise: effect of mode of carbohydrate administration. J Appl Physiol 66:720–726, 1989

89. Zawadski KM, Yaspelkis BB III, Ivy JL: Carbohydrate-protein complex increases the rate of muscle glycogen storage after exercise. J Appl Physiol 72:1854–1859, 1992

90. Tarnopolsky MA, Dyson K, Atkinson SA, et al: Mixed carbohydrate supplementation increases carbohydrate oxidation and endurance exercise performance and attenuates potassium accumulation. Int J Sport Nutr 6:323–336, 1996

91. Burke LM, Collier GR, Beasley SK, et al: Effect of coingestion of fat and protein with carbohydrate feedings on muscle glycogen storage. J Appl Physiol 78:2187–2192, 1995

THERAPEUTICS IN SPORTS MEDICINE

Physical Therapy Management of the Injured Athlete

ANITA GROSS ▪ LIZ HARRISON ▪ BERT CHESWORTH ▪ ANITA SYMONDS PERRIGO

The physical therapy management of sports injuries integrates knowledge and skills from a number of physical therapy areas, including orthopedics, and neuromuscular, cardiovascular, and respiratory therapy. The unique aspect of physical therapy for athletes is to assess and manage individuals who are performing activities at many kinematic and kinetic levels above what is considered normal. Thus evaluation in sports injuries is multifaceted and integrative and includes the following clinical judgments:

1. Diagnosis/Cause
   a. Arrive at a clinical diagnosis, identify the tissue at fault (pathophysiologic entity), determine the immediate predisposing and maintaining factors
   b. Determine whether further evaluation by a physician or other professional is required
2. Prognosis: Estimate the outcome of the disorder and plan the appropriate course of therapy with specific short-term and long-term goals, for the athlete
3. Measurement: Establish outcome measures responsive to treatment effect
4. Therapy/Harm
   a. Determine whether therapy may be of benefit
   b. Determine cautions and contraindications to therapy
   c. Decide which therapy technique to use
   d. Judge the parameters of the therapy technique
   e. Determine links with other management strategies

Many assessment tools and techniques may not have the properties necessary to accurately detect relevant differences in this population. In addition, the detection of abnormality is further compromised by lack of normal values for athletic activities. A simple example is the evaluation of range of motion and flexibility. A gymnast must have extreme spinal range of motion to successfully perform certain events. The ranges obtained by many athletes are in excess of the normal values required for activities of daily living such as walking or stair climbing.

These high levels of function require that the physical therapist develop or adapt assessment and treatment techniques or tools to fit these tasks. In addition, there is a need to determine reasonable normative values for various athletes. To date, there is little published information on normative data related to sports.

The area of functional evaluation must address the muscle and connective tissue structures, as well as the physiologic systems that move the body. In addition, the physical therapist must assess the individual within very challenging and changing environments. Many activities expose the athlete to external forces that cannot be controlled or even predicted. Determining the probability that certain outcomes will occur as part of the natural history of a disorder is a further challenge to the physical therapist. Risk of injury and the opportunity for recovery are determined in part by the type of sport, and this must be considered when developing prevention or rehabilitation programs. A clinician must address these risk factors if the goal is to return an athlete to his or her sport. This may be one of the most serious flaws in therapeutic programs that do not match the individual to the environment.

Psychological factors relative to the athlete and the sport influence the physical therapist's interaction with the individual and affect outcomes. Methods for evaluating these factors and addressing them within a rehabilitation program add to the multifaceted approach to treatment. Working with other health professionals such as psychologists, physicians, nutritionists, and pharmacists is essential to providing comprehensive management. In addition, it is essential that physical therapists have a working knowledge of sports, and wherever possible a formal link to the coaches, trainers, sports organizations, and parents of child athletes.

To determine the best evidence on which to manage athletic injuries or conditions, one must search a variety of areas linking basic science and clinical science in such fields as physical therapy, orthopedics, sports medicine, sports physical therapy, and exercise physiology.

There are many traditions in sports and sports medicine. Although traditions must not be neglected, since in some cases they are the basis for the art of practice, it is essential that diagnostic and assessment procedures and techniques, prognostic indicators, and treatments be critically appraised to ensure that time, energy, and resources are used to enhance an athlete's health and performance. In many cases the lack of research in sports injury management has propagated use of less effective and poorly based treatments. This chapter evaluates the evidence for diagnosis, measurement, prognosis, and therapy in some common areas of sports physical therapy practice.

DIAGNOSIS AND MEASUREMENT

Evaluation Methods

Properties of evaluation methods or tools depend on the goals of the measurement. The following questions should be posed when the appropriateness of test procedures in athletic populations is evaluated:

1. Is there evidence of reliability testing?
   a. Test-retest (intrarater), between raters (interrater), and internal consistency of components of the test (eg, in questionnaires or physical examinations that include various tests).
   b. Components of function (eg, mobility, muscle strength, flexibility, aerobic and anaerobic capacity) vary among athletes in different types of sports. Athletes may demonstrate more extremes of change because of training, season, and level of competition or practice.
2. How has validity been investigated? Was the population being investigated relevant to the problem (eg, athletic population, age specific)? Were testers and clinicians blind to the condition? Was there a comparison reference (gold standard)? Normal values or gold standards may be difficult to obtain for sports owing to the large variation in athletes. An impairment or disability for an athlete may be defined differently depending on the physical requirements of a sport.
3. Is it feasible (cost, facility, equipment) to perform this test in your setting? Consideration of protective equipment is important relative to effect on results of testing. Some testing procedures require expensive equipment or specialized facilities that may not be available.
4. Can you determine what a clinically relevant finding would be? Relevant change is not simply the ability to compete or not compete. In evaluating relevant change, one must consider all aspects of the activity. In addition to examining physical components of the activity, change related to other factors should be investigated, eg, level of activity (training, practice, competition), length of time that an athlete can participate, and quality of performance.
5. Will the test findings affect management of the client? Measures that do not appropriately represent the physical requirements of the athlete will not provide useful information on which to base treatment.

It is important to define the role of evaluation and testing procedures and understand measurement properties. Diagnostic tests such as ligamentous stress testing are used to identify the specific structure or organ involved. Although useful for diagnosis, these tests may not be appropriate for evaluation of treatment programs.

Measurement properties that should be evaluated when selecting clinical tests include sensitivity and specificity. *Sensitivity* is the ability of a test to accurately detect the presence of a condition or injury, ie, a positive finding. *Specificity* is the ability of a test to correctly identify when there is no injury or disorder, ie, negative findings.[1]

Outcome measures must be reliable, valid, and have the capacity to detect relevant clinical change. Prognostic testing is used to predict long-term function. The degree of importance of the various properties depends on whether the test is focused primarily on diagnosis, outcome evaluation, or prognosis. It is imperative that clinicians determine the goal of testing before interpreting test results. Finally, and perhaps most important to their validity, measurement tools and methods must be easy to administer and record; otherwise, clinicians will not incorporate them into busy clinical settings. This is more challenging in sports injury management because the clinician is often in a nonclinical, less controlled environment, and tests and evaluation methods may not be feasible. None of the studies reviewed investigated the effect of the sports environment on the validity of measurement.

Diagnostic and Outcome Measures

The literature on musculoskeletal evaluation methods is extensive. For the purpose of this chapter, we gathered evidence on evaluation methods relevant to clinical diagnosis and outcome measures in sports physical therapy by performing a hand search of five journals (1995–1998): *The American Journal of Sports Medicine, The Clinical Journal of Sports Medicine, The Journal of Orthopedic and Sports Physical Therapy, Physiotherapy,* and *Physical Therapy*. The search was limited to research articles related to evaluation of the shoulder, knee, and ankle. Of the 77 articles considered, the majority (47) investigated the knee, 16 evaluated the shoulder, and 14, the ankle. The studies varied from literature searches to clinical trials. Of those articles reviewed, the majority (58) reported findings based on nonathlete populations. Both male and female subjects were well represented in the studies. The most common age of populations studied was young adult to middle age (20–40

years), and a few studies were done in younger or older populations. The relevance of this finding is that specific diagnostic tests and outcome measures may not be applicable in athletic, pediatric, or senior populations.

Based on this review, it is apparent that the focus on evaluation continues to be primarily in the area of diagnostic testing, which is aimed at arriving at a clinical diagnosis, identifying the structure at fault, identifying predisposing or contributing factors, and determining referral or treatment. Research into outcome measures, which are used to monitor and evaluate treatment effectiveness and change in a condition over time, is increasing as clinicians become more interested in function and disability versus impairment alone. However, the limited number of studies specific to athletic populations decreases the potential validity and application to sports injury management. Evidence supports the need to consider revision of tools for physically active populations.[1–3]

Taken from our 5-year review, examples of investigations on impairments and functional measures for the ankle, knee, and shoulder are presented in Table 9–1. These studies evaluated various measurement properties of musculoskeletal diagnostic methods and outcome measures. Those that investigated primarily athletic populations are identified.

There is moderate evidence to support reliability, as well as reasonable sensitivity and specificity, of several diagnostic tests. Components of physical examinations of the knee and ankle have shown good reliability and validity. Fewer studies have investigated shoulder diagnostic testing; thus less evidence is available to support validity of physical examination. Glenoid labral tears have been diagnosed effectively with physical examination compared with magnetic resonance imaging (MRI).[4,5] Similarly Muellner et al[6] found good results for clinical evaluation of meniscal tears in comparison with MRI. In regard to outcome measures, there is potential for more variability depending on the populations evaluated. As noted, there are few studies on athletes. Mohtadi[7] described a quality-of-life measurement scale that may have promise for athletic populations after anterior cruciate ligament (ACL) reconstruction, based on early results. Other tools, such as the patient-specific functional scale,[3] have yet to be investigated in

TABLE 9–1. Summary of Recent Studies Evaluating Common Impairment and Functional Outcome Measures for Ankle, Knee, and Shoulder Regions

DIAGNOSTIC OR IMPAIRMENT TEST	AUTHOR	OUTCOME MEASURE	AUTHOR
Ankle		**Ankle**	
Ligamentous stress tests	Kumbhare[9] Liu et al[4,5]	Motor activity score	*Wilson et al[11]
MRI	Liu et al[4,5]		
Ottawa ankle rules	Leddy et al[10]		
Physical examination	*Wilson et al[11] Kumbhare[9] Liu et al[4,5]		
Knee		**Knee**	
Arthroscopy	Stanitski[13]	Cincinnati	*Sgaglione et al[8]
Clinical meniscal test	*Muellner et al[6]	Functional lower extremity assessment questionnaires	Hoher et al[37] Juris et al[38] Pincivero et al[19] Neeb et al[39] Harrison et al[40] MacIntyre et al[17]
Cyriax selective tissue tension	Franklin et al[14]	Hop test	Sekiya et al[18] Petchnig et al[41]
Inclined squat strength test	Munich et al[15]	KOOS (knee injury and osteoarthritis outcome)	*Roos et al[42]
Limb girth measures	Ross and Worrell[46]	Lysholm knee injury scoring questionnaire	*Demirdjian et al[43] Hoher et al[37] *Sgaglione et al[8]
McGill pain questionnaire	MacIntyre et al[17]	Noyes questionnaire	*Demirdjian et al[43]
MRI	Stanitski[13]	Patient-specific functional scale	Chatman et al[3]
Muscle strength	Sekiya et al[18] Pincivero et al[19]	Quality of life scale	Montadi[7]
Patellofemoral alignment	Tomsich et al[20] Fitzgerald and McClure[21]	SF-36 health assessment	Shapiro et al[44]
Physical examination	Stanitski[13] O'Shea et al[22]	Step test	Harrison et al[28]
Proprioception	Kramer et al[23] *Shiraishi et al[24]	Tegner knee rating system	*Sgaglione et al[8]
Stress tests	Eakin and Cannon[25] Hewett et al[26] Adler et al[27]		
Subjective knee complaints using VAS (visual analogue scale, pain)	Harrison et al[28]		

TABLE 9–1. Summary of Recent Studies Evaluating Common Impairment and Functional Outcome Measures for Ankle, Knee, and Shoulder Regions *Continued*

DIAGNOSTIC OR IMPAIRMENT TEST	AUTHOR	OUTCOME MEASURE	AUTHOR
Shoulder		**Shoulder**	
Anterior slide test	Wright and Hawkins[29]	DASH (disability of arm, shoulder, hand)	Hudak et al[45]
Cyriax differential diagnosis	Pellecchia et al[30]	Rowe and UCLA scale for shoulder conditions	Romeo et al[16]
End-feel/movement diagrams	Chesworth et al[31]	SPADI (shoulder pain and disability index)	Heald et al[2]
Glenoid labral tears	Berg and Ciullo[32]		
Physical examination	Liu et al[4,5]		
Impingement relief	Corso[33]		
Strength	*Scoville et al[34] Hutchinson et al[35] Burnham et al[36]		

MRI, magnetic resonance imaging.
*Study performed in athletic population.

athletic populations. Heald et al[2] found the Sickness Impact Profile (SIP)–36 to be inadequate for evaluation of shoulder disorders. Scales that provide global health ratings may not discriminate higher level functional activities, thus limiting their use in athletic injury management. Sgaglione et al[8] recommended that outcome after ACL surgery is best reported using individual components (ie, subjective, objective, functional) versus overall rating and that symptoms and function should be stratified according to patient activity demands.

Injury Continuum

Evaluation of injuries must be considered on a continuum from acute onset to return to activity. Table 9–2 describes common areas of assessment reported in the literature, including impairment and function relevant to sport performance. Timing of assessment procedures is primarily determined by the theoretical stage of the injury and presentation of signs and symptoms.

On-field or on-site evaluation most commonly involves acute, traumatic episodes involving one or more of the major systems or structures of the body. Evidence on which to promote the most appropriate PT management

of acute injuries is primarily focused on injuries of the musculoskeletal system, which commonly present with inflammation, damage of muscle or soft tissue, fracture of bone, and signs and symptoms of pain. The PT must have a knowledge of and basic skills to provide on-site emergency care for neurovascular, thoracoabdominal, or other system trauma. However, these are most appropriately referred to and managed by a medical practitioner after appropriate first-aid, stabilization, and transportation.

Owing to the nature of sport and injury it is difficult to research the acute problems. Access to patient populations, ethical considerations, and patient compliance are issues that limit this type of study. Most studies evaluating diagnostic tests and outcome measures involve conditions after resolution of the acute stage. Those studies that have investigated acute injury evaluation of the musculoskeletal system focus on identification of impairments through diagnostic testing. Not all studies standardize or report the stage of injury (ie, acuity), which makes it more difficult to interpret results.

In the evaluation of acute injury management and diagnosis a definition of the components of acute injury is helpful. In addition to the definition of acute injury as occurring in the past 24 to 48 hours, further categorization or

TABLE 9–2. Continuum of Impairment and Functional Evaluation: Onset of Injury to Return to Activity

	ACUTE ONSET	SUBACUTE ONSET	RETURN TO ACTIVTY	RETURN TO SPORT
Impairment Evaluation				
Flexibility		x	x	x
Ligament stress test	x	x		
Muscle strength		x	x	x
Pain	x	x	x	
Range of motion	x	x	x	
Sensory or proprioception	x	x		
Selective tissue integrity	x	x		
Vascular	x	x		
Functional Evaluation				
Accuracy			x	x
Agility			x	x
Alignment		x	x	x
Endurance or repetitions			x	x
Power			x	x
Skill			x	x
Speed			x	x
Stability		x	x	x

definition can include variables such as observed or not observed, emergent or urgent, area involved (organ or structure), time of injury (training, practice, competition), and presence of signs and symptoms. Injuries are observed only by clinicians who provide on-site service, and no evidence was found related to the study of this component. Emergent care is most commonly managed on-site by attention to ABCs (airway, breathing, circulation), primary and secondary scans, identification of appropriate first-aid, and coordination of transportation for further medical management. Evaluation techniques applied in emergent situations focus on identification of life-threatening conditions, possible complications, and risk of further injury.

Although extremely important, evidence for emergent evaluation techniques was not reviewed. Urgent care most commonly involves acute injuries resulting in structural damage of the neuromusculoskeletal system. Of those studies that evaluated acute injury, most tests focused on the area involved, and signs and symptoms associated with the injury; other variables were not specified. Most information on vari-

ables such as time of injury are found in the sports injury epidemiology literature. Sports epidemiology knowledge should be more closely linked to the management of injuries, including the development of evaluation methods.

Evidence to validate evaluation of acute injury management is found in the research on sprains. Sprain injuries are common in sport, and perhaps most sports injury research has focused on sprains. Depending on the joint involved, degree of sprain is most commonly assessed clinically by determining the amount of movement palpated during a stress test.[9,13,25,27,29] Depending on the methods of testing and the joint of interest, reliability of tests has been shown to be reasonable. A commonly referenced categorization of ligament sprain defining amount of joint displacement is as follows:

- First degree (mild), <5 mm
- Second degree (moderate), 5 to 10 mm
- Third degree (severe), >8 mm, complete rupture,[26] or >10 mm[39]

Even within this categorization there are some differences because it often is difficult to isolate injuries to a single ligamentous structure.[47]

Validation of diagnostic methods for sprains has commonly used gold standards of imaging techniques or arthroscopy.[12,13] In comparison, outcome measures commonly do not have previously established gold standards.[3] Development of valid outcome measures is challenging and often less applicable across populations.

The range of functional limitations due to an injury depends on the nature and level of the sport and the area and extent of the injury. For example, with an acute ankle sprain an athlete can move quickly from an inability to bear weight to normal ambulation. Although this recovery is significant, the clinician must remember that the functional requirements of sporting activities such as running, jumping, landing, and cutting produce high forces at the ankle joint. It is important that evaluation techniques and treatment programs consider these advanced requirements and build them into testing and exercise programs.[39] Evaluation of joint structures around the ankle should consider the type and intensity of forces that will be applied to contractile and inert structures. Many of the traditional stress tests and analysis of impairments and function of the ankle region do not adequately test the functional requirements.[1] Monitoring of compensatory movements that may occur, especially at the surrounding joints and hip and knee, must also be emphasized to prevent secondary injury or chronic conditions.

Neeb et al[39] reviewed the use of common clinical tests and questionnaires used with ACL reconstruction. The study suggests caution in application of the anterior drawer test because of lack of sensitivity and shows that pivot-shift testing also lacks sensitivity. We also studied the type of questionnaires using disability rating scales and, similar to a study by Heald et al[2] on shoulder problems, found that disability questionnaires must be appropriately designed for athlete populations. Table 9–3 presents examples of measurement properties reported for common diagnostic tools and outcome measures from selected studies of the shoulder, knee, and ankle.

Challenges in Evaluating Athletes

Determining the ability of an athlete to return to practice or competition can be difficult. Often diagnostic tests are used, but they inadequately evaluate function. Typically it is recommended that impairments be resolved before sports activities are resumed. In reality, this is not common practice because many athletes continue to complain of symptoms or have impairments throughout their competitive life. For example, Sekiya et al[18] described the lack of correlation between anterior laxity of the knee and single-leg hopping as a functional activity in ACL reconstructed knees. The mistake commonly made is to consider that the athlete should be either in or out of activity. Return to activity must not be considered "all or none." Components of the sport should be introduced into the program, and testing performed at frequent intervals. The following questions should be addressed:

- Do signs and symptoms subside within a reasonable time?
- Does the tissue or structure appear to be adapting, as evaluated with increased stress?
- Are there other compensatory movements?
- Do the benefits of the activity outweigh the risks?

Research has focused on the impairment level (diagnostic tests); however, comprehensive evaluation measures must continue to be developed relevant to the athletic environment and unique requirements of sporting activities.

Athletes most commonly participate in activities that take place in noncontrolled environments. Development of functional outcomes specific to the area of injury and the activity will enhance the ability to more effectively assess the effect of treatments. Athletic activites include skill, agility, speed, power, and accuracy of movement. To date there is poor evidence to support the link between level of impairment and return to functional levels. However, one must be cautious in the interpretation of poor correlation between the diagnostic test results and outcomes because impairments are measures of structural loss or abnormality and are only one aspect of physical function.[39] The evidence to date suggests that a clinician should not stop at measurement of impairment; however, it would also be foolish to throw out valid clinical tests, as they provide essential information in some cases on which to base treatment. It is important that clinicians consider the purpose

TABLE 9–3. Review of Selected Studies of Common Clinical Evaluation Methods for Shoulder, Knee, and Ankle Regions

AUTHOR	TEST	TYPE OF TEST	PROPERTIES	COMMENTS
Shoulder				
Heald et al[2]	Shoulder pain and disability	Outcome measure	Moderate validity	Not so useful in occupational and recreational population
Chesworth et al[31]	Movement diagram and end-feel in shoulder rotation	Diagnostic measure	Intrarater reliability moderate: ICC = .58–.89, κ = .48–.59 Interrater reliability moderate: ICC = .85–.91, κ = .62–.76	
Knee				
Muellner et al[6]	Clinical examination vs MRI meniscal tears	Diagnostic measure	Clinical examination: Sensitivity = 97% Specificity = 87% Positive predictive value = 92% Negative predictive value = 99% MRI: Sensitivity = 98% Specificity = 86% Positive predictive value = 92% Negative predictive value = 97%	Clinical examination as effective as MRI in diagnosing meniscal tear
Chatman et al[3]	Patient-specific functional scale for knee dysfunction	Outcome measure	Test-retest R = .84 Reasonable sensitivity to change demonstrated	Requires investigation in athlete populations
Sekiya et al[18]	Single-legged hop test, anterior laxity, and muscle strength in ACL reconstruction	Outcome measure	No significant correlation between hop and anterior laxity, and low correlation values with quadriceps muscle strength	
Sgaglione et al[8]	Hospital for Special Surgery Lysholm Score, Tegner Activity Score, Cincinnati	Outcome measure	Cincinnati scale appears better for active and athletic populations	
Zachazewski et al[47]	Literature review of common knee scales	Outcome measure	No specific scale identified as the most useful for athletic population	Reviews a number of scales and provides a comprehensive overview
Neeb et al[39]	Literature review of common knee scales	Outcome measure	Sport Activity Rating System (SARS)	Intrarater reliability moderate
			Factor Occupational Rating System Scale (FORSS) Lysholm Score, Tegner Activity Score One-legged hop: Sensitivity = 52% Specificity = 97% Timed hop test: Sensitivity = 49% Specificity = 94%	Intrarater reliability good
		Diagnostic measure	Lachman test: Sensitivity = 99% Anterior Drawer Test: Sensitivity = 74% KT-1000 ACL Test: Sensitivity = 67%–90% ICC = .83–.88 Pivot-shift test: Sensitivity = 0–98% Specificity = 82%	
Ankle				
Liu et al[12]	Comparison of MRI and clinical examination in anterolateral impingement	Diagnostic measure	Clinical examination: Sensitivity = 94% Specificity = 75% MRI: Sensitivity = 39% Specificity = 50%	

TABLE 9–3. Review of Selected Studies of Common Clinical Evaluation Methods for Shoulder, Knee, and Ankle Regions *Continued*

AUTHOR	TEST	TYPE OF TEST	PROPERTIES	COMMENTS
Leddy et al[10]	Ottawa Ankle Rules	Diagnostic measure	Sensitivity = 100% Specificity = 37%–42%	Clinical practice guidelines based on Ottawa Rules
Wilson et al[11]	Disablement measures following acute ankle sprain	Diagnostic measure	Volumetric measure of swelling responsive to change; ROM not responsive to change; perceived athletic ability and observed motor activity scores responsive to change	

ACL, anterior cruciate ligament; ICC, internal conversion coefficient; ROM, range of motion.

of the test when interpreting the measurement properties.

Diagnostic tests must have reasonable levels of sensitivity and specificity, and outcome measures must demonstrate not only evidence of reliability but also validity, including the ability to detect relevant change. Evidence supports validity of diagnostic tests for evaluation of common sports injuries of the knee and ankle, with less support for shoulder evaluation techniques. Although the majority of outcome measures have not been evaluated in athletic populations, there appears to be great interest in the development of and need for these tools.

PROGNOSIS

Prognosis is the relative probability that a certain outcome will occur as part of the natural history of an illness or disease.[48] Major gaps exist in the sports medicine literature with regard to prognostic issues. This section reviews the evidence regarding prognosis in a common sports injury, rupture of the ACL. The literature review was performed from the perspective of a full-time clinician, who would have computer access to the more commonly used databases for literature searches but limited direct access to sports injury–related journals.

Methods

Two common databases were used in the search strategy: Medline from 1966 to September 1998 and CINAHL abstracts from 1982 to September 1998. The search was conducted using *anterior cruciate ligament* and *prognosis related* medical subject heading (MeSH) terms and *text word* (tw) as search terms. Articles were limited to those that used human subjects and were written in the English language. In addition, a hand search was performed of the *Journal of Orthopaedic and Sports Physical Therapy* and the *American Journal of Sports Medicine* for the 10-year period 1988 to 1998. Articles from our personal files were included. Only studies with 60% or more athletes or sport-related injuries were included.

To guide the review of articles pertaining to prognosis, six questions adapted from Sackett et al[48] were used:

1. Did the authors study an inception cohort?
2. Did the authors describe the referral pattern to your satisfaction?
3. Were all subjects in the inception cohort followed up?
4. Were objective outcomes used?
5. Were study outcomes blindly evaluated?
6. Were other prognostic factors controlled with statistical methods?

Each study was also graded for "level of evidence," as proposed by Sackett et al[49]:

Level I
    Randomized trials
    Significant benefit or no-difference finding
    Large sample size
Level II
    Randomized trials
    Positive trend but no statistical significance or no-difference finding
    Small sample size
Level III
    Concurrent comparisons between treatment groups (nonrandom)

Level IV

Retrospective comparisons: current "treated" vs former "untreated" (nonrandom)

Level V

Case series (no control subjects)

Results

Search Strategy

Table 9–4 summarizes the studies obtained in the above search strategy for ACL-injured athletes. Different study designs were utilized, giving varied levels of evidence; relatively small sample sizes were studied in most cases; subgroups of patients with combined ligamentous injuries were commonly included; and the age of the study cohorts was relatively consistent among investigations. The various study designs reflect different research objectives, which may be one explanation for the varied prognostic findings.

For example, Andersson et al[50,51] compared surgical with nonsurgical ACL treatment and in a quasi-random fashion allocated patients to two treatment groups. Randomization and the significant treatment benefits give their study a level of evidence of I. Alternatively, in a cross-sectional study, Lephart et al[56] recruited athletes with a confirmed ACL injury and grouped subjects into "those who could" and "those who could not" return to preinjury levels of activity. Clinically relevant variables were evaluated to determine their association with return to preinjury activity. Because there were no controls in the study group, we assigned a level of evidence of V. Louden et al[57] used a classic case-control design to determine the relationship between postural variables and ACL injury. Although control subjects were used, treatment comparison was not a study objective; therefore this study was assigned a level of evidence of V. Lundberg and Messner[58] used a similar design to determine whether isolated medial collateral ligament (MCL) injuries (ie, controls) or combined ACL-MCL injuries (ie, cases) yielded a different prognosis. For the same reason, this study was assigned a level of evidence of V. The majority of studies used a case-series approach to document the prognosis for patients with an

TABLE 9–4. Summary of Studies From Prognosis Search Strategy: Anterior Cruciate Ligament Injuries in Athletes

AUTHOR	DESIGN	LEVEL OF EVIDENCE	SAMPLE		MEAN AGE (RANGE)
			TOTAL (N)	SUBGROUP (N)	
Andersson et al[50]	Randomized	I	111	ACL (20), ACL+ (91)	25 (13–49)
Andersson and Gillquist[51]	Randomized	I	107	ACL (55), ACL+ (52)	NR
Barrack et al[52]	Retrospective	V	72	ACL (72)	25 (16–45)
Casteleyn and Handelberg[53]	Retrospective	V	228	ACL (48), ACL+ (180)	33 (16–66)
Daniel et al[54]	Prospective	V	292	Stable (56), unstable (236)	NR (15–44)
Finsterbush et al[55]	Retrospective	V	98	ACL only (98)	26 (13–45)
Lephart et al[56]	Cross-sectional	V	41	Unstable (41)	23 (16–32)
Louden et al[57]	Case-control	V	40	Surgery: yes (8), no (12), controls (20)	26 (16–41)
Lundberg and Messner[58]	Case-control	V	40	ACL (20), ACL + MCL (20)	24 (15–36)
Puddu et al[59]	Prospective	V	62	Meniscectomy (37), ACL + meniscus (25)	22 (16–38)
Robins et al[60]	Retrospective	V	20	ACL + MCL (20)	23 (16–35)
Sommerlath et al[61]	Retrospective	V	22	Partial ACL (22)	29 (13–53)

ACL, anterior cruciate ligament; MCL, medial collateral ligament; +, ACL injury combined with other ligamentous injury of the knee; NR, not reported.

ACL injury, receiving a level of evidence of V.[52-55,59-61] The articles summarized in Table 9–5 consist mainly of level V evidence, which according to Sackett et al[48,49] may provide useful prognostic information. However, caution must be exercised in drawing strict conclusions when interpreting level V evidence.

Small sample sizes may have limited the statistical power to find a significant difference, should one truly exist. This is particularly relevant given the variety of subgroups of ligamentous and meniscal injuries. Furthermore, these subgroups may make generalization of findings more difficult. Therefore, readers should review the study of interest to determine whether the study cohort is comprised of injuries that mirror their clinical setting. The age of patients in a given setting should also be similar. In this regard, it is noted the consistency of patient age in Table 9–4 suggests ACL injuries occur in a reasonably well-defined age group.

Prognosis Evaluation

Table 9–5 summarizes the application of the six prognostic questions outlined by Sackett et al.[48] The study by Puddu et al[59] was not included because their cohort of interest was comprised of high-level semiprofessional and professional athletes. The article by Finsterbush et al[55] was excluded because no prognosis findings were reported. The study by Sommerlath et al[61] was removed because only descriptive information

TABLE 9–5. Summary of Findings After Applying the Six Prognostic Questions Outlined by Sackett et al[48]*

STUDY	INCEPTION COHORT	REFERRALS	FOLLOW-UP (%)	OBJECTIVE OUTCOME CRITERIA	PROGNOSTIC FINDING
Andersson et al[50]	Injury to scope: ≤5 d	96% sports	96	Manual stress tests, function scores, arthrometer, meniscal injury, late surgery	Better return to preinjury sport with augmentation
Andersson and Gillquist[51]	Acute injury	76% sports	93	One-legged hop test, figure-of-8 run, function scores, arthrometer	Better figure-of-8 run time and return to sports with repair
Barrack et al[52]	Acute injury	≥80% sports	82	Function score, late surgery	Meniscal tear at time of injury predicts late ACL surgery
Casteleyn and Handelberg[53]	Injury to scope: ≤3 wk (83%)	60% recreation	48	Age, function score, late surgery, activity modification	No significant prognostic variables
Daniel et al[54]†	Injury to assessment: mean = 4 d	74% sports	75	Arthrometer, sport participation, occupation, symptoms, impairments, one-legged hop test, late surgery	Age, preinjury hours of sports per year, and arthrometer displacement predict late surgery
Lephart et al[56]	Subacute injury	100% athletes	NR	Arthrometer, Cybex, girth, return to activity, ROM, function score, side-step semicircle, lateral cross-over, shuttle run	Return to preinjury athletic activity with higher scores on functional rating scale
Louden et al[57]†	NR	100% athletes	100	Pelvic position, femoral anteversion, hamstring length, standing knee extension, navicular drop, subtalar position	Standing knee extension, navicular drop, and subtalar position significant predictors of ACL-injured group
Lundberg and Messner[58]	Acute injury	93% sports	100	Return-to-work and previous activities, function score, arthrometer, x-rays, reinjury	Combined ligament ruptures predict reinjuries
Robins et al[60]	Injury to surgery: ≤1 wk	90% sports	100	ROM	Slower return of knee extension ROM with proximal MCL lesions

ACL, anterior cruciate ligament; MCL, medial collateral ligament; ROM, range of motion; NR, not reported; d, days; wk, weeks; y, years; mo, months.

*There was no "blind" outcome assessment in any of these studies.

†Performed multivariate analysis.

was provided with no statistical procedures in the results. The remaining nine articles are listed alphabetically.

Columns 2 to 5 in Table 9–5 correspond to the first four questions recommended by Sackett et al.[48] The fifth requirement, regarding "blind" outcome assessment, was not met by any of the studies. The sixth concern, regarding adjustment for additional prognostic factors, is noted by a daggar. Only Daniel et al[54] and Louden et al[57] performed a multivariate analysis.

Prognostic findings reported by each study are included in column 6.

For the studies we reviewed, the six prognostic questions of Sackett et al[48] were answered as follows.

1. **Was an inception cohort studied?** As a group, it appears that the patients studied were identified soon after injury. Half of the studies reported the time between injury and assessment or surgery; others noted more generally that patients were in the acute or subacute phase of injury. Louden et al[57] recruited patients who had undergone arthroscopic examination of an ACL rupture within 2 years of the test date. However, for a number of studies, the extent to which the study samples consisted of first-time ACL or knee injuries is not known. Only three studies[52,54,56] explicitly stated that patients with a prior history of knee surgery were excluded.

2. **Was the referral pattern described?** Noting the referral pattern is important so that readers know if they can generalize findings to their own clinical practice. Since athletes with an ACL injury were the patient group of interest, the proportion of athletes or sports-related injuries has been summarized. Although the proportion varied, it appears to be relatively high. The facilities where patients were recruited were primarily tertiary care hospitals, with the exceptions of a military setting,[52] a U.S. health plan,[54] and a sports medicine facility.[56] This may be important because specialized health care centers, may attract more severe and technically challenging cases, creating a negative bias for prognosis, or because specialized services available from highly trained health care providers may inflate prognostic outcomes.

3. **Was there complete follow-up of the inception cohort?** Follow-up status was determined for the majority of subjects in most of the studies in Table 9–5. The exception was a 48% follow-up achieved by Casteleyn and Handelberg,[53] which may account for the lack of prognostic findings in their study. Follow-up was not applicable for the study by Lephart et al[56] because of the cross-sectional nature of the study design.

4. **Were objective outcomes used?** For the most part, objective outcome criteria were used. Table 9–5 illustrates that a variety of outcomes were used, from manual stress tests (less objective) to mechanical measures with an arthrometer and the Cybex dynamometer (more objective).

Functional scores were derived by some authors in the form of tests and questionnaires. In these instances the content of the test or questionnaire could be easily reproduced from the text or the citations that were provided. No studies performed "blind" assessment of their outcomes.

5. **Was there statistical adjustment for other prognostic factors?** Both papers by Andersson et al[50,51] indicated that surgery provided a better prognosis for return to sport. Although no multivariate analysis was provided, the reader should note that randomization is a means of controlling for extraneous variables in the study design. Therefore the absence of statistical control may not be an issue in these two studies. The level I evidence regarding the effects of surgery compared with conservative treatment supports the use of surgical treatment to facilitate return to preinjury sports activity.

Only two studies used multivariate statistics to control for other possible prognostic variables. Daniel et al[54] performed a stepwise discriminant analysis to identify factors predictive of late surgery in unstable knees. The most important variable for predicting meniscal or ligament surgery was total hours of participation per year in sporting activities that involved jumping, pivoting, or lateral motion. Anterior tibial displacement and patient age were also significant variables in the final discriminant function.

Louden et al[57] used conditional stepwise logistic regression to identify clinical measures of posture that were significantly related to ACL injury. Three variables contributed significantly to the multivariate model: knee extension in standing, forefoot pronation, and rearfoot pronation. The results were strengthened by high intrarater reliability statistics. Although the study design makes it difficult to establish that postural findings were present prior to the ACL injury, the theoretical construct proposed by the authors has biologic plausibility and is consistent with current clinical perspective. A prospective design is warranted to confirm the authors' hypothesis.

The guide proposed by Sackett et al[48] can be helpful in determining how much subjective confidence can be placed in the prognostic findings. For example, we summarize below our findings in two subgroups of articles: those reporting multivariate findings and those reporting less complex bivariate statistical results.

Multivariate Findings. For the two studies that controlled for other prognostic factors, increased age, higher preinjury hours of sports per year, and larger values for mechanically measured anterior displacement of the knee are predictive of late surgery.[54] These inferences are limited only by the lack of a blind assessment of outcome. The prognostic value of postural faults in predicting ACL injury[57] is limited by the lack of a clearly defined inception cohort and the lack of a blind assessment of outcome. Although specific screening programs were not evaluated, prognostic findings by Daniel et al[54] and Louden et al[57] may have practical relevance to physical therapists involved in preseason screening.

Bivariate Findings. For the remainder of the studies, there was no statistical control of other possible prognostic variables. Three authors provided a general description of their cohort at the time of recruitment.[52,56,58] Accordingly, results from these studies should be interpreted with more caution. The study with a more detailed description of their cohort has revealed that ACL-injured patients with MCL lesions regain extension range of motion (ROM) more slowly when their MCL injury is located in the proximal portion of the ligament.[60] This may be relevant to physical therapists because of the importance of ROM in the subacute phase of treatment.

Conclusion

The literature reviewed demonstrated that most studies consist of **grade V level of evidence yielding grade C recommendations**. The excep-

tion is the grade A recommendation that prognosis for return to sport is improved with surgical intervention. While the grade C recommendations may be viewed as a limitation, it should be emphasized that level V studies may contain useful prognostic information.[49]

THERAPY

Objective

The objective of our review of the literature was to determine whether physical therapy treatment methods change important clinical outcomes in the injured athlete.

A broad spectrum of treatment techniques and methods are available to the sports physical therapist. In searching the available literature, we first reviewed previously published systematic reviews of ankle, knee, and shoulder soft tissue disorders available in the orthopedic literature. Since there was sparse evidence of effectiveness in the orthopedic literature and even less in athletes with soft tissue injuries, we used a systematic review method to identify and synthesize literature on soft tissue injuries in athletes. Three regions in which sports injuries commonly occur, the knee, ankle, and shoulder, were chosen as the area of interest for this review.

Methods
Inclusion Criteria

Type of Study. Three types of study designs were used: systematic review, randomized controlled trials (RCT), and controlled clinical trials (CCT).

Type of Participants. Athletes with soft tissue or musculoskeletal injuries to the knee, ankle, or shoulder were the targeted group. (An athlete is anyone participating in sports activities.) An athlete sample was accepted if it met the following criteria:

1. **Definite athletic sample:** at least 50% of the reported sample was involved in sports activities.
2. **Probable athletic sample:** outcome measures relating to return to sport was used, although the sample was not clearly described as being involved in sports.

3. **Possible athletic sample**: the article's introduction specifically discussed sport-related injuries or therapies, and the authors were from athletic institutions; the soft tissue disorder was a common sports-associated injury.

Type of Intervention. Treatment methods used by physical therapists are listed in Table 9–6.

Types of Outcomes Measures. Important clinical outcomes, such as pain, function (return to sports), patient satisfaction, and other measures of impairment or disability, were used.

Search Strategy

The Medline database was searched for English language systematic reviews, meta-analyses, and RCTs for a 10-year period to December 1997. By limiting the search with the design term (RCT), level I and II evidence was ensured. To locate systematic reviews and meta-analyses, the strategy of Hunt and McKibbon[62] was used. To search for RCTs the terms *randomized controlled trial* (pt) and *random* (tw) were used. These terms were combined with anatomic (eg, shoulder, ankle, knee), disorder (eg, knee injury), and therapy MeSH terms and related text words.

In addition, a hand search of three sports medicine journals, the *American Journal of Sports Medicine, Journal of Orthopaedic and Sports Physical Therapy,* and *Clinical Journal of Sport Medicine,* was conducted to find articles published from January 1997 to March 1998. The annotated bibliography entitled "Outcomes Effectiveness of Physical Therapy," presented by the American Physical Therapy Association, was hand searched.[63] Articles in our personal files

---

TABLE 9–6. Clinical Therapeutic Processes Used by Physical Therapists

Exercise
  Acquatic, flexibility, strengthening and endurance (open kinetic vs closed kinetic, isometric, isotonic, isokinetic, plyometric, sport-specific functional progression), reestablishment of proprioception, kinesthesia, joint position sense, neuromuscular control
Therapeutic heat or cold
  Pulsed electromagnetic field, ultrasound, laser, cryotherapy, heat packs, infrared, paraffin, fluid therapy, hydrotherapy, microwave, short-wave diathermy, vasocoolant, spray
Biofeedback
  Electromyelography, pressure biofeedback
Electrotherapy
  Neuromuscular stimulation, transcutaneous electrical nerve stimulation, infrared, electroacupuncture, microcurrent
Acupuncture
Traction
  Mechanical, manual
Orthotics
  Cervical collar
Manual therapies
  Manipulation, mobilization, massage, neuromuscular techniques, various complementary manual therapies (eg, craniosacral, fascial release)
Complementary therapies
  Mind-body interventions, movement awareness, traditional Chinese medicine, herbal treatments
Education
  Instructional strategies (individual, group), instructional media (verbal, written, audiotapes, audiovisual material, computer-assisted instruction), type of learning activity (lecture, discussion, demonstration, practice, reinforcement), structure (planned instruction vs haphazard question-and-answer sessions), teaching content
Pharmacologic considerations
Psychological considerations

were also included. Identification of relevant citation postings and selection of articles meeting inclusion criteria were conducted by one of us (A.G.).

Assessment of Method Quality and Validity

In reading literature reviews, a clinician can be misled if the conclusions reached in the review are not based on sound methods. The 10 criteria from Oxman and Guyatt[64] were used to assess the general quality of each review article:

Search methods (maximum score, 4):
1. The search methods used to find evidence (primary studies) on the primary question(s) were stated.
2. The search for evidence was reasonably comprehensive.

Selection methods (maximum score, 4):
3. The criteria used for deciding which studies to include in the review was reported.
4. Bias in the selection of articles was avoided.

Validity assessment (maximum score, 4):
5. The criteria used for assessing the validity of the studies reviewed were reported.
6. The validity for each study cited was assessed using appropriate criteria (either in selecting studies for inclusion or in analyzing the studies that are cited).

Synthesis (maximum score, 6):
7. The methods used to combine the findings for the relevant studies (to reach a conclusion) was reported.
8. Findings of the relevant studies were combined appropriately relative to the primary question the review addresses.
9. The conclusions made by the author(s) were supported by the data or analysis reported in the review.

Scoring (maximum score, 9):
10. How would you rate the scientific quality for this review? Overall method quality score equals the sum of all of the above scored criteria divided by 2. Descriptive terms correspond to the arithmetic sums.*

The following three criteria are associated with evidence of bias in estimating treatment

---

*Modified from Oxman AD, Guyatt GH: Guidelines for reading literature reviews. Can Med Assoc J 138:697–703, 1988.

effects[65] and were used to assess the validity of the RCT or CCTs meeting selection.

1. Is there evidence of adequate concealment of randomization of subjects entering the trials? (maximum score, 2)
2. Were all noncompleters accounted for at the trial's conclusion? (maximum score, 2)
3. Were all patients, outcome assessors, and clinicians blinded to treatment allocation? (maximum score, 2)*

Validity (method quality) assessment of systematic reviews was conducted by one reviewer (A.P.) and of the RCTs and CCTs by two reviewers (A.G., A.P.) independently. The total validity score for systematic reviews follows the citation posting in the bibliography. The criterion scores for validity assessment of the RCTs and CCTs are noted in Table 9–7 as are the corresponding levels of evidence (previously defined in the Prognosis discussion).

Data Extraction

Raw data on means and standard deviations for all outcomes, as well as the author's report of the study results, were extracted from the full manuscripts by one of us (A.G.). Demographic data extracted included the disorder, sport, athlete description, and treatment.

Data Analysis

Agreement between investigators was calculated for study validity assessment using the PC-Agree program.[82,83] It was performed prior to consensus, and was used to measure potential bias inherent in this process. The kappa or quadratic weighted kappa statistic was used to assess agreement.[84] Results <0 reflect poor agreement; 0 to 0.20, slight agreement; 0.21 to 0.40, fair agreement; 0.41 to 0.60, moderate agreement; 0.61 to 0.80, substantial agreement; and 0.81 to 1.00, almost perfect agreement.[84]

Details of analyses specific to each therapy are reported in Table 9–7. For simplicity, the Direction of Effect is noted for each outcome. Using a fixed effects model, effect sizes of standard mean difference (SMD) (95% confidence

---

*Data from Schultz KF, Chalmer I, Hayes RJ, et al: Empirical evidence of methodological quality associated with estimates of treatment effects in controlled trials. JAMA 273:408–412, 1995.

Text continued on page 151

TABLE 9–7. Physical Therapy: Evidence-based Practice During Three Phases of Treatment for Musculoskeletal or Soft Tissue Disorders in Athletes

THERAPY (TIMING OF OUTCOME)	AUTHOR	SAMPLE DESCRIPTION	OUTCOME MEASURE	EFFECT SIZE	DIRECTION OF EFFECT	LEVEL OF EVIDENCE	VALIDITY A	B	C
Preinjury/Prevention									
Orthosis vs no treatment control (1 season to 2 y)	Sitler et al[66]	Sample: definite athlete (recreational) Disorder: ankle sprain (grade 1, 2 or 3) Sport: basketball Expt n = 789 Ctrl n = 812	Incidence of ankle sprain in previously injured ankle at 2 y of treatment	Peto OR 0.24 (95% CI: 0.05,1.07)	Benefit: favors treatment	I	0	2	0
			Incidence of ankle sprain in previously uninjured ankle at 2 y of treatment	Peto OR 0.38 (95% CI: 0.20,0.71)	Benefit: favors treatment	I			
	Surve et al[67]	Sample: definite athlete (recreational) Disorder: ankle sprain (grade 1, 2 or 3) Sport: soccer Expt n = 244 Ctrl n = 260	Incidence of ankle sprain in previously injured ankle at 1 playing season	Peto OR 0.21 (95% CI: 0.10,0.44)	Benefit: favors treatment	I	0	2	0
			Incidence of ankle sprain in previously uninjured ankle at 1 playing season	Peto OR 1.23 (95% CI: 0.50,3.02)	No evidence of benefit	II			
	Tropp et al[68]	Sample: definite athlete (recreational) Disorder: ankle sprain Sport: senior soccer teams Expt n = 124 Ctrl n = 171	Incidence of ankle sprain in previously injured ankle at 6 mo of treatment	Peto OR 0.19 (95% CI: 0.07,0.52)	Benefit: favors treatment	I	0	0	0
			Incidence of ankle sprain in previously uninjured ankle at 6 mo of treatment	Peto OR 0.61 (95% CI: 0.11,3.50)	No evidence of benefit	II			

Intervention	Study	Sample/Disorder/Sport	Outcome	Statistic	Conclusion				
Wobble board training vs control (3 to 6 mo follow-up)	Tropp et al[68]	Sample: definite athlete (recreational) Disorder: ankle sprain Sport: senior soccer team Expt n = 142 Ctrl n = 171	Incidence of ankle sprain in previously injured ankle	Peto OR 0.21 (95% CI: 0.09,0.53)	Benefit: favors treatment	I	0	0	0
			Incidence of ankle sprain in previously uninjured ankle	Peto OR 0.56 (95% CI: 0.20,1.56)	No evidence of benefit	II			
	Wester et al[69]	Sample: definite athlete Disorder: ankle sprain (grade: not specified) Sport: soccer, handball, volleyball, other Expt n = 24 Ctrl n = 24	Incidence of ankle sprain in previously injured ankle	Peto OR 0.30 (95% CI: 0.10,0.95)	Benefit: favors treatment	I	0	2	0

During Sport and Immediately After Injury

Intervention	Study	Sample/Disorder/Sport	Outcome	Statistic	Conclusion				
Elastic wrap + elevation vs elevation (1 treatment)	Rucinski et al[70]	Sample: possible athlete Disorder: ankle sprain (grade 1 or 2) Sport: not specified Expt n = 10 Ctrl n = 10	Volumetric measurement after 1 treatment	SMD 1.3 (95% CI: 0.3,2.2)	Evidence of benefit: favors control	II	0	2	0
Pneumonic compression + elevation vs elevation (1 treatment)	Rucinski et al[70]	Sample: possible athlete Disorder: ankle sprain (grade 1 or 2) Sport: not specified Expt n = 10 Ctrl n = 10	Volumetric measurement after 1 treatment	SMD 2.0 (95% CI: 0.9,3.1)	Evidence of benefit: favors control	II	0	2	0

Table continued on following page

TABLE 9–7. Physical Therapy: Evidence-based Practice During Three Phases of Treatment for Musculoskeletal or Soft Tissue Disorders in Athletes *Continued*

THERAPY (TIMING OF OUTCOME)	AUTHOR	SAMPLE DESCRIPTION	OUTCOME MEASURE	EFFECT SIZE	DIRECTION OF EFFECT	LEVEL OF EVIDENCE	VALIDITY A	B	C
Air-stirrup vs compression bandage (3 wk of treatment)	Leanderson and Wredmark[71]	Sample: possible athlete; Disorder: ankle sprain (grade 2 or 3); Sport: not specified; Expt n = 39; Ctrl n = 34	SIP: all measures at 5 d, 2 wk, 4 wk, 10 wk	More mobile in first week after injury; $P < .05$ (Mann-Whitney)	Benefit: favors treatment	I	0	0	0
			Sick leave from work	$P < .05$ (students t-test)	Benefit: favors treatment	I			
			Ankle function (Karlsson's score)	Not significant (ANOVA) at all follow-up points	No evidence of benefit	II			
			AROM (DF/PF)	Not significant (ANOVA) at all follow-up points	No evidence of benefit	II			
			Cost saving	USD 237 (SEK 1750) per patient per injury	Benefit: favors treatment	II			
Cold vs heat (3 d of treatment)	Coté et al[72]	Sample: possible athlete; Disorder: ankle sprain (grade 1 or 2); Sport: not specified; Expt n = 10; Ctrl n = 10	Volumetric measure (edema)		Benefit: favors treatment	I	0	2	1
			Day 1	SMD -1.05 (95% CI: $-1.99, -0.10$)					
			Day 2	SMD -0.37 (95% CI: $-1.25, -0.52$)					
			Day 3	SMD -1.72 (95% CI: $-2.78, -0.66$)					

Intervention	Study	Sample/Disorder	Outcome measure	Effect size	Benefit	Level			
							1	0 2	1
Cold vs contrast bath (3 d of treatment)	Coté et al[72]	Sample: possible athlete Disorder: ankle sprain (grade 1 or 2) Sport: not specified Expt n = 10 Ctrl n = 10	Volumetric measure Day 1	SMD −1.28 (95% CI: −2.26,−0.30)	Benefit: favors treatment	I			
			Day 2	SMD −0.40 (95% CI: −1.28,−0.49)					
			Day 3	SMD −1.33 (95% CI: −2.32,−0.34)					
							0	2	0
Wobble board training vs usual treatment (12 wk of treatment)	Wester et al[69]	Sample: definite athlete (recreational) Disorder: ankle sprain (grade: not specified) Sport: soccer, handball, volleyball, other Expt n = 24 Ctrl n = 24	Volumetric measure (edema)	SMD 0.13 (95% CI: −0.44,0.70)	No evidence of benefit	II			
			Pain at rest	Peto OR 0.11 (95% CI: 0.02,0.58)	Benefit: favors treatment	I			
			Pain with walking	Peto OR 1.00 (95% CI: 0.32,3.11)	No evidence of benefit	II			
			Pain during sport	Peto OR 0.50 (95% CI: 0.13,1.90)	No evidence of benefit	II			
			Instability	Peto OR 0.11 (95% CI: 0.02,0.58)	Benefit: favors treatment	I			

Rehabilitation and Maintenance

Intervention	Study	Sample/Disorder	Outcome measure	Effect size	Benefit	Level			
							0	2	1
Supervised rehabilitation vs home rehabilitation program (6 wk standard treatment + 12 wk expt treatment + 6 wk follow-up)	Beard and Dodd[73]	Sample: definite athlete Disorder: ACL reconstruction Sport: not specified Expt n = 10 Ctrl n = 11	Function (Lyshom score)	SMD 0.24 (95% CI: −0.62,1.10)	No evidence of benefit	II			
			Activity level (Tegner score + VAS sport/ADL)	SMD 0.40 (95% CI: −0.47,1.26)	No evidence of benefit	II			
			Anterior tibial translation (KT-1000 arthrometer)	SMD −0.64 (95% CI: −1.52,0.25)	No evidence of benefit	II			
			Muscle strength (Kin Com dynamometer) quadriceps	SMD 0.64 (95% CI: −0.25,1.52)	No evidence of benefit	II			

Table continued on following page

TABLE 9–7. Physical Therapy: Evidence-based Practice During Three Phases of Treatment for Musculoskeletal or Soft Tissue Disorders in Athletes *Continued*

THERAPY (TIMING OF OUTCOME)	AUTHOR	SAMPLE DESCRIPTION	OUTCOME MEASURE	EFFECT SIZE	DIRECTION OF EFFECT	LEVEL OF EVIDENCE	VALIDITY A	B	C
Supervised rehabilitation vs home rehabilitation program (continued) (all outcomes measured at 4.5 wk of treatment + 4 wk follow-up)	Jokl et al[74]	Sample: possible athlete Disorder: medial menesectomy Sport: not specified Expt n = 15 Ctrl n = 15	Hamstring	SMD 0.70 (95% CI: −0.19,1.59)	No evidence of benefit	II	0	0	1
			No report of pain	Peto OR 1.36 (95% CI: 0.29,6.60)	No evidence of benefit	II			
			Return to normal activities	Peto OR 1.00 (95% CI: 0.13,7.92)	No evidence of benefit	II			
			Return to work	Peto OR 0.25 (95% CI: 0.04,1.64)	No evidence of benefit	II			
			Return to sports	Peto OR 0.77 (95% CI: 0.19,3.18)	No evidence of benefit	II			
			Overall knee function (4-point scale)	Peto OR 1.00 (95% CI: 0.13,7.92)	No evidence of benefit	II			
			Knee gives away	Peto OR 1.00 (95% CI: 0.06,16.79)	No evidence of benefit	II			
			Difficulty with stairs	Peto OR 2.06 (95% CI: 0.20,21.36)	No evidence of benefit	II			
			Difficulty with crouching	Peto OR 0.34 (95% CI: 0.06,1.79)	No evidence of benefit	II			
			Limping	Not significant: $\rho = 0.678$ (Fisher's exact test)	No evidence of benefit	II			
			Mean % deficit strength, power, endurance, ROM	Not significant: $\rho \geq 0.037$ to $\rho \leq 0.986$ (least square means method)	No evidence of benefit	II			

Intervention	Study	Sample	Outcome	Result	Conclusion	Level		
Protonic exercise + rehabilitation program vs rehabilitation program (6 mo of treatment)	Timm[75]	Sample: possible athlete Disorder: ACL reconstruction Sport: not specified Expt n = 30 Ctrl n = 30	Return to unrestricted activity	SMD −3.3 (95% CI: −3.54, −3.06)	Benefit: favors treatment	I	0	0
			Cost	SMD −6.87 (95% CI: −8.24, −5.50)	Benefit: favors treatment	I	2	1
Closed kinetic chain exercises vs open kinetic chain exercise (12 mo of treatment)	Bynum et al[76]	Sample: probable athlete Disorder: ACL repair Sport: not specified Expt n = 32 Ctrl n = 32	Function (Lyshom score)	Not significant: ρ = 0.55 (paired t-test or chi-square test used)	No evidence of benefit	II	2	2
			Activity level (Tegner activity level)	Not significant: ρ = 0.25	No evidence of benefit	II		
			Satisfaction survey	Significant: P <.007	Benefit: favors treatment	I		
			Ligament laxity (KT-1000 arthrometer)	Significant: @ 20 lb P = .051 @ max P = .018	Benefit: favors treatment	I		
			Manual testing Ligament laxity Lachman Pivot shift	Not significant: ρ = 0.60 / ρ = 0.82	No evidence of benefit	II	2	2
			Presence of patellofemoral tenderness	Not significant: ρ = 0.48	No evidence of benefit	II	2	1
			ROM Extension deficit Flexion deficit	Not significant: ρ = 0.50 / ρ = 0.25	No evidence of benefit	II		

Table continued on following page

TABLE 9–7. Physical Therapy: Evidence-based Practice During Three Phases of Treatment for Musculoskeletal or Soft Tissue Disorders in Athletes *Continued*

THERAPY (TIMING OF OUTCOME)	AUTHOR	SAMPLE DESCRIPTION	OUTCOME MEASURE	EFFECT SIZE	DIRECTION OF EFFECT	LEVEL OF EVIDENCE	VALIDITY A	B	C
CPM + standard protocol vs standard protocol (3 d of treatment)	McCarthy et al[77]	Sample: probable athlete Disorder: ACL repair Sport: not specified Expt n = 15 Ctrl n = 15	Pain (amount of narcotic delivered from patient-controlled analgesia pump)	SMD −1.16 (95% CI: −1.94, −0.38)	Benefit: favors treatment	I	0	0	0
			Oral pain medication intake	SMD −0.74 (95% CI: −1.49, 0.00)	Benefit: favors treatment	I			
			Pain intensity (12-point scale)						
			Day 1	SMD −0.21 (95% CI: −0.93, 0.51)	No evidence of benefit	II			
			Day 2	SMD −0.64 (95% CI: −1.37, 0.10)					
			Day 3	SMD 0.14 (95% CI: −0.58, 0.85)					

Intervention	Study	Sample/Disorder/Sport	Outcome measure	Result	Conclusion	Level			
Taping + exercise vs exercise (4 wk of treatment)	Kowall et al[78]	Sample: probable athlete Disorder: patellofemoral syndrome Sport: not specified Expt n = 12 Ctrl n = 13	Pain: frequency, severity, effect on athletic activity, ADL (VAS)	Not significant	No evidence of benefit	II	2	2	0
			Strength (Cybex II dynamometer)	Not significant	No evidence of benefit	II			
			EMG activity of quadriceps	Not significant	No evidence of benefit	II			
EMG biofeedback for motor control training + exercise vs exercise (isokinetic strengthening + endurance) (duration treatment not clear, 52 wk[?])	Reid et al[79]	Sample: definite athlete (elite) Disorder: subluxing shoulder Sport: hockey, football, swimming, basketball, volleyball, racquetball, baseball, tennis Expt n = 9 Ctrl n = 11	Functional ability	Not significant	No evidence of benefit	II	0	2	0
			Pain intensity at rest (3 point scale)	Not significant	No evidence of benefit	II			
			Pain with activity (3 point scale)	Not significant	No evidence of benefit	II			
			Strength (Cybex 340 dynamometer)	Not significant	No evidence of benefit	II			
Deep friction massage + rest + ice + stretching + US vs rest + ice + stretching + US (2 wk of treatment)	Schwellnus et al[80]	Sample: definite athlete (recreational or elite) Disorder: iliotibial band friction syndrome Sport: long distance runners Expt n = 9 Ctrl n = 8	Daily pain recall (VAS)	SMD −0.29 (95% CI: −1.25,0.67)	No evidence of benefit	II	0	2	1
			Total pain experienced during running (VAS)	SMD −0.21 (95% CI: −1.17,0.75)	No evidence of benefit	II			

Table continued on following page

TABLE 9–7. Physical Therapy: Evidence-based Practice During Three Phases of Treatment for Musculoskeletal or Soft Tissue Disorders in Athletes *Continued*

THERAPY (TIMING OF OUTCOME)	AUTHOR	SAMPLE DESCRIPTION	OUTCOME MEASURE	EFFECT SIZE	DIRECTION OF EFFECT	LEVEL OF EVIDENCE	VALIDITY A	B	C
Iontophoresis + exercise vs "established protocol" (heat, friction massage, phonophoresis, ice) + exercise (2 to 3 wk of treatment + about 2 d follow-up)	Pellecchia et al[81]	Sample: probable athlete Disorder: infrapatellar tendonitis Sport: not reported Expt n = 11 Ctrl n = 13	Pain (VAS)	No between group analysis reported Expt median 1.4 (min 0, max 6.4) Ctrl median 2.6 (min 0, max 7.1)	Not clear		0	2	0
			Functional index questionnaire	Expt median 9.5 (min 4, max 14) Ctrl median 8.5 (min 4, max 14)	Not clear				
			Number of step-ups	Expt median 26 (min 3, max 30) Ctrl median 13.5 (min 1, max 30)	Not clear				
			Palpation of tenderness	Expt median 2 (min 1, max 3) Ctrl median 2 (min 1, max 1)	Not clear				

Key: expt = experimental group; ctrl = control group; n = sample size analyzed; level of evidence: I, randomized controlled trial (RCT) with significant benefit or no-difference finding and large sample size; II, RCT with positive trend but no significant difference and small sample size; CPM, continuous passive movement; validity: A, adequate concealment of randomization of subjects (max = 2); B, noncompleters accounted for at trial conclusion (max = 2); C, patient, outcome assessor, and clinician were blind to treatment allocation (max = 2); OR, odds ratio; SMD, standard mean difference; CI, confidence interval; SIP, sickness impact profile; AROM, active range of motion; DF/PF, dorsiflexion to plantar flexion; USD, US dollars; SEK, Swedish krown; US, ultrasound; ADL, activities of daily living; VAS, visual analogue scale; ANOVA, analysis of variance; ρ, population correlation coefficient; EMG, electromyography; ACL, anterior cruciate ligament.

interval [CI]) were calculated when continuous data were available. The SMD is a unitless measure reported in units of standard deviation. Depending on the outcome measure, a negative effect size may indicate a decrease in the outcome of interest (eg, decreased pain, reduced volumetric measure for edema, shorter time to unrestricted activity, smaller cost), and a positive effect size may indicate an increase in the outcome of interest (eg, increased function, increased anterior tibial translation, increased muscle strength). Generally, an effect size can be interpreted as small (± 0.20), medium (± 0.50), or large (± 0.80), as defined by Cohen.[85] All results reported were based on the sample size analyzed, ie, the sample completing the study.

When dichotomous data were present, *Peto's odds ratio (OR)* was calculated. The OR is the odds that subjects in the experimental treatment have a positive outcome over the odds that subjects in the control have a positive outcome. That is, for the outcome "return to work," an OR >1 favors the treatment, and for the outcome "incidence of ankle sprain," an OR <1 favors the treatment.

Before calculation of a pooled effect measure, the trials were assessed for clinical and biologic sensibility of pooling. This assessment was based on clinical judgment regarding the similarity of the intervention, the similarity in duration of treatment, and the disorder type. Statistical homogeneity was tested and is reported in Table 9–8 for the respective comparison.

Results

Eight of seventeen systematic review articles related in part to orthopedic medicine for the shoulder, knee, and ankle region.[86–93] The total quality assessment score follows their respective citations in the reference section. One poor quality review was retrieved that related to physical therapy, prevention, and sports medicine.[93]

Sixteen controlled trials (RCT/CCTs) were selected from some 46 citations identified as being possibly relevant. Four[66–69] included therapies for an athlete's "preinjury or prevention program," four[69–72] for their "during sport and immediately postinjury management program," and nine[73–81] for their "rehabilitation and maintenance program." Table 9–7 details the findings.

Validity Assessment

The estimated agreement (se) between investigators in validity assessment for criterion A was $\kappa = 0.43$ (se: 0.25), for criterion B $\kappa = 0.13$ (se: 0.21), and for criterion C $\kappa(w) = 0.87$ (se: 0.21). Different internal decision rules and understanding of methods used to ensure adequate concealment resulted in the lower agreement level for criterion A. Oversight (eg, details given in tables or as footnotes to tables) was the primary reason for disagreement in criterion B. The mean total method score was 2.2 (SD: 1.3) across the 16 studies. The maximum score was 5/6.[76]

Preinjury or Prevention Program

Three studies[66–68] evaluated the incidence of ankle sprain in subjects with previously sprained ankles: two for recreational soccer[68] and one for recreational basketball.[66] The pooled Peto OR 0.21 (95% CI: 0.12, 0.36) demonstrated that the use of orthosis during sport was beneficial in reducing the incidence of ankle sprain in subjects with a previously injured ankle (Table 9–8, Comparison A). In the previously uninjured ankle the pooled Peto OR 0.57 (95% CI: 0.34, 0.93), demonstrated less benefit, albeit continued benefit in favor of using an ankle orthosis (Table 9–8, Comparison B). Furthermore, training on a wobble board was beneficial in reducing the incidence of ankle sprain in the previously injured ankle in two studies[68,69]: pooled Peto OR 0.24 (95% CI: 0.24) (Table 9–8, Comparison C). No side effects were reported in the use of an orthosis or wobble board training. (Poor systematic tracking and reporting of treatment side effects were noted for all remaining studies.) Method limits included inadequate concealment and blinding for all trials. An overestimate of the effect's magnitude therefore may be present.

During Sport Management Program

Five comparisons in three studies[69,70,72] evaluated treatment method that may influence inflammation or the presence of edema. Rucinski et al[70] provided evidence in favor of elevation alone (the control intervention) when it was compared to elastic wrap plus elevation [SMD 1.3 (95% CI: 0.3, 2.2)] or pneumonic compression plus elevation [SMD 2.0 (95% CI: 0.9, 3.1)] after one treatment. In other words, there was evidence of harm in elastic wrap plus elevation

TABLE 9–8. Meta-Analysis of Orthosis or Wobble Board vs No Treatment for Ankle Sprain in the Previously Injured and Uninjured Ankle

STUDY (3 mo–2 y FOLLOW-UP)	EXPT n/N	CTRL n/N	PETO OR (95% CI Fixed)	WEIGHT (%)	PETO OR (95% CI FIXED)
Comparison A: Orthosis vs No Treatment Control					
Outcome: Incidence of Ankle Sprain in Previously Injured Ankle					
Sitler et al[66]	1/87	6/90		13.2	0.24 (0.05, 1.07)
Surve et al[67]	5/127	28/131		56.2	0.21 (0.10, 0.44)
Tropp et al[68]	1/45	19/75		30.7	0.19 (0.07, 0.52)
Total (95% CI)	7/259	53/296		100.0	0.21 (0.12, 0.36)
Chi-square 0.05 (df = 2)					
z = 5.63					

.01 .1 1 10
Favors treatment   Favors control

Comparison B: Orthosis vs No Treatment Control					
Outcome: Incidence of Ankle Sprain in Previously Uninjured Ankle					
Sitler et al[66]	10/702	29/722		61.0	0.38 (0.20, 0.71)
Surve et al[67]	11/117	10/129		30.9	1.23 (0.50, 3.02)
Tropp et al[68]	1/15	11/96		8.1	0.61 (0.11, 3.50)
Total (95% CI)	22/834	50/947		100.0	0.57 (0.34, 0.93)
Chi-square 4.47 (df = 2)					
z = 2.24					

.01 .1 1 10
Favors treatment   Favors control

Comparison C: Wobble Board vs No Treatment Control					
Outcome: Incidence of Ankle Sprain in Previously Injured Ankle					
Tropp et al[68]	3/65	19/75		61.3	0.21 (0.09, 0.53)
Wester et al[69]	6/24	13/24		38.7	0.19 (0.10, 0.95)
Total (95% CI)	9/89	32/99		100.0	0.24 (0.12, 0.50)
Chi-square 0.23 (df = 1)					
z = 3.89					

.01 .1 1 10
Favors treatment   Favors control

EXPT, experimental group; CTRL, control group; OR, odds ratio; CI, confidence interval; df, degrees of freedom; z, z score; n, number of events; N, number of participants.

and pneumonic compression plus elevation. A replication of these findings in studies with larger sample sizes is required (low power). Additionally, method issues may limit interpretation of the findings. Not surprisingly, cold was beneficial in reducing edema when it was compared to the use of heat [SMD (at day 3) −1.72 (95% CI: −2.78, 0.66)] or contrast bath [SMD (at day 3) −1.33 (95% CI: −2.32, 0.34)] at day 1 through 3 of treatment after injury.[72] The sample size was small (n = 20), thus suggesting that this study should be replicated to ensure a true effect. The use of a wobble board demonstrated no evidence of benefit [SMD 0.13 (95% CI: −0.44, 0.70)] in reducing edema after 12 weeks of treatment.[72]

The wobble board showed evidence of benefit in reducing pain at rest and instability following ankle sprain [Peto OR 0.11 (95% CI: 0.02, 0.58) for both measures][69]; It showed no evidence of benefit for managing pain with walking or sport. Again the study failed to demonstrate the latter factors definitively.

Finally, the use of an air-stirrup improved the mobility score in the sickness impact profile (SIP), reducing sick leave from work and costs (see Table 9–7). There was no evidence that ankle function or ROM improved with 3 weeks of treatment. Low power and an extremely low method score limit confidence in these results.

Rehabilitation and Maintenance Program

Four studies[73-76] investigated exercise methods, often within a **multimodal rehabilitation management** strategy: three after ACL reconstruction and one after medial menisectomy. Two studies[73,74] evaluated supervised rehabilitation programs with structured home rehabilitation programs; one after 18 weeks of treatment plus 6 weeks of follow-up[73] and the second after $4\frac{1}{2}$ weeks of treatment and 4 weeks of follow-up.[74] Both trials demonstrated no evidence of benefit across all outcome measures (see Table 9-7, Rehabilitation and Maintenance). Low power limits the confidence the reader can place on these results. A further trial demonstrated that a protonic exercise program plus a rehabilitation program was beneficial in returning the person to unrestricted activities [SMD −3.3 (95% CI: −3.54, −3.06)] and in terms of cost [SMD −6.87 (95% CI: −8.24, 5.50)] when compared to a rehabilitation program alone. Method quality was low in this trial. In one well-designed RCT,[76] closed kinetic chain exercises were more beneficial than standard open kinetic chain exercises in reducing ligament laxity but were not more beneficial in improving function or activity level.

Three further trials investigated therapies seen to be **adjunctive to exercise therapies**: taping for patellofemoral syndrome,[78] electromyographic biofeedback (EMG-BF) for motor control in shoulder subluxation disorders,[79] and iontophoresis in patellar tendinitis.[81] For two (taping and EMG-BF) of the three studies, there was no evidence that pain was lessened nor that functional activity or strength improved. Unfortunately the iontophoresis trial did not report group comparisons, although it does appear from the posttreatment median data presented that pain was lessened and the number of step-ups increased more with iontophoresis than with the "established protocol." No clear determination of the direction or magnitude of the effect can be made with the reported data. Again, all three trials had small samples, and there is not enough power to definitively state that no benefit exists.

One RCT evaluated **continuous passive movement (CPM)** in ACL repair. It reduced the amount of narcotics delivered from a patient controlled analgesic pump [SMD −1.16 (95% CI: −1.94, −0.38)] and the number of oral analgesics taken by the subject [SMD −0.74 (95% CI: −1.49, 0.00)]; however, there was no evidence that it reduced the patient-perceived pain intensity from day 1 through 3 after surgery (see Table 9-7). An extremely low method score may suggest that the noted effect has been overestimated. Thus replication of this trial is warranted.

Finally, deep friction massage was evaluated for iliotibial band friction syndrome with 2 weeks of treatment.[80] No evidence was noted for reduction of daily pain recall [SMD −0.29 (95% CI: −1.25, 0.67)] or pain with running [SMD −0.21 (95% CI: −1.17, 0.75)]. Low power limits conclusive interpretation from these findings.

Discussion

A structured approach to the identification, selection, and validity assessment of the literature was used in this overview. The validity (method quality) scoring system used in this overview had acceptable measurement properties. The method limitations of this review included a limited search strategy. Thus some potential exists for language bias or publication bias. Selection bias may be a further limitation, although criteria set a priori should in part control for it.

In general, all therapies have not been studied in enough detail to adequately assess either efficacy or effectiveness. Primarily, single trials were retrieved in each subcategory.

There is reasonable support for advising individuals with previous ankle sprains to use an orthosis or wobble board training during the prevention phase of physical therapy. Not enough scientific testing exists to reasonably determine if other therapies are truly of benefit, are of no benefit, or are harmful. Replication of small positive studies is needed.

The best available evidence suggests benefit with elevation, air stirrup, cold, and wobble board training during the postinjury phase of physical therapy and protonic exercise, closed kinetic chain exercise, and CPM in the rehabilitation phase. No evidence of benefit exists for the supervised vs home rehabilitative program, taping, EMG-BF for motor control, deep friction massage, or iontophoresis. In one small trial a higher volumetric measurement following elastic wrap plus elevation or pneumonic compression plus elevation suggests some potential for harm. Considering the varied treatment approaches to sports injury, with their potential risks and costs, further work is needed to determine optimal treatment approaches.

A limitation of many trials evaluated in this review is that the magnitude of treatment effects could not be determined from data presented in the study. The studies reviewed in this section commonly used combinations of treatment in designs that did not allow for measures of individual or interaction effects. Since these effects may be important in the delivery of care, future studies should consider the use of factorial designs to measure them.

Future designs should also consider consistent use of valid and reliable outcome measures for pain, function (disability), and patient satisfaction so that their results and the magnitude of the trials effect can be judged. Additionally, study designs with high method rigor are essential.

SUMMARY

The synthesis of the currently available literature in diagnosis, measurement, prognosis, and therapy provides some foundation for an evidence-based approach to practice.

Although there is extensive literature in the area of diagnostic testing, studies have focused on nonathletic populations. More recently outcome measures for the general musculoskeletal population have been developed, and some validation studies are being carried out. Again, athletic populations are not studied as frequently, which limits the generalizability of study results. The majority of studies evaluating diagnostic and outcome measures investigate peripheral joint injuries. Ligamentous structures are the primary focus of diagnostic procedures, and many stress tests and components of physical examination have been shown to be valid. To date, outcome measures relevant for sports populations are limited, but recent work has shown promise.

Reviewing the literature to determine the prognosis for a sports injury has demonstrated that **most studies consist of grade V level of evidence yielding grade C recommendations.**

When applied to a common sports injury such as an ACL rupture, factors that make sense from a clinical perspective emerge from the literature as significant prognostic factors. Grade C recommendations have limitations, but level V studies contain important prognostic information.[49]

Not surprisingly, the therapies have not been studied in enough detail to provide definitive answers of therapy benefit, no benefit, and harm. Reasonable support exists for advising persons with previous ankle sprains to use an orthosis and wobble board training during the prevention phase of physical therapy.

REFERENCES

1. Oberg U, Oberg T: Discriminatory power, sensitivity and specificity of a new assessment system (FAS). Physiother Can 49:40–47, 1997
2. Heald SL, Riddle DL, Lamb RL: The shoulder pain and disability index: the construct validity and responsiveness of a region-specific disability measure. Phys Ther 77:1079–1089, 1997
3. Chatman AB, Hyams SP, Neel JM, et al: The patient-specific functional scale: measurement properties in patients with knee dysfunction. Phys Ther 77:820–829, 1997
4. Liu S, Henry MH, Nuccion S, et al: Diagnosis of glenoid labral tears: a comparison between MRI and clinical examinations. Am J Sports Med 24:149–154, 1996
5. Liu SH, Henry MH, Nuccion SL: A prospective evaluation of a new physical examination in predicting glenoid labral tears. Am J Sports Med 24:721–725, 1996
6. Muellner T, Weinstabl R, Schabus R, et al: The diagnosis of meniscal tears in athletes: a comparison of clinical and MRI investigations. Am J Sports Med 25:7–12, 1997
7. Mohtadi N: Development and validation of the quality of life outcome measure questionnaire for chronic ACL deficiency. Am J Sports Med 26:350–359, 1998
8. Sgaglione N, Del Pizzo W, Fox JM, et al: Critical analysis of knee ligament rating systems. Am J Sports Med 23:660–667, 1995
9. Kumbhare DA: Delayed physical examination for detecting ankle ligament lesions. Clin J Sports Med 7:230, 1997
10. Leddy JJ, Smolinski RJ, Lawrence J, et al: Prospective evaluation of the Ottawa ankle rules in a university sports medicine center: with a modification to increase specificity for identifying malleolar fractures. Am J Sports Med 26:158–165, 1998

11. Wilson RW, Gieck JH, Gansneder BM, et al: Reliability and responsiveness of disablement measures following acute ankle sprains among athletes. J Orthop Sports Phys Ther 27:348–355, 1998

12. Liu SH, Nuccion SL, Finerman G: Diagnosis of anterolateral ankle impingement: comparison between MRI and clinical examination. Am J Sports Med 25:389–393, 1997

13. Stanitski CL: Correlation of arthroscopic and clinical examinations with MRI findings of injured knees in children and adolescents. Am J Sports Med 26:2–6, 1998

14. Franklin ME, Conner-Kerr T, Chamness M, et al: Assessment of exercise induced minor muscle lesions: the accuracy of Cyriax diagnosis by selective tension paradigm. J Orthop Sports Phys Ther 24:122–129, 1996

15. Munich H, Cipriani D, Hall C, et al: The test-retest reliability of an inclined squat strength test protocol. J Orthop Sports Phys Ther 26:209–213, 1997

16. Romeo AA, Bach BR Jr, O'Halloran KL: Scoring systems for shoulder conditions. Am J Sports Med 24:472–476, 1996

17. MacIntyre DL, Hopkins PM, Harris SR: Evaluation of pain and functional activity in patellofemoral pain syndrome: reliability and validity of two assessment tools. Physiother Can 47:164–172, 1995

18. Sekiya I, Muneta T, Ogiuchi T, et al: Significance of the single-legged hip test to the ACL reconstructed knee in relation to muscle strength and anterior laxity. Am J Sports Med 26:384–388, 1998

19. Pincivero DM, Lephart SM, Karunakara RG: Relation between open and closed kinematic chain assessment of knee strength and functional performance. Clin J Sports Med 7:11–16, 1997

20. Tomsich DA, Nitz AJ, Threlkeld AJ, et al: Patellofemoral alignment: reliability. J Orthop Sports Phys Ther 23:200–208, 1996

21. Fitzgerald GK, McClure PW: Reliability of measurements obtained with four tests for patellofemoral alignment. Phys Ther 75:84–92, 1995

22. O'Shea KJ, Murphy KP, Heekin RD, et al: The diagnostic accuracy of history, physical examination, and radiographs in the evaluation of traumatic knee disorders. Am J Sports Med 24:164–167, 1996

23. Kramer J, Handfield T, Kiefer G, et al: Comparisons of weight-bearing and non-weightbearing tests of knee proprioception performed by patients with PFPS and asymptomatic individuals. Clin J Sports Med 7:113–118, 1997

24. Shiraishi M, Mizuta H, Kubota K, et al: Stabilometric assessment in the ACL reconstructed knee. Clin J Sports Med 6:32–39, 1996

25. Eakin CL, Cannon WD Jr.: Arthrometric evaluation of PCL injuries. Am J Sports Med 26:96–102, 1998

26. Hewett TE, Noyes FR, Lee MD: Diagnosis of complete and partial PCL ruptures: stress radiography compared with ICT-IDOG arthrometer and posterior drawer testing. Am J Sports Med 25:648–655, 1997

27. Adler GG, Hockman RA, Beach DM: Drop leg Lachman test: a new test of anterior knee laxity. Am J Sports Med 23:320–323, 1995

28. Harrison E, Quinney H, Magee D, et al: Analysis of outcome measures used in the study of PFPS. Physiother Can 47:264–272, 1995

29. Wright SA, Hawkins RJ: The anterior slide test for identifying superior glenoid labral tears. Clin J Sports Med 6:64, 1996

30. Pellecchia G, Paolina J, Connell J: Intertester reliability of the Cyriax evaluation in assessing patients with shoulder pain. J Orthop Sports Phys Ther 23:34–38, 1996

31. Chesworth BM, MacDermid JC, Roth JH, et al: Movement diagram and "end-feel" reliability when measuring passive lateral rotation of the shoulder in patients with shoulder pathology. Phys Ther 78:593–601, 1998

32. Berg E, Ciullo J: A clinical test for superior glenoid labral or "SLAP" lesions. Clin J Sports Med 8:121–123, 1998

33. Corso G: Impingement relief test: an adjunctive procedure to traditional assessment of shoulder impingement syndrome. J Orthop Sports Phys Ther 22:183–192, 1995

34. Scoville CR, Arciero RA, Taylor DC, et al: End range eccentric antagonistic/concentric agonist strength ratios: a new perspective in shoulder strength assessment. J Orthop Sports Phys Ther 25:203–207, 1997

35. Hutchinson B, Linney M, McFarland CJ, et al: Reliability and predictability of traditional single plane shoulder movement strength values to more functional diagonal pattern strength when measured on a Cybex isokinetic dynamometer. Physiother Can 48:41–46, 1996

36. Burnham RS, Bell G, Olenic L, et al: Shoulder abduction strength measurement in football players: reliability and validity of two field tests. Clin J Sports Med 5:90–94, 1995

37. Hoher J, Bach T, Munster A, et al: Does the mode of data collection change results in a subjective knee score? Self-administrations interview. Am J Sports Med 25:642–647, 1997

38. Juris PM, Phillips EM, Dalpe C, et al: A dynamic test of lower extremity function following ACL reconstruction and rehabilitation. J Orthop Sports Phys Ther 26:184–191, 1997

39. Neeb TB, Aufdemkampe G, Wagener JHD, et al: Assessing ACL injuries: the association and differential value of questionnaires, clinical tests and functional tests. J Orthop Sports Phys Ther 26:324–331, 1997

40. Harrison E, Magee D, Quinney H: Development of a clinical tool and patient questionnaire for evaluation of patellofemoral pain syndrome. Clin J Sports Med 6:163–170, 1996

41. Petchnig R, Baron R, Albrecht M: The relationship between isokinetic quadriceps strength test and hop tests for distance and one legged vertical jump test following anterior cruciate ligament reconstruction. J Orthop Sports Phys Ther 28:23–31, 1998

42. Roos EM, Roos HP, Lohmaner LS, et al: Knee injury and osteoarthritis outcome score (KOOS): development of a self-administered outcome measure. J Orthop Sports Phys Ther 28:88–96, 1998

43. Demirdjian AM, Petrie SG, Givanche CA, et al: The outcomes of two knee scoring questionnaires in a normal population. Am J Sports Med 26:46–51, 1998

44. Shapiro ET, Richmond JC, Rockett SE, et al: The use of a generic, patient-based health assessment (SF-36) for evaluation of patients with anterior cruciate ligament injuries. Am J Sports Med 24:196–200, 1996

45. Hudak PL, Amadeo PC, Bombardier C, et al: Development of an upper extremity outcome measure: the DASH (disabilities of the arm, shoulder and hand). Am J Industrial Med 29:602–608, 1996

46. Ross M, Worrell TW: Thigh and calf girth following knee injury and surgery. J Orthop Sports Phys Ther 27:9–15, 1998

47. Zachazewski J, Magee D, Quillen W: Athletic injuries and rehabilitation, W.B. Saunders, Philadelphia, 1996

48. Sackett DL, Haynes BR, Guyatt GH, et al: Making a prognosis. In: Clinical Epidemiology: A Basic Science For Clinical Medicine, 2nd ed. Little Brown, Boston, 1991, pp. 173–185

49. Sackett DL: Levels of evidence and clinical decision making in rehabilitation. In Basmajian JV, Banerjee SN (eds): Clinical Decision Making In Rehabilitation. New York, 1996, Churchill Livingstone, pp. 1–4

50. Andersson C, Odensten M., Good L, et al: Surgical or nonsurgical treatment of acute rupture of the anterior cruciate ligament. J Bone Joint Surg 71A:965–974, 1989

51. Andersson C, Gillquist J: Treatment of acute isolated and combined ruptures of the anterior cruciate ligament: a long-term follow-up study. Am J Sports Med 20:7–12, 1992

52. Barrack RL, Bruckner JD, Kneisl J, et al: The outcome of nonoperatively treated complete tears of the anterior cruciate ligament in active young adults. Clin Orthop 259:192–199, 1990

53. Casteleyn PP, Handelberg F: Non-operative management of anterior cruciate ligament injuries in the general population. J Bone and Joint Surg 78B:446–451, 1996

54. Daniel DM, Stone ML, Dobson BE, et al: Fate of the ACL-injured patient: a prospective outcome study. Am J Sports Med 22:632–644, 1994

55. Finsterbush A, Frankl U, Matan Y, et al: Secondary damage to the knee after isolated injury of the anterior cruciate ligament. Am J Sports Med 18:475–479, 1990

56. Lephart SM, Perrin DH, Fu FH, et al: Relationship between selected physical characteristics and functional capacity in the anterior cruciate ligament-insufficient athlete. J Orthop Sports Phys Ther 16:174–181, 1992

57. Louden JK, Jenkins W, Louden KL: The relationship between static posture and ACL injury in female athletes. J Orthop Sports Phys Ther 24:91–97, 1996

58. Lundberg M, Messner K: Ten-year prognosis of isolated and combined medial collateral ligament ruptures: a matched comparison in 40 patients using clinical and radiographic evaluations. Am J Sports Med 25:2–6, 1997

59. Puddu G, Ferretti A, Mariani P, et al: Meniscal tears and associated anterior cruciate ligament tears in athletes: course of treatment. Am J Sports Med 12:196–198, 1984

60. Robins AJ, Newman AP, Burks RT: Postoperative return of motion in anterior cruciate ligament and medial collateral ligament injuries: the effect of medial collateral ligament rupture location. Am J Sports Med 21:20–25, 1993

61. Sommerlath K, Odenstein M, Lysholm J: The late course of acute partial anterior cruciate ligament tears: a nine to 15-year follow-up evaluation. Clin Orthop 281:152–158, 1992

62. Hunt DL, McKibbon KA: Locating and appraising systematic reviews. Ann Intern Med 126:532–538, 1997

63. American Physical Therapy Association: Outcomes effectiveness of physical therapy: an annotated bibliography. Alexandria, Va, 1995, APTA publications

64. Oxman AD, Guyatt GH: Guidelines for reading literature reviews. Can Med Assoc J 138:697–703, 1988

65. Schulz KF, Chalmer I, Hayes RJ, et al: Empirical evidence of methodological quality associated with estimates of treatment effects in controlled trials. JAMA 273:408–412, 1995

66. Sitler M, Ryan J, Wheeler B, et al: The efficacy of a semirigid stabilizer to reduce acute ankle injury in basketball: a randomized clinical study at West Point. J Sports Med 22:453–461, 1994

67. Surve I, Schwellnus MP, Noakes T, et al: A five-fold reduction in the incidence of recurrent ankle sprains in soccer players using the sport-stirrup orthosis. Am J Sports Med 22:601–606, 1994

68. Tropp H, Askling C, Gillquist J: Prevention of ankle sprains. Am J Sports Med 13:259–262, 1985

69. Wester JU, Jespersen SM, Nielsen KD, et al: Wobble board training after partial sprains of the lateral ligaments of the ankle: a prospective randomized study. J Orthop Sports Phys Ther 23:332–336, 1996

70. Rucinski TJ, Hooker DN, Prentice WE, et al: The effect of intermittent compression on edema in postacute ankle sprains. J Orthop Sports Phys Ther 14:65–69, 1991

71. Leanderson J, Wredmark T: Treatment of acute ankle sprain: comparison of a semirigid ankle brace and compression bandage in 73 patients. Acta Orthop Scand 66:529–531, 1995

72. Coté DJ, Prentice WE, Hooker DN, et al: Comparison of the three treatment procedures for minimizing ankle sprain swelling. Phys Ther 68:1072–1076, 1988

73. Beard DJ, Dodd CAF: Home or supervised rehabilitation following anterior cruciate ligament reconstruction: a randomized controlled trial. J Orthop Sports Phys Ther 27(2):134–143, 1998

74. Jokl P, Stull PA, Lynch K, et al: Independent home versus supervised rehabilitation following arthroscopic knee surgery: a prospective randomized trial. J Arthroscop 5:298–305, 1989

75. Timm KE: The clinical and cost-effectiveness of two different programs for rehabilitation following ACL reconstruction. J Orthop Sports Phys Ther 25:43–48, 1997

76. Bynum BE, Barrack RL, Alexander AH: Open versus closed chain kinetic exercises after anterior cruciate ligament reconstruction: a prospective randomized study. Am J Sports Med 23:401–406, 1995

77. McCarthy MR, Yates CK, Anderson MA, et al: The effect of immediate continuous passive motion on pain during the inflammatory phase of soft tissue healing following anterior cruciate ligament reconstruction. J Orthop Sports Phys Ther 17:96–101, 1993

78. Kowall MG, Kolk G, Nuber GW, et al: Patellar taping in the treatment of patellofemoral pain: a prospective randomized study. Am J Sports Med 24:61–66, 1996

79. Reid DC, Saboe LA, Chepeha JC: Anterior shoulder instability in athletes: comparison of isokinetic resistance exercise and an electromyographic biofeedback reeducation program—a pilot program. Physther Can 3:251–256, 1996

80. Schwellnus MP, Mackintosh L, Mee J: Deep transverse frictions in the treatment of iliotial band friction syndrome in athletes: a clinical trial. Physiotherapy 78:564–568, 1992

81. Pellecchia GL, Hamel H, Behnke P: Treatment of infrapatellar tendonitis: a combination of modalities and transverse friction massage versus iontophoresis. J Sport Rehabil 3:135–145, 1994

82. Walter SD, Cook R: PC-Agree (version 3.0). A PC program for the analysis of observer variation. Department of Clinical Epidemiology and Biostatistics, McMaster University, Hamilton, ON, Canada L8N 3Z5

83. Holman CD: Epidemiologic programs for computers and calculators: analysis of interobserver variation on a programmable calculator. Am J Epidemiol 120:154–160, 1984

84. Landis RJ, Koch GG: The measurement of observer agreement for categorical data. Biometrics 33:159–174, 1977

85. Cohen J: Statistical power analysis for the behavioral sciences, 2nd ed. Hillsdale, NJ, 1988, Lawrence Erlbaum

86. Gam AN, Johannsen F: Ultrasound therapy in musculoskeletal disorders: a meta-analysis. Pain 63:85–91, 1995 [OQA: 7.5/9]

87. Holmes MA, Rudland JR: Clinical trials of ultrasound treatment in soft tissue injury: a review and critique. Physiother Theory Pract 7:163–175, 1991

88. Shrier I, Matheson GO, Kohl HW: Achilles tendinitis: are corticosteroid injections useful or harmful? Clin J Sport Med 6:245–250, 1996 [OQA: 5.5/9]

89. Arroll B, Ellis-Pegler E, Edwards A, et al: Patellofemoral pain syndrome: a critical review of the clinical trials on nonoperative therapy. Am J Sports Med 25:207–212, 1997 [OQA: 5.5/9]

90. Beckerman H, Bouter LM, Van der Heijden GJ, et al: Efficacy of physiotherapy for musculoskeletal disorders: what can we learn from research? Br J Gen Pract 43:73–77, 1993 [OQA: 8/9]

91. Ogilvie-Harris DJ, Gilbart M: Clin J Sport Med 5:175–186, 1995 [OQA: 7/9]

92. Shrier I: Treatment of lateral collateral ligament sprains of the ankle: a critical appraisal of the literature. Clin J Sports Med 5:187–195, 1995 [OQA: 4/9]

93. Cipriani DJ, Swartz JD, Hodgson CM: Triathlon and the multisport athlete. J Orthop Sports Phys Ther 27:42–50, 1998 [OQA: 1/9]

10

Chiropractic Management of the Injured Athlete

EDWARD R. CROWTHER ▪ JAROSLAW P. GROD

BACKGROUND

Chiropractic is currently the third largest primary contact health care profession in North America behind medicine and dentistry.[1] It is estimated that between 10% and 12% of the population receive chiropractic treatment each year for a variety of health-related complaints.[2] Most patients, 94%, do so for assessment and treatment of head, neck and back pain.[2] Increasingly, both recreational and professional athletes are accessing chiropractic treatment for sports-related injuries. Recent surveys of practice profile and patterns of chiropractors in North America suggest that between 19% and 22% of patients attending chiropractors are professional or amateur athletes.[3,4] It is now commonplace for sports teams and organizations to include chiropractors among their health care consultants.[1]

The clinical management of sports injuries by physicians and allied health care practitioners has significant common ground. Common treatment domains utilized by all types of practitioners, including chiropractors, typically include cold and heat modalities, electrical modalities, exercise, rehabilitation, and nutrition.[5] Adjunctive therapies available for use by chiropractors are diverse and include bracing, taping, nutritional counseling, acupuncture, and orthotics appliances. Table 10–1 highlights the varied types and frequency of therapeutic interventions utilized by chiropractors in the treatment of musculoskeletal injuries including sports-related injuries.[4] These common domain therapies, their clinical applications, scientific rationale, and indications and contraindications for use are covered in detail in other chapters of this text. Sections of this chapter dealing with contraindications, complications, and the research status of manipulative therapy are meant to better inform all health care practitioners of the clinical issues surrounding manipulative therapy when they are considering its use in the injured athlete.

Manipulation as a form of therapy is thought to predate most other procedures employed by the healing arts.[6] It is well accepted that early Old and New World societies routinely practiced various forms of therapeutic manipulation.[7] Hippocrates and Galen, the Prince of Physicians, advocated manipulation of the spine.[7] During the middle ages the art of manipulation was kept alive, often being passed down from one generation of folk healers to the next.

Not until the late nineteenth century was the practice of manipulation formalized when Andrew Taylor Still developed the concepts of osteopathy. By 1968 the American Medical Association had initiated the amalgamation of osteopathy with medicine, and although manipulation is a component of training, it no longer remains a primary treatment modality of most osteopathic physicians.[8]

In 1895, Daniel David Palmer, a self-styled magnetic healer, postulated that "spinal subluxation" and secondary nerve pressure were responsible for all human ailments, historically categorized into type O (organic or visceral disorders) and type M (musculoskeletal disorders) conditions. Although research into the effects

TABLE 10–1. Types and Frequency of Common Therapeutic Interventions Utilized by Chiropractors

INTERVENTION	FREQUENCY (%)
Manipulation	100
Corrective therapy or exercise	95.8
Cryotherapy	92.6
Bracing	90.8
Nutritional counseling	83.5
Bed rest	82.0
Orthotics	79.2
Heat	78.5
Traction	73.8
Ultrasound	68.8
Taping	42.0
Interferential current	36.7
Diathermy	26.7
Hydrotherapy	12.7
Acupuncture	11.8

of spinal manipulative therapy on type O conditions increasingly suggests a lack of efficacy,[9] investigations centered around type M or musculoskeletal conditions (primarily head, neck, and back pain) continue to support its effectiveness.[10,11] It is estimated that 94% of all manipulative procedures in the United States are delivered by chiropractors, with the remaining 6% provided by medical and osteopathic physicians and physical therapists.[12]

Description of Manipulative Therapy

Manipulation is generally defined as manual therapy in which loads are applied to a joint (usually the spine), using short or long lever methods, to move the selected joint through its range of voluntary motion, after which impulse loading is applied.[13] More specifically, Haldeman defines manipulation as "all procedures in which the hands are used to mobilize, adjust, stimulate, or otherwise influence the spinal and paraspinal tissues with the aim of influencing the patient's health."[14] These include, but are not limited to, long-amplitude, nonspecific manipulation; specific, short-amplitude, high-velocity spinal manipulation; active or functional manipulation; mobilization; manual traction; soft tissue massage; and point pressure manipulation.[14]

Of these procedures it is the specific, short-amplitude, high-velocity spinal manipulation that is most often associated with chiropractic interventions. Sandoz[15,16] has described this form of manipulation as a passive manual maneuver during which a synovial joint is carried beyond the normal physiologic range of movement without exceeding the boundaries of anatomical integrity. Figure 10–1 demonstrates the three stages of joint manipulation. Initially the joint is moved within its active range of movement and subsequently into the passive range. Stage 3 moves the joint beyond its end range into the paraphysiologic space. The negative pressure developed within the joint during stage 3 often creates a cavitation of dissolved gases within the synovial joint, creating the characteristic "crack" associated with manipulative therapy[17] (Fig. 10–2). Movement into the pathologic zone carries with it the potential for disruption of the integrity of the holding elements of the joint. Properly trained, skilled practitioners of manipulative therapy can provide safe manipulative procedures up to and within the paraphysiologic space without injury to the joint and its associated structures.

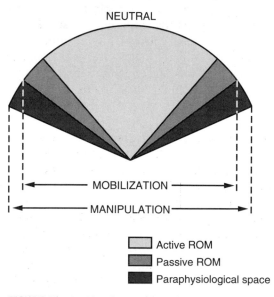

FIGURE 10–1. The three stages of joint mobilization and manipulation as described by Sandoz. (Adapted from Sandoz R: Some physical mechanisms and effects of spinal adjustments. Ann Swiss Chiropract Assoc 6:91–141, 1976.)

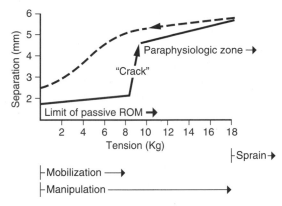

FIGURE 10-2. A load separation curve demonstrating the degree of joint separation of a metacarpophalangeal joint under increasing tension. (Adapted from Sandoz R: Some physical mechanisms and effects of spinal adjustments. Ann Swiss Chiropract Assoc 6:91–141, 1976.)

Physiologic Effects of Manipulation

Practitioners of manipulative therapy (MT) historically have described the focus of their therapeutic efforts in a variety of different terms. Osteopaths describe the target of treatment as the **osteopathic lesion**, which is hypothesized to be the site of vascular compression due to osseous dysrelationships. Traditionally, chiropractors refer to similar neurologic compressive lesions as **subluxations**. Over time, and with the influence of various philosophies and the emergence of scientific evidence, chiropractors have endeavored to be more descriptive in their terminology relating to manipulable lesions. Other terms used include *dyskinesia, vertebral subluxation complex, aberrant mechanics, bony maladjustment, spinal irritation, segmental dysfunction, and joint dysfunction.*

Segmental or joint dysfunction is currently the most common term used to characterize a manipulable lesion. Leach defines joint dysfunction as:

> *A common basic spinal lesion recognized by lessened or otherwise altered mobility, altered pressure threshold to pain, and signs of neuromuscular dysfunction.*[18]

Clinically, joint dysfunction is characterized by point tenderness or altered pain threshold to pressure in the adjacent paraspinal musculature or over the spinous process, loss of normal motion in one or more planes, and abnormal contraction or tension within the adjacent paraspinal musculature. Mennell[19] has proposed that MT may be effective in relieving pain associated with joint dysfunction by restoring normal joint movement. This clinical observation is consistent with the proposed neurobiologic and neurochemical effects of MT.

There are a number of possible reasons why manipulation of joints may have a therapeutic effect, and these are considered in both a biochemical and neurobiologic perspective.[20] A number of recent studies suggest both an immediate and longitudinal effect of serial manipulation that includes both improved range of motion and reduction in pain in patients with acute and chronic low back pain.[11] The possible mechanism for this observation may lie in foundational work conducted by Wyke.[21,22] The articular capsules of the spinal zygapophyseal joints contain numerous mechanoreceptors that relay proprioceptive information on joint position and mobility through myelinated fibers to the substantia gelatinosa of the spinal cord. Increased proprioceptive input through type I and II receptors associated with spinal mobility is thought to diminish the transmission of nociceptive afferent input through type IV receptors. Manipulation of painful, restricted joints beyond their usual range may initiate stimulation of type I and II receptors, thereby inhibiting type IV nociceptors and reducing nociceptive input at the anterior spinothalamic tract. This concept was further supported and developed by Melzack and Wall[23] through their research into the gate theory of pain modulation. The gate theory proposes that the central transmission of sensory information including pain can be inhibited and blocked by increased proprioceptive input and conversely facilitated by a reduction in proprioceptive input. Although it is clear that the majority of pain reduction, improved range of motion, and functional status is a result of the natural history of mechanical spine pain, manipulation may provide greater palliative benefits and enhance earlier recovery over other conservative interventions.

More recently investigators have begun to consider the role of manipulation in the endogenous opiate system as a possible mechanism in pain relief. Vernon et al[24] demonstrated a rise in plasma beta-endorphin levels within minutes of a single spinal manipulation. Other investigators have identified an impact of manipulation on the immune system. Brennan and colleagues in a series of studies[25-27] have demonstrated that the immune system responds in a variety of ways to spinal manipulation. Although these and other studies document the transient effects of MT, larger controlled studies are required to determine whether any of these effects have any positive impact on the recovery and health status of any patient.

CHIROPRACTIC EVALUATION OF THE INJURED ATHLETE

The chiropractic approach to the clinical evaluation of the injured athlete is consistent with what is done by other health care providers: a thorough history and complete physical examination. Initial off-site evaluation of the injured athlete often begins with a series of intake forms. Pain diagrams, neck disability indices, low back disability indices, and visual analogue scales can provide a valuable objective measure of pain, functional impairment, and disability. A complete history detailing the presenting complaint, mechanism of injury, aggravating and relieving factors, history of similar injury, and past health history is necessary in establishing a differential diagnosis.

Physical assessment of the injured athlete begins with recording standard vital signs: blood pressure, heart rate, temperature, and respirations. The area of primary complaint should be inspected for any signs of abnormality, deformity, bruising, or discoloration. Palpatory assessment will reveal areas of tenderness, pain, and increased muscle tone.

Range of motion of all affected joints must be assessed. Goniometers can provide objective, reliable, and angular measures of the joints of the limbs. Cervical and lumbar range of motion instruments (CROM and BROM) can provide reliable measures of cervical and lumbar range of motion.

Where **neurologic insult** is suggested, a thorough neurologic evaluation is needed. Deep tendon reflexes, muscle strength testing, and sensory deficit assessment can help differentiate injuries associated with peripheral nerve, nerve root, or spinal cord insult.

Orthopedic evaluation helps identify sites of articular or osseous injury. Chiropractic palpatory examination can help identify joint dysfunction in spinal and extremity injuries. When necessary, investigation such as plain film radiography, advanced imaging, and nuclear medicine may be required to confirm the diagnosis. Figures 10–3 and 10–4 demonstrate algorithms useful in the assessment of traumatic neck and low back injuries.[28]

TREATMENT COMPLICATIONS AND CONTRAINDICATIONS

Although MT is considered a safe procedure, adverse reactions to treatment can and do occur. Side effects can range from transient, short-term, discomfort to death. Dvorak et al[29] have developed a useful classification system based on both chronologic and clinical criteria (Table 10–2):

1. Adequate reaction
2. Exceeding reaction
3. Reversible complication
4. Irreversible complication

Adequate Reaction. This has been defined as transient discomfort of the patient developing within hours of a manipulation and resolving spontaneously within 2 days. It is usually characterized by regional soreness, light-headedness, and fatigue. Complaints are typically subjective.

Exceeding Reaction. Less commonly patients may experience a more pronounced reaction to a manipulative procedure resulting in an exacerbation of the presenting complaint. Unlike an adequate reaction, exceeding reactions demonstrate clear objective signs of a worsening clinical picture. Signs and symptoms typically develop within 6 to 12 hours of the treatment and resolve without treatment within 2 days.

Reversible Complication. Rarely a manipulation may result in an exacerbation, complication, or iatrogenic injury that mandates an immediate change in management and that may require additional diagnostic procedures. This may include the development of a radiculopathy, rib fracture, articular derangement, or vertebral artery insult leading to transient vertebral basilar artery symptoms. Depending on the nature of the injury, treatment options can range

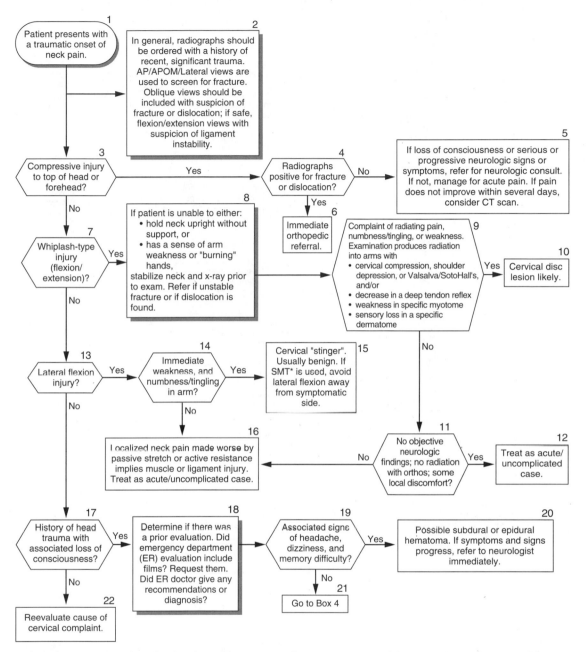

FIGURE 10–3. Algorithms for the clinical assessment of traumatic injury of the cervical spine. AP, anteroposterior; APOM, anteroposterior open mouth; LBP, lumbar puncture; SLR, straight leg raising; WLR, weak leg raising; SI, sacroiliac joint; SMT, spinal manipulative therapy. (From Souza T: Differential Diagnosis for the Chiropractor, p. 45, © 1997, Aspen Publishers, Inc.)

from conservative treatment through surgical interventions. Chronologic criteria range from immediate reaction to days, with complete recovery depending on type of insult.

Irreversible Complication. Rarely, MT can result in permanent injury with subsequent im-

pairment and disability. This can include regional weakness associated with radiculophty to paraplegia and tetraplegia subsequent to vertebral basilar artery injury. Chronologic criterion is immediate or within 48 hours. Table 10–2 categorizes Dvorak's four subclassifications of chronologic and clinical criteria.

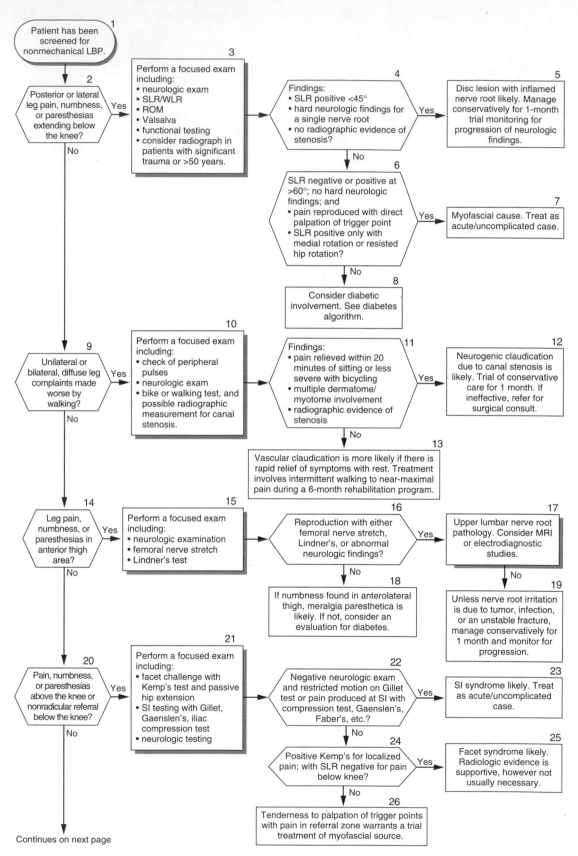

FIGURE 10-4. Algorithm for the clinical assessment of the lumbar spine. (Adapted with permission from K. McCarthy, *Topics in Clinical Chiropractic*, Vol. 1, pp. 79–80. © 1994, Aspen Publishers, Inc.)

Continues on next page

Illustration continued on opposite page

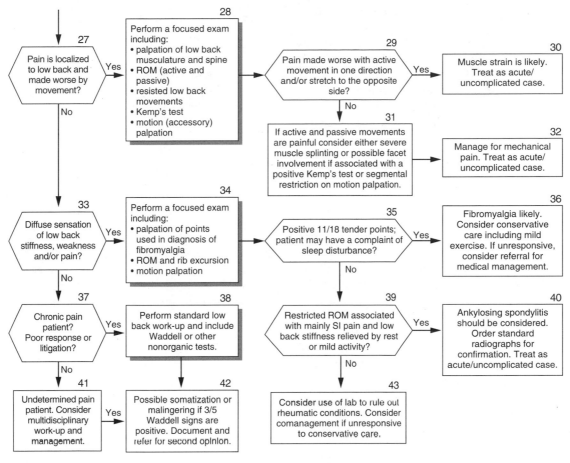

FIGURE 10–4 *Continued*

Incidence

Although complications thought to be related to MT are often reported in the popular press, the actual frequency of documented injury in the scientific literature is small and more accurately reflects the rarity of such events. Serious vascular side effects following cervical spine injury are thought to occur in between 1 per 1 million and 1 per 3 million manipulations.[12] Cauda equina syndrome following manipulation is even less common, with a rate of occurrence of 1 per 10 million lumbar spine manipulations. Manipulation remains a safe procedure for treatment of spinal and extremity injuries and when compared to other forms of interventions is exem-

TABLE 10–2. Chronologic and Clinical Criteria for the Classification of Complications From Manipulative Therapy

REACTION TYPE	ONSET	RESOLUTION	INJURY
Adequate reaction	Hours	2 d	Subjective pain
Exceeding reaction	Hours	2 d	Objective injury
Reversible injury	Days	Injury dependent	Full resolution
Irreversible complication	Immediate	Permanent	Impairment or disability

Adapted from Dvorak J, Kranzlin P, Muhlemann D, Walchli B: Musculoskeletal complications. In Haldeman S (ed): Principles and Practices of Chiropractic, 2nd Ed. Appleton & Lange, East Norwalk, Conn, 1992, pp 549–577.

plary. A recent Rand study[10] comparing relative risks of serious complications associated with common treatment options for spinal conditions reports a complication rate of 15,600 per 1 million for cervical spine surgery and 1000 per 1 million for serious gastrointestinal hemorrhage associated with nonsteroidal anti-inflammatory drug (NSAID) use. MT maintained a relative risk of 1 per 1 million. Table 10–3 provides an outline of relative risk of common therapeutic interventions for neck injuries.

Risk Factors

The safety of any therapy can be enhanced by identifying those risk factors thought to be associated with the development of side effects and complications. Factors thought to predispose to vascular injury were thought initially to be history of vascular disease, cigarette use, oral contraceptive use, osteoarthritis, increasing age, and migraine headache. Terrett,[12] in a review of 183 cases of cerebral vascular accidents, was unable to correlate any historical factors or comorbidities associated with increased risk of cerebral vascular accident following manipulation. Additionally, traditional physical examination procedures such as blood pressure, arterial auscultation, and functional vascular tests failed to identify those at risk. This notwithstanding, the prudent practitioner continues to be sensitive to such proposed risk factors until further research more clearly defines their role in the injured athlete and general population.[30]

When considering the implementation of MT in the management of the injured athlete, one should consider the presence of both absolute

TABLE 10–3. Relative Risk of Serious Complication from Customary Interventions for Cervical Spine Injuries

TREATMENT	RISK
Surgery	15.6/1000
NSAID	1/1000
Manipulation	1/1,000,000

From Hurwitz EL, Aker PD, Adams AH, et al: Manipulation and mobilization of the cervical spine: a systematic review of the literature. Spine 21:1746–1759, 1996.

TABLE 10–4. Contraindications to Spinal Manipulative Therapy

Primary bone tumors
Metastatic bone disease
Osteomyelitis
Inflammatory arthritides
Osteoarthritis
Trauma
Progressive neurologic disorders
Congenital abnormalities
Osteoporosis
Blood clotting disorders

and relative contraindications to MT. Since the recreational athlete is more likely to span all decades of life and more likely to present with known or unknown comorbidities, it is in this group that the clinician must be most sensitive to the possibility of contraindications to manipulation (Table 10–4).

Tumors. Because bone tumors negatively affect the structural integrity of bone, they represent an absolute contraindication to regional manipulation and a relative contraindication when removed from the area. Primary bone tumors are more common in those in the second and third decades of life and are increasingly rare with age. Primary bone tumors beyond age 40 are those most likely associated with multiple myeloma and its variants.[31] More common in the second half of life are those metastatic bone diseases associated with primary tumors of colon, breast, prostate, and thyroid.

Infection. Osteomyelitis represents both a contraindication to manipulation and an urgent medical condition. Osteomyelitis is not typically visualized on plain film radiographs until at least 25% to 30% of focal bone destruction occurs, a time frame of approximately 3 weeks. Clinicians must be sensitive to the presence of atypical musculoskeletal pain and fever and consider laboratory testing and advanced imaging in this patient profile.

Arthritides. Generally, inflammatory joint disease is an absolute contraindication to manipulation in the affected joint.[32] The most serious sequela is rupture of the transverse ligament with dislocation of the atlas in individuals with systemic arthritides.[33] Rheumatoid and psoriatic arthritis are those arthritides most often associated with this phenomenon. Cervical spine radiographs with flexion-extension views will detail the degree of instability at the atlas-axis joint. Amounts greater than 3 mm in adults and 5 mm in children are suggestive of cervical instability. In athletes with clinical signs of cord compression a neurosurgical consult should be requisitioned. Conversely the spinal ankylosis associated with the seronegative arthritides such as Reiters, psoriatic arthritis, and ankylosing spondylitis represents an absolute contraindication.

Osteoarthritis. Degenerative joint disease is not considered an absolute contraindication to manipulation, although it remains an important consideration in the decision tree.[34] Degenerative changes in the cervical spine have not been shown to increase the risk of vertebral basilar or carotid artery injury,[12] nor are there any studies suggesting the corelation between manipulation and degenerative joint disease and other adverse reactions. When prescribing manipulative procedures in the older recreational athlete in whom degenerative joint disease is a consideration, the best approach is a cautious, slow mobilization with increasing force and progression over time to manipulation.

Trauma. Trauma in athletes remains both an indication and contraindication to manipulation. Thorough assessment is necessary to determine which individuals require MT as a result of their injuries and those who are precluded from MT as a result of the nature of their injuries and who require a different approach to treatment. Trauma in sports can be classified into two domains: macrotrauma, which is caused by external mechanical forces exerted on the spine or extremities such as fracture and dislocation, and microtrauma, which is a result of prolonged, repetitive movement, classic examples being stress fractures and lateral epicondylitis.[29] Significant trauma such as fracture and dislocation is easily documented through radiographic evaluation and advanced imaging techniques such as CT and MRI.

Although such injuries represent absolute contraindications to manipulation, manual procedures can be instituted to improve range of motion and decrease pain when adequate healing has occurred.[29] In the athlete experiencing soft tissue injuries and mechanical joint pain without evidence of fracture and dislocation, MT can be prescribed early. Considerable discussion and debate has centered about the clinical phenomenon of joint hypermobility and its implication for MT.[35-37] White and Panjabi[38] defined clinical instability as:

> loss of the ability of the spine under physiologic loads to maintain relationships between vertebrae in such a way as neither damage nor subsequent irritation to the spinal cord or nerve roots, and, in addition, no development of incapacitating deformity or pain due to structural changes.[38]

Spinal Instability. The question remains whether this represents a contraindication to manipulation. Some authors suggest that repeated forceful manipulation may in fact cause or increase the magnitude of preexisting spinal instability.[39,40] Indeed the Standards of Practice Guidelines[30] developed through consensus advise that segmental hypermobility of the spine remains a relative contraindication. Other authors suggest that manipulation may be of benefit in the acute stage of injury.[29] With the exception of significant spinal instability associated with complete destruction of the holding element of a joint the diagnosis of such clinical instability is difficult. Clinical evaluation of instability is frought with issues surrounding the validity and reliability of customary palpatory, stress, and provocative testing. Stress views incorporated in standard radiographic evaluation can more accurately detect instability, but in the end it is difficult to confirm whether the athlete's ongoing complaints are a direct result of the instability or a result of other factors.

Neurologic Disorders. Signs and symptoms associated with acute myelopathy and cauda equina represent an absolute contraindication to manipulation.

Congenital Abnormalities. Although difficult to detect in otherwise healthy, asymptomatic athletes, congenital abnormalities, such as agenesis of the dens of C2 leading to atlantoaxial instability and spondylolysis with listhesis, in the injured athlete may represent a contraindication to MT.

Osteoporosis. Any condition affecting the mineralization and subsequent strength of bone, such as age-related osteoporosis in the older recreational athlete, remains a concern. Recreational athletes with a history of oral or inhaled corticosteroid use associated with chronic conditions such as asthma may be at risk for structural bone failure following manipulation.

Hematologic Considerations. Although such athletes are unlikely to be encountered, athletes with a history of blood clotting disorders or use of anticoagulant therapy should not undergo MT because of the risk of intraspinal hemorrhage.

EVIDENCE FOR MANIPULATIVE THERAPY IN MANAGEMENT OF SPORTS-RELATED INJURIES

The concept of evidenced-based medicine and best practice methods in health care has significantly altered the way in which all health disciplines view the value and validity of the care they provide. It has ushered in a new age of professional introspection and self-doubt as each profession begins to review the scientific evidence in support of its therapeutic interventions. Historically in areas of therapy that have inherent safety risks such as pharmacologic interventions, legislation has ensured that products be tested for safety, efficacy, and effectiveness before they are introduced to the health care arena. This has not been the case when conservative management of musculoskeletal injuries and, even more so, sports-related injuries are under consideration.

Conservative care provided by the medical and allied health professions with a long history of apparent safety and anecdotal claims of effectiveness has not been the focus of rigorous testing. For example, the Agency for Health Care Policy and Research commissioned a multidiscipline expert panel to review the scientific evidence of conservative management of acute low back pain.[41] Following a critical review of the literature it was the opinion of the panel that only manipulation and NSAIDs were deemed efficacious and effective in the management of acute low back pain in adults. Usual and customary treatments such as ultrasound, back school, bed rest, traction, and mobilization were not recommended. Increasingly there is a demand that all therapies be tested for safety and effectiveness in an effort to differentiate between useful and useless therapies and to identify interventions with similar effectiveness but with significant variations in safety.[42]

In the scientific evidence for efficacy and effectiveness there is a clear hierarchy of quality of research. Randomized, double-blind, placebo, controlled clinical trials remain the gold standard of clinical research. Less structured are the observational trials, or case control or cohort studies. Descriptive studies such as cross-sectional, correlational studies, case series, and case reports provide methods of documenting clinical observations. Finally, expert opinion based on clinical experience may often be the only rationale for the use of a particular therapy.

There is little clinical evidence in the literature to support the use of MT in the management of sports-related injuries. The current evidence consists primarily of expert opinion and case reports relating to the management of spine and extremity injuries.[41] There is, however, a significant body of research relating to manipulation for neck pain, head pain, and back pain in the general population. There is some concern about whether the results of these studies can be generalized to populations with spinal injuries acquired through sports. It would seem reasonable that spinal injuries would respond to MT much as neck, head, and back pain do regardless of the mechanism of injury. An argument could be made that athletes, both recreational and professional, may respond better to all forms of therapy in view of the motivation to recover, lack of secondary gain, compliance to treatment recommendations, elevated health status at time of injury, and other possible factors known to affect recovery times.[41] On this basis we will review the current status of the research in spinal MT in general with the sincere belief that similar treatment results should be expected in athletes.

Low Back Pain

The epidemiology of low back pain in sports has not been extensively studied, but Williams[43] estimates that spinal injuries may account for up to 15% of all sports-related injuries. Keene et al[44] reviewed the frequency and types of lumbar injuries in intercollegiate athletes over a 10-year period and determined a lumbar injury rate of

7%. Interestingly only 6% of injuries occurred in competition, with the other 94% sustained during practice. Not unexpectedly, the majority of injuries occurred in football and gymnastics. Acute back injuries were the most frequent types of injuries with the majority diagnosed as muscle strain, a condition thought to respond well to MT.

There is a wealth of randomized clinical trials comparing spinal MT for acute and chronic low back pain with a variety of conservative therapies. Recently, thorough systematic reviews of the literature have helped categorize the clinical trials for all conservative interventions for low back pain.[11] Reviewing the literature relative to acute low back pain revealed at least 12 quality studies. Of these, 11 trials reported greater improvement with MT in all subjects or within subgroups when it was compared to other treatment interventions such as diathermy, infrared heat, massage, electrical stimulation, and the control group.[45-54] The evidence in subacute and chronic low back pain includes 12 quality studies also, of which eight reflect better outcomes for MT when compared to various forms of treatment including bed rest, analgesics, massage, back education, and usual care provided by a family physician.[55-62] On the strength of evidence it is appropriate to consider spinal MT a front line therapy for uncomplicated low back, sports-related injuries.

Cervical Spine Injuries

Sports-related cervical spine injuries run a broad spectrum from mild sprain or strain injuries to life-threatening cervical spine fracture with spinal cord compression. For illustration, Albright[63] in a retrospective study of 342 college football players recorded 60 neck injuries. Of these, 55% were deemed soft tissue or skeletal injuries without neurologic involvement. In those patients experiencing neurologic involvement (45%), most followed a course of transient neck pain and nerve root dysfunction with subsequent neck stiffness and reduced range of motion before experiencing full recovery. Three players experienced permanent neurologic deficit of the fracture.

The literature pertaining to the efficacy of spinal manipulative therapy for cervical spine pain is less voluminous than that for low back pain. Hurwitz et al[10] in a systematic review of the literature were unable to locate any randomized clinical trials of manipulation for acute cervical spine injuries. For subacute and chronic neck pain, two randomized clinical trials demonstrated improvements in both pain scores and range of motion following MT.[64,65] Two other studies assessed the efficacy of the cointerventions of MT and muscle relaxants versus muscle relaxants alone.[66,67] Both studies suggested a greater degree of improvement in the manipulation and medicated group versus the manipulation group alone. The authors suggest that manipulation is probably more effective than mobilization or traditional physical therapy in the management of cervical spine pain.

Extremity Injuries

Chiropractors are engaged extensively in the management of a wide variety of sports-related injuries including injuries to the extremities, and they report effectiveness in this area. There remains, however, little quality evidence to support these claims, and certainly investigations have developed beyond the case report and case control level. There are numerous case reports outlining the successful chiropractic management of hip injuries,[68-71] shoulder injuries,[72-74] knee injuries,[75,76] and ankle injuries.[77,78] These case studies serve to highlight the often diverse, multimodal therapeutic approach, including MT by chiropractors, in the rehabilitation of the injured athlete. Since there are numerous cointerventions in each case report it is difficult to determine the degree to which MT alone is responsible for resolution of complaints. Randomized control trials are needed to understand the proposed efficacy and effectiveness of manipulation of the injured extremity.

REFERENCES

1. Chapman-Smith D: The Chiropractic Report. 11(2):2, 1997
2. Aker PD: Ontario Health Survey. 1990
3. Christensen MG, Delle Morgan MG: Job analysis of chiropractic in Canada. National Board of Chiropractic Examiners, Greeley, Colo, 1993
4. Christensen MG, Delle Morgan MG: Job analysis of chiropractic in the United States. National Board of Chiropractic Examiners, Greeley, Colo, 1993

5. DeLee JC, Drez D: Orthopedic sports medicine. WB Saunders, Philadelphia, 1994

6. Gatterman MI: Chiropractic management of spine related disorders. Williams & Wilkins, Baltimore, 1990

7. Schafer RC: Chiropractic health care. Foundation for Chiropractic Education and Research, Des Moines, 1976, pp 10–14

8. Schiotz EH, Cyriax J: Manipulation past and present. William Heinemann Medical Books, London, 1975, pp 5–45

9. Balon J, Aker PD, Crowther ER, et al: A comparison of active and simulated chiropractic manipulation as adjunctive treatment for childhood asthma. N Engl J Med 339:1013–1020, 1998

10. Hurwitz EL, Aker PD, Adams AH, et al: Manipulation and mobilization of the cervical spine: a systematic review of the literature. Spine 21:1746–1759, 1996

11. van Tulder MW, Koes BW, Bouter LM: Conservative treatment of acute and chronic low back pain: a systematic review of randomized controlled trials of the most common interventions. Spine 22:2128–2156, 1997

12. Terrett AGJ: Vertebral basilar stroke following manipulation. Des Moines National Chiropractic Mutual Insurance Company, Des Moines, 1996

13. Haldeman S: Spinal manipulative therapy: a status report. Clin Orthop Rel Res 179:63, 1983

14. Haldeman S: Spinal manipulative therapy in the management of low back pain. In Finneson BE (ed): Low Back Pain. JB Lippincott, Philadelphia, 1980

15. Sandoz R: Some physical mechanisms and effects of spinal adjustments. Ann Swiss Chiropract Assoc 6:91, 1976

16. Sandoz R: Some reflex phenomena associated with spinal derangements and adjustments. Ann Swiss Chiropract Assoc 7:45, 1981

17. Mierau D: Manipulation and mobilization of the third metacarpophalangeal joint: a quantitative radiographic and range of motion study. Manual Med 3:135–140, 1988

18. Leach RA: The Chiropractic Theories, 3rd Ed. Williams & Wilkins, Baltimore, 1994, p 18

19. Mennell J McM: The musculoskeletal system: differential diagnosis from symptoms and physical signs. Aspen, Gaithersburg, Md, 1992, p 30

20. Dhami SID, DeBoer KF: Systemic effects of spinal lesions. In Haldeman S (ed): Principles and Practices of Chiropractic, 2nd Ed. Appleton & Lange, East Norwalk, Conn, 1992, pp 115–135

21. Wyke BD: The neurology of joints. Ann R Coll Surg Engl 41:25–58, 1967

22. Wyke BD: The neurology of low back pain. In Jason MIV (ed): The Lumbar Spine and Back Pain, 3rd Ed. Churchill Livingstone, New York, 1987

23. Melzack R, Wall PD: Pain mechanisms: a new theory. Science 150:971–979, 1965

24. Vernon HT, Dhami MSI, Howlet TP, Annett R: Spinal manipulation and beta-endorphins: a controlled study of the effect of a spinal manipulation on plasma endorphin levels in normal males. J Manipulative Physiol Ther 9:115–123, 1986

25. Brennan PC, Graham MA, Triano JJ, et al: Lymphocytic profiles in patients with chronic low back pain enrolled in a controlled trial. J Manipulative Physiol Ther 4:219–227, 1994

26. Brennan PC, Hondras MA: Priming neutrophils for an enhanced respiratory burst by manipulation of the thoracic spine. In Work S (ed): Proceedings of the 1989 Conference on Spinal Manipulation, Washington DC. Foundation for Chiropractic Education and Research, Des Moines, 1989, pp 160–183

27. Graham MA, Brennan PC: Functional ability of natural killer cells as an outcome measure for treatment efficacy. In Work S (ed): Proceedings of the 1991 Conference on Spinal Manipulation, Arlington, Va. Foundation for Chiropractic Education and Research, Des Moines, 1991, pp 84–86

28. Souza T: Differential Diagnosis for the Chiropractor. Aspen, Gaithersburg, Md, 1997

29. Dvorak J, Kranzlin P, Muhlemann D, Walchli B: Musculoskeletal complications. In Haldeman S (ed): Principles and Practices of Chiropractic, 2nd Ed. Appleton & Lange, East Norwalk, Conn, 1992, pp 549–577

30. Henderson D, Chapman-Smith DA, Mior S, Vernon H (eds): Clinical Guidelines for Chiropractic Practice in Canada. Canadian Chiropractic Association, Toronto, 1994

31. Yochum RT, Rowe LJ: Essentials of Skeletal Radiology. Williams & Wilkins, Baltimore, 1987

32. Greenman PE: Principles of Manual Medicine. Williams & Wilkins, Baltimore, 1989, p 99

33. Kleynhans AM: Complications of and contraindications to spinal manipulative therapy. In Haldeman S (ed): Modern Developments in the Principles and Practice of Chiropractic. Appleton-Century-Croft, East Norwalk, Conn, 1980, pp 359–384

34. Stoddard A: Manual of Osteopathic Practice. Hutchinson, London, 1969, p 279

35. McGregor M, Mior S: Anatomical and functional perspectives of the cervical spine. Part III: The "unstable" cervical spine. J Can Chiropract Assoc 34:145–152, 1990

36. Rifkinson-Mann S, Mormino J, Sahcdev VP: Subacute cervical spine instability. Surg Neurol 26:413–416, 1986

37. Kirkaldy-Willis WH, Farfan HF: Instability of the lumbar spine. Clin Orthop 165:110–123, 1982

38. White AA, Panjabi MM: Clinical Biomechanics of the Spine. JB Lippincott, Philadelphia, 1978, p 192

39. Stoddard A: Manual of osteopathic medicine, 2nd Ed. Hutchinson, London, 1983, pp 290–291

40. Grieve GP: Lumbar spine instability. Physiotherapy 68:2–8, 1982

41. U.S. Department of Health and Human Services Public Health Service, Agency for Health Care Policy and Research: Acute Low Back Problems in Adults. Clinical Practice Guideline number 14. AHC PR Publication no. 95-0642. Rockville, Md, 1994

42. Sackett DL, Richardson WS, Rosenberg W, Haynes RB: Evidenced-Based Medicine. Churchill Livingstone, New York, 1997

43. Williams RW: Biomechanical factors in spinal injuries. Br J Sports Med 14:14, 1980

44. Keene JS, Albert MJ, Springer SL, et al: Back injuries in college athletes. J Spinal Dis 2:190–195, 1989

45. Bergquist-Ullman M, Larrson U: Acute low back pain in industry: a controlled prospective study with special reference to therapy and confounding factors. Acta Orthop Scand 170(suppl):1–17, 1977

46. Blomberg S, Svardsudd K, Mildenberger F: A controlled multicentre trial of manual therapy in low back pain. Scand J Prim Health Care 11:83–90, 1993

47. Delitto A, Cibulka MT, Erhard RE, et al: Evidence for use of an extension-mobilization category in acute low back syndrome: a prescriptive validation pilot study. Phys Ther 73:216–228, 1993

48. Farrell JP, Twomey LT: Acute low-back pain: comparison of two consecutive treatment approaches. Med J Aust 1:160–164, 1982

49. Hadler NM, Curtis P, Gillings DB, Stinnett S: A benefit of spinal manipulation as adjunctive therapy for acute low-back pain: a stratified controlled trial. Spine 12:703–705, 1987

50. MacDonald RS, Bell CMJ: An open controlled assessment of osteopathic manipulation in nonspecific low-back pain. Spine 15:364–370, 1990

51. Mathews W, Morkel M, Mathews J: Manipulation and traction for lumbago and sciatica: physiotherapeutic techniques used in two controlled trials. Physiother Pract 4:201–206, 1988

52. Nwaga VCB: Relative therapeutic efficacy of vertebral manipulation and conventional treatment in back pain management. Am J Phys Med 61:273–278, 1982

53. Rasmussen GG: Manipulation in treatment of low back pain: a randomized clinical trial. Manual Med 1:8–10, 1979

54. Wreje U, Nordgren B, Aberg H: Treatment of pelvic dysfunction in primary care: a controlled study. Scand J Prim Care 10:310–315, 1992

55. Arkuszewski Z: The efficacy of manual medicine in low back pain: a clinical trial. Manual Med 2:68–71, 1986

56. Evans DP, Burke MS, Lloyd KN, et al: Lumbar spinal manipulation on trial. Part 1: Clinical assessment. Rheumatol Rehabil 17:46–53, 1978

57. Gibson T, Grahame R, Harkness J, et al: Controlled comparison of short-wave diathermy treatment with osteopathic treatment in nonspecific low-back pain. Lancet pp 1258–1261, 1981

58. Herzog W, Conway PJW, Willcox BJ: Effects of different treatment modalities on gait symmetry and clinical measures for sacro-iliac joint patients. J Manipulative Physiol Ther 14:104–109, 1991

59. Koes BW, Bouter LM, Mameren H van: Randomised clinical trial of manual therapy and physiotherapy for persistent back and neck complaints: results of a one year follow-up. Br Med J 304:601–605, 1992

60. Postachini F, Facchini M, Palieri P: Efficacy of various forms of conservative treatment in low back pain: a comparative study. Neuro Orthop 1:28–35, 1988

61. Triano JJ, McGregor M, Hondras MA, Brennan PC: Manipulative therapy versus education programs in chronic low back pain. Spine 20:948–955, 1995

62. Waagen GN, Haldeman S, Cook G, et al: Short term trial of chiropractic adjustments for the relief of chronic low-back pain. Manual Med 2:63–67, 1986

63. Albright J, McAuley E, Martin R, et al: Head and neck injuries in college football: an eight year analysis. Am J Sports Med 13:147–152, 1985

64. Cassidy JD, Lopes AA, Yong-Hing K: The immediate effects of manipulation versus mobilization on pain and range of motion in the cervical spine: a randomized controlled trial. J Manipulative Physiol Ther 15:570–575, 1992

65. Vernon HT, Aker PD, Burns S, et al: Pressure pain threshold evaluation of the effect of spinal manipulation in the treatment of chronic neck pain: a pilot study. J Manipulative Physiol Ther 13:13–16, 1990

66. Sloop DR, Smith DS, Goldenberg E, Dore C: Manipulation for chronic neck pain: a double blind controlled study. Spine 7:532–535, 1987

67. Howe DH, Newcombe RG, Wade MT: Manipulation of the cervical spine: a pilot study. J R Coll Gen Pract 33:564–579, 1983

68. Bartlinski J, Tarquini F: Conservative care of iliotibial band syndrome: a short report. J Sports Chiropract Rehab 12:163–164, 1998

69. Russell B: A study of lumbopelvic dysfunction/psoas insufficiency and its role as a major cause of dance injuries. Chiropract Sports Med 5:9–17, 1991

70. Horrigan J: Resolution of a groin injury in a professional hockey player by soft tissue mobilization: a case report. Chiropract Sports Med 6:151–154, 1992

71. Baker G: Iliotibial band syndrome and tibialis posterior syndrome resulting from a fixated talus: a case report. Chiropract Sports Med 9:119–121, 1995

72. Jaffe MP, Bonsall WB: A traumatic osteolysis of the distal clavicle: a case report. J Sports Chiropract Rehab 12:65–70, 1998

73. Leahy P: Synoviochondrometaplasia of the shoulder: a case report. Chiropract Sports Med 6:5–9, 1992

74. Buchberger D: Scapular-dysfunctional syndrome as a cause of grade 2 rotator cuff tear: a case study. Chiropract Sports Med 7:38–45, 1993

75. Souza T: Treatment of common knee disorders. Part II: Specific conditions. Chiropract Sports Med 4:119–128, 1990

76. Meyer J, Zachman Z, Keating J, Traina A: Effectiveness of chiropractic management for patellofemoral pain syndrome: a single subject experiment. J Manipulative Physiol Ther 13:539–549, 1990

77. Carter S, Carter A: Chiropractic management of Achilles tendonopathy. Sports Exercise Manage 3:108–110, 1997

78. Bratingham J, Silverman J, Deliman A, et al: Chiropractic management of Achilles tendonitis. J Neuromusc Sys 2:52–55, 1994

SUGGESTED READING

Eisenberg DM, Davis RB, Ettner SL, et al: Trends in alternative medicine use in the United States, 1990–1997: the results of a follow-up national survey. JAMA 280:1569–1575, 1998

Eisenberg DM, Kessler RC, Foster C, et al: Unconventional medicine in the United States: prevalence, costs, and patterns of use. N Engl J Med 328:246–252, 1993

Herkowitz HN, Rothman RH: Subacute instability of the cervical spine. Spine 9:138–157, 1985

Kopansky DR, Popadopoulos C: Canadian chiropractic resource databank. J Can Chiropract Assoc 41:157–191, 1997

Shekelle P: What role for chiropractic in health care. N Engl J Med 339(1):1074, 1998

Tamulaitis CM, Auerbach GA, Chance MA, et al: Chiropractic growth outside North America. In Haldeman S (ed): Principles and Practices of Chiropractic, 2nd Ed. Appleton & Lange, East Norwalk, Conn, 1992, pp 599–619

11

Appraisal of Alternative Treatment Methods in Sports Medicine Rehabilitation

DINESH A. KUMBHARE ■ JOHN V. BASMAJIAN

Sports medicine, in its widest sense, carries a heavy overload of unproved methods to treat the residual disabilities arising from acute and chronic insults to the bodies of professional and amateur players of all ages. We hasten to add: many appear to respond well to a wide range of methods favored by practitioners ranging from trainers and coaches to specialized therapists, physiatrists, and orthopedic surgeons. Some of these treatments have a rational linkage to established physiologic, biomechanical, and pathologic processes. For example, common sense suggests that an ice pack compress to a traumatized area may reduce bleeding and tissue reaction, hence promoting earlier recovery. But common sense also led earlier generations of well-meaning physicians to incarcerate millions of heart attack victims with complete bed rest for 5 weeks. If they died of pulmonary embolism either in bed or shortly after mobilization, this outcome was accepted as the natural history of cardiac damage. Today we know better. The ideal treatment was dead wrong.

CONCISE SURVEY OF ALTERNATIVE THERAPIES

Alternatives to conventional medical treatment methods, including allied health practices are numerous. They boast individual histories that began before recorded history, on the one hand, and only a decade or two on the other. What they have in common is that most conventional physicians and surgeons view them with skepticism and rejection. Even when they are tolerant of complementary therapies, they almost never perform or prescribe them. Physical therapists and athletic trainers dabble in one or two procedures, sometimes enthusiastically, but rarely embrace a system to the exclusion of accepted conventional therapies. Some of the conventional therapies are no more "proved" by research than the unconventional therapies are.

The following, in alphabetical order, is a broad but incomplete list of alternative therapies, excluding osteopathic medicine, which has become the accepted foster sibling of conventional (allopathic) medicine. Much more detail may be found in the book by Fulder.[1]

Acupuncture and Acupressure (Shiatsu). These ancient Chinese treatments are too well known to require explanation. *Electrical stimulation* through a needle and *ear acupuncture* are variations, as is moxibustion, in which smoldering mugwort leaves are placed at the insertion point.

Alexander Technique. Invented by an Australian Shakespearean actor in 1869 when he began to have difficulty vocalizing, the Alexander technique teaches proper posture of the vertebrae, head, and neck to minimize stress and its consequences. The technique has received wide acclaim and some inconclusive research support.

Anthroposophic Medicine. This system, invented by Rudolf Steiner, has three subdivisions: eurythmy, speech therapy, and art therapy. It aims to achieve harmony between people and their environment through self-awareness and homeopathic remedies.

Aromatherapy. In aromatherapy, essential aromatic oils from plants are applied to the skin, and massage is used to relieve various symptoms.

Autogenics. This technique of autosuggestion, taught by psychotherapists, enhances relaxation and reduces stress.

Biofeedback. Various electronic displays are used to train subjects to alter otherwise unsensed internal activities, especially of muscles and vessels. This is the only method in nonconventional medicine that is based on medical research and has been validated with multiple double-blind research studies in rehabilitation.

Bone Setting. Bones and joints of the limbs are restored after injury.

Breathing Therapies. These include *Pranayama* (Indian yogic breathing).

Chiropractic. This technique requires no description, being well known (see Chapter 10).

Cranial Therapy. The bones of the cranium are manipulated.

Electrical Therapies. These include *magnetic field therapy, diathermy,* and *ion generators* to influence deeper tissues.

Feldenkrais Technique. Related to the Alexander retraining technique, the Feldenkrais technique concentrates on motion and awareness, similar to *Tai chi.*

Healing. Healing techniques utilize "psychic energy" and include *faith healing, spiritual healing, magnetic healing, mental healing, laying on of hands, absent healing (at a distance), prayer healing, spirit healing (exorcism), auric healing (employing a body's "aura"), homeopathy, biochemic remedies (employing tiny doses of drugs), and Bach flower remedies or salts.*

Jin Shin Do. Jin Shin Do is a form of acupressure. The practioner tries to establish a "safe place" where the recipient can, with gentle specific touch, become aware of and relive the original feeling in slow motion to the intensity that he or she desires. This is done to make adjustments to the "alignment" of yin-yang polarity, the five elements (fire, earth, metal, water, wood), and qi (chi) energy.

Kinesiology (Applied Kinesiology). Not to be confused with the scientific use of this term, kinesiology is a diagnostic and therapeutic approach advocated by chiropractor George Goodheart since 1965 that is widely used in sports. Finger pressure is believed to strengthen weakened muscles, but no reliable research has confirmed efficacy.

Massage. A well-known therapy, massage is believed to stimulate the circulation and tissues. Variations include *postural integration, reflexology, rolfing,* and *polarity therapy.*

Noncontact Therapeutic Touch. Noncontact therapeutic touch is a learned process by which the practitioner centers his or her mind or induces a state of consciousness similar to a meditative state, becomes clear about the intent to help or heal, and moves the palms of the hands slowly as if to form a silhouette around the body of the recipient in an effort to assess or influence the individual's energy system. The assumption is that all living things generate vibratory fields.

Polarity Therapy. This is a combination of massage and instruction of *body alignment.*

Reflexology (Reflex Zone Therapy). This therapy utilizes foot massage for organ symptoms.

Relaxation and Meditation. These self-explanatory methods are taught by trained psychotherapists to restore health.

Rolfing, Hellerwork, and Soma. Originated by Dr. Ida Rolf, who was an associate at Rockefeller Institute, rolfing is concerned with improving well-being and overall health. Dr. Rolf taught that physical relationships of the body's tissues (its structure) determine how the body functions. In the optimal structure (and, hence, function), the body has a vertical relationship to gravity. The body is balanced ("rolfed") so the force of gravity can flow through. Then, spontaneously, the body heals itself.

Trager Approach. This approach stresses the communication between the quality of feelings to the nervous system. Using a series of gentle, noninvasive movements of joints, muscles, and the entire body through full available (pain-free) range of motion to convey positive, pleasurable feelings, which enter the central nervous system and begin to trigger tissue changes by means of many sensorimotor feedback loops between the mind and the muscles.

OUTCOME MEASURES

Rarely are the outcomes in sports medicine rehabilitation as dramatic as in cardiology. Nevertheless, the acceptance of commonsense approaches is routine and natural against a background of virtually no gold standard research in sports medicine and therapy. We believe the professions must take the leadership in developing outcome measures that are valid and reproducible.

Outcome measures have three purposes: discriminative, predictive, and evaluative. Evaluation is the most relevant in sports medicine decision making. The recommendations of the conference organized by the National Center for Medical Rehabilitation Research and the Agency for Health Care Policy and Research are extremely relevant in discussions of values, cross-domain issues measurements, controlled studies, and therapeutic efficacy. Their report[2] is an excellent beginning for all who care about outcome measures. Here we concentrate on the special focus of both this book and this chapter and offer a sample template of how one might clarify the issues of efficacy.

As Kronenberg et al[3] proclaim, with apparent glee, alternative medicine is now being embraced by medical practitioners "as an exciting new area for investigation." They point out that conventional rehabilitation professionals "have had a long and productive relationship with so-called 'simple unconventional' therapies including massage, biofeedback, acupuncture, physical manipulation, exercise, and relaxation techniques." But they do not mention therapeutic touch, rolfing, mesmerism, vital energy, chan-

neling, homeopathy, herbalism, naturopathy, hypnosis, holism, and vitalism, among other therapies, which are considered the real, unconventional approaches. In fact, biofeedback and relaxation therapy have been studied in *double-blind* studies quite thoroughly at medical schools.

Eisenberg et al[4] define alternative medicine as "medical interventions not taught widely in US medical schools or generally available in US hospitals." They found in a survey that "roughly 1 in 4 Americans who see their medical doctors for a serious health problem may be using unconventional therapy in addition to conventional medicine for that problem." Many of us would not accept the breadth of Eisenberg's definitions of "alternative," but that quarrel will never end so long as we accept and understand that much of what healers do has a nonspecific or "debonafide" positive outcome, or what used to be called the placebo effect. While we condemn the deliberate use of deception as the basic method of any treatment, we should be thankful that many of our therapies, old and new, have a strong debonafide healing effect. We have compelling evidence that debonafide (placebo) effects are a common, almost essential, part of both good and poor results in pharmacologic and physical realms. Why not also in complementary therapies?[5]

Intensive research to determine the specific effects of everything we do remains a top priority because, although we admire the debonafide effects of any treatment, science and plain honesty cannot be ignored. They demand that we learn as much about debonafide effects as possible while also learning more about the powerful tool of their nonspecific response.

Some would say that having a naive or ignorant or suggestible subject is important for the success of a debonafide treatment or advice. In an editorial *The Lancet*[6] described a remarkable experiment in a class of medical students asked to cooperate in a study of sedatives and stimulants. Participants were to take one of two capsules, half of which were blue and half were pink. In fact, all of the capsules were inert placebos. The medical students were more susceptible to debonafide effect than other people were. They became sedated with the blue capsules and elated with the pink capsules. More striking, there were marked changes in blood pressure in at least 65% of the students; that is, an actual morphologic or physiologic change occurred.

A scathing editorial by Tannock and Warr[7] in the Canadian Medical Association Journal sums up our conclusions about blind acceptance of unconventional therapies: "The treatment recommendations that physicians make are founded ideally on some understanding of the scientific basis . . . and high quality evidence with regard to efficacy and safety." We concur with their recommendation that physicians and, we would add, all healing and training professions "should become knowledgeable about unconventional treatments in vogue," so that they can discuss them wisely. Unless the professional personally has seen or experienced convincing evidence of substantial efficacy beyond the 50% placebo response,[8] caution is essential. A recommendation of any "complementary therapy" delivered with conviction and "hype" is a placebo, as efficacious as placebo often is.

PLACEBO EFFECT OF MACHINES

Many sports medicine professionals are smug because they use techniques and machines rather than drugs. They should know about the placebo effect of machines, too. In 1968, Schwitzgebel and Traugott[9] reported experiments with normal subjects who were attached by arm electrodes to electronic machines. It was implied that their performance on special tasks would be improved when the current was on, and would decrease when it was off. In all cases, however, no current was ever turned on, and the hypothesis was borne out. When the subjects thought the current was on, their performance increased markedly. In a rehabilitation setting the surroundings, equipment, and assured way in which clinicians and trainers handle the equipment have a strong influence on the patient.

There is no question that approaches other than chemotherapy have strong debonafide influences. Byerly[10] pointed out that placebos seemed to work like magic incantations. Both require an object of concentration, and virtually anything can function as an object. Further, the improvement need not be simply subjective. Byerly cites a rheumatoid arthritis study in which placebos achieved the same level of effectiveness as aspirin in objective improvement in the swelling of the joints. Physical agents other than ingested chemicals may have the same powerful debonafide response, as difficult as it is for people in rehabilitation to accept.

A research study on the treatment of back problems[11] found that the electronic gear of the recording devices (inserted electrodes, electromyographic equipment, various electronic devices, and a computer) raised the placebo response in almost 200 patients with back problems to about 50%, from about 30% with sugar pills. The superiority under these circumstances of treatment with diazepam (Valium) for painful spasms of the back is hard to interpret; in another double-blind study using impressive recording apparatus, we found that diazepam succeeds at only about 60% level.[12] Is the special effect of diazepam only 10%? We cannot give a final answer. But clinicians who do various complex things to patients, with and without machines, should be aware that physical and psychosocial procedures must surely have a strong debonafide effect that is urgently in need of clarification in sports medicine and therapy.

THE THERAPIST IS VITAL

Despite everything said here, the therapist, whether a physical therapist, occupational therapist, trainer, psychotherapist, or physician, is vital. A human being surrounded by the mystique of a profession has the strongest influence. If that clinician is knowledgeable about the procedures and confident, and, above all, comes in close contact with the patient, almost any treatment is successful in 30% to 50% of patients. A confident trainer or clinician who touches and manipulates the patient greatly enhances the effectiveness of therapy regardless of whether the current fad is carried out correctly or incorrectly. Hence, many patients will recover from disabilities of the musculoskeletal system even with "improper" manipulation or traction rather than "proper" manipulation advocated by some charismatic healer. It doesn't seem to matter whether transcutaneous electrical nerve stimulation (TENS) or acupuncture is done absolutely "correctly"; many patients will achieve substantial success or cure. The important element seems to be a close contact between the patient and the therapist. This is at least as important as the specific effect, if any, of the treatment.

TREATMENT VERSUS TRAINING

Therapists in their clinical practice perform many training procedures that are highly effective, for example, gait training for amputees, and patients with stroke and cerebral palsy. But this is not really "therapy"; it is assisting patients who are doing the therapy themselves with the assistance of a trained person. It is education or reeducation, not therapy in the classic medical model. When physical therapists are engaged, there still is some overlay of debonafide effect, but the main effect is one of learning or adaptation.

In contrast is the complex of modalities in which the clinician does something to the patient, eg, heat and cold treatments, manipulation, massage, noninvasive internal deep therapies such as ultrasound and radiant energy in general, vibration, and electrical stimulation. These are treatments, not training, and here the debonafide factor becomes an overwhelmingly important feature of the relationship between clinician and patient. Here the personality flows from one to the other and enhances the specific effect of the treatment.

What specific effects do these various therapeutic conditions have that exceed the debonafide, or nonspecific, effect? These areas require intensive exploration by the several rehabilitation professions.

Placebos have always been with us and always will be. They certainly are important in both Eastern and Western medicine. Anything can act as a placebo, whether chemical, electrical, mechanical, radiant, verbal and transmitted, or internal such as thought and faith. It is difficult to properly identify and study this important effect.

MODEL DESIGN FOR A CONTROLLED PILOT STUDY

Against the above background, any research would be welcome, but a well-controlled double-blind study would be the most useful for proving the efficacy of old or new therapeutic methods in sports and exercise rehabilitation. We offer unsophisticated readers our model for a pilot clinical trial using a factorial design to compare the effectiveness of *anti-inflammatory medication plus physical therapy,* with *physical therapy alone* in *the functional recovery of acute ankle sprains in athletes.* It is based on an approved master's thesis (McMaster University, 1995) by Dr. Kumbhare as a model for a full-scale trial employing the model.

Rationale For Study

Ankle sprains are one of the most common problems in sports medicine. Conservative management of acute nonsurgical sprains has not been subjected to methodologically rigorous study. Nonsteroidal anti-inflammatory drugs (NSAIDs) are commonly prescribed for sprains. This study would examine the analgesic and anti-inflammatory effects of these medications in conjunction with physical therapy in the treatment of ankle sprains.

Statement of Problem

The proposed study used a factorial design to compare the effectiveness of NSAIDs and a physical therapy program in the management of acute (less than 48 hours) nonsurgical ankle sprains. The selected outcome measures would be used to quantitate function.

The Question

Does the use of NSAIDs or participation in a comprehensive physical therapy program (singly or in combination) reduce the number of days to return to sport? Specifically, the study will attempt to test the following three hypotheses (Ho):

Ho 1. (NSAID): Number of days for return to sport is the same in groups who do and who do not take NSAIDs.

Ho 2. (PT): Number of days for return to sport is the same in groups who do and who do not participate in a comprehensive physical therapy program.

Ho 3. (PT + NSAID): The combination of physical therapy and NSAIDs has no advantage over the summed individual treatment effects.

Clinical Presentation

While ankle sprains are usually caused by a combination of plantar flexion and inversion, other mechanisms such as dorsiflexion, rotation, and direct trauma can also contribute to injury. Signs and symptoms will vary depending on the severity of the injury. Tenderness and swelling are localized over the injured structures. With minimal damage, when the examiner applies a mild tension force, there is slight pain and no ligamentous laxity, and no other structures are injured. As the severity of injury increases, more structures are damaged, and signs and symptoms are more diffuse. For example, with severe ankle injury, tenderness and swelling are generalized; stressing the injured areas is extremely painful; and the anterior drawer test indicates some laxity. The anterior drawer test is used to measure the amount of anteroposterior accessory movement at the ankle joint. With complete rupture of the ligaments, the ankle is unstable with diffuse tenderness and swelling, a definite anterior drawer test without an end point, and *absence* of pain when stressing the joint. Also, other structure such as the interosseous membrane, peroneal retinaculum, talus, tibia, fibula, and os calcis may be injured. Physical examination should be used to evaluate the extent of injury and the presence of associated injury.

Radiologic Evaluation

Stiell et al[13] proposed "rules" for radiologic evaluation of acute ankle injuries. They reported that more than 85% of patients arriving at an emergency department with an ankle sprain were sent for x-ray studies but that fewer than 15% of those patients had significant fractures. In an effort to avoid unnecessary x-ray studies while still feeling confident that a fracture is not missed, Steill et al[13,13a] proposed the Ottawa Ankle Rules. These are clinical decision aids to help physicians decide definitively, from the clinical examination, which patients do not have fractures:

A. An ankle x-ray series is only required if there is any pain in the malleolar zone and any of these findings:
   1. Bone tenderness at the posterior edge or tip of the lateral malleolus
   2. Bone tenderness at the posterior edge or tip of the medial malleolus
   3. Inability to weight bear both immediately and in the emergency department
B. A foot x-ray series is only required if there is any pain in the midfoot zone and any of these findings:
   1. Bone tenderness at the base of the fifth metatarsal
   2. Bone tenderness at the navicular bone
   3. Inability to weight bear both immediately and in the emergency department

Literature Review of Conservative Management of Ankle Sprains

This review focuses on various components of the conservative management of ankle sprains. Surgical interventions for ankle sprains are not included.

Choice of NSAID

There are no clear guidelines to assist the clinician in selecting the most appropriate agent for a specific patient. Therefore, the NSAID used in this study would be chosen on the basis that it has a short duration and rapid onset of action and that it has few side effects and is relatively inexpensive.

Physical Therapy

There are few studies that examine the role of physical therapy in ankle sprains. A Medline search would be conducted in an attempt to find studies that examined the effects of physical therapy on ankle sprains. After searching back to 1966, only one trial was identified that looked at a complete physical therapy program. Brooks et al[14] observed 21 patients with acute ankle sprains for 5 weeks. The patients received an iced foot bath, "mobilization," and "instruction" on normal gait. This group was compared with 27 patients who received no treatment. There was no significant difference between treatment and comparison groups with respect to the average number of days off work. This small study was randomized but not double-blinded, and the physical therapy program did not include a strengthening or proprioceptive component. The outcome measures did not include assessments of pain or function.

Eiff et al[15] conducted a cohort study of 82 patients who had first-time ankle sprains to determine whether early immobilization or mobilization was associated with early return to military work. The patients were randomly assigned to two groups: (1) an early mobilization group who underwent an active rehabilitation program 2 days after injury and (2) an immobilization group who underwent an active rehabilitation program 10 days after injury. At one-year follow-up, the early mobilization group had less pain at 3 weeks, but otherwise there was no difference between the two groups in the frequency of residual symptoms. Patients in the early mobilization group were more likely to return to full work.

There were only two other studies dealing with physical therapeutic modalities. The first study was a nonblinded, nonrandomized case series that examined cryotherapy. Hocutt et al[16] showed that cryotherapy was better tolerated than hot packs by 37 patients with acute ankle sprains. Williamson et al,[17] in a randomized, double-blinded trial involving 154 patients with acute ankle sprains, showed that ultrasound was not helpful in managing swelling.

Proprioception

Three trials examined proprioceptive deficits and functional instability. Freeman et al[18–20] used the modified Romberg test to demonstrate that patients with functional instability had proprioceptive deficits. Study samples were small and poorly described, and there was a high dropout rate (54%). Preinjury estimates of proprioception and functional instability were not documented. Without this information it is difficult to interpret the results.

Tropp[21] used a force platform and stabilometry to measure the area of body sway. Tropp's results must be interpreted with caution because the sample sizes were small. The study lacked sufficient power to detect a statistically significant difference even if one existed. Insufficient statistical detail was provided, and it is unclear whether differences between or within subjects were detected. The measured areas were not compared with normal values.

Gross[22] reported the effects of recurrent lateral ankle sprains on active and passive judgment of joint position. A two-way analysis of variance (ANOVA) for repeated measures was used to indicate that ankle sprains have no significant effect on judgment of ankle position. Passive judgment was significantly better than active judgment in patients without injured ankles. No statistical significance was found between injured and uninjured ankles.

Goldie et al[23] studied 48 athletes at least 8 weeks after an inversion ankle injury. A three-way ANOVA was used to show that in untrained subjects postural lateral steadiness was significantly worse on the injured than the uninjured legs with the eyes open and with the eyes closed, whereas no postural deficit was found on the injured leg in trained subjects with the eyes open or closed. It was concluded that rehabilitation following inversion injury of the ankle should include balance retraining.

Gross[22] proposed a model for joint position sense that suggested that joint receptors act as a major contributor to joint position sense. Muscle receptors contribute to the perception of joint movement more than joint position.

Based on these case series, it is difficult to arrive at a clear conclusion regarding proprioception and its role in functional instability. Clinically, it is believed that proprioceptive abnormalities contribute to initial and recurrent ankle sprains by contributing to an increase in functional instability. It is also believed that retraining can reduce any proprioceptive abnormalities and therefore functional instability.

Modalities

Two articles[24,25] examined the effects of pulsed shortwave therapy in the treatment of ankle sprain. Barker et al[24] examined 73 patients with ankle sprains less than 36 hours old. A randomized, double-blind study design was used to assess the efficacy of a commercial lower power pulsed shortwave therapy machine in the treatment of lateral ligament sprain. An active treatment group and control group were observed. No statistical difference between the two groups was detected, and the authors concluded that there was no sound evidence for the efficacy of pulsed shortwave therapy in the treatment of acute ankle sprain.

Another study, by McGill,[25] examined the effects of pulsed shortwave therapy on lateral ligament ankle sprains. Thirty-seven patients were allocated to active and treatment groups in a double-blind but not randomized study. No statistically significant difference between the two groups was detected in relation to the average pain score, the amount of analgesia taken, and the time to full weight bearing. No consistent treatment effect was detected. Based on the results of these two studies, it would seem that pulsed shortwave therapy for acute lateral ligament sprains of the ankle does not provide any significant treatment benefit.

Laba and Roestenburg[26] examined the efficacy of ice therapy for acute inversion ankle sprain. Thirty patients were randomly assigned to active and control groups. No statistical difference was detected in the level of pain or the amount of swelling in patients treated with or without ice. These results were likely influenced by the small number of patients and insensitive methods for the measurement of pain and swelling.

Paris et al[27] examined the effects of the neuroprobe on the treatment of second-degree ankle inversion sprains in 16 patients. A neuroprobe is a type of acupuncture-mediated transcutaneous electrical nerve stimulation. No statistically significant difference was detected between groups for rehabilitation time relative to edema and pain. This study was not double blinded, which may have resulted in attention bias toward the active treatment group. The investigators did not use an objective method of evaluating pain, and their sample size was too small. Nonetheless, it was concluded that neuroprobe treatment may enhance the rehabilitation process in ankle sprains.

Cote et al[28] compared cold, heat, and contrast baths on the amount of edema in first- and second-degree sprains during the subacute (48 hours post injury) phase of rehabilitation. Cold treatment was found to be significantly different from treatment with heat and contrast baths. No significant difference was detected between heat and contrast baths, and it was therefore concluded that cold therapy was the most appropriate of the three treatments for minimizing edema from the third through fifth days after injury.

Four other studies identified in the literature all concluded that application of cold in acute ankle sprains is safe and "therapeutically sound" for controlling pain, loss of motion, and edema. These studies were low in power, were not randomized or double blinded, and did not use objective measurement techniques. The results should therefore be interpreted with caution.

Roycroft and Mantgani[29] examined early active management of inversion injuries of the ankle. Thirty-seven patients were entered into the initial conservative treatment study arm, which called for application of a wool and Elastoplast bandage or plaster of Paris backslab and crutches to maintain non-weight-bearing status. In first-degree ankle sprains, the recovery period in the active treatment arm was up to a maximum of 15 days, compared with up to 30 days in the initial conservative treatment arm. For second-degree injury, the recovery period was 30 days in the immediate active treatment arm and up to 50 days in the initial conservative treatment arm. It was concluded that these differences were statistically significant and that active treatment results in an early return to normal functional activities. Of the study subjects, 46% were lost to follow-up.

Conclusion from Literature Search

There is lack of acceptable evidence for the efficacy of the use of analgesics, NSAIDS, and the various components of physical therapy in the treatment of acute ankle sprains. Health professionals usually use a combination of these treatments. However, it is not known which of these are most effective or when to use them most efficaciously. There is a need to examine analgesics, NSAIDS, and physical therapy of acute ankle sprains in a comprehensive manner. All the various components such as modalities, compressive dressings, strengthening, proprioception, and progressive return to sport need to be examined. The resultant pilot study incorporated these components. However, conclusions could only be drawn about the whole program, not its component parts. The following pages are transcribed from the thesis that resulted. It is provided as a practical model for those who do appropriate research on the efficacy of alternative treatment methods.

SCALE TO GRADE SEVERITY OF ANKLE SPRAINS

Item Selection

The types of items required are difficult to measure with conventional quantitative methods; therefore, a six-point *modified Likert scale* (Table 11–1) is used. It is important that the scale adequately cover the domain of clinical evaluation of ankle sprains. This is achieved by clinical observation, literature review, and expert opinion by a specialist in sports medicine, rheumatology, or physiatry and a research physical therapist. The scale is applied to various

---

TABLE 11–1. Scale for Grading Severity of Ankle Sprains

---

*Pain**
None, minimal, moderate, severe, exquisite, unbearable

Swelling
None, trace, localized minimal, localized moderate, generalized with no effusion, generalized with ankle effusion, toe involvement

Contusion/discoloration
None, trace, <5 cm, 5–10 cm, >10 cm; involves toes, whole foot

Soft tissue tenderness
None, trace, localized minimal, localized moderate, generalized moderate, generalized severe

Bone tenderness
None, trace, localized minimal, localized moderate, generalized moderate, generalized severe

Squeeze test (compress distal fibula and tibia)
None, trace, localized minimal, localized moderate, generalized moderate, generalized severe

Range of motion[†] (ROM; compared with unaffected side)
Plantar flexion
   Full, 75%–100%, 50%–75%, 25%–50%, <25%, 0% (no movement)
Dorsiflexion
   Full, 75%–100%, 50%–75%, 25%–50%, <25%, 0% (no movement)
Inversion
   Full, 75%–100%, 50%–75%, 25%–50%, <25%, 0% (no movement)
Eversion
   Full, 75%–100%, 50%–75%, 25%–50%, <25%, 0% (no movement)

Power (compared with unaffected side)
Inversion
   Grade 5, grade 4+, grade 4, grade 4−, grade 3, <grade 2
Eversion
   Grade 5, grade 4+, grade 4, grade 4−, grade 3, <grade 2

Anterior drawer test (compared with unaffected side)
0–2 mm (normal range), 2–5 mm, 5–7 mm, 7–10 mm, 10–15 mm, >15 mm

Talar tilt (compared with unaffected side)
0–5 degrees (normal), 5–10 degrees, 10–15 degrees, 15–20 degrees, 20–30 degrees, >30 degrees

Ability to bear weight on injured foot[‡]
Full, 75%–100%, 50%–75%, 25%–50%, <25%, 0%

Flamingo stance on the injured foot[§]
>30 s (normal), 20–30 s, 10–20 s, 5–10 s, 1–5 s, unable

---

*Rater records his or her perception of the patient's pain.
[†]The rater compares the ROM of the affected side with that on the other side to determine the percentage of ROM *lost*.
[‡]Performed using a standard bathroom type scale, as follows: First, obtain the patient's total weight, then measure how much weight he or she is able to tolerate through the unaffected limb standing on both feet but with the injured foot on the bathroom scale. Divide this weight into the patient's total weight to determine the percentage of weight bearing.
[§]With the second hand of a wristwatch, the rater times how long the patient is able to stand on the injured foot with the eyes closed.

types of ankle sprains to determine whether the items appear to measure what they are supposed to. All items on the scale are assigned a weight of 1. The modified Likert scale is scored from 0 to 5. A maximum score of 0 implies no ankle impairment, and a maximum possible score of 80 reflects severe impairment.

Experimental Design

To account for possible systematic changes in patients with each consecutive rating, a Latin square design with order of raters and time as variables was used when the scale was applied.

Training sessions, involving raters and one or two patients, were used to help familiarize the raters with the scale items. Prior to each session, raters were sent a copy of the scale and given 3 weeks to familiarize themselves with it. Questions about scale administration were clarified before the start of the reliability study.

The scale was administered by seven raters, all of whom regularly assess ankle sprains. The raters administered the scale at time 1 and again at time 2 (a day later) in the same patients.

RESULTS

Seven patients, with a mean age of 27 years, were enrolled in the pilot study. The duration of symptoms ranged from 24 hours to 26 years. The patient with an ankle sprain for 26 years had permanent residual effects.

The data were analyzed with a repeated measures analysis of variance (ANOVA) on *BMDP statistical software,* as summarized in Table 11–2. Data were calculated using absolute, not relative, error terms. These are reasonable because they represent the worst possible value for an estimate comparing rater 1 time 1 with rater 2 time 2, for example. Homogeneity of items by the Cronbach alpha is approximately 0.98.

FULL-SCALE STUDY DESIGN PROPOSAL

We concluded that a full-scale study is warranted. A 2×2 factorial design should be used to evaluate four groups: NSAIDs plus physical therapy; NSAIDs alone; physical therapy and acetaminophen (used as placebo); and acetaminophen without NSAIDs or physical therapy.

The factorial study design is used to make two or more different therapeutic comparisons in the same trial without increasing the required number of patients, which is quite large in any case. An advantage of this design is that it allows the study of interactions between treatments (eg, whether NSAIDs plus physical therapy produces earlier return to sports than NSAIDs or physical therapy alone).

Inclusion Criteria

Active university and professional athletes in our community will be included in the study if they meet the following inclusion criteria:

1. Acute ankle sprain less than 48 hours old.
2. Sprain is unilateral or bilateral.
3. Grade 1 or 2 sprain. Sprains will be classified into three types: grade 1, mild stretching of the ligament with the fibers still intact; grade 2, more severe injury with partial disruption of the ligament fibers; and grade 3, complete disruption of the ligament.[30]
4. Pain score ≥ 4 on the visual analogue scale (VAS).
5. No abnormality on plain or stress x-ray studies of the ankle.
6. Informed consent.

Exclusion Criteria

The following exclusion criteria will apply:

1. Previous intolerance to NSAIDS (eg, dyspepsia, hematemesis, melena, renal insufficiency).
2. Currently active medical problems involving the gastrointestinal tract that are contraindications to NSAID administration (eg, peptic ulcer disease, gastritis, gastroesophageal reflux).
3. Previous sensory abnormalities such as peripheral neuropathy, and reduced proprioception from any cause.
4. Ankle sprain resulting in instability as defined by a positive anterior drawer test (>1 cm movement, no end point) and stress x-ray studies, with a talar tilt >15 degrees. Grade 3 ankle sprains are, by convention, first treated with a below-knee walking cast for 6 weeks before physical therapy is started.

TABLE 11–2. Results of Pilot Study* (Data Analysis Combining Time 1 and Time 2 Using Repeated Measures ANOVA)

SOURCE	DEGREES OF FREEDOM	SUM OF SQUARES	MEAN SUM OF SQUARES	F STATISTIC	PROBABILITY	ESTIMATE OF VARIANCE COMPONENT
Mean	1	24515.31	24515.31			
Patient	6	5929.26	988.21			68.45
Time	1	0.65	0.65			0.00 (actually, −0.49)
Rater	6	597.98	99.66			5.44
Patient + time	6	111.63	18.60	3.29	0.0111	1.85
Patient + rater	36	612.45	17.01	3.01	0.0007	5.68
Rater + time	6	72.92	12.51	2.15	0.0716	0.93
Patient + rater + time	36	203.80	5.661			5.661

ANOVA, analysis of variance.
*Intraclass correlation coefficient: Intrarater, 0.84; interrater, 0.80; interrater as intrarater, 0.78.

5. Plain x-ray abnormalities (eg, fractured tibia, fibula, talus, or os calcis; degenerative changes).
6. Other diagnosis (eg, acute peroneal retinaculum rupture, distal fibular fracture, osteochondral fracture of the talus, fracture of the os calcis [anterior process]).
7. Refusal to provide informed consent.

There will be no need clinically to exclude patients on the basis of age or gender because these factors do not influence treatment. Also, it will not be necessary to exclude recurrent ankle sprains because these are usually treated essentially the same as initial lesions and there is usually no significant clinical difference in the rate of recovery.

Physical Therapy Program

The physical therapy program used for this study will consist of methods and exercises that can be performed at most facilities by most physical therapists. The protocol will be reviewed as uniformly as possible.

An important component of any comprehensive program is patient education, to help patients understand their problem and the factors that may have contributed to it. It may also improve their motivation and compliance. Therefore, before entrance to the study, patients will be given a standardized educational session and reading material on ankle sprains and the purpose of the study.

The physical therapy protocol will contain three phases: acute (first 24 to 48 hours after injury), early mobilization, and intensive rehabilitation. Throughout the program, appropriate aerobic activity will be performed by the athlete to maintain cardiovascular fitness. This will be accomplished by stationary cycling without tension and using only the uninvolved leg for pedaling, although both legs may be used when tolerated. A program to maintain strength and flexibility of the upper body and unaffected leg will also be performed during the formal rehabilitation program.

Acute Phase

The acute phase will be implemented during the first 24 to 48 hours after injury, as follows:

1. *"Rest"*: Avoiding movement and activities that aggravate pain. Use crutches, with or without weight bearing as tolerated.
2. *Cryotherapy*: Submersion in a slush tank for 20 minutes, three or four times a day. If available, a cryoboot may also be used.
3. *Compression*: Wear three socks, one on top of the other. This works better than wrapping with a tensor bandage because it conforms to the foot almost perfectly and does not cause

constriction. Taping or pressure splinting will also be used.

4. *Elevation:* Place the injured limb above the level of the heart. While the patient is asleep, the leg should be placed atop three pillows. This same position is required while the patient is awake, sitting with the leg on a stool or chair is not true elevation. This position needs to be maintained for 1 hour three times daily.

Early Mobilization

Early mobilization will be promoted as follows:

1. *Range of motion:* ROM will include a combination of active and passive ROM, with pain as the limiting factor. This process will begin while the limb is submerged in the slush tank. Passive ROM will be achieved by placing surgical tubing around the forefoot, stirrup fashion. The athlete will slowly pull straight back and to either side within the limits of pain. Active ROM will be achieved by asking the athlete to dorsiflex, plantar flex, invert, and draw letters of the alphabet while the foot is submerged. These exercises will be performed with compression of the foot and ankle using the technique described earlier. The regimen will be performed three times daily.

2. *Progressive weight bearing as tolerated:* To minimize pain, this will be performed three times daily, as soon as the limb is removed from the slush tank. As pain diminishes, progressive weight bearing will be phased into progressive gait training. This will be accomplished using crutches at first and then quickly progressing to the use of a cane and then an ankle brace.

3. *Strength:* This will require the use of surgical tubing three times daily, with four repetitions of dorsiflexion, plantar flexion, eversion, and inversion, holding each repetition for 20 seconds.

4. The next phase begins when weight bearing is painless, approximately 75% active ROM has been regained, and the swelling has virtually resolved.

Intensive Rehabilitation

The intensive rehabilitation phase will consist of the following exercises:

1. *Stretching:* For gastrocnemius and soleus muscles, a slant board will be used. The quadriceps and hamstring muscles will be stretched using prone knee flexion and supine toe touching, respectively. These exercises will be performed three times daily.

2. *Strengthening:* Plantar flexion strengthening will be achieved using toe curling with a towel, and standing heel raises, first using both legs and progressing to one leg. Dorsiflexion strengthening will be achieved using a 1-pound weight suspended from the forefoot. Inversion and eversion strengthening exercises will be performed using tubing. Each exercise will be performed three times daily in four sets of 10 repetitions.

3. *Bicycling:* Bicycling will start with no resistance, and then progressive resistance will be applied as tolerated for 10 to 15 minutes daily.

4. *Proprioception training:* This will be achieved initially by single-leg weight bearing with the eyes closed. The process will begin as soon as the athlete can bear weight. If available, a wobble board and a ski trainer will be phased in as soon as tolerated. These activities will be performed three times daily in four repetitions.

5. *Impact loading:* This will be achieved by having the athlete jump on a small trampoline, with progression to running on the spot and jumping to a squat position (half squat, then full squat).

6. *Progressive functional activities:* When tolerated, fast walking, straight running, running and cutting at approximately 45 degrees and then 90 degrees, and running in a figure-of-eight will be attempted. These routines will be introduced once the athlete has full ROM and strength and is essentially pain free.

7. *Progressive return to sport:* This will be attempted once the athlete has the ability to tolerate fast walking, straight running, running and cutting at approximately 45 and 90 degrees, and running in a figure-of-eight with minimal exacerbation of symptoms.

OUTCOME MEASUREMENT

Primary Outcome

The primary outcome of interest for the present study would be the number of days to return to sport. The measurement will record the number of days from injury, including the day of injury, to return of the athlete to the original sport.

Secondary Outcome

The secondary outcome measures are as follows:

1. Number of days for pain relief. Pain will be measured using the VAS. The VAS also provides a continuous data set that is helpful for analysis purposes, and is easy to administer once patients are familiar with its format. It is known to detect large changes (about 20 mm), but there is ongoing debate on whether it is sensitive to small changes in pain status.[28] For this study, a 50% reduction in VAS score will be regarded as significant change in pain. An ANCOVA will be used for statistical analysis, with pretreatment VAS score as the covariate.
2. Ability to participate at best sport will be graded with the following scale: (1) able to play pain free and at preinjury ability, (2) able to play at preinjury level but with pain, (3) substandard play without pain, (4) substandard play with pain and (5) unable to play. This arbitrary scale is rather crude, but it represents an attempt to stratify functional outcome retrospectively. Owing to the nature of acute sports injuries and the methodologic design of the current study, it will be impossible to make preinjury functional assessments. It is also difficult to accurately assess all athletes (from different sports).
3. Ankle sprain scale.
4. Recurrence of ankle sprain on injured leg.
5. Number of days to commencement of training.

These secondary outcome measures are designed to quantitate the athlete's activity level and so allow a correlation to be made between activity and return to sport. The main drawback of this approach is the measurement of preinjury ability. This is impossible after the athlete suffers an ankle sprain. The purpose of this study is to evaluate NSAIDS and a physical therapy program, and thus it is more important to correctly

measure the level of activity soon after the time of injury than to assess preinjury abilities.

METHODS

Once the patients have been selected, based on inclusion and exclusion criteria, informed consent will be obtained. Informed consent will be obtained from a parent or guardian if the athlete is younger than 16 years.

Compliance

Compliance with a maneuver is an important component of effectiveness. Although an effectiveness trial attempts to reflect the clinical situation, simple strategies to improve compliance affect study analysis and generalizability. Patients will be asked to keep a log book to record their intake of NSAIDS and any drug side effects. Attendance at physical therapy will be recorded by the clinic. The project coordinator will review these log books weekly. Athletes who have low compliance will be contacted to determine their reasons, and they will be encouraged to improve their performance.

Contamination and Cointervention

Contamination occurs when the control group inadvertently receives the experimental maneuver, thereby diluting the anticipated differences between interventions.[31] Cointervention is the performance of additional acts or strategies in the experimental group but not in the control group, resulting in more reported outcomes in the experimental group. This observed difference cannot be attributed to the study maneuver alone. Cointervention is more likely when the study is unblinded.[29] In this study, knowledge of an individual athlete will permit the investigators or others involved with the trial to pay more attention to the experimental group. This will allow those with an expectation bias to affect the study results. Such effects can be minimized by double blinding.

Patients will be asked not to participate in any other physical therapy program for the lower extremity or take any analgesic medications not provided by the investigators. Patients will be provided a list of the common analgesics (prescription and over-the-counter) that need to be avoided. They will be excluded from the trial if a change in their medical status requires treatment with analgesics or renders them unable to participate in the physical therapy program.

Stratification

Patients will be stratified among the groups for recurrent sprains, severity of sprain, and type of sport. The type of sport will be classified as (1) sports that place a high demand on the ankle and (2) sports that do not place a high demand on the ankle. Stratification will ensure that each group has an equal number of patients with recurrent ankle sprains and an equal proportion of patients with variable severity of sprain.

Maneuver

Patients (or their parent or guardian) who have given informed consent will be provided with a standard educational session on the VAS by the project coordinator and with a diary for recording their daily VAS scores. Every effort will be made to motivate patients to mark their diaries and to elevate the injured foot as much as possible.

Patients will be randomly assigned to one of four groups. The assignment will be known only to the principal investigator. Variable block randomization, with a block size of 4, will be used. To maintain uniformity of the groups, the randomization will also stratify patients according to grade of ankle sprain, recurrent injury, and sport type. The four groups will consist of (1) physical therapy plus placebo medication (acetaminophen), (2) NSAID alone, (3) NSAID plus physical therapy, and (4) no treatment (neither medications nor physical therapy). Groups 1 and 4 will be given a placebo oral medication (acetaminophen).

All oral medications will look alike. The NSAID will be chosen based on short duration of action, rapid onset of action, fewest side effects, and least expense. Patients will be given enough medication to last until the next therapy session, which should help motivate patients to attend therapy sessions. There will be no delay in receiving physical therapy; if possible, patients will receive therapy on the same day or at the latest by the following day.

Compliance will be determined by correlating the number of pills left with the number of pills the patient said were consumed. Each patient will be asked on a weekly basis about side effects of the medications. Compliance with therapy will be assessed by taking attendance at physical therapy sessions. Also at each session the patients will be asked how many hours they elevated the injured foot.

All patients entered into the study will be followed up. Patients who choose to withdraw or are lost to follow-up will be contacted and their reasons recorded.

All groups will be assessed by an independent assessor who does not know the treatment regimen received by the athlete. Every effort will be made to have no contact between the assessor and the physical therapists and the principal investigator. Assessments will be carried out at daily intervals for 2 weeks, followed by weekly assessment for 4 weeks. The time for follow-up may require lengthening, depending on the data obtained. The assessor will have a predetermined number of items, ie, outcome measures, to record at each assessment, including number of days to return to sport, commencement of training, ability to participate in best sport, ankle sprain scale score, and recurrence of ankle sprain.

Statistical Considerations
Sample Size Calculation

To estimate sample size, we should assume an α and β level of 0.05 and 0.20, respectively. Also, assume that we wish to detect a change of 1 day. The mean number of days to return to work according to Muckle[32] was 5.3 days. The mean square error within subjects, obtained from their data, was 1.44. After making these assumptions and calculations, an estimate of sample size per group is 431. Further, assuming a 10% dropout rate, a total of 1,896 patients will be required.

Analysis

Statistical analysis will require using tables and graphs of mean number of days to return to sport, patients' mean age, mean VAS score, mean number of days to pain relief and to commencement of training, and average amount of time to single-leg stance (proprioception) and secondary outcome measures.

The primary analysis will be on an intention-to-treat basis, and every patient entered into the trial must be accounted for. Patients who are lost to follow-up, are noncompliant, or receive cointervention will be considered study failures.

The results of the mean number of days to return to sport, to pain relief, and to commencement of training, and recurrence of ankle sprains will be analyzed using one-way ANOVA. The ankle sprain scale score will be analyzed using a repeated measures ANOVA. The factors will include severity of ankle sprain, recurrence of ankle sprain, and sport. The variable sport will be broken down to sports that place a high demand on the ankle, and sports that do not place a high demand on the ankle. This method should analyze for possible interactions between the two treatments.

An additional, secondary analysis will be performed on an efficacy basis. Patients will be removed from the analysis if they do not attend physical therapy for three consecutive sessions or do not take medications for three consecutive doses (based on the half-life).

If statistical significance has been achieved, the results will be examined from the clinical point of view to determine whether significance also exists. The literature does not provide any consensus on how much of a difference is clinically different. To determine this, local experts in sports medicine, orthopedic surgery, rheumatology, physical medicine, and rehabilitation and physical therapy will be polled. These results will be compared with answers to similar questions posed to patients; then consensus opinion may be approached. These results will be compared with the statistically obtained results of the study to determine clinical and statistical significance.

Ethical Considerations

Informed consent will be obtained from patients before their entry into the formal study. No preamble will be used to explain the study before the patients read the informed consent form, but questions will be answered afterward. This should reduce any feelings of coercion that patients may have. For patients younger than 16 years, written informed consent will be obtained from a parent or guardian, and verbal informed consent will be obtained from the patient.

This study places its participants under minimal to no risk, since acetaminophen, NSAIDS, and physical therapy are standard therapeutic interventions for ankle sprain and other conditions. Acetaminophen can cause nausea, vomiting, abdominal pain, and very rarely (in overdose amounts) hepatic necrosis. These serious side effects are usually dose related and require drug ingestion in the overdose range (eg, 10–15 g). This study will use acetaminophen in small doses within the recommended range.[33]

Physical therapy involves techniques to reduce pain and inflammation and to improve stretching, strengthening, and aerobic fitness. When administered by a registered therapist, as in the proposed study, no side effects are expected. Physical therapy is not experimental, but it is an innovative technique for ankle sprains, as described in this study protocol.

Patients will be reminded that they are free at any time to withdraw from the study or refuse further treatment at any time. They will also be reminded that confidentiality will be maintained at all times.

We believe this study proposal provides a practical example of how to evaluate important clinical issues in sports medicine. The methodology of this proposal demonstrates that it is theoretically possible to evaluate variables that have traditionally been thought to be difficult or impossible to examine quantitatively. The ICC values of the pilot study show the statistical "power" available with this method.

CONCLUSIONS

Many techniques are used by a variety of health professionals to treat sports injuries. Some of these are summarized in this chapter. Most remain unproved, and to our knowledge have not been examined rigorously. Much work needs to be done in this rapidly expanding field. This chapter discusses the importance of the debonafide effect and its possible ramifications. The effect should not be underestimated. We provide an example of how study methods may be used to study variables previously thought to be difficult to evaluate rigorously.

Finally, we propose that those using complementary medicine continue to embrace what all physicians are pledged to do:

1. Do no harm.
2. Take an appropriate history, do a good physical examination, and perform investigations relevant to the diagnosis.
3. Be sure the patient is aware of the prevailing conventional approach to treatment, and refer the patient as required or requested.
4. Advise the patient that the clinician is practicing a complementary form of diagnosis or therapy usually not considered in the conventional scope of practice.
5. Inform the patient of what to expect in the diagnosis and treatment and give a time frame in which the therapy should be assessed.
6. Monitor the therapy within the parameters of patient compliance and cooperation and institute other interventions when necessary.
7. Document the procedures that have been undertaken.

REFERENCES

1. Fulder S: The Handbook of Alternative and Complementary Medicine, 3rd Ed. Oxford University Press, New York, 1996
2. Fuhrer MJ: Conference report: an agenda for medical rehabilitation outcomes research. Am J Phys Med Rehabil 74:243, 1995
3. Kronenburg F, Mallery B, Downey JA: Rehabilitation medicine and alternative therapies: new words, old practices. Arch Phys Med Rehabil 75:928–929, 1994
4. Eisenberg D, Kessler RC, Foster C, et al: Unconventional medicine in the United States. Natl English J Med 328:246–252, 1993
5. Basmajian JV: A new look at the placebo effect. Med Post 35:13, 1999
6. Drug or placebo? [editorial]. Lancet 2:122, 1972
7. Tannock IF, Warr DG: Unconventional therapies for cancer: a refuge from the rules of evidence? [editorial]. Can Med Assoc J 159:801–802, 1998
8. Basmajian JV: Many challenges remain. In: Basmajian JV, Banerjee SN: Clinical Decision Making in Rehabilitation. Churchill Livingstone, New York, 1996
9. Schwitzgebel RK, Traugott M: Initial note on the placebo effect of machines. Behav Sci 13:267, 1968
10. Byerly H: Explaining and exploring placebo effects. Perspect Bio Med 19:423, 1976
11. Basmajian JV: Effects of cyclobenzeprine HCl on skeletal muscle spasm in the lumbar spine region and back. Two double-blinded controlled clinical studies. Arch Phys Med Rehabil 60:59–63, 1978
12. Basmajian JV: Reflex cervical muscle spasm: treatment by diazepam, phenobarbital or placebo. Arch Phys Med Rehabil 64:121, 1983
13. Steill IG, Greenberg GH, McKnight RD, Wells GA: The "real" Ottawa ankle rules [letter, comment]. Ann Emerg Med 27(1):103–104, 1996
13a. Laupacis A, Steill IG, Stewart D, Anis A: Using the Ottawa ankle rules [letter, comment]. Ann Emerg Med 28(6):730–731, 1996
14. Brooks SC, Potter BT, Rainey JB: Treatment for partial tears of the lateral ligament of the ankle: a prospective trial. Br Med J 282:606, 1981
15. Eiff MP, Smith AT, Smith GE: Early mobilization in the treatment of lateral ankle sprains. Am J Sports Med 22:1, 83–88, 1994
16. Hocutt JE, Jaffe R, Rylander R, et al: Cryotherapy in ankle sprains. Am J Sports Med 10:316, 1982
17. Williamson JB, George TK, Simpson DC, et al: Ultrasound in the treatment of ankle sprains. Injury 17:176, 1986
18. Freeman MAR: Treatment of ruptures of the lateral ligament of the ankle. J Bone Joint Surg 47B:661–668, 1965
19. Freeman MAR: Instability of the foot after injuries to the lateral ligament of the ankle. J Bone Joint Surg 47B:669–677, 1965
20. Freeman MAR, Dean MRE, Hanham IWF: The etiology and prevention of functional instability of the foot. J Bone Joint Surg 47B:678–685, 1965
21. Tropp H: Functional Instability of the Ankle Joint. Linkoping University Medical Dissertations, No. 202, Linkoping, Sweden, 1985
22. Gross MT: Effects of lateral ankle sprains on active and passive judgements on joint position. Phys Ther 67:1505–1509, 1987
23. Goldie PA, Evans OM, Bach TM: Postural control following inversion injuries of the ankle. Arch Phys Med Rehabil 75:969–975, 1994
24. Barker AT, Barlow PS, Porter J, et al: A double-blind clinical trial of low power pulsed shortwave therapy in the treatment of soft tissue injury. physiotherapy 71:500–504, 1985
25. McGill SN: The effects of pulsed shortwave therapy on lateral ligament sprain of the ankle. N Z J Physiol 16:21–24, 1988
26. Laba E, Roestenburg M: Clinical evaluation of ice therapy for acute ankle sprain injuries. N Z J Physiol 7:9, 1989
27. Paris DL, Baynes F, Gucker B: Effects of the neuroprobe in the treatment of second degree ankle inversion sprains. Phys Ther 63:35–40, 1983
28. Cote DJ, Prentice WE, Hooker DN, et al: Comparison of three treatment procedures for minimizing ankle sprain swelling. Phys Ther 68:1072–1076, 1988
29. Roycroft S, Mantgani AB: Treatment of inversion injuries of the ankle by early active management. Physiotherapy 69:355–356, 1983

30. Sheon RP, Moskowitz RW, Goldberg VM: Soft Tissue Rheumatic Pain, Recognition, Management, Prevention, 2nd Ed. Lea & Febiger, Philadelphia, 1987

31. Sackett DL, Haynes RB, Tugwell P: Clinical Epidemiology: A Basic Science for Clinical Medicine. Little, Brown & Company, Toronto, 1985, p 171

32. Muckle DS: Comparative study of ibuprofen and aspirin in tissue injuries. Rheum Rehabil 13:141–147, 1977

33. Hutson MA: A double-blind study comparing ibuprofen 1800 mg and 2400 mg daily and placebo in sports injuries. J Int Res 14:142, 1986

SPECIAL
CONSIDERATIONS

12

Exercise Physiology in the Mature Athlete

PER-OLOF ÅSTRAND

BACKGROUND

The mature athlete has a favorable lifestyle because there is a pronounced plasticity and adaptability in the structural and functional properties of cells, tissues, and organ systems in the human body when exposed to various stimuli. While there is unanimous agreement that regular physical activity is essential for optimal function of the human body, it is evident that extrinsic factors such as diet, smoking, and exercise are reflected in the morbidity and mortality statistics, especially in the elderly.

Aging is obligated to be associated with reduced maximal aerobic power and reduced muscle strength, ie, with reduced physical fitness. As a consequence of diminished exercise tolerance, a large and increasing number of elderly persons will be living below, at, or just above normal "thresholds" of physical ability. They need only a minor intercurrent illness to render them completely dependent. Physical training can readily produce a profound improvement in functions essential for physical fitness in old age.

Adaptability to regular physical activity causes less disruption of the cells' *milieu interieur* and minimizes fatigue, thereby enhancing performance and the economy of energy output during physical demands of daily activities. Regular physical activity reduces the risk of premature mortality, in general, and of coronary heart disease, hypertension, colon cancer, and diabetes mellitus in particular. Physical activity also improves mental health and is important for the health and optimal function of muscles, bones, and joints.

The most recent recommendations advise people of all ages to include a minimum of 30 minutes of physical activity of moderate intensity, such as brisk walking, on most, if not all, days of the week. Mature athletes are much more active and thereby accrue greater health benefits than less active persons.

A Historic Note

I am a veteran of meetings devoted to papers and discussions dealing with the effects of physical exercise on human performance, organ function, and health. Sooner or later at such meetings a pertinent question arises: What is the role of habitual physical activity in the primary and secondary prevention of diseases, particularly cardiovascular diseases?

A quite typical flux of presentations and thoughts was as follows. At one stage, almost everyone was enthusiastic about the many positive effects of training on various functions. Then the epidemiologists presented data in favor of the beneficial effects of regular exercise but claimed that so far there is no conclusive proof that physical training per se can prevent disease. In the third phase of the meeting, many harmful effects of exercise were discussed.

The result was often confusion and a sort of despair on the part of those who at the beginning participated in the love songs devoted to regular exercise. The final recommendation was that anyone, particularly those no longer young and the untrained, should undergo a careful medical examination, including a so-called stress test, to get some sort of certification to join an exercise program without risk.

My standard comments were:

1. If a drive to stimulate people to exercise is successful, there are not enough physicians qualified to execute stress tests.

2. There is so far no medical examination that, in a foolproof manner, can exclude hazardous effects of vigorous exercise on the cardiovascular organs in a particular individual. Even advanced examinations can result in too many false-positive and false-negative diagnoses to be absolutely reliable.

3. From a psychological point of view, emphasis on the importance of a health examination to evaluate whether exercise can be recommended gives a definite impression that exercise is more a threat to health than a sedentary life style is.

Therefore, sometime in the 1960s, I presented the following recommendation: "The question is frequently raised whether a medical examination is advisable before commencing a training program. Certainly anyone who is doubtful about her/his state of health should consult a physician. In principle, however, there is less risk in activity than in continous inactivity. In a nutshell, my opinion is that it is *more advisable to pass a careful medical examination if one intends to be sedentary* in order to establish whether one's state of health is good enough to stand the inactivity."[1]

When asking a physician whether there are scientific data to prove that physical training is beneficial, it is apparently inevitable that she or he concentrate on the question of whether such training is useful in the primary and secondary prevention of disease in his or her speciality. Many physicians still state that epidemiologic studies are inconclusive.

For this reason, many physicians do not actively recommend exercise, and I shall add, provocatively, that too many of them know too little about exercise physiology. If you research the standard basic textbooks in physiology for medical students, you will find one explanation of this lack of knowledge: very few pages of the text are devoted to a discussion of the acute and chronic effects of exercise on different structures and functions.

In many ways, this almost total exclusion of exercise physiology in the textbooks is remarkable, considering that physiologic analysis of an exercise situation gives a unique opportunity to learn how different functions are coordinated and integrated. The definite trend is that new scientific frontiers such as molecular biology, genetics, immunology, development biology, and neuroscience dominate both in research and in teaching medical students. It is, however, the physiologist's responsibility to convert the lifeless pieces of molecular and cellular biology into whole living organisms.

In my opinion, "exercise physiology" is from these viewpoints particularly important because an exercise situation in various environments provides a unique opportunity to study how different functions are regulated and integrated. In fact, most functions and structures are in one way or another affected by acute and chronic (ie, in a training program) exercises. Therefore, exercise physiology is to a high degree an integrated science with the goal of identification of the mechanisms of overall body function and its regulation. There is total, unanimous agreement among exercise physiologists that regular exercise is essential for optimal function of the human body.

One reason for this introduction is that at one stage of a discussion on the effects of training it is important to separate physiologic from clinical aspects. Thereby some of the confusion mirrored in the mass media can be avoided. Then, of course, it is essential that the physiologists and clinicians join in the discussions. This publication serves an important purpose with its integration of different disciplines in human biology, treated as both basic and applied sciences. For instance, by exposing the cardiologist who does not believe that physical inactivity is a risk factor for coronary heart disease, it is hoped that he or she will prescribe exercise because of its many positive effects on body structures and functions.

When prescribing pills, many physicians do not demand so much scientific proof that the medicine is justified for a particular patient as when it is a question of influencing the patient's life style. However, now there are numerous publications in epidemiology that emphasize many health hazards of a sedentary life style. The mature athlete is someone of middle age or older who is physically active to prepare for a competition. However, I will in this discussion also include mature individuals who have the ambition to conquer the "lazy dog," apparently an innate characteristic of the elderly.

HEALTH BENEFITS OF HABITUAL PHYSICAL ACTIVITY

Haskell[2] argues that quantity and quality of exercise to obtain health-related benefits may differ from what is recommended for physical fitness benefits. He points out that the view taken by advocates of the physical activity–health paradigm is that for many people, especially those inclined not to perform more vigorous exercise—and they are in the majority—some benefit is better than none. "The greatest health benefits from an increase in physical activity appear to occur when very sedentary persons begin a regular program of moderate intensity, endurance type activity. Further increases in intensity or amount of activity appear to produce further benefits in some, but not all, biological or clinical parameters. The magnitude of benefits becomes less for similar increase in intensity and/or amount of activity"[2] (Fig. 12–1).

A similar message is presented in the 1996 report by the US Surgeon General,[3] which points out that during the past few years the American College of Sports Medicine, the Centers for Chronic Disease Control and Prevention, the National Center for Chronic Disease Prevention and Health Promotion, the American Heart Association, the President's Council on Physical Fitness and Sports, and the National Institutes of Health have all recommended regular, moderate-intensity physical activity as an option for those who get little or no exercise. And they are many: more than 60% of American adults are not regularly physically active. In fact, 25% of all adults are not active at all.

Haskell[2] points out that many Americans may be surprised at the extent and strength of the evidence linking physical activity to numerous health improvements. Most significantly, regular physical activity greatly reduces the risk of dying of coronary heart disease, the leading cause of death in most Western industrialized countries. Habitual physical activity also reduces the risk of diabetes, hypertension, and colon cancer and fosters healthy muscles, bones, and joints.

Regular participation in physical activity also appears to reduce depression, improve mood, and enhance ability to perform daily tasks throughout life. In other words, it helps to maintain function and preserve independence in older adults. This report grew out of an emerging consensus among epidemiologists, experts in exercise science, and health professionals that physical activity need not be of high intensity to improve health. Moreover, health benefits appear to be proportional to the amount of activity. Thus every increase in activity adds some benefits.

Emphasizing the amount rather than the intensity of physical activity offers more options for people to select from in incorporating physical activity into their daily lives. Experts advise previously sedentary people embarking on a physical activity program to start with short du-

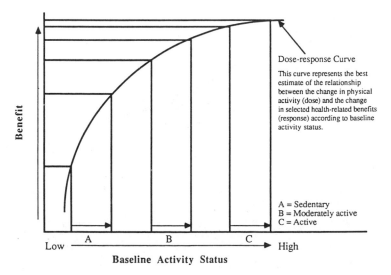

FIGURE 12–1. Health benefits of physical activity. (From Haskell WL: Health consequences of physical activity: understanding and challenges regarding dose-response. Med Sci Sports Exerc 26:649, 1994.)

Dose-response Curve

This curve represents the best estimate of the relationship between the change in physical activity (dose) and the change in selected health-related benefits (response) according to baseline activity status.

A = Sedentary
B = Moderately active
C = Active

Benefit

Low — High

A B C

Baseline Activity Status

rations of moderate-intensity activity and gradually to increase the duration or intensity until the goal is reached.

The most recent recommendations advise people of all ages to include a minimum of 30 minutes of moderate physical activity, such as brisk walking, on most, if not all, days of the week.[3] It is also acknowledged that for most people, greater health benefits can be obtained by engaging in physical activity of more vigorous intensity or of longer duration. Here the mature athlete enters the picture!

It should be pointed out that some of the positive effects of exercise vanish after a few days. Therefore, regularity in activity is important. When the purpose is to train the oxygen transport system, the intensity of the exercise should be approximately 75% or more of the maximal oxygen uptake.

Maximal Oxygen Uptake (Aerobic Power)

The highest oxygen uptake a person can attain when exercising large muscle groups at sea level is by definition her or his maximal oxygen uptake or aerobic power. There is good support for the hypothesis that the central circulation is the limiting factor for this power. In other words, the potential of the skeletal muscles to consume oxygen in their mitochondria exceeds the capacity of the oxygen transport system to deliver oxygen.[4,5]

In many laboratories, maximal aerobic power has been measured in unselected persons of different ages. A common finding is a peak at 15 to 20 years of age, with the lower range in women (Fig. 12–2). It should be pointed out that oxygen uptake gives quite accurate information about the aerobic energy output (1 L O_2 consumed in the tissue yields approximately 20 kJ), and the oxygen uptake, expressed in liters per minute, is highly correlated with cardiac output. In most studies there is a gradual decline in maximal oxygen uptake from the age of approximately 20 years onward,[6] with a decrease of approximately 10% per decade. When oxygen uptake is related to body weight ($\dot{V}O_2$ ml $\cdot$ kg^{-1} $\cdot$ min^{-1}), this peak appears at still lower ages.[4]

On the basis of an extensive literature review, Shwartz and Reibold[7] concluded that between the ages of 50 and 75 years, the decline is actually 15% per decade (peak oxygen uptake in liters per minute). However, for *master athletes a decline of just some 5% per decade in this maximum* has been reported.[8] One important factor behind the decline in peak oxygen uptake with age is a reduction in maximal heart rate and therefore in cardiac output.

Training will not significantly modify this reduction in heart rate. It is well documented that training over several months can improve maximal aerobic power by a few percent up to 100%; however, there are large individual variations in

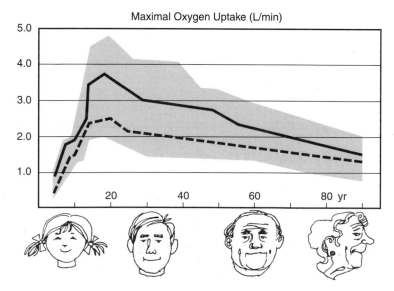

Maximal Oxygen Uptake (L/min)

FIGURE 12–2. Mean values for maximal oxygen uptake (aerobic power) measured during exercise on treadmill or cycle ergometer in 350 female (*dashed line*) and male (*solid line*) relatively well-trained subjects 4 to 65 years of age. Shadowed area covers +2 SD for male subjects to −2 SD for women. The lines and areas beyond 65 years of age are extrapolated. (From Åstrand P-O, Rodahl K: Textbook of work physiology. McGraw-Hill, New York, 1986, p. 333.)

the response to a standardized training protocol.[9] The adaptation of the oxygen transport system to training is of the same relative magnitude in ages ranging from 20 to 70 or 80 years, and the response is independent of gender.[4] Therefore, it is not surprising that athletes in endurance disciplines at any age have significantly higher maximal aerobic power than is found in the population in general.

In addition to the effect of training on aerobic power, athletes are usually genetically endowed with a relatively high maximal aerobic power. For the general population, it is interesting that recent attention has been drawn to findings from studies showing that gains in cardiorespiratory fitness are similar when physical activity occurs in several short sessions (eg, 10 minutes) as when the same total amount and intensity of activity occurs in one longer session (eg, 30 minutes).[3]

Although, strictly speaking, the health benefits of such intermittent activity have not yet been demonstrated, it is reasonable to expect them to be similar to those of continuous activity. Moreover, for people who are unable to set aside 30 minutes for physical activity, shorter episodes are clearly better than none. Indeed, one study has shown greater adherence to a walking program among those walking several times a day than among those walking once a day, when the total amount of walking time was kept the same.[3]

It is interesting that young athletes tested when they have just qualified for a national team in endurance events have a high maximal aerobic power. In the years that follow they train daily and intensively. There are seasonal fluctuations in this power, but usually the highest value recorded in those years is not significantly different from the one first observed.

No doubt there is a definite maximum dependent on the individual's natural aerobic power. Data obtained in the laboratory and statistics of world records and personal best performances reveal that after the age of 30 to 35 years, there is an inevitable decline in maximal aerobic power (in individuals who were well-trained before). The best times in the marathon distance are noted in the range from 23 to approximately 35 years of age (Fig. 12–3). A high maximal aerobic power per kilogram of body weight is important, but a somewhat low maximum can be compensated for by good running efficiency, ability to maintain high speed with energy

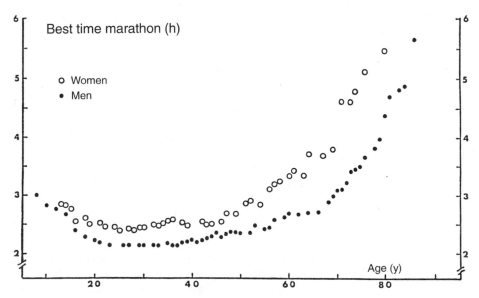

FIGURE 12–3. Best times recorded for marathon runners of different ages. It should be noted that the profile for the courses and weather conditions can be different among races.

demands close to maximal aerobic power, an optimal utilization of substrates, and smart tactics.

It is interesting to note that mature athletes perform very well at older ages, even beyond 60 years. At approximately 60 years, average maximal aerobic power of 1.6 L/min in women and 2.5 L/min in men has been reported in healthy but sedentary individuals (24 and 30 ml · kg^{-1} · min^{-1} respectively). That is in contrast to approximately 2.2 and 3.6 L/min, respectively, found in master athletes in endurance events (36 ml and 58 ml · kg^{-1} · min^{-1}, respectively).[6]

The stress on various functions when exercising at submaximal intensity (eg, when walking) is related to the ratio of submaximal aerobic power to maximal aerobic power. The same is true for perceived exertion. A person weighing 65 kg needs approximately 1 L of oxygen per minute when walking at a speed of 5 km/h. For the average man, that is moderate exercise intensity but close to maximal oxygen uptake for a 70-year-old woman. With a body weight of 100 kg, that walk for many persons will tax the aerobic power up to or even beyond the maximum.

It is evident that it is important for the aging individual to try to keep fit and slim. At our department we have a longitudinal study that includes former students of physical education. Maximal oxygen uptake, lung function, and some other parameters were measured first in 1949, then again in 1970 and 1982. For one male subject a reduction in maximal oxygen uptake from 3.95 to 3.56 L/min was noted during the first 21-year period. When studied again 12 years later, he was back to the 3.95 L/min level, probably as a result of intensified training (age then 61 years). In contrast, in one subject, maximal oxygen uptake decreased from 4 to 2 L/min when he was gradually forced into a relatively sedentary life style owing to rheumatoid arthritis (age 65 years)[6] (Fig. 12–4). These two cases illustrate how critical lifestyle can be to the aging effect on the oxygen transport system.

With age there is a gradual decline in maximal heart rate. With unchanged stroke volume and arteriovenous oxygen difference (a − vO_2), this reduction will result in decreased maximal cardiac output and therefore in maximal aerobic

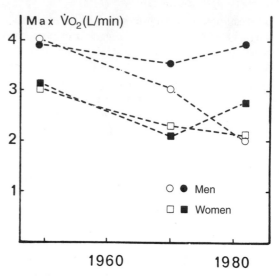

FIGURE 12–4. Maximal oxygen uptake measured in 4 subjects in 1949, 1970, and 1982, respectively. In 1949 they were students in physical education, approximately 25 years old. (From Åstrand P-O, Bergh U, Kilbom Å: A 33-year follow-up of oxygen uptake and related variables of former physical education students. J Appl Physiol 82:1844, 1997.)

power.[8] Hagberg et al[10] report that the oxygen pulse during maximal exercise was identical in masters endurance athletes and young athletes. Evidently the stroke volume and a − vO_2 difference were similar in the two groups. The decline in maximal heart rate could explain the masters' lower maximal aerobic power. In the subject with similar maximal oxygen uptake in 1949 and 1982 (Fig. 12–4) the maximal heart rate had declined from 200 to 188 to 182 in 1982. The calculated oxygen pulse was 19.7 ml in 1949 and 21.7 ml in 1982.

On echocardiographic evaluation, endurance athletes of any age have significantly greater left ventricular volume and mass than untrained people of the same age.[10–12]

Anaerobic Power

Measurement of oxygen uptake gives a good estimate of aerobic power. In contrast, there is no method available to measure accurately anaerobic power and capacity. "Anaerobic tests" available include maximal 30- to 60-s sprint bouts on a cycle ergometer or track. Most common is the 30-s Wingate test.[13] With highly motivated subjects such tests are quite reproducible. However, the time is not long enough to test anaerobic capacity, and it is presently impossible to measure an aerobic contribution to the energy yield, eg, with oxygen delivered from myoglobin.

Lactate

A high concentration of lactate in exercising muscle and in the blood is only a signal indicating that there has been substantial anaerobic breakdown of glycogen. A high degree of motivation is essential to attain high concentrations of lactate. It is typical that an athlete reaches a higher lactate level after an important competition than after an all-out test in the laboratory, exercise time being the same. There is a trend after maximal effort that the peak blood lactate concentration is higher after a period of training, and this peak concentration is lower at older ages.

It is well documented that at a given submaximal but relatively high work rate, trained individuals have a lower blood lactate concentration than when untrained. Also, when subjects exercise at a given percentage of maximal aerobic power, training can reduce the lactate level. As a consequence, the trained individual can run, bicycle, ski, or swim at a relatively high speed without a continuous accumulation of lactate in muscles and blood. At least two factors can explain this finding: an increase in maximal oxygen uptake and the ability to exercise at a higher percentage of this maximum without lactate production. In addition, improved technique will reduce the energy cost to maintain a given speed.

Training can reduce (normalize) the pulmonary ventilation at a given relatively high oxygen uptake (subject age was 63 ± 2 years).[14] One factor behind such an effect could be reduced metabolic hydrogen ion (H^+) production after training.

MUSCLE MASS AND STRENGTH

After the age of approximately 50 years there is a significant reduction in muscular strength. Peak muscle strength is usually reached at age 20 to 30 years for men and a few years earlier for women. At older ages, there is a loss of motoneurons and therefore motor units, muscle mass,

and strength, events which in cross-sectional studies accelerate between age 50 to 60 years. By age 80, nearly half of these tissues and functions have been lost. Certainly, there are also large individual variations, and different states of training can highly influence test results. The individual muscle fibers have a relatively normal cross-sectional area during adult life, up to the age of 80 years, with some diminution in the area of the fast-twitch fibers (type II).[15,16] It is not surprising that older individuals have a relatively poor power potential for the performance of a vertical jump.

Muscle fibers that have been deprived of their nerve supply can be reinnervated by the process of fiber sprouting. Nearby intact nerve terminals can sprout and form new synapses. As a consequence, with age there can be an increase in the number of muscle fibers in a motor unit (motoneuron plus the muscle fibers it innervates). It is an open question whether activation or training of a muscle group can promote fiber sprouting and thereby minimize the reduction of muscle mass in old age.

During the first weeks of strength training, the improvement is not associated with an increase in the cross-sectional area of the muscle groups involved. Then there is often a gradual increase in both strength and the cross-sectional area, particularly of the type II fibers. There is also a specificity in the training so that improved strength is more pronounced in the type of activity that was trained than in other exercises.

Both of these phenomena can be explained by the fact that the activity in the central nervous system (CNS) is of decisive importance to the number of motor units and the frequency at which they are activated at a given time. As a result of training, the CNS can apparently command more muscle cells to activity by removing inhibitions, and the same muscle mass can then produce more strength.[4]

Fiatarone et al[17] studied nine frail, institutionalized volunteers aged 86 to 96 years (mean, 90 years) who undertook 8 weeks of high-intensity resistance training. They used an adaptation of standard rehabilitation principles of progressive resistance training with concentric (lifting) and eccentric (lowering) activation of knee extensor muscles. Three times a week the subjects performed three sets of eight repetitions with each leg with a 1- to 2-minute rest period between sets. Except for the first week, the load was 80% of the one-repetition maximum.

Before training began, the maximal weight they could lift once was on average 7.6 kg, and after the 8 weeks of training it was on average 19.3 kg. Midthigh muscle area increased 9%. Mean tandem gait speed improved 48% after training. The activation of the muscles involved lasted only some 10 minutes per week.

These findings suggest that age does not appear to affect the trainability of skeletal muscle.

TECHNIQUE AND COORDINATION

Once one has learned bicycling, or a swim stroke, tennis serve, or golf swing, it is remarkable how well the skill is maintained even if not practiced for years. However, without training, one tires quickly and the technique may deteriorate (eg, in swimming or playing the piano or the guitar).

What about well-maintained agility in old age? Many musicians demonstrate that remarkable performances are possible in later years. Artur Rubenstein brilliantly played technically demanding Chopin compositions when almost 90 years old. Andrés Segovia still gave classic guitar concerts at age 93 years. These are just two examples.

Musicians usually practice several hours daily. Apparently such training can maintain agility. Most aging individuals do not include agility in their daily activities, and their movements become slow and clumsy. We believe that this is an inevitable consequence of aging, but it may not be so. It may be the result of inactivity. Perhaps hours of muscle activity can promote fiber sprouting and maintain the muscle mass and a high-level CNS-muscle function.

It should be mentioned that efficiency in walking and running at a given speed is similar from the age of approximately 15 years up to at least the age of 70 years in individuals without medical problems in the locomotor organs.

NUTRITIONAL ASPECTS

Many masters endurance runners run 50 to 200 km/wk.[11,18,19] They are high energy consumers, and of necessity their food intake is high. The substrates for active muscles are carbohydrate and free fatty acids (FFA). One effect of

endurance training is increased utilization of FFA during exercise at a given percentage of maximal aerobic power. This shift in the utilization of substrates is glycogen saving, and it will take longer time to empty a given store of glycogen, thereby improving the potential for good performance in endurance events. A reasonable daily energy intake for the 50 km/wk runner is 12.5 MJ, and for the 200-km runner, 20 MJ (body weight approximately 70 kg). With a well-balanced diet, 10 MJ should be enough to cover the demand for essential nutrients. Well-nourished runners are apparently on the safe side.

In contrast, sedentary individuals with little physical activity in their job and leisure time must restrict their energy intake to less than 10 MJ to prevent obesity. They are in the risk zone of malnutrition. With age there is a reduced resting metabolism, but the demand for essential nutrients seems to be the same as at younger ages. If physically inactive, the older individual is therefore particularly at risk of malnutrition with respect to some essential nutrients. There are reports that malnutrition is the most common immunodeficiency world wide.[20] Regular exercise can prevent undernutrition and therefore enhance positive phagocytic function. One conclusion is that chronic exercise may enhance resting levels of the immune system and thus abrogate age-related immunodeficiency.[20]

It should be emphasized that an individual with a high energy output certainly needs more carbohydrate, fat, and water, but the demand for other nutrients is essentially the same as for sedentary individuals. A high energy output must be balanced by a high energy intake if the body weight is to stay constant. With a well-balanced diet, the mature athlete can secure an adequate intake of essential nutrients. Therefore, supplementation of vitamins and other nutrients in mature athletes seems not so important as in sedentary elderly individuals.

RISKS OF PHYSICAL ACTIVITY

The risks associated with physical activity must be considered. The most common health problems that have been associated with physical activity are musculoskeletal injuries, which can occur with excessive intensity and volume of activity for which the body is not conditioned.

Much more serious associated health problems, ie, myocardial infarction, and sudden death are much rarer, occurring primarily among sedentary people with advanced atherosclerotic disease who engage in strenuous activity to which they are unaccustomed. Sedentary people, especially those with preexisting health problems, who wish to increase their physical activity should therefore gradually build up to the desired level. Even among people who are regularly physically active, the risk of myocardial infarction or sudden death is somewhat increased during physical exertion, but their overall risk of those outcomes is lower than that among people who are sedentary.[3,21] Siscovick[22] reports that among habitually vigorous men, the overall risk of primary cardiac arrest calculated on a 24-hour basis was only 40% of that for sedentary men.

Vuori's[23] estimation of the incidence of sudden cardiovascular death in all recreational exercise and sports in the total Finnish male population is as follows: one death in 11.5 million exercise sessions in 20- to 39-year-old men, one death in 2.6 million sessions in 40- to 49-year-old men, and one death in 2.2 million sessions in 50- to 69-year-old men.

As a group, master athletes are healthier and physiologically younger than sedentary controls. It can be expected that their life expectancy will be longer than that of the general population because their level of training is comparable to that of the former elite athlete.[24]

NEW FIELDS OF STUDY

Endorphins

An interesting new field of study is *endorphins* and their effects on the CNS. There are many supporters of the statement that "exercise is the best tranquilizer." It is well established that the release of β-endorphins is elevated after prolonged, strenuous exercise.[25] These neurohormones (β-endorphin, encephalin, and dynorphin), which have an effect resembling that of certain opiates, play an important role in general physiologic stress reactions. They serve to reduce pain and enhance the feeling of well-being.

The increased release of endorphins during strenuous exercise may thus, at least in part, explain the feeling of well-being commonly experienced at the end of a training session. As a matter of fact, attachment of endorphins to specific receptors in the brain has been demonstrated in individuals after long-distance running. It is also of interest to note that the endorphin antagonist naloxone has the opposite effect.[26]

Immune System

The immune system was briefly discussed above. It is not possible to conclude whether endurance training can alter an age-related decline in immune function. Klarlund Pedersen and Bruunsgaard[20] point out that the major reason for this uncertainty is related to the scarcity of data addressing the issue of exercise and immune function in the elderly. There is primarily a lack of studies in humans. The available data suggest that although age-related decline in immune function can be retarded, the greatest effect will be seen only in highly conditioned subjects, ie, in mature athletes.[20]

Oxygen Free Radicals

Growing evidence indicates that oxygen free radicals are important mediators of skeletal muscle damage and inflammation after strenuous exercise. The generation of free radicals is increased during exercise as a consequence of increases in mitochondrial oxygen consumption and electron transport flux.[27,28] However, in trained individuals, scavanger and antioxidant enzyme activity increase markedly.[27] In this way, the increased oxidative stress induced by exercise may be compromised by increased antioxidant activity. There is no convincing evidence that supplements of antioxidant vitamins in well-nourished athletes can meaningfully mitigate free radical formation.[29]

Diabetes

Habitual physical activity can markedly reduce the risk of non-insulin-dependent (type II) diabetes. It is interesting to note that muscle contractions not only increase muscle insulin sensitivity and responsiveness, but they also stimulate glucose transport independent of insulin.[30]

CONCLUSIONS

The history of hominids covers millions of years. During more than 99% of our existence we have been hunters and food gatherers. For survival, brisk daily walking of 5 to 15 km was essential. I believe that running was an exceptional event in the daily activities, not as essential for survival as the more economical walking.[4] Conclusion: habitual brisk walking is a basic activity to promote optimal function.

However, it is still an open question as to how critical the intensity and duration of habitual physical activity need be to promote optimal function and positive health effects summarized in Table 12–1. Presently we cannot evaluate the effects of 2 hours at a moderate work rate compared with 1 hour at twice that energy demand on vital functions. Additional factors influence the performance of master athletes.[31]

At any rate, regular physical activity is essential for optimal physical fitness and health. Therefore, go out and walk or run with your dog—even if you don't have one!

TABLE 12–1. Effects of Habitual Physical Activity

Increase in maximal oxygen uptake and cardiac output
Reduced heart rate at given oxygen uptake
Reduced blood pressure
Reduced heart rate · blood pressure product
Improved efficiency of heart muscle
Favorable trend in incidence of cardial morbidity and mortality
Increased capillary density in skeletal muscle
Increased mitochondrial density in skeletal muscle
Reduced lactate production at given percentage of maximal oxygen uptake
Reduced perceived exertion at given oxygen uptake
Enhanced ability to utilize free fatty acids as substrate during exercise; glycogen saving
Improved endurance during exercise
Increases metabolism; advantageous from a nutritional viewpoint
Counteracts obesity
Increased high-density lipoprotein concentrations in blood
Improved structure and function of ligaments, tendons, and joints
Increased muscle strength
Increased production of endorphins
Enhanced nerve fiber sprouting to reinnervate muscle fibers?
Enhanced tolerance to hot environment; increased sweat production
Reduced platelet aggregation
Counteracts osteoporosis
Can normalize glucose tolerance
Can reduce risk for some types of cancer

From U.S. Department of Health and Human Services: Physical Activity and Health: A Report of the Surgeon General, GA, Superintendent of Documents, PO Box 371954, PA 15250-7954, S/N 017-023-00196-5, 1996

REFERENCES

1. Åstrand P-O, Rodahl K: Textbook of Work Physiology. McGraw-Hill, New York, 1970, p. 608
2. Haskell WL: Health consequences of physical activity: understanding and challenges regarding dose-response. Med Sci Sports Exerc 26:649, 1994
3. US Department of Health and Human Services: Physical Activity and Health: A Report of the Surgeon General, GA, Superintendent of Documents, PO Box 371954, PA 15250-7954, S/N 017-023-00196-5, 1996
4. Åstrand P-O, Rodahl K: Textbook of Work Physiology. McGraw-Hill Book Co, New York, 1986
5. Saltin B: Cardiovascular and pulmonary adaptation to exercise. In Bouchard C, Shephard RJ, Stephens TS, et al (eds): Exercise, Fitness, and Health. Human Kinetics Books, Champaign, Ill, 1990, p. 187
6. Åstrand P-O, Bergh U, Kilbom Å: A 33-year follow-up of oxygen uptake and related variables of former physical education students. J Appl Physiol 82:1844, 1997
7. Shwartz E, Reibold RC: Aerobic fitness norms for males and females aged 6 to 75 years: a review. Aviat Space Environ Med 61:3, 1990
8. Hagberg JM: Physical activity, fitness, health, and age. In Bouchard C, Shephard RJ, Stephens, T (eds): Physical Activity, Fitness, and Health. Human Kinetics Publishers, Champaign, Ill, 1994, p. 993
9. Bouchard C, Boulay MR, Simoneau J-A, et al: Heredity and trainability of aerobic and anaerobic performances. Sports Med 5:69, 1988
10. Hagberg JM, Allen WK, Seals DR, et al: A hemodynamic comparison of young and older endurance athletes. J Appl Physiol 58:2041, 1985
11. Child JS, Barnard RJ, Taw RL: Cardiac hypertrophy and function in master endurance runners and sprinters. J Appl Physiol 57:176, 1984
12. Scott Green J, Crouse SF: Endurance training, cardiovascular function and the aged. Sports Med 16:331, 1993

13. Bar-Or O: The Wingate anaerobic test: an update on methodology, reliability, and validity. Sports Med 4:381, 1987

14. Yerg JE II, Seals DR, Hagberg JM, et al: Effect of endurance exercise training on ventilatory function in older individuals. J Appl Physiol 58:791, 1985

15. Grimby G, Saltin B: The aging muscle. Clin Physiol 3:209, 1983

16. Booth FW, Thomason DB: Molecular and cellular adaptations of muscle in response to exercise: perspectives of various models. Physiol Rev 71:541, 1991

17. Fiatarone MA, Marks EC, Ryan ND, et al: High-intensity strength training in nonagenarians. JAMA 263:3029, 1990

18. Barnard RJ, Grimditch GK, Wilmore J: Physiological characteristics of sprint and endurance master runners. Med Sci Sports 11:167, 1979

19. Kavanagh T, Shephard RJ: The effects of continued training on the aging process. Ann N Y Acad Sci 301:656, 1977

20. Klarlund Pedersen B, Bruunsgaard H: Nutrition, age and immunity in exercise. In Klarlund Pedersen B (ed): Exercise Immunology. R G Landes Co, Austin, Texas, 1997, p. 149

21. Thompson PD, Fahrenbach MC: Risks of exercising: cardiovascular including sudden cardiac death. In Bouchard C, Shephard RJ, Stephens T (eds): Physical Activity, Fitness, and Health. Human Kinetics Publishers, Champaign, Ill, 1994, p. 1019

22. Siscovick DS: Risks of exercising: sudden death and injuries. In Bouchard C, Shephard RJ, Stephens S, et al (eds): Exercise, Fitness, and Health. Human Kinetics Publishers, Ill, 1990, p. 707

23. Vuori I: The cardiovascular risks of physical activity. Acta Med Scand Suppl 711:205–214, 1986

24. Sarna S, Kaprio J: Life expectancy of former elite athletes. Sports Med 17:149, 1994

25. Goldfarb AH, Jamurtas AZ: Beta-endorphin response to exercise: an update. Sports Med 24:8, 1997

26. Janal MN, Colt EWD, Clark WC, et al: Pain sensation, mood, and plasma endocrine levels in man following long-distance running: effects of naloxone. Pain 19:13, 1984

27. Dekkers JC, van Doornen LJP, Kemper HCG: The role of antioxident vitamins and enzymes in the prevention of exercise-induced muscle damage. Sports Med 21:213, 1996

28. Sjödin B, Hellsten Westling Y, Apple FS: Biochemical mechanisms for oxygen free radical formation during exercise. Sports Med 10:236, 1990

29. Kanter M: Free radicals and exercise: effects of nutritional antioxidant supplementation. Exerc Sport Sci Rev 23:375, 1995

30. Cortright RN, Dohm GL: Mechanisms by which insulin and muscle contraction can stimulate glucose transport. Can J Appl Physiol 22:519, 1997

31. Maharam LG, Bauman PA, Kalman D, Skolnik H, Perle SM: Masters athletes: factors affecting performance. Sports Med 28:273, 1999

13

Validation of Guidelines for Aerobic Exercise in Pregnancy

LARRY A. WOLFE ■ MICHELLE F. MOTTOLA

Before the early 1980s, both traditional medical advice and common practice in North American society were for women to avoid strenuous exertion throughout pregnancy. Such advice was based on the belief that pregnancy is a delicate process that can be undermined easily by physiologic stress and the idea that contracting maternal skeletal muscle may deprive the developing fetus of oxygenated blood flow and energy substrates for normal growth. Early studies of hard physical work combined with undernutrition[1] and forced exercise in laboratory animals[2] tended to support this viewpoint.

Over the past 20 years, there has been a substantial increase in the participation of women in strenuous sports and fitness and recreational activities, as well as greater involvement in nontraditional occupations (eg, police work, firefighting, military service, construction work) that require strenuous exertion or heavy manual labor. When women become pregnant, medical guidelines are needed to make informed judgments on safe limits for exertion at different stages of pregnancy, requirements for occupational leave or job modifications, or changes in physical conditioning programs, as well as for the timing of return to prepregnant physical activity levels after childbirth.

This chapter has *three main purposes*: to summarize current information about the risks and benefits of exercise in pregnancy, to examine scientific support for existing guidelines for exercise in pregnancy, and to explore the use of exercise for the prevention and treatment of important maternal-fetal diseases. Particular emphasis is placed on validation of exercise prescription guidelines published by the Canadian Society for Exercise Physiology[3] as part of the Physical Activity Readiness Medical Examination for Pregnancy (PARmed-X for Pregnancy).

RISKS OF EXERCISE DURING PREGNANCY

Much has been written about the hypothetical risks of both acute and chronic exercise during pregnancy.[4–9] With reference to acute bouts of strenuous exercise, these have included exercise-induced reductions in uterine blood flow, leading to transient fetal hypoxia[10]; postexercise hypoglycemia, causing a temporary reduction in fetal glucose availability[11]; fetal hyperthermia[4,12]; and induction of premature labor.[13] The most important concern about chronic exercise has been that repeated bouts of strenuous exercise may have an additive effect on fetal oxygen delivery and substrate availability, causing intrauterine growth restriction and low birth weight.[13] These early concerns were based in large part on studies of exercising laboratory animals or retrospective studies of pregnant recreational athletes.

As described in our recent review,[14] substantial knowledge now exists on fetal response to exercise. The most common fetal reaction to sustained submaximal exercise is increased heart rate at baseline, which appears to be related to the intensity and duration of exertion.[15] Recent studies involving both submaximal[16] and maximal graded exercise testing[17] of healthy women in late gestation demonstrated temporary reduction followed by a delayed rise in fetal heart rate baseline after exercise.

Some studies have also reported transient fetal bradycardia (fetal heart rate <120 beats per minute [bpm]) in association with maximal exercise testing,[18,19] whereas there appears to be a much lower incidence of transient fetal bradycardia in association with bouts of submaximal exercise.[18,20] In either case, fetal bradycardia has been observed most commonly in the immediate post-exercise period when vascular beds in maternal skeletal muscle are still vasodilated and cardiac output is rapidly falling, possibly resulting in maternal hypotension and a temporary reduction in uterine blood flow.[21] Recent studies also suggest that the incidence of postexercise bradycardia may be lower in pregnant women who are physically active.[17]

Other fetal reactions to strenuous exercise testing have included transient reductions in fetal movements and reactivity,[19] fetal heart rate variability,[17,19] and breathing movements.[22,23] It seems probable that all of the fetal responses cited above are protective reactions to exercise-induced reductions in uterine blood flow, increased fetal temperature, transfer of maternal catecholamines across the placenta,[24] or a combination of these factors. However, it is important to note that no published studies have reported fetal injury or mortality as a result of strenuous exercise testing or physical conditioning in healthy pregnant women.[14,25]

Concern about the possibility of exercise-induced fetal hyperthermia has been based on reports of neural tube and facial defects caused by chronic heating in laboratory animals, maternal fever, and sauna or hot tub exposure during closure of the neural tube in the first trimester.[26] However, to our knowledge, no published studies have reported such teratogenic effects in relation to maternal exercise exposure. In addition, physiologic studies[27–29] have shown that human pregnancy is accompanied by enhanced peripheral vasodilation and a lower threshold for sweating, resulting in blunted increases in core temperature during exercise compared with the nonpregnant state.

Several laboratories[29–32] have reported reductions in maternal blood glucose concentration following strenuous exercise in late gestation.[30] In light of recent evidence that glucose transport in maternal skeletal muscle may be reduced in late pregnancy,[33] the most likely mechanism to explain this effect is blunted catecholamine-mediated liver glycogenolysis,[31] reduced liver glycogen storage,[34] or a combination of these effects. Since maternal blood glucose is the main substrate for fetal growth, such reductions would tend to reduce fetal glucose availability in the postexercise period. However, there is evidence that regular aerobic-type exercise reduces insulin resistance,[35] increases liver glycogen storage,[34] and helps prevent reductions in maternal blood glucose levels following strenuous exercise testing in late gestation.[32] Thus regular exercise would tend to protect rather than jeopardize fetal glucose availability.

Traditional concerns about exercise-induced induction of premature labor were reinforced by an early investigation by Clapp and Dickstein.[13] The authors reported that a group of pregnant recreational athletes who continued to exercise at preconception levels in the third trimester had lighter babies (−500 g), gained less weight (−4.6 kg), and delivered at a significantly earlier gestational age (−8 days) than subjects who discontinued exercise after week 29. However, subsequent studies from the same laboratory confirmed that regular exercise does not increase the incidence of either early miscarriage[36] or premature labor.[37]

There is some scientific support for the idea that very high volumes or intensities of maternal physical conditioning are associated with low birth weight.[13,38] However, a substantial body of evidence now confirms that regular moderate aerobic conditioning in well-nourished pregnant women has no significant effect on fetal growth.[39–41]

HYPOTHETICAL RISKS OF PHYSICAL INACTIVITY IN PREGNANCY

A major focus of research over the past three decades has been to examine the validity of postulated risks of exercise in pregnancy. Many of these risks have been found to be either nonexistent or overstated in terms of their seriousness, and the presence of effective maternal mechanisms and fetal reflexes to protect the fetus from hypoxic stress has often been overlooked. At the same time, a substantial body of evidence has accumulated to demonstrate the physiologic ill effects and health risks of bed rest and very

TABLE 13–1. Hypothetical Risks of Maternal Bed Rest and Inactivity in Human Pregnancy

Loss of cardiovascular and muscular fitness

Greater risk for gestational glucose intolerance

Higher susceptibility to excessive maternal weight gain

Higher risk for varicose veins and deep vein thrombosis

Higher risk for pre-eclampsia

Higher incidence of physical complaints such as dyspnea and low back pain

Poor psychological adjustment to normal physical changes in pregnancy

---

low levels of physical activity.[42] Many of these existing studies did not include female subjects, and even less information is available from pregnant women. However, it is reasonable to speculate, based on available evidence, that an abrupt reduction in physical activity will lead to a loss of physical fitness, and may contribute to excessive maternal weight gain,[43] vascular problems such as varicose veins[44] or deep vein thrombosis,[45] a greater risk for developing serious maternal-fetal disease such as gestational diabetes,[46] pre-eclampsia,[47,48] and musculoskeletal and postural problems including bone loss[49] and low back pain,[50] poor psychological adjustment to physical changes in pregnancy,[51] and a higher incidence of other physical discomforts and complaints[51-53] (Table 13–1).

DOSE-RESPONSE RELATIONSHIP FOR EXERCISE IN PREGNANCY

In view of the fact that too much exercise and very low levels of physical activity both appear to be associated with increased maternal-fetal health risks, there must be an optimal quantity and quality of exercise that maximizes the benefits and minimizes the risks of physical activity in pregnancy. The existence of such a dose-response relationship (Fig. 13–1) is illustrated by published studies that have examined varying intensities and durations of leisure time physical activity and their effects on birth weight. As summarized in a recent review by Pivarnik,[41] the meta-analytic study of Lokey et al[40] reported no significant effect of moderate aerobic conditioning on birth weight, whereas Hatch et al[54] reported that women who participate in "heavy exercise" (approximately 2000 kcal/wk) delivered babies who were significantly heavier (+276 g)

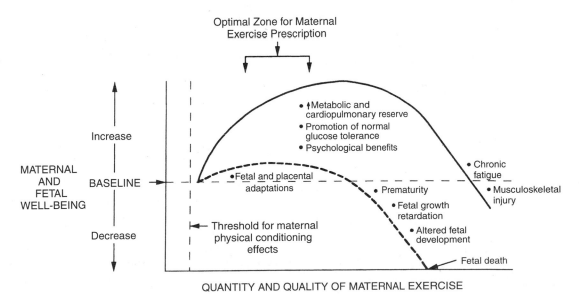

FIGURE 13–1. Postulated dose-response relationship between quantity and quality of prenatal exercise and maternal-fetal well-being. *Solid line,* maternal dose-response curve; *dashed line,* fetal dose-response curve. (From Wolfe LA, Brenner IKM, Mottola MF: Maternal exercise, fetal well-being and pregnancy outcome. Exerc Sport Sci Rev 22:145–194, 1994. Used with permission.)

than did women who were classified as nonexercisers. From a mechanistic viewpoint, such an effect could be mediated by a training-induced increase in placental volume[55] or other fetal and placental adaptations. However, studies by Clapp et al,[13,56] which involved recreational athletes who probably had higher weekly energy expenditures than the subjects of Hatch et al,[54] reported that subjects who continued strenuous exercise until term delivered significantly lighter babies than others who discontinued exercise in late gestation. This was attributed to a reduction in fetal adiposity rather than an overall effect on fetal growth.[56] Similarly, Bell et al[38] reported that subjects who participated in a high volume of exercise (5–7 days a week) delivered lighter offspring (−315 g) than did sedentary control subjects.

VALIDITY OF CURRENT GUIDELINES FOR EXERCISE IN HEALTHY PREGNANT WOMEN

From a historical perspective, numerous review articles, books, book chapters, and technical bulletins have been published by physicians, exercise scientists, and medical and scientific organizations to provide guidelines for safe and effective exercise in human pregnancy. Early versions of these guidelines were based on unproved theoretical concepts and common sense because of a lack of scientific information. As a result, these early guidelines were necessarily conservative and tended to create limits and barriers to exercise.[6,10] A good example of this was the first version of exercise and pregnancy guidelines published by the American College of Obstetricians and Gynecologists.[57] While these guidelines were a good first attempt to provide guidance, they also included limits for exercise intensity (maternal heart rate should not exceed 140 bpm) and duration (strenuous exercise should not exceed 15 minutes) that had no scientific basis and have since been shown to be unnecessarily restrictive. Accordingly, these limits were replaced in a revised version of the guidelines,[57] with general advice to stop exercising when fatigued and not to exercise to exhaustion. However, specific advice on methods to monitor aerobic exercise intensity and to avoid overexertion was not provided. Guidelines for aerobic exercise duration, rate of progression for aerobic exercise, and detailed advice for muscle conditioning were also not included.

PARmed-X for Pregnancy

The original version of the Physical Activity Readiness Medical Examination for Pregnancy (PARmed-X for Pregnancy) was developed in the mid-1980s to screen pregnant subjects for research in the Clinical Exercise Physiology Laboratory at Queen's University. It included a checklist of absolute and relative contraindications for physicians to use to clear their pregnant patients for involvement in a prenatal exercise program. It also included advice for safe and effective exercise prescription and exercise safety based on earlier publications from Fitness Canada[59] and the Fitness Ontario Leadership Program.[60] A key concept was that pregnancy is an excellent time for previously inactive women to begin a new exercise program and develop other healthy lifestyle habits.

The PARmed-X for Pregnancy was further developed by the Ontario Fitness Safety Standards Committee (N. Gledhill, PhD, Chairperson).[61] Another key concept introduced at this stage was that use of the form by physicians and midwives would help to familiarize them with methods for safe and effective exercise prescription for their pregnant patients. The form was further refined by an Expert Committee of the Canadian Society for Exercise Physiology (CSEP) prior to its publication in 1996.[3] Of particular importance was the addition of safety precautions for muscle conditioning (by Dr Michelle Mottola, School of Kinesiology, University of Western Ontario) and advice for active living, healthy eating, and maintenance of positive self and body images.[3] The PARmed-X for Pregnancy in its current form (Appendix) was recently endorsed in a position statement published by the Canadian Academy of Sports Medicine (L.M. Stevenson, MD, Committee Chair) for medical screening and exercise prescription for healthy pregnant women[62] based on an exhaustive review of current medical and scientific literature by Stevenson.[25,63] Finally, a companion booklet from CSEP for pregnant and postnatal exercise participants has been published and is available to the general public.[63a]

Indexes of Exercise Intensity

Prescription of exercise intensity in pregnancy is complicated by changes in the control of heart rate, which are established early in the first trimester.[64] These changes include an increase of 10 to 15 bpm in resting heart rate and a moderate reduction in peak heart rate during maximal exercise testing.[65,66] Recent studies support the hypothesis that the higher resting heart rate is due to a reduction in cardiac parasympathetic activity,[67,68] and the lower and maximal heart rate is caused by blunted sympathoadrenal responses to strenuous exercise.[31,67] Since maximal heart rate reserve is reduced[32] (Fig. 13–2), use of conventional heart rate target zones to prescribe and monitor exercise intensity is therefore less dependable in the pregnant compared with the nonpregnant state.

To ensure safe and effective monitoring of exercise intensity, the PARmed-X for Pregnancy employs a combination of intensity prescriptional methods. First, a modified version of the conventional age-corrected heart rate target zone has been formulated. Since maximal heart rate reserve is reduced and maximal heart rate is lower in pregnancy, the target heart rate zone for each age decade has been reduced from 20 to 15 bpm and the high end of the zone has been reduced by 5 bpm in accordance with the cardiac autonomic changes cited above (Appendix).

Since the relationship between absolute work rate or oxygen uptake with ratings of perceived exertion (RPE) is not significantly altered in healthy human pregnancy,[69,70] it is recommended that RPE be used in addition to the modified heart rate target zone. A target RPE zone of 12 to 14 on Borg's 15-point (6 to 20) scale is useful for this purpose. Finally, as recommended originally by Fitness Canada,[59] the "talk test" (ability to carry on a verbal conversation while exercising) is recommended as a final check to prevent overexertion. Since respiratory sensitivity is augmented in pregnancy,[71] this test is more sensitive than when it is used in healthy nonpregnant subjects.

Research Support for PARmed-X for Pregnancy

Aerobic exercise guidelines continued in the PARmed-X for Pregnancy (Table 13–2) were first formulated in the mid-1980s based on a current survey of existing literature[7,8] and review of earlier guidelines from other sources. Since

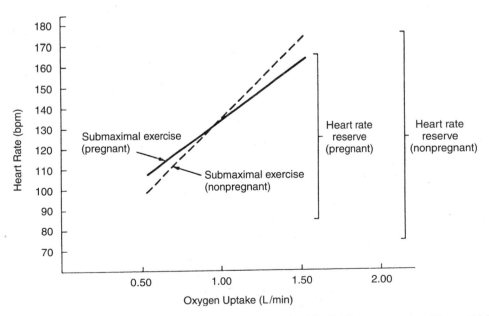

FIGURE 13–2. Maximal heart rate reserve during exercise in healthy human pregnancy. (From Wolfe LA, Mottola MF: Aerobic exercise in pregnancy: an update. Can J Appl Physiol 18:117–147, 1993. Used with permission.)

TABLE 13–2. Summary of PARmed-X for Pregnancy Recommendations for Aerobic Exercise in Pregnancy

Pregnancy is a good time to adopt permanent healthy life style habits (including regular exercise).

Pregnant women should not begin a new exercise program or increase the intensity or duration of regular exercise prior to the 14th week or after the 28th week of gestation.

The best time to begin a new program or increase exercise intensity and/or duration is during the second trimester, since the risks of exercise and discomforts of pregnancy are lowest.

Non-weight-bearing or low-impact exercise modalities are usually better than weight-bearing modalities.

Aerobic exercise should be conducted regularly (minimum of 3 d/wk, 15 minutes per session).

Aerobic exercise should be increased gradually up to a maximum of approximately 30 minutes per session and 4–5 session per week during the second trimester.

Use modified pulse rate target zone and rating of perceived exertion (12–14 on Borg's 6.20 RPE scale) to monitor exercise intensity.

Use "talk test" as a final check to avoid overexertion.

Avoid exercising in warm or humid environments.

Maintain adequate hydration and nutrition; drink liquids before and after exercise.

Know reasons to discontinue exercise and consult a qualified physician.

Reprinted with permission from Canadian Society for Exercise Physiology (CSEP): Physical activity readiness medical examination for pregnancy (PARmed-X for Pregnancy). Available from CSEP, 185 Somerset St. W, Suite 202, Ottawa, ON, K2P OJ2, Canada, 1996

that time, two controlled prospective studies have been conducted to test the efficiency and safety of these guidelines. Both studies used the same experimental design, and both required approximately 3 years to complete.

Both studies used healthy, nonsmoking, previously inactive pregnant women as subjects. After medical screening using a form similar to that used as part of the current PARmed-X for Pregnancy, subjects entered the study between the 16th and 20th weeks of gestation and chose voluntarily to participate as members of the experimental (exercising) group or a control group who remained physically inactive. This approach was used instead of a randomized design, to promote compliance with the assigned treatment and to minimize dropout. However, subjects were recruited from a homogeneous middle socioeconomic population and were allowed to choose group assignments only after meeting the specific entry criteria. In both studies, this resulted in experimental and control groups that were similar with respect to maternal age, parity, body height, adiposity (as reflected by skinfold thickness), and aerobic fitness.[70,72]

The experimental group in both studies participated in an aerobic exercise program (stationary cycling) during the second and third trimesters in accordance with guidelines described in the current PARmed-X for Pregnancy document. Exercise intensity was prescribed on an individual basis using modified pulse rate target zones (approximately 140–150 bpm in most cases) and a target RPE zone of 12 to 14 on Borg's 15-point (6 to 20) scale. The "talk test" was also employed as a general safety measure. Supervised exercise classes were conducted by a qualified instructor 3 days a week. Aerobic exercise duration began at 15 minutes per session and increased by 2 minutes per week for the first 4 weeks followed by 1 minute per week to reach 25 minutes per session by the end of the second trimester. Exercise intensity and duration were held constant during the third trimester. Individual exercise logs were kept by the instructor to document steady-state exercise heart rate, exercise duration, and class attendance. Subjects detrained during the immediate 3 to 4 months postpartum.

Physiologic testing was conducted at study entry (16–20 weeks of gestation) and near the end of both the second (~27 weeks) and third (~37 weeks) trimesters, and 3 to 4 months postpartum in both groups. In the first study, this included basic anthropometric measures, a resting echocardiogram,[71] metabolic cardiorespiratory and perceptual responses to a three-stage submaximal cycling test,[70,73] and fetal responses to 15 minutes of steady-state cycling.[20]

In the second study, testing involved basic anthopometric measures,[73a] maternal metabolic cardiorespiratory, and perceptual responses to a graded submaximal cycling test,[72,73b] and fetal responses to a graded submaximal cycling test.[16] In both studies, information on labor and delivery was collected by qualified medical personnel. This included birth weight, gestational age at delivery, duration of labor (three stages), Apgar scores, use of medications and analgesics, and labor complications (eg, need for cesarean delivery, episiotomy, meconium-stained amniotic fluid).

Both studies demonstrated the efficacy of the PARmed-X for Pregnancy guidelines (Table 13–3) for the improvement of aerobic fitness. In the first study, moderate increases in physical work capacity of a heart rate of 150 or 170 bpm (PWC_{150} or PWC_{170}) were observed in the con-

---

TABLE 13–3. Controlled Prospective Physical Conditioning Studies That Have Used PARmed-X for Pregnancy Guidelines: Summary of Major Findings

Study 1 (Involving Steady-State Exercise Testing)

Aerobic fitness (as reflected by PWC_{150}) increased 38% in the experimental (exercise) group; PWC_{150} also increased 10% in the control group.[70]

Aerobic conditioning attenuates respiratory responses to heavy steady-state exercise in late gestation.[70]

Aerobic conditioning in pregnancy does not reduce resting heart rate; conditioning effects to reduce heart rate unmasked during exercise and become evident at higher exercise heart rates.[71]

Ratings of perceived exertion (RPE) are not significantly altered by pregnancy or advancing gestational age; aerobic conditioning during pregnancy reduces RPE during steady-state cycling at standard steady-state work rates.[70]

Moderate aerobic conditioning does not significantly augment pregnancy-induced increases in cardiac dimensions.[71]

The most common fetal response to sustained steady-state exercise (stationary cycling) is a gradual increase in fetal heart rate, with recovery to pre-exercise baseline within 20–30 minutes; fetal bradycardic responses are rare and transient and usually occur in the immediate postexercise period.[20]

Maternal aerobic conditioning may allow pregnant women to exercise at higher work rates without inducing fetal hypoxic stress.[20]

Study 2 (Involving Graded Submaximal Exercise Testing)

Aerobic fitness (as reflected by oxygen pulse at a maternal exercise heart rate of 170 bpm) increased 17%; oxygen pulse at 170 bpm decreased 4% in the control group.[72]

The work rate at the ventilatory anaerobic threshold (T_{vent}) is not altered significantly by pregnancy or advancing gestational age; T_{vent} increases significantly following maternal aerobic conditioning.[72]

Maternal aerobic conditioning may help preserve the ability to use carbohydrate and produce lactate during heavy non-steady-state exercise.[72]

RPE during graded exercise is not significantly altered by pregnancy or advancing gestational age; maternal aerobic conditioning reduces RPE at standard work rates during graded exercise.[73b]

Postexercise reduction in maternal plasma glucose concentration in late gestation may be prevented by maternal aerobic conditioning.[32]

Maternal aerobic conditioning may help to preserve maternal energy stores (as reflected by skinfold thickness) in late gestation.[73a]

The most common fetal response following strenuous graded exercise is a reduction in fetal heart rate baseline, followed by a delayed increase in the postexercise period.[16]

Both Studies (Pooled Labor and Delivery Data)

Aerobic conditioning in accordance with PARmed-X for Pregnancy guidelines had no effect on birth weight; mean values in the exercise group (3,539 ± 70 g) and control group (3,592 ± 77 g) were similar to those predicted from age- and sex-corrected norms for the Canadian population.[76]

Aerobic conditioning had no significant effect on the length of gestation (39.9 ± 0.2 vs 39.5 ± 0.4), length of labor (three stages), and Apgar scores; use of medications or analgesics; or the incidence of labor and delivery complications.[39]

trol group, and may have reflected a conditioning effect of carrying a greater body mass during activities of daily living in late gestation. However, changes in the experimental (exercise) group were much larger. In the second study, significant increases were observed for both aerobic fitness, as reflected by the oxygen pulse at a heart rate of 170 bpm, and the work rate at the ventilatory anaerobic threshold (T_{vent}).

In both studies, there was no significant reduction in resting heart rate after aerobic conditioning in pregnancy. However, the expected reductions in heart rate were observed during heavy exercise at standard work rates, suggesting that conditioning effects are "masked" during pregnancy in the resting state.[70,71] Other beneficial effects of aerobic conditioning in pregnancy included significant reductions in overall RPE, the ventilatory equivalent for oxygen,[70] and respiratory perception of effort of standard submaximal work rates.

Results of publications from other laboratories,[66,74,75] have suggested that with advancing gestational age there may be a reduction in the ability to utilize carbohydrate and produce lactate during strenuous exercise. This was confirmed in both studies,[70,72] but the findings also suggested that this effect is attenuated by maternal aerobic conditioning. Similarly, a significant reduction in plasma glucose level was observed following a graded cycle ergometer test in late gestation in the sedentary control group but not in subjects who were aerobically conditioned.[32]

Results from study 1[20] confirmed that the most common response to sustained submaximal maternal aerobic exercise in a healthy fetus is a gradual increase in fetal heart rate baseline, followed by a gradual return to pre-exercise fetal heart rate baseline in the immediate 20 to 30 minutes after exercise. In contrast, data from study 2 indicated that graded maternal exercise testing (peak heart rate +170 beats/min) results in a modest reduction in fetal heart rate immediately after exercise, followed by a delayed increase.[16] It was postulated that the reduction in fetal heart rate was a reflex response to mild fetal hypoxia related to transient venous pooling, maternal hypotension, and reduced uterine blood flow in the immediate postexercise period. The delayed rise in fetal heart rate may be a compensatory reaction to restore fetal oxygen availability where not significantly altered by

maternal aerobic conditioning. However, conditioned subjects may be able to exercise at higher absolute power outputs without causing significant fetal hypoxic responses.[16,20]

Pooled results of the two studies[39] indicated that maternal physical conditioning had no significant effect on birth weight, duration of labor (three stages), 1- and 5-minute Apgar scores, gestational age at delivery, medication use (analgesic and oxytocic drugs), or incidence of labor complications (eg, need for cesarean delivery, meconium-stained amniotic fluid). It is important to note that pregnancy and labor outcomes were favorable in both the experimental (exercise) and control (nonexercise) groups and that the number of dropouts for medical reasons was low in both groups and did not differ between the two groups. Also, mean birth weight in both groups was close to that predicted using sex- and gestational age–corrected norms for the Canadian population.[76] Finally, none of the dropouts for medical reasons in the exercise groups were attributed to involvement in the exercise program.

EXERCISE FOR PREVENTION AND TREATMENT OF MATERNAL-FETAL DISEASE

Gestational Diabetes Mellitus

Gestational diabetes mellitus (GDM) may be present in as many as 12.3% of North American pregnancies.[77] A significant number of affected women are unable to maintain glycemic control through dietary means alone and subsequently will need insulin injections for the duration of the pregnancy.[78] While GDM generally resolves after delivery, some studies report an incidence of up to 60% conversion to true diabetes (type II, non-insulin-dependent) within the first year postpartum, with higher risk of conversion in obese women with early onset of GDM.[81] Multiparous women and women requiring insulin who gave birth to a macrosomic infant are also at risk for type II diabetes postpartum.[81–83] In addition, recent evidence suggests that the risk of type II diabetes increases with the number of GDM pregnancies.[84] Of equal concern is the increased risk that the offspring of mothers with GDM will have diabetes, childhood obesity, hypertension, and intellectual impairment.[85] Thus, pregnancies complicated by GDM are associated with significant maternal and fetal risk, including problems with labor and delivery owing to macrosomia and shoulder dystocia.[86]

In GDM, it is essential to achieve and maintain normal metabolic control. This must be accomplished through a regulated diet without compromising maternal nutritional status, thereby ensuring optimal fetal development.[87] Ingestion of frequent small meals (3 meals plus 3 or more snacks) may change insulin secretion patterns and may decrease need for insulin.[88] The total amount of calories ingested daily (38 kcal/kg ideal body weight during pregnancy) as well as the way in which carbohydrates are distributed throughout the day are also important in women with GDM.[88]

Exercise may be a safe and effective intervention as adjunctive therapy in women with GDM.[46] The Third International Workshop Conference on GDM suggested that future research should include clinical trials to test aggressive therapies such as reduced calories, exercise, and insulin.[89] In addition, Jovanovic[80] recently suggested that exercise may be better treatment for GDM than insulin.

Jovanovic-Peterson et al[90] randomized 20 GDM women to a dietary therapy group and a group receiving the same dietary therapy plus an exercise program 3 times per week, 20 minutes per session, using an arm ergometer. After 6 weeks, the women with GDM in the exercise program had normalized their glycosylated hemoglobin (Hb A1c) values and their fasted plasma glucose levels. Measurement of Hb A1c has been considered an objective account of chronic glycemic control (reflecting the preceding 6 weeks[87]) in diabetes.[91] Bung et al[92] studied 41 patients with GDM-A2 (1-week failure of intensive dietary therapy) by randomizing them to a group of exercise and diet or a group receiving insulin and diet. The exercise program consisted of recumbent cycling at 50% of maximum aerobic capacity for 45 minutes (3 bouts of 15 minutes, interspersed with two 4-minute rest periods) 3 times per week. No differences were found between the groups in blood glucose values or in delivery complications and neonatal outcomes. They suggested that exercise may enable avoidance of insulin therapy by promoting decreases in blood glucose values through increasing insulin sensitivity.[92]

In contrast, Avery et al[93] randomized 33 women with GDM to an exercise group or a nonexercise group. Exercise consisted of moderate exercise (70% of estimated maximum heart rate) on a stationary cycle for 30 minutes 3 and 4 times weekly. They found that this exercise program did not change blood glucose levels, Hb A1c, and incidence of newborn hypoglycemia but did result in a modest increase in cardiovascular fitness compared with no-exercise intervention. Lesser et al[94] failed to find a change in glycemic excursion in women with GDM (n = 6) compared with pregnant women without GDM (n = 5) after an acute bout of moderate intensity exercise (60% maximum oxygen uptake) on a stationary cycle for 30 minutes after a mixed nutrient meal. They suggested that a single bout of moderate intensity exercise did not blunt the glycemic response observed after a mixed nutrient meal. The differing results in these studies may be attributed to exercise intensity; mild intensity exercise (in which changes in glucose metabolism were noted) may be better than moderate intensity exercise (in which no changes in glycemic control were observed) for promoting glucose uptake by tissues.

Intensity of aerobic conditioning may be an important factor in altering glucose metabolism. A 3-year study recently completed in our laboratory showed that mild intensity exercise (30% of peak oxygen uptake) on a stationary cycle promoted glucose uptake from the blood of normal pregnant women when an oral glucose load (75 g) was administered immediately after mild steady-state exercise in the third trimester.[95] The blood glucose values were not different from those in age- and fitness-matched nonpregnant controls, which suggests that mild intensity exercise may promote glucose clearance from the blood. This same effect was not found when pregnant women engaging in moderate intensity exercise (70% of peak oxygen uptake) on a stationary cycle also underwent oral glucose tolerance testing immediately after the steady-state exercise: a glucose sparing effect was apparent. In addition, when glucose transporter *GLUT 4* was measured from a muscle biopsy from the vastus lateralis muscle of these women, mild exercise training promoted a significant increase in *GLUT 4* values, compared with moderate intensity training.[95]

From our results, it would appear that mild intensity exercise promotes glucose uptake from the blood to the tissues of healthy pregnant women.[95] These observations are important because women at risk for GDM and women with GDM who have high blood glucose levels may be able to use a mild exercise program in conjunction with a dietary regimen to help control and perhaps normalize blood glucose levels by promoting insulin sensitivity and glucose uptake in skeletal muscle, which may also be a key component in prevention of GDM or delaying the onset of GDM in women at risk.

Pre-Eclampsia

Even though pre-eclampsia or pregnancy-induced hypertension, is observed in approximately 10% of all pregnancies worldwide,[96] its causes have not been clearly identified. Sometimes labeled as the "disease of theories,"[97] pre-eclampsia is accompanied by increased blood pressure ($>140/90$ mm Hg), renal dysfunction (including proteinuria), and altered cardiac autonomic function.[98] The endocrine abnormalities may be caused by endothelial cell dysfunction. Abnormal placental trophoblastic invasion of the uterine spiral arteries is an essential feature of pre-eclampsia,[99] and there also appears to be a genetically based tendency to develop the disease.[100] As a result of these pathologic changes, pre-eclampsia is associated with increased perinatal mortality and intrauterine growth retardation.

Little research exists on the possible relationship between regular exercise in pregnancy and the incidence of pre-eclampsia. An early study by Erdelyi[101] reported a significantly lower incidence of toxemia in a group of 172 pregnant Hungarian athletes compared with a control group of 150 pregnant nonathletes. More recently, Marcoux et al[47] performed a retrospective study of leisure time physical activity during the first 20 weeks of pregnancy in a group of hospital patients that included 172 women with pre-eclampsia, 254 women with GDM, and 505 healthy pregnant controls. All women were primiparas. Subjects who performed regular leisure time exercise had reduced incidence of pre-eclampsia and pregnancy-induced hypertension, and the relative risk for these conditions decreased with increasing estimated energy expenditure in physical activity.

Some evidence is also available from animal studies to support the hypothesis that regular exercise may be useful to prevent or treat pregnancy-induced hypertension. Jones et al[102] studied the effects of regular voluntary exercise on resting cardiovascular function and reproductive tissue blood flow in pregnant normotensive Wistar-Kyoto (WKY) rats and pregnant spontaneously hypertensive rats (SHR). Nonexercising pregnant rats of both strains were also studied. No differences were observed for fetal number, fetal weight, or the number of fetal resorptions among the groups, but exercise appeared to enhance reproductive tissue blood flow in exercised SHR rats compared with nonexercising SHR controls.

It seems clear that more research is warranted on the relationship between maternal physical activity and the incidence of pre-eclampsia. Such studies could, using a prospective randomized design, investigate the effects of regular aerobic exercise on the incidence of pre-eclampsia, as well as the physiologic functions (eg, autonomic control, cardiovascular function, blood volume, renal function, endocrine factors) that are altered in pre-eclampsia. Subjects could include primiparas with a family history of pre-eclampsia or women with a history of pre-eclampsia in previous pregnancies, and should be assigned randomly to exercising or control groups. The effects of different exercise intensities and durations also need to be examined.[102]

SUMMARY AND CONCLUSIONS

Research over the past two decades has demonstrated that moderate aerobic conditioning, as outlined in the PARmed-X for Pregnancy document, is safe and effective in preventing many of the physical ill effects of bed rest or physical inactivity in healthy women undergoing uncomplicated pregnancies. There also appears to be a dose-response effect, and an optimal quantity and quality of maternal physical conditioning for the promotion of fetal growth.

Existing studies of the effects of acute and chronic exercise on maternal glycemic control have produced varying findings, perhaps because of differences in the subject populations studied and the intensity and duration of exercise.

Recent evidence suggests that mild exercise may be more effective than more strenuous exertion to promote glucose uptake by maternal tissues.

Findings from both human epidemiologic studies and investigations in laboratory animals suggest that regular exercise may help prevent pre-eclampsia. However, controlled randomized clinical trials are needed to confirm or refute the value of regular maternal exercise to prevent GDM and pre-eclampsia.

REFERENCES

1. Tafari N, Naeye RL, Gobeze A: Effects of maternal undernutrition and heavy physical work during pregnancy on birth weight. Br J Obstet Gynaecol 87:222–226, 1980
2. Terada M: Effect of physical activity before pregnancy on fetuses of mice exercised forcibly during pregnancy. Teratology 10:141–144, 1974
3. Canadian Society for Exercise Physiology: Physical Activity Readiness Medical Examination for Pregnancy (PARmed-X for Pregnancy). Available from CSEP, 185 Somerset St W, Suite 202, Ottawa, ON, K2P 0J2, Canada, 1996
4. Lotgering FK, Gilbert RD, Longo LD: Exercise responses in pregnant sheep: blood gases, temperatures and fetal cardiovascular system. J Appl Physiol 55:834–841, 842–850, 1983
5. Paolone AM, Worthington M: Caution and advice on exercise during pregnancy. Contemp Obstet Gynecol 25:150–162, 1985
6. Gauthier MM: Guidelines for exercise during pregnancy: too little or too much? Physician Sports Med. 14:162, 164–169, 1986
7. Wolfe LA, Ohtake PJ, Mottola MF, McGrath MJ: Physiological interactions between pregnancy and aerobic exercise. Exerc Sport Sci Rev 17:295–351, 1989
8. Wolfe LA, Hall P, Webb KA, et al: Prescription of aerobic exercise during pregnancy. Sports Med 8:273–301, 1989
9. McMurray RG, Mottola MF, Wolfe LA, et al: Recent advances in understanding maternal and fetal responses to exercise. Med Sci Sports Exerc 25:1305–1321, 1993
10. Lotgering FK, Gilbert RD, Longo LD: Exercise responses in pregnant sheep: oxygen consumption, uterine blood flow and blood volume. J Appl Physiol 55:834–841, 1983
11. Treadway JL, Young JC: Decreased glucose uptake by the fetus after maternal exercise. Med Sci Sports Exerc 21:140–145, 1989
12. Edwards MJ: Hyperthermia as a teratogen: a review of experimental studies and their clinical significance. Teratog Carcinog Mutagen 6:563–582, 1986
13. Clapp JF III, Dickstein S: Endurance exercise and pregnancy outcome. Med Sci Sports Exerc 16:556–562, 1984
14. Wolfe LA, Brenner IKM, Mottola MF: Maternal exercise, fetal well-being and pregnancy outcome. Exerc Sport Sci Rev 22:145–194, 1994
15. Clapp JF III, Little CD, Capeless EL: Fetal heart rate response to sustained recreational exercise. Am J Obstet Gynecol 168:198–206, 1993
16. Brenner IKM, Wolfe LA, Monga M, McGrath MJ: Physical conditioning effects on fetal heart rate responses to graded maternal exercise. Med Sci Sports Exerc 31:792–799, 1999
17. MacPhail A, Davies GAL, Victory R, Wolfe LA: Fetal heart rate responses to strenuous exercise in late gestation [abstract]. Am J Obstet Gynecol 18(vol 1, part 2):79, 1999
18. Carpenter MW, Sady SP, Hoegsborg B, et al: Fetal heart rate response to maternal exertion. JAMA 259:3006–3009, 1988
19. Manders MA, Sonder GJ, Mulder EJ, Visser GH: The effects of maternal exercise on fetal heart rate and movement patterns. Early Hum Dev 48:237–247, 1997
20. Webb KA, Wolfe LA, McGrath MJ: Effects of acute and chronic maternal exercise on fetal heart rate. J Appl Physiol 97:2207–2213, 1994
21. Morton MS, Paul MS, Compos GR, et al: Exercise dynamics in late gestation: effects of physical training. Am J Obstet Gynecol 152:91–97, 1985
22. Maršál K, Lofgren O, Gennser G: Fetal breathing movements and maternal exercise. Acta Obstet Gynecol Scand 58:197–201, 1979
23. Maršál K, Gennser G, Lofgren O: Effects on fetal breathing movements of maternal challenges. Acta Obstet Gynecol Scand 58:335–342, 1979
24. Sodha RJ, Proegler M, Schneider H: Transfer and metabolism of norepinephrine studied from maternal-to-fetal and fetal-to-maternal sides of the in vitro profused human placental lobe. Am J Obstet Gynecol 148:474–481, 1984
25. Stevenson L: Exercise in pregnancy. Part 1: Update on pathophysiology. Can Fam Physician 73:97–104, 1997
26. McMurray RG, Katz VL: Thermoregulation in pregnancy. Sports Med 10:146–158, 1990
27. Jones MT, Norton KI, Dengel DR, Armstrong RB: Effects of training on reproductive tissue blood flow in exercising pregnant rats. J Appl Physiol 69:2097–2103, 1990
28. Clapp JF III, Wesley M, Sleamaker RH: Thermoregulatory and metabolic responses prior to

and during pregnancy. Med Sci Sports Exerc 19:124–180, 1987

29. Clapp JF III: The changing thermal response to endurance exercise in pregnancy. Am J Obstet Gynecol 165:1684–1689, 1991

30. Platt LD, Artal R, Semel J, et al: Exercise in pregnancy. II: Fetal responses. Am J Obstet Gynecol 147:487–491, 1983

31. Bonen A, Campagna P, Gilchrist L, et al: Substrate and endocrine responses during exercise at selected stages of pregnancy. J Appl Physiol 73:134–142, 1992

32. Wolfe LA, Mottola MF: Aerobic exercise in pregnancy: an update. Can J Appl Physiol 18:119–147, 1993

33. Mottola MF, Bonen A, Hammond JMS, et al: Effects of moderate aerobic conditioning on glucose tolerance and GLUT 4 expression in human pregnancy [abstract]. Med Sci Sports Exerc 31:567, 1999

34. Mottola MF, Christopher PD: Effects of maternal exercise on liver and skeletal muscle glycogen storage in pregnant rats. J Appl Physiol 71:1015–1019, 1991

35. López-Luna P, Iglesias MA, Muñoz C, Herrera E: Aerobic exercise during pregnancy reverses maternal insulin resistance in rats. Med Sci Sports Exerc 30:1510–1514, 1998

36. Clapp JF III: The effect of maternal exercise on early pregnancy outcome. Am J Obstet Gynecol 161:1453–1457, 1989

37. Clapp JF III: The course and outcome of labor following endurance exercise during pregnancy. Am J Obstet Gynecol 163:1799–1805, 1990

38. Bell RJ, Palma SM, Lumley JM: The effect of vigorous exercise during pregnancy on birthweight. Austr N Z J Obst Gynaecol 35:46–51, 1995

39. Brenner IKM, Monga M, Webb K, et al: Controlled prospective study of aerobic conditioning effects on pregnancy outcome [abstract]. Med Sci Sports Exerc 23:S169, 1991

40. Lokey EA, Tran ZU, Wells CL, et al: Effects of physical exercise on pregnancy outcomes: a meta-analytic review. Med Sci Sports Exerc 23:1234–1239, 1991

41. Pivarnik JM: Potential effects of maternal physical activity on birth weight: a brief review. Med Sci Sports Exerc 30:400–406, 1998

42. Convertino VA, Bloomfield SA, Greenleaf SE: An overview of the issues: physiological effects of bed rest and restricted physical activity. Med Sci Sports Exerc 29:187–190, 1997

43. Clapp JF III, Little KD: Effect of recreational exercise on pregnancy weight gain and subcutaneous fat deposition. Med Sci Sports Exerc 27:170–177, 1995

44. Berwin BR, Roddie JC: Venous distensibility during pregnancy determined by graded venous congestion. Am J Obstet Gynecol 125:921–923, 1976

45. Laros RK Jr: Thromboembolic disease. In: Creasy RK, Resnik R (eds): Maternal-Fetal Medicine: Principles and Practice, 2nd Ed. WB Saunders, Toronto, 1989, pp. 763–776

46. Bung P, Artal R: Gestational diabetes and exercise: a survey. Semin Perinatol 20:328–333, 1996

47. Marcoux S, Brisson J, Fabra J: The effect of leisure time physical activity on the risk of preeclampsia and gestational hypertension. J Epidemiol Commun Health 73:147–152, 1989

48. Roberts JM: Pregnancy-related hypertension. In: Creasy RK, Resnik R (Eds): Maternal-Fetal Medicine: Principles and Practice, 2nd ed. WB Saunders, Toronto, 1989, pp. 777–823

49. Bloomfield SA: Changes in musculoskeletal structure and function with prolonged bed rest. Med Sci Sports Exerc 29:197–206, 1997

50. Berg G, Hammer M, Moeller-Neilson J: Low back pain during pregnancy. Obstet Gynecol 71:71–75, 1988

51. Wallace AM, Boyer DB, Holm K: Aerobic exercise, maternal self-esteem and physical discomforts during pregnancy. J Nurse Midwifery 31:255–262, 1986

52. Hall DC, Kaufmann DA: Effects of aerobic and strength conditioning on pregnancy outcomes. Am J Obstet Gynecol 157:1199–1203, 1987

53. Varassi G, Bazzono C, Edwards T: Effects of physical activity on maternal plasma β-endorphin levels and perception of labor pain. Am J Obstet Gynecol 160:707–712, 1989

54. Hatch MC, Shu XO, McLean DE, et al: Maternal exercise during pregnancy, physical fitness and fetal growth. Am J Epidemiol 137:1105–1114, 1993

55. Clapp JF III, Rizk KD: Effect of recreational exercise on midtrimester placental growth. Am J Obstet Gynecol 167:1518–1521, 1992

56. Clapp JF III, Capeless E: Neonatal morphometrics following endurance exercise during pregnancy. Am J Obstet Gynecol 163:1803–1811, 1990

57. American College of Obstetricians and Gynecologists: Exercise during pregnancy and the postnatal period. ACOG, Washington, DC, 1985

58. American College of Obstetricians and Gynecologists: Exercise during pregnancy and the postpartum period. ACOG Tech Bull 189:2–7, 1994

59. Fitness and Pregnancy. Fitness Canada, Ottawa, 1982

60. Fitness Ontario Leadership Program: Pre/Post Natal Fitness. Ontario Ministry of Tourism and

Recreation, Sports and Fitness Branch, Toronto, 1983

61. Gledhill N, for the Fitness Safety Standards Committee: Final Report to the Minister of Tourism and Recreation on the Development of Fitness Safety Standards in Ontario, Toronto, 1990

62. Canadian Academy of Sports Medicine: Position statement on exercise and pregnancy—1999. Available from CASM, 1600 James Naismith Dr., Gloucester, Ontario, K1B 4N4

63. Stevenson L: Exercise in pregnancy. Part 2: Recommendations for individuals. Can Fam Physician 43:107–111, 1997

63a. Canadian Society for Exercise Physiology: Active Living During Pregnancy—1999. Available from CSEP, 185 Somerset St W, Suite 202, Ottawa, Ontario, K2P OJ2

64. Capeless EL, Clapp JF III: Cardiovascular changes in early phase of pregnancy. Am J Obstet Gynecol 161:1449–1453, 1989

65. Clapp JF III: Maternal heart rate in pregnancy. Am J Obstet Gynecol 132:659–660, 1985

66. Lotgering FK, Van Doorn MK, Struijk PC, et al: Maximal aerobic exercise in pregnant women: heart rate, O₂ consumption, CO₂ production, and ventilation. J Appl Physiol 70:1016–1023, 1991

67. Avery ND, Wolfe LA, McGrath MJ: Effects of human pregnancy on heart rate variability (HRV) above and below the ventilatory anaerobic threshold [abstract]. Can J Appl Physiol 23:462, 1998

68. Avery ND, Wolfe LA, McGrath MJ: Effects of human pregnancy on spontaneous baroreflex (SBR) function above and below the ventilatory anaerobic threshold [abstract]. Can J Appl Physiol 23:463, 1998

69. Pivarnik JM, Lee W, Miller JF: Physiological and perceptual responses to cycle and treadmill exercise during pregnancy. Med Sci Sports Exerc 23:470–475, 1991

70. Ohtake PJ, Wolfe LA: Physical conditioning attenuates respiratory responses to exercise in late gestation. Med Sci Sports Exerc 30:17–27, 1998

71. Wolfe LA, Preston RJ, Burggraf GW, McGrath MJ: Effects of pregnancy and chronic exercise on maternal cardiac structure and function. Can J Physiol Pharm 77:909–917, 1999

72. Wolfe LA, Walker RM, Bonen A, McGrath MJ: Effects of pregnancy and chronic exercise on respiratory responses to graded exercise. J Appl Physiol 76:1928–1936, 1994

73. Oktake PJ, Wolfe LA, Hall P, McGrath MJ: Physical conditioning effects on heart rate and perception of exertion in pregnancy [abstract]. Can J Sports Sci 13:71P, 1988

73a. Greer FA, Wolfe LA: Chronic exercise effects on subcutaneous adiposity in pregnancy [abstract]. Med Sci Sports Exer 25:S119, 1994

73b. Wolfe LA, VonRaay AM, Dumas GA, McGrath MJ: Perception of exertion in pregnancy: aerobic conditioning effects [abstract]. Med Sci Sports Exerc 25:573, 1992

74. Artal R, Wiswell R, Romen Y, Dorey F: Pulmonary responses to exercise in pregnancy. Am J Obstet Gynecol 154:378–383, 1986

75. McMurray RG, Katz VL, Berry MJ, Cefalo RC: The effect of pregnancy on metabolic responses during rest, immersion and aerobic exercise in the water. Am J Obstet Gynecol 158:481–486, 1988

76. Arbuckle TE, Wilkins R, Sherman GJ: Birth weight percentiles by gestational age in Canada. Obstet Gynecol 81:39–48, 1993

77. Magee MS, Walden CE, Beredetti TJ: Influence of diagnostic criteria on the incidence of gestational diabetes and perinatal morbidity. JAMA 270:324, 1993

78. Coustan DR, Imarah J: Prophylactic insulin treatment of gestational diabetes reduces the incidence of macrosomia, operative delivery and birth trauma. Am J Obstet Gynecol 150:836–842, 1984

79. Langer O, Berkus M, Brustman L: Rationale for insulin management in gestational diabetes mellitus. Diabetes 40(suppl 12):186–190, 1991

80. Jovanovic L: Management of diet and exercise in GDM. Prenat Neonat Med 3:534–541, 1998

81. Damm P, Kuhl C, Bertelsen A: Predictive factors for the development of diabetes in women with previous GDM Am J Obstet Gynecol 167:607–610, 1992

82. Weller KA: Diagnosis and management of gestational diabetes. Am Fam Physician 53:2053–2057, 1996

83. Coustan DR: Gestational diabetes: a continuum of risk. Eur J Endocrin 137:13–14, 1997

84. Peters R, Kjos S, Xiang A, et al: Effect of a second pregnancy on the risk of NIDDM in women with recent gestational diabetes. Diabetes 44(suppl 1):14A, 1995

85. Pettitt DJ, Aleck KA, Baird HR, et al: Congenital susceptibility to NIDDM: role of intrauterine environment. Diabetes 37:622–624, 1988

86. Freinkel N, Ellenberg P, Rifkin H: The mother in pregnancies complicated by diabetes. In: Rifkin H, Porte D (eds): Diabetes Mellitus, Theory and Practice. Elsevier, Amsterdam, 1990

87. Canadian Diabetes Association: Guidelines for the nutritional management of diabetes in pregnancy: position statement. Beta Release 15:75–82, 1995

88. Gunderson EP: Intensive nutrition therapy for gestational diabetes. Diabetes Care 20:221–226, 1997

89. Metzger BE: Summary and recommendations of the Third International Workshop: Conference on Gestational Diabetes Mellitus. Diabetes 40(suppl 2):197–201, 1991

90. Jovanovic-Peterson L, Durak EP, Peterson CM: Randomized trial of diet vs. diet plus cardiovascular conditioning on glucose levels in gestational diabetes. Am J Obstet Gynecol 161:415–419, 1989

91. Homko CJ, Khandelwal M: Glucose monitoring and insulin therapy during pregnancy. Obstet Gynecol Clin North Am 23:47–74, 1996

92. Bung P, Bung C, Artal R, et al: Therapeutic exercise for insulin-requiring gestational diabetics: results from a randomized prospective longitudinal study. J Perinatol Med 21:125–137, 1993

93. Avery MD, Leon AS, Kopher RA: Effects of a partially home-based exercise program for females with gestational diabetes. Obstet Gynecol 89:10–15, 1997

94. Lesser KB, Gruppuso PA, Terry RB, Carpenter MW: Exercise fails to improve postprandial glycemic excursion in females with gestational diabetes. J Maternal Fetal Med 5:211–217, 1996

95. Mottola MF, Weis CA, Lewis NT, et al: Effect of mild versus moderate maternal exercise on glucose metabolism [abstract]. Med Sci Sports Exerc 30:S259, 1999

96. Consensus report: National High Blood Pressure Education Program Working Group report on high blood pressure in pregnancy. Am J Obstet Gynecol 163:1689–1712, 1990

97. Broughton Pipkin F, Rubin PC: Pre-eclampsia: the disease of theories. Br Med Bull 50:381–396, 1994

98. Eneroth-Grimfors E, Westgren M, Ericson M, et al: Autonomic cardiovascular control in normal and pre-eclamptic pregnancy. Acta Obstet Gynecol 73:680–687, 1994

99. Pijnenborg R, Anthony J, Davey DA, et al: Placental bed spiral arteries in the hypertensive disorders of pregnancy. Br J Obstet Gynaecol 98:648–655, 1991

100. Arngrimsson R, Bjornsson J, Greirsson RT, et al: Genetics and familial predisposition to eclampsia and pre-eclampsia in a defined population. Br J Obstet Gynaecol 97:762–769, 1990

101. Erdelyi GJ: Gynecological survey of female athletes. J Sports Med Phys Fitness 2:174–179, 1962

102. Jones RL, Botti JS, Anderson WM, Bennett NL: Thermoregulation during aerobic exercise in pregnancy. Obstet Gynecol 65:340–345, 1985

Physical Activity Readiness Medical Examination for Pregnancy

Physical Activity Readiness
Medical Examination for
Pregnancy (1996)

PARmed-X for PREGNANCY PHYSICAL ACTIVITY READINESS MEDICAL EXAMINATION

PARmed-X for PREGNANCY is a guideline for health screening prior to participation in a prenatal fitness class or other exercise.

Healthy women with uncomplicated pregnancies can integrate physical activity into their daily living and can participate without significant risks either to themselves or to their unborn child. Postulated benefits of such programs include improved aerobic and muscular fitness, promotion of appropriate weight gain, and facilitation of labour. Regular exercise may also help to prevent gestational glucose intolerance and pregnancy-induced hypertension.

The safety of prenatal exercise programs depends on an adequate level of maternal-fetal physiological reserve. PARmed-X for PREGNANCY is a convenient checklist and prescription for use by physicians to evaluate pregnant patients who want to enter a prenatal fitness program and for ongoing medical surveillance of exercising pregnant patients.

Instructions for use of the 4-page PARmed-X for PREGNANCY are the following:

1. The patient should fill out the section on PATIENT INFORMATION and the PRE-EXERCISE HEALTH CHECKLIST (PART 1, 2, 3, and 4 on p. 1) and give the form to the physician monitoring her pregnancy.

2. The physician should check the information provided by the patient for accuracy and fill out SECTION C on CONTRAINDICATIONS (p. 2) based on current medical information.

3. If no exercise contraindications exist, the HEALTH EVALUATION FORM (p. 3) should be completed, signed by the physician, and given by the patient to her prenatal fitness professional.

In addition to prudent medical care, participation in appropriate types, intensities and amounts of exercise is recommended to increase the likelihood of a beneficial pregnancy outcome. PARmed-X for PREGNANCY provides recommendations for individualized exercise prescription (p. 3) and program safety (p. 4).

NOTE: Sections A and B should be completed by the patient before the appointment with the physician.

A PATIENT INFORMATION

NAME _____

ADDRESS _____

TELEPHONE _____ BIRTHDATE _____ HEALTH INSURANCE No. _____

NAME OF
PRENATAL FITNESS PROFESSIONAL _____

PRENATAL FITNESS
PROFESSIONAL'S PHONE NUMBER _____

B PRE-EXERCISE HEALTH CHECKLIST

PART 1: GENERAL HEALTH STATUS

In the past, have you experienced (check YES or NO):

	YES	NO
1. Miscarriage in an earlier pregnancy?	❏	❏
2. Other pregnancy complications?	❏	❏
3. I have completed a PAR-Q within the last 30 days.	❏	❏

If you answered YES to question 1 or 2, please explain:

_____

Number of previous pregnancies? _____

PART 2: STATUS OF CURRENT PREGNANCY

Due Date: _____

During this pregnancy, have you experienced:

	YES	NO
1. Marked fatigue?	❏	❏
2. Bloody discharge from the vagina ("spotting")?	❏	❏
3. Unexplained faintness or dizziness?	❏	❏
4. Unexplained abdominal pain?	❏	❏
5. Sudden swelling of ankles, hands or face?	❏	❏
6. Persistent headaches or problems with headaches?	❏	❏
7. Swelling, pain or redness in the calf of one leg?	❏	❏
8. Absence of fetal movement after 4th month?	❏	❏
9. Failure to gain weight after fourth month?	❏	❏

If you answered YES to any of the above questions, please explain:

PART 3: ACTIVITY HABITS DURING THE PAST MONTH

1. List only regular fitness/recreational activities:

_____
_____

INTENSITY	FREQUENCY (times/week)			TIME (minutes/day)		
	1-2	2-4	4+	<20	20-40	40+
Heavy	___	___	___	___	___	___
Medium	___	___	___	___	___	___
Light	___	___	___	___	___	___

2. Does your regular occupation (job/home) activity involve:

	YES	NO
Heavy Lifting?	❏	❏
Frequent walking/stair climbing?	❏	❏
Occasional walking (>once/hr)?	❏	❏
Prolonged standing?	❏	❏
Mainly sitting?	❏	❏
Normal daily activity	❏	❏
3. Do you currently smoke tobacco?*	❏	❏
4. Do you consume alcohol?*	❏	❏

PART 4: PHYSICAL ACTIVITY INTENTIONS

What physical activity do you intend to do?

_____

Is this a change from what you currently do? ❏ YES ❏ NO

> ***NOTE: PREGNANT WOMEN ARE STRONGLY ADVISED NOT TO SMOKE OR CONSUME ALCOHOL DURING PREGNANCY AND DURING LACTATION.**

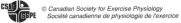

© *Canadian Society for Exercise Physiology*
Société canadienne de physiologie de l'exercice

Supported by: Health Santé
Canada Canada

1

Physical Activity Readiness
Medical Examination for
Pregnancy (1996)

PARmed-X for PREGNANCY PHYSICAL ACTIVITY READINESS MEDICAL EXAMINATION

C CONTRAINDICATIONS TO EXERCISE: to be completed by physician

Absolute Contraindications			Relative Contraindications		
Does the patient have:	YES	NO	*Does the patient have:*	YES	NO
1. Ruptured membranes, premature labour?	☐	☐	1. History of spontaneous abortion or premature labour in previous pregnancies?	☐	☐
2. Persistent second or third trimester bleeding/placenta previa?	☐	☐	2. Mild/moderate cardiovascular or respiratory disease (e.g., chronic hypertension, asthma?)	☐	☐
3. Pregnancy-induced hypertension pre-eclampsia or toxemia?	☐	☐	3. Anemia or iron deficiency? (Hb < 10 g/dl)?	☐	☐
4. Incompetent cervix?	☐	☐	4. Very low body fatness, eating disorder (anorexia, bulimia)?	☐	☐
5. Evidence of intrauterine growth retardation?	☐	☐	5. Twin pregnancy after 28th week?	☐	☐
6. Multiple pregnancy (e.g., triplets)?	☐	☐	6. Other significant medical condition?	☐	☐
7. Uncontrolled Type I diabetes, hypertension or thyroid disease, other serious cardiovascular, respiratory or systemic disorder?	☐	☐	Please specify: _____		

NOTE: Risk may exceed benefits of regular physical activity. The decision to be physically active or not should be made with qualified medical advice.

PHYSICAL ACTIVITY RECOMMENDATION: ☐ Recommended/Approved ☐ Contraindicated

Prescription for Aerobic Activity

RATE OF PROGRESSION: The best time to progress is during the second trimester since risks and discomfort of exercise are lowest at that time. It is not advisable to begin a new exercise program or increase the amount of exercise prior to the 14th week of pregnancy or after the 28th week. Aerobic exercise should be gradually and progressively increased during the second trimester from a minimum of 15 minutes per session to a maximum of approximately 30 minutes per session.

WARM-UP/COOL-DOWN: Aerobic activity should be preceded by a brief (10-15 min.) warm-up and followed by a short (10-15 min.) cool-down. Low intensity calesthenics, stretching and relaxation exercises should be included in the warm-up/cool-down.

PRESCRIPTION/MONITORING OF INTENSITY: The best way to prescribe and monitor exercise is by combining the heart rate and rating of perceived exertion (RPE) methods.

F	**I**	**T**	**T**
FREQUENCY	**INTENSITY**	**TIME**	**TYPE**
Begin at 3 times per week and progress to four or five times per week	Exercise within an appropriate RPE range and/or target heart rate zone	Attempt 15 minutes, even if it means reducing the intensity. Rest intervals may be helpful	Non weight-bearing or low-impact endurance exercise using large muscle groups (e.g., walking, stationary cycling, swimming, aquatic exercises, low impact aerobics)

"TALK TEST" - A final check to avoid overexertion is to use the "talk test". The exercise intensity is excessive if you cannot carry on a vertbal conversation while exercising.

TARGET HEART RATE ZONES

The heart rate zones shown below are appropriate for most pregnant women. Work during the lower end of the HR range at the start of a new exercise program and in late pregnancy.

	Heart Rate
Age	Range
< 20	140-155
20-29	135-150
30-39	130-145
≥ 40	125-140

RATING OF PERCEIVED EXERTION (RPE)

Check the accuracy of your heart rate target zone by comparing it to the scale below. A range of about 12-14 (somewhat hard) is appropriate for most pregnant women.

6	
7	Very, very light
8	
9	Somewhat light
10	
11	Fairly light
12	
13	Somewhat hard
14	
15	Hard
16	
17	Very hard
18	
19	Very, very hard
20	

The original PARmed-X for PREGNANCY was developed by L.A. Wolfe, Ph.D. of Queen's University, Kingston, Ontario. The muscular conditioning component was developed by M.F. Mottola, Ph.D. of The University of Western Ontario, London, Ontario. It has been revised by an Expert Advisory Committee assembled by the Canadian Society for Exercise Physiology and the Fitness Program-Health Canada (1996).

Translation and reproduction in its entirety is encouraged

Disponible en français sous le titre «Examination medicale sur l'aptitude à l'activité physique pour les femmes enceintes (X-AAP pour les femmes enceintes)»

To order additional printed copies of the PARmed-X for PREGNANCY, the PARmed-X and/or the PAR-Q, (for a nominal charge) contact the:

Canadian Society for Exercise Physiology
185 Somerset St. West, Suite 202
Ottawa, Ontario CANADA K2P 0J2
tel. (613) 234-3755 FAX (613) 234-3565

2

Physical Activity Readiness
Medical Examination for
Pregnancy (1996)

PARmed-X for PREGNANCY
PHYSICAL ACTIVITY READINESS MEDICAL EXAMINATION

Prescription for Muscular Conditioning

It is important to condition all major muscle groups during both prenatal and postnatal periods.

WARM-UPS & COOL DOWN:
Range of Motion: neck, shoulder girdle, back, arms, hips, knees, ankles, etc.
Static Stretching: all major muscle groups
(DO NOT OVER STRETCH!)

EXAMPLES OF MUSCULAR STRENGTHENING EXERCISES

CATEGORY	PURPOSE	EXAMPLE
Upper back	Promotion of good posture	Shoulder shrugs, shoulder blade pinch
Lower back	Promotion of good posture	Modified standing opposite leg & arm lifts
Abdomen	Promotion of good posture, prevent low-back pain, prevent diastasis recti, strengthen muscles of labour	Abdominal tightening, abdominal curl-ups, head raises lying on side or standing position
Pelvic floor ("Kegels")	Promotion of good bladder control, prevention of urinary incontinence	"Wave", "elevator"
Upper body	Improve muscular support for breasts	Shoulder rotations, modified push-ups against a wall
Buttocks, lower limbs	Facilitation of weight-bearing, prevention of varicose veins	Buttocks squeeze, standing leg lifts, heel raises

Precautions for Muscular Conditioning During Pregnancy

VARIABLE	EFFECTS OF PREGNANCY	EXERCISE MODIFICATIONS
Body Position	• in the supine position (lying on the back), the enlarged uterus may decrease the flow of blood returning from the lower half of the body as it presses on a major vein (inferior fena cava)	• past 4 months of gestation, exercises normally done in the supine position should be altered • such exercises should be done side lying or standing
Joint Laxity	• ligaments become relaxed due to increasing hormone levels • joints may be prone to injury	• avoid rapid changes in direction and bouncing during exercises • stretching should be performed with controlled movements
Abdominal Muscles	• presence of a rippling (bulging) of connective tissue along the midline of the pregnant abdomen (diastasis recti) may be seen during abdominal exercise	• abdominal exercises are not recommended if diastasis recti develops
Posture	• increasing weight of enlarged breasts and uterus may cause a forward shift in the centre of gravity and may increase the arch in the lower back • this may also cause shoulders to slump forward	• emphasis on correct posture
Precautions for Resistance Exercise	• emphasis must be placed on continuous breathing throughout exercise • exhale on exertion, inhale on relaxation • Valsalva Manoevre (holding breath while working against a resistance) causes a decrease in blood pressure and therefore should be avoided • avoid exercise in supine position past 4 months gestation	

Health Evaluation Form
(to be completed by patient and given to the prenatal fitness professional after obtaining medical clearance to exercise)

I, _____ PLEASE PRINT (patient's name), have discussed my plans to participate in physical activity during my current pregnancy with my physician and I have obtained his/her approval to begin participation.

Signed: _____
(patient's signature)

Date: _____

PHYSICIAN'S COMMENTS:

Name of Physician: _____ M.D.

Address: _____

Telephone: _____

_____

_____

_____

_____ M.D.
(physician's signature)

3

Physical Activity Readiness
Medical Examination for
Pregnancy (1996)

Advice for Active Living During Pregnancy

Pregnacy is a time when women make beneficial changes in their health habits to protect and promote the healthy development of their unborn babies. These changes include adopting improved eating habits, abstinence from smoking and alcohol intake, and participating in regular moderate physical activity. All of these changes can be carried over into the postnatal period and many health experts believe that pregnancy is a very good time to adopt healthy lifestyle habits that are permanent by integrating physical activity with enjoyable healthy eating and a positive self and body image.

Active Living:

➤ see your doctor before increasing your activity level during pregnancy

➤ exercise regularly but don't overexert

➤ exercise with a pregnant friend or join a prenatal exercise program

➤ follow FITT principles modified for pregnant women

➤ know safetey considerations for exercise in pregnancy

Healthy Eating:

➤ the need for calories is higher (about 300 more per day) than before pregnancy

➤ follow Canada's Food Guide to Healthy Eating and choose healthy foods from the following groups: whole grain or enriched bread or cereal, fruits and vegetables, milk and milk products, meat, fish, poultry and alternatives

➤ drink 6-8 glasses of fluid, including water, each day

➤ salt intake should not be restricted

➤ limit caffeine intake i.e., coffee, tea, chocolate, and cola drinks

➤ dieting to lose weight may be harmful

Positive Self and Body Image:

➤ remember that it is normal to gain weight during pregnancy

➤ accept that your body shape will change during pregnancy

➤ enjoy your pregnancy as a unique and meaningful experience

Enjoy eating well, being active and feeling good about yourself. That's VITALIT ®

SAFETY CONSIDERATIONS

◆ Avoid prolonged or strenuous exertion during the 1st trimester

◆ Avoid isometric exercise or straining while holding your breath

◆ Maintain adequate nutrition and hydration - drink liquids before and after exercise

◆ Avoid exercising in warm/humid environments

◆ Avoid exercise while lying on your back past the 4th month of pregnancy

◆ Avoid activities which involve physical contact or danger of falling

◆ Periodic rest periods may help to minimize possible low oxygen or temperature stress to the fetus

◆ Know the reasons to stop exercise and consult a qualified physician immediately if they occur

** CAUTION **   It is important to monitor the temperature of heated pools. Maternal body temperature during exercise may be increased more by exercising in a warm environment.

REASONS TO CONSULT A PHYSICIAN

◆ Persistent uterine contractions (more than 6-8 per hour)

◆ Bloody discharge from vagina

◆ Any "gush" of fluid from vagina (suggesting premature rupture of the membranes)

◆ Unexplained pain in abdomen

◆ Sudden swelling of extremities (ankles, hands, face)

◆ Swelling, pain and redness in the calf of one leg (suggesting phlebitis)

◆ Persistent headaches or disturbances of vision

◆ Unexplained dizziness or faintness

◆ Marked fatigue, heart palpitations or chest pain

◆ Failure to gain weight (less than 1 kg per month during last two trimesters)

◆ Absence of usual fetal movement

Supported by:

Health   Santé
Canada   Canada

4

14

The Pediatric Athlete

DINESH A. KUMBHARE

Children are not little adults and should not be treated as such. They have important physical differences; eg, their bones absorb more energy than adult bones do. Their long bones have cartilaginous growth plates near the ends for longitudinal growth, apophyses with their own growth plates for attachment of musculotendinous structures, and growing articular cartilage. The porosity of the bone, the presence of growth plates, and other biomechanical differences lead to a different spectrum of injuries in children and growing adolescents compared with those in adults.

Despite concerns about sports injuries in children, participation in organized sports is safer than free play at home or on the playground.[1] A classic study performed in 1966 of emergency room visits for treatment of trauma, only 4.3% of injuries were caused by sports. Bicycling injuries accounted for another 4.5% of injuries. Of all injuries reported, 71.3% occurred either at home or in the yard.[2] Lenaway et al[3] reported in 1992 that of school-related injuries sustained by children from elementary school through high school, 53% were sports-related.

Although injuries sustained by young athletes are always of concern, children who participate in organized sports and fitness activities have opportunities to develop self-discipline, self-confidence, independence, and interpersonal skills. Appropriate strengthening and flexibility exercises and training methods can decrease chance of incurring an injury.[4] The introduction of an active lifestyle in youth may influence a child's desire and ability to maintain a high level of activity in subsequent years.[5]

MUSCULOSKELETAL CONSIDERATIONS IN CHILDREN AND ADOLESCENTS

Longitudinal Growth Plate Injury

Longitudinal growth occurs between apophyses and metaphyses of long bones and at the joint surface. The load on these growth regions is primarily compressive, although shear and torsional loads are also present. Growth plates have decreased strength during puberty.[6] Some physes that contribute to longitudinal growth seem particularly susceptible to injury during sports activity, including the distal femur, distal tibial, and distal radial physes. Injury to a physis may mimic the signs and symptoms that typically indicate a sprain or strain in an adult. Therefore, it is recommended that during physical examination the growth plates in the injured areas be carefully palpated and that radiographs generally should be obtained before manipulating or stressing the region. In any child with knee or anteriomedial thigh pain, slipped capital femoral apophysis or other hip injuries should be considered in the differential diagnosis.

Apophyseal Injury

The apophyseal growth plates are at sites of insertion of musculotendinous structures and are subjected to traction in a young athlete whose muscles are too tight relative to the adjacent long bones and joints. Repeated trauma to the apophysis also can occur through load injuries. If the pain resulting from inflammation is ignored, a single rapid, forceful contraction of the inserting musculotendinous unit may avulse the apophysis.[7,8] Chronic repetitive avulsion stress may lead to marked enlargement of the apophysis or to spur formation (eg, break-dancer hip, Osgoode-Schlatter disease).[9]

Physeal Versus Ligament Injury

Growth plate injuries occur because of the difference in the strength of the physis compared with that of the ligament supporting a joint. A period of most rapid growth (peak height velocity) near puberty is usually when the physis seems more likely to fail.[10] For girls, the peak age for physeal injury is about 11 years, and for boys, 12 to 14 years.[11] The site of insertion of ligamentous structures also influences whether the injury will result in failure of the ligament or physis.[12]

Diaphysis and Metaphysis

Immature bone is more porous than adult bone. Generally speaking, porosity is greatest at the regions undergoing the most rapid remodeling, particularly at the metaphysis. Increased porosity has been suggested as the etiologic factor resulting in metaphyseal buckle (torus) fractures. These injuries may result from relatively minor trauma.[13,14] Torus fractures often leave one cortex completely intact and the opposite cortex minimally buckled or overlapping.

Plastic deformation of the bone occurs, and the long bone may bend rather than break. The deformed bone may return nearly to its original shape because of the elastic recoil of the surrounding soft tissue.[15] If this occurs, the limb may have significantly injured structures on physical examination but no obvious radiologic abnormality, or it may be plastically deformed, with no radiologically apparent discrete fracture line. Marked plastic deformity may require manipulation to complete the fracture and allow the injured bone to be reduced to a more anatomic position.[5]

Periosteum

The bones of children have thicker, stronger, and more vascular periosteal envelopes. The intact periosteum can provide stability to a torus fracture, which can lead health care providers to the false impression that the fracture may be stable, and the injured child and parents may

believe the injury is a simple bruise or sprain when in fact it is a fracture.[5] However, a flap of periosteum may become entrapped in the fracture gap and prevent closed reduction. Periosteum provides a remarkable regenerative path because of its vascularity, and because it is so reactive to growth-enhancing hormones and other circulating growth factors, new bone may be formed rapidly within an empty periosteal sleeve. This may account for the re-formation of a normally shaped clavicle following what may appear to be a severe acromioclavicular separation.[5]

Articular Cartilage

The articular cartilage of a skeletally immature individual is thicker than in an adult and contains growth cartilage. Frequently injured regions include the proximal humerus, the distal femur, and the radiocapitellar joint.

Osteochondritis Dissecans

Murabarnk and Carroll[16,17] proposed endogenic factors as predisposing an individual to osteochrondritis dissecans, including generalized tissue laxity, family history, other apophyseal abnormalities, and possible endocrine dysfunction. They found no difference between the activity levels of patients with osteochrondritis dissecans compared with a control group. With this hypothesis in mind, osteochrondritis dissecans of the distal femur, often found bilaterally, may already be present because of the endogenous factors, and symptoms may be brought on by such activities as jumping.[16,11]

Berndt and Harty[18] reported that trauma to articular cartilage may result in partial or complete separation of the articular fragment from the remainder of the apophysis. Chondral or osteochondral injuries of the talus are consistent with this theory. These injuries are most frequently seen when athletes have sustained one or more ankle sprains in the past. An athlete can have permanent chondral and osteochrondral injuries, most frequently affecting the radiocapitellar joint, without recalling any significant traumatic events. Small articular fragments are thought to become completely separated from the joint surface, and, as they are nourished by the synovial fluid, grow until they are large enough to produce symptoms.[5]

Fractures Through Nonossified Cartilage

Some injuries must be suspected on the basis of the clinical setting and radiologic findings of soft tissue swelling and abnormal alignment rather than on visible fracture lines seen on x-ray films. These principles are especially important when evaluating an injury to a child's elbow because of the relatively high frequency of bone injury relative to ligamentous injury in the 5- to 13-year-old age group. Just before ossification occurs, it can be difficult to visualize fracture lines through unossified regions of the elbow joint.[19]

Menisci

The meniscus of a young child has vascular channels that frequently extend inward to or even beyond the halfway mark. Adult menisci generally have vessels in only the outer (peripheral) third.[20] This property may have implications for the types of injuries sustained at different ages. Children younger than 10 years rarely tear menisci, and the incidence of symptomatic meniscal lesions of all types was approximately 2 in 10,000 children younger than 19 years in one report.[21] Another study of acute knee hemarthroses performed by Steaniski et al[23] found that 7 of 15 children aged 7 to 12 years had meniscal tears.[22]

ACUTE INJURIES

Age-Related Fractures

There is an increased incidence of fractures in children and adolescents during periods of most rapid growth, or peak height velocity. Typical patterns and locations of fractures vary somewhat by age. Fractures of the growth plate vary according to how much of the physis is fused at the time of injury.[23] Also, children are more likely than adults to sustain fractures and less likely to sustain ligamentous sprains. Ekeland et al[24] in 1993 reported a study of recreational alpine skiers and found that children younger than 10 years had nine times the incidence of lower leg fractures compared with skiers older than 20 years, who were more likely to sustain knee sprains.

Physeal Fractures

Salter and Harris[25,25a] in their classic paper of 1963 described fractures through the growth plates at the ends of long bones. Their classification has remained because of its importance to prognostication of potentially abnormal growth subsequent to fracture.

Type I: Type I fracture involves only the physis. If it is nondisplaced, it may be innocuous; however, complete displacement may cause marked deformity as a result of arrested growth with or without avascular necrosis.

Type II: Type II fracture involves a portion of the physis and usually exits the opposite side of the bone through the metaphysis. These fractures are usually displaced, and even with accurate reduction of the fracture, growth may slow or stop in the injured portion of the physis.

Type III: Type III fracture traverses the physis, crosses the epiphysis, and enters the joint. The displaced fracture usually involves the articular surface, and if there is significant articular surface malalignment, premature osteoarthritis can develop.

Type IV: Type IV fracture crosses the metaphysis and epiphysis, and enters the articular surface. Increased bony deformity may occur if the bone of the epiphysis on one side unites with the bone of the metaphysis on the other side of the fracture line, and just as in type III fractures, premature development of osteoarthritis is likely if there is significant articular surface malalignment.

Type V: Type V fracture involves the physis only. Cells of the growth plate are thought to be crushed. Occasionally, there is no radiographic evidence of fracture. The existence of a pure type V fracture has been questioned by Peterson and Burkhart[26] and Ogden.[27] These researchers believe that the injury to the physis, which is initially invisible on x-ray films but causes growth arrest, is actually an injury to the vascularity of the physis itself or to the perichondrial ridge rather than a compressive injury, which gradually injures the growth chondrocytes of the physis directly.

Salter and Harris additionally described type VI fracture, involving only the zone of Ranvier; type VII fracture, which is completely intraepiphyseal; type VIII, which is a metaphyseal fracture that significantly injures the peripheral vascular supply; and type IX, involving only the diaphyseal appositional new bone formation.

Sprains

Child and adolescent athletes may sustain sprains, just as adult athletes do. It is generally accepted that the course of healing, however, is more rapid.[16] A subtle difference is that the same force that might cause a sprained ligament in an adult may cause a fracture in a child. It is also possible that both a sprain and a fracture may be present in combination.[28,29]

Meniscal Injury

The presentations and mechanisms of injury are similar in children, adolescents, and adult athletes. The clinical presentation is described in Chapter 22 and therefore is not repeated here. The difference between growing individuals and adults is that there is believed to be increased vascularity in the child's meniscus, which results in a better prognosis for healing of a torn meniscus, and the time for healing is also generally accepted to be shorter.[16]

OVERUSE INJURIES

Inflexibility and Injury

The elongation of adjacent muscles appears to follow the growth of long bones. It is generally accepted that the muscles respond to the stimulus of stretch. If a muscle is not stretched routinely through its entire range of motion, it becomes short relative to adjacent bones. This problem is particularly apparent in muscles that cross two joints, eg, gastrocnemius, hamstring, and rectus femoris. Relatively tight muscles can

lead to bony injury by several postulated mechanisms[16]:

1. Traction from muscle contraction or excessive stretch
2. Compression causing mechanical abnormality within the joint or on the opposite side of the joint
3. Rubbing or snapping over a bony prominence

Hypermobility

Athletes with marked laxity of joint ligaments and capsular structures require strong surrounding muscles to support the joint and provide satisfactory balance of strength and flexibility. Lysens et al[30] describe traits that are most likely to be associated with overuse injuries: being tall and having an endomorphic habitus, little static strength but high explosive strength, and poor muscle flexibility with high ligamentous laxity. Researchers have also described a relationship between gastrocnemius tightness and calcaneal epiphysitis,[31] and rectus femoris tightness and Osgood-Schlatter's disease and jumper's knee.[32] Orava and Puranen[33] described Osgood-Schlatter's disease and calcaneal apophysitis as the most common overuse injuries in athletes younger than 16 years. These comprised 16% of overuse injuries sustained in this population of athletes.[33]

Overuse injuries are also sports specific. Gymnasts typically injure their wrists, pitchers their shoulders, and field hockey players their forearms. These findings are not surprising given the sport specific adaptations that occur. These have been described in detail by Kibler et al[34]: decreased flexibility of the legs in athletes who participate in sports that primarily exercise the lower body and increased external rotation but decreased internal rotation of the dominant shoulder compared with a nondominant shoulder in athletes in sports that primarily exercise the upper body.[34]

Patellofemoral Pain Syndrome
Terminology

Patellofemoral pain syndrome (PFPS) is one of the most common problems encountered in sports medicine. In the healthy adolescent, PFPS refers to pain that is presumed to originate from the patellofemoral articulation without gross anatomic changes in the articular cartilage or bone of the patella or femur. The causes of PFPS in an adolescent differ from those of degenerative arthritis in the adult knee. There is ongoing debate regarding the cause of PFPS, and it has been called by many names,[35] which usually describe clinical variants, eg, patellagia, patellofemoral compression syndrome, chondromalacia patellae, and patellar malalignment syndrome.[36] The growing body of literature seems to have adopted PFPS in an attempt to cover all of the possible causes and clinical variants.[36]

Clinical Presentation

Patellofemoral pain syndrome commonly occurs between the ages of 12 and 35 years, with insidious onset of retropatellar or peripatellar knee pain for months to years. The pain is commonly characterized as a dull ache with an occasional sharp component that is brought on by activities such as running, jumping, or ascending or descending stairs. The pain is generally relieved by rest and application of ice. Prolonged sitting may also cause worsening of pain (positive theatre sign), which can be relieved by straightening the knee. Physical findings suggestive of PFPS include increased Q angle, genu recurvatum, femoral anteversion, patella alta, tight hamstring muscles, poorly developed vastus medialis obliquus, painful resisted knee ex-

tension, tenderness of the medial or lateral patellar facets, and a positive Clarke sign. The Clarke sign is positive if pain is elicited when the examiner presses the patella against the femur during quadriceps contraction in full knee extension.[35-37] A clinical variant of PFPS is miserable malalignment syndrome, with excessive internal rotation of the femur and secondary external tibial rotation with pronation of the foot.[37]

To date there are no generally accepted criteria for diagnosing PFPS; therefore most clinicians use a combination of signs and symptoms detailed above and in Table 14–1. Other painful conditions are excluded, eg, osteoarthritis, quadriceps rupture, patellar tendonitis, Sinding-Larson-Johanson syndrome, osteochondral fractures, and reflex sympathetic dystrophy, to name a few.

Radiologic Evaluation

Practically speaking, x-ray studies are not much help in the diagnosis of PFPS. Merchant et al[38] described an axial view with the knee flexed 45 degrees over the end of the table. From these views, he was able to measure a congruence angle with a normal angle of 16 degrees. Hughston[39] described a sunrise view: with the patient prone and the knee flexed 55 degrees, the intercondylar notch should have an angle of 125 degrees. Unfortunately, occult changes in

---

TABLE 14–1. Diagnosis of Patellofemoral Pain Syndrome

Since there are no generally accepted diagnostic criteria for patellofemoral pain syndrome (PFPs), 10 regional clinical experts were questioned to establish regional consensus. They included rheumatologists, physiatrists, orthopedic surgeons, and physiotherapists, all of whom had an interest in PFPS. These experts believed that PFPS is a significant component of their practices. To diagnose PFPS, the following consensus was reached:

1. The history should include the insidious onset of anterior knee pain and four of the following:
   a. Retropatellar or peripatellar pain
   b. Pain exacerbated by jumping or ascending or descending stairs
   c. Positive theater sign
   d. History of crepitus
2. The physical examination should reveal a poorly developed vastus medialis obliquus and two of the following:
   a. Increased Q angle (>20 degrees)
   b. Excessive genu recurvatum (>10 degrees of hyperextension)
   c. Patella alta
   d. Femoral anteversion
   e. External tibial torsion
   f. Hamstring muscle contracture
   g. Positive Clarke sign
   h. Tenderness of the medial or lateral patellar facet

position and variation of quadriceps tone have rendered these techniques unreliable.

Insall and Salvati[40] compared the length of the patella and the ligamentum patellae on lateral roentgenographs of normal knees. Measurements were approximately equal, and normal variation did not exceed 20%. They suggested that the diagnosis of patella alta could be made with a ratio of less than 1:1. Lancourt and Cristini[41] used the Insall-Salvati criteria to evaluate patellofemoral disorders. They found an index of 0.8 in patients with patellar dislocation, 0.86 in patients with chondromalacia of the patella, and 1.2 in those with apophysitis of the tibial tubercle. They noted that patellar length to patellar ligament was 1.0 in normal patients.

Based on these studies, it can be concluded that these x-ray changes are not specific for PFPS. X-ray studies are usually used to verify a clinical suspicion of osteoarthritis or osteochondral fractures. Therefore, in the proposed study, x-ray studies will be used only to rule out clinically suspected conditions. These are infrequent in the study sample of healthy, skeletally mature adolescents.

Management

Most authors agree that conservative treatment helps the patient with PFPS.[37] As early as 1937, Fairbanks[42] advised against early operation in young patients with knee problems, because of the low incidence of pathologic conditions. Common opinion has not changed since then. Steadman[43] described his nonoperative treatment and strongly suggested it be tried before operation. DeHaven et al,[44,45] in their conservative exercise program, found that only 8 of 75 patients subsequently required operative intervention. Review of the various components of conservative management follows. The numerous surgical treatments are not reviewed here.

To determine whether an intervention is effective, the natural history of the disorder must be known. The true effects of the intervention will only be known if they can be separated from the natural history. To date there is only one study of the natural history of PFPS. Sandow and Goodfellow[46] followed a cohort of 65 female patients aged 10 to 20 years (average age 15.5 years) with anterior knee pain. Fifty-four patients returned their questionnaires after 4 years and 4 months (range, 2–8 years). Results indicate that nearly all the patients (94.4%) continued to experience some pain, but that its severity had diminished in many (46.3%) and worsened in only a few (13%). The frequency of pain was not high. Most (81.5%) reported that they felt pain about once a week or even less frequently; 87% of the patients reported using analgesics never or only rarely. Knee pain severely restricted sports activities in 16.7%, but 48.1% of patients, though still complaining of some pain, participated in sports. Approximately half the patients had bilateral knee pain; in the others there was no predominance of left (29.6%) or right (22.3%) knee pain. Some patients who had improvement on one side subsequently developed pain on the other side. Sandow and Goodfellow concluded that the disorder tended to improve with time and was a serious source of continuing disability and handicap in very few. They also concluded that clinical examination and standard radiographs are adequate to exclude serious pathologic disorders in young female patients with anterior knee pain syndrome (PFPS). They believed that arthrography, arthroscopy, and computed tomography were usually not necessary.

Medication

There are no clinical studies available that examine the analgesic or anti-inflammatory effects of medications used in patellofemoral disorders. Most of the literature has examined the effects of nonsteroidal anti-inflammatory medications (NSAIDs) on the progression of chondromalacia. Although important, this is not relevant for a review of PFPS. To date there is only one study that examines pain relief in the knee joint. Bradley et al[47] compared an anti-inflammatory dose of ibuprofen, an analgesic dose of ibuprofen, and acetaminophen in the treatment of chronic osteoarthritic knee pain in 184 patients (mean age, 56 years). They concluded after 4 weeks of treatment that there was no clinically or statistically significant difference between acetaminophen and ibuprofen, whether the latter was administered in analgesic or anti-inflammatory dosages.

Therefore, one may conclude that in the short term, ibuprofen does not offer any advantages over acetaminophen for the treatment of knee pain due to osteoarthritis. Analgesic medications and NSAIDs probably have a role in the management of PFPS, but clear evidence is lacking at this time. All medications have side effects that must be carefully considered before prescribing them. These medications must be considered in the present study because they are important confounders.

Physical Therapy

Accepted components of most comprehensive treatment programs include decreasing exacerbating activities, analgesic methods such as ice or ultrasound, stretching and strengthening of the quadriceps and especially the vastus medialis obliquus and hamstring muscles, orthotics if required, and ice after workouts and at other times during the day when symptoms are present. The literature contains many different physical therapy programs, but unfortunately no clinical trials exist that examine the effectiveness of physical therapy for pain reduction in PFPS.

Using a cohort study design, DeHaven et al[45] investigated the effects of physical therapy on chondromalacia patellae in 100 university athletes. Symptomatic control was achieved with salicylates (600 mg four times daily for 4 weeks) and elimination of exacerbating activity. The reader was not told how patients who developed side effects to salicylates were treated. A progressive resistance and graduated running program was initiated when symptoms were controlled at rest and while lifting 30 pounds with the quadriceps. The maintenance program consisted of unrestricted activity, a progressive resistance exercise program two to three times per week, and adjunctive measures such as knee pads, patellar braces, and shoe orthotics. The duration of each phase was not clearly outlined. In all physical therapy programs, measurement of patient compliance is critical when determining effectiveness; this was not discussed by the authors.

All patients participated in this program; there was no control group. Follow-up was after 11.5 months (range, 6–22 months) by history and physical examination in 75 of 100 athletes; no explanation was provided for nonparticipants. Fifty athletes (66%) resumed unrestricted activities, and 17 (23%) returned to restricted activities. The authors considered these two groups as successful results of their conservative treatment program, yielding a total success rate of 82%. They explained that the patients who

could resume only restricted activities without disability during or afterward were pleased to be participating at all and were willing to accept some limitations rather than consider surgical treatment in the hope of regaining unrestricted activity.

DeHaven et al[45] reported that eight patients (11%) were unable to resume any athletic activities, and these patients were referred for surgical treatment, the results of which were not provided. The reader was not told why the athletes could not resume activities, but presumably this was secondary to pain. Also, we were not told about the full extent of these athletes' disabilities or handicaps. The study sample was not homogeneous, since postoperative knee patients were included with patients with "idiopathic" PFPS. The study design did not include a control group, and expectation and observer biases were not taken into account. The primary outcome measure was return to sport, and pain or activities of daily living were not measured. These design flaws make it difficult to accept the results.

Grana and Yates[48] studied 67 knees in a cohort of 49 patients with a mean age of 21 years (range, 11–48 years) for an average of 14.9 months (range, 8–19 months). The diagnosis of PFPS was not outlined; 76% were female, and 37% had bilateral symptoms. Associated trauma was reported in 33% of patients. All patients were placed on a program of NSAIDs (type and dosage not specified) and activity restriction. The exercise component consisted of stretching and isometric or isotonic quadriceps strengthening and normalizing the quadriceps-hamstring muscle ratio.[49] Follow-up was accomplished via telephone questionnaire, and examination was not repeated; 57% of patients reported subjective improvement, 25% were unchanged, and 18% were worse. Function in 54% was considered satisfactory, and in 45% was unsatisfactory.

Grana and Yates[48] did not define the sample precisely; there was no control group. Follow-up was by telephone questionnaire, and patients were not reexamined. Observer and expectation bias were not considered. The experimental methods were not defined sufficiently. The type of nonsteroidal medication that each patient received was not specified. Pain, an essential feature of PFPS, was not assessed. Also, there was a high noncompliance rate, with no explanation offered. Could the noncompliance have been due to side effects from the NSAIDs? Did physical therapy worsen the symptoms? For all of these reasons, the study results are difficult to interpret.

Henry and Crosland[50] studied recurrent patellar subluxation in 145 patients for an average of 3.1 years (range, 2–5 years). There were approximately equal numbers of male and female patients. The mean age of patients was 23 years. The conservative program consisted of a patellar stabilizing brace and isometric quadriceps strengthening exercises three times a day for 6 weeks. Results of this program were classified as successful if patients participated in all activities without symptoms or with some symptoms. The rest of the patients were classified as unsuccessful; 76% of patients thought exercises "helped." Expectation bias was not controlled for. The rehabilitation program was not comprehensive, since it did not include patient education, activity restriction, NSAIDs, selective vastus medialis obliquus strengthening, or progressive activation. For these reasons, the results are difficult to accept.

Strengthening the vastus medialis obliquus has been an important part of physical therapy. Two studies examined this issue. In 1986, Moller et al[50a,b] examined the role of the vastus medialis obliquus and lateralis in the alignment of the patella during maximal isometric quadriceps contraction in 28 patients by electromyography (EMG). Patients were divided into three groups on the basis of history, physical examination, and arthroscopic findings. Group A consisted of 28 unaffected knees that served as controls; group B included 11 knees with patellar subluxation; and group C consisted of 17 knees with idiopathic chondromalacia patellae. The muscular activity pattern was the same in groups B and C and was reduced compared with the control group. There was no difference between the activity of the vastus medialis obliquus and lateralis muscles, and it was therefore inferred that there was no muscle imbalance.

Sousa and Gross[51] compared the integrated EMG activity ratio of vastus medialis obliquus and lateralis muscles between healthy subjects and patients with PFPS. They divided their patients into three groups: group 1 consisted of seven patients with no previous knee pathology serving as the control group; group 2 included nine patients with unilateral PFPS; and group 3 consisted of the same nine patients, but the unaffected knee was tested. EMG activity ratio of the vastus medialis obliquus and lateralis muscles were recorded with the patients ascending and descending stairs, with submaximal and maximal isometric contraction. EMG activity in the control group was significantly greater than in the other two groups. Patients with PFPS had abnormal activation patterns.

There are many sources of error in these studies, eg, surface electrode placement and gain setting on the EMG machine. Both studies contained small samples, and the diagnosis of PFPS was not defined. Taken together, the results of these studies should be viewed with caution. Most authors believe that selective vastus medialis obliquus strengthening makes sense in PFPS, but the literature does not contain enough evidence to support or contradict this view.

The literature indicates that considerable controversy exists regarding physical therapy in the treatment of PFPS.

Overuse Injuries of Bone

Overuse injuries of bone are caused by repetitive compressive forces. Gymnasts develop a stress reaction of the distal radial growth plate that causes permanent growth disturbance and deformity of the distal radius.[52–55] Similar injuries have been described that affect the distal radius and ulna in break-dancers.[56] The usual treatment includes relative rest, ie, allowing only those activities that do not cause pain or swelling at the site of the injury and the use of a wrist brace that prevents full dorsiflexion. If overuse injuries of bone are diagnosed in the early phase of epiphyseolysis, full recovery generally occurs.

Unusual Stress Fractures

Athletes who have sustained unusual or multiple stress fractures should be questioned regarding their nutritional practices, and female athletes should be questioned about their menstrual status. The female athlete triad of disordered eating, amenorrhea, and osteoporosis should be considered and ruled out, since it increases the susceptibility to fractures.[31]

Unusual stress fractures have been reported in young athletes, which include scaphoid waste fracture in weight lifters,[57] first rib fracture in gymnasts,[58] and second metacarpal fracture in tennis players.[59] Strong muscles in a limb provide protection from stress fractures to adjacent bones by reducing joint reaction forces and by sharing load with the adjacent bones. Therefore, a strength training exercise program should be considered an important part of any training program. However, stress fractures may occur in children if there are marked changes in training patterns. Less strength training may help prevent overuse injuries.[16]

SPECIAL DIAGNOSTIC CONSIDERATIONS

The skeletally immature athlete may present with a symptom whose cause may be completely different from the diagnostic possibilities usually considered in a skeletally mature athlete. For example, knee pain may not reflect local injury at all but an injury to the hip, eg, anterior dislocation or slipped capitofemoral epiphysis. These alternative diagnoses should be taken into account during an on-field examination.

Strong consideration should be given to obtaining plain radiographs before performing stress maneuvers to prevent possible displacement of a nondisplaced fracture. For example, in a skeletally immature athlete with an obvious knee injury, valgus stress applied to test for possible medial collateral ligament injury may displace a distal femoral physeal fracture; similarly, access motion with the Lachman test could be related to a torn anterior cruciate ligament from evulsion of the ligament and its osteochondral insertion from the remainder of the tibia.

ETIOLOGIC FACTORS

Training Error

Children may be more likely than adults to make training errors because they often have less patience to follow a plan of gradually increasing intensity, speed, distance, and complexity of activity. Training errors often occur when an injured athlete returns to an activity at his or her former level of competition or complexity. Prevention of recurrent injury therefore requires careful counselling and monitoring of the athlete.

Equipment

Sports equipment is expensive, and few families can afford appropriate equipment for their rapidly growing children. Most expensive equipment, such as helmets, skates, and ski boots, usually is purchased used. Footwear is often suboptimal, chosen by the child or adolescent to be fashionable, but this type of footwear is usually poorly cushioned and nonsupportive. Also, few families can afford to buy appropriate footwear for different sports. Court sports, distance running, and aerobic dance require different types of footwear. Most young athletes participate in a variety of sports for many hours per week with one pair of sneakers not specific for any of the sports engaged in.

Changes in Coordination

Temporary changes in coordination during growth spurts and weight gain compound other problems already present, such as inflexibility. Coordination changes are particularly apparent in sports that involve extreme body awareness, such as gymnastics, ballet, figure skating, and diving.

Team Matching

In most organized sports, children are matched simply by age. Matching by height, weight, or Tanner sexual maturity stage is likely to be more appropriate for most contact and collision sports, because of differences in rates of growth, maturation, and emotional development.[60] The best method for appropriate matching has not been defined as yet.

Coaches

Coaches in many organized sports are either volunteers or school coaches who have had little education in the principles of appropriate training methods, equipment maintenance, safety rules, and child and adolescent psychology. The coach is important to the practicing and competition exposure that young athletes experience. Education is critical for prevention of injury in the skeletally immature athlete.

CHRONIC DISEASE IN THE YOUNG ATHLETE

The purpose of this section is to discuss four common chronic diseases of childhood—asthma, diabetes, anemia, and obesity—and to point out how these diseases can be managed for optimal athletic performance (Table 14–2). Discussion of definition, clinical signs and symptoms, and standard medical management is beyond the scope of this chapter and therefore is not discussed. It is assumed that the reader has a good working knowledge of each of these conditions.

Asthma

Athletes with appropriately managed and controlled asthma are able to participate at elite levels. In the 1984 Summer Olympics, 10% of

TABLE 14–2. Specific Training-Related Benefits Reported in the Child With a Chronic Disease

DISEASE	POSSIBLE BENEFITS
Asthma	Reduced intensity and frequency of exercise; reduced bronchoconstriction
Cerebral palsy	Prevention of contractures in the hands; reduction in spasticity with ambulation
Coronary risk	Improved lipoprotein profile; reduced adiposity and blood pressure
Cystic fibrosis	High respiratory muscle endurance; enhanced clearance of bronchial mucus
Diabetes mellitus	Better diabetic control
Hypertension	Reduction of blood pressure at rest
Myopathies	Strengthening of residual muscle; prolongation of ambulation status; prevention of contractures; weight control
Obesity	Weight and adiposity controlled; improved lipoprotein profile; enhanced socialization and self-esteem

athletes had exercise-induced asthma, yet more than half of these athletes with asthma were unaware of their diagnosis.[61,62] Success in sport depends on continuous appropriate management of asthma. It is important to involve young athletes and their parents, since appropriate knowledge of pharmacologic treatment is necessary. The young athlete with asthma should also be aware of stimuli that trigger an asthma attack, eg, upper respiratory infection, cold weather, allergies (ragweed, dust, pollen), emotional stress, and environmental pollution.

Training may benefit the patient with asthma. Studies in swimmers with asthma revealed that swimming training can improve fitness.[63–65] Exercise can also lessen the severity of asthma symptoms, as evidenced by decreased number of emergency room visits, frequency of attacks, rate of hospitalization, and school absenteeism.[66]

Training Recommendations

Short (4–10 minutes), intense bouts of exercise before any athletic event are generally recommended. Athletes with asthma should perform appropriate warm-up. Exercise in cold, dry air, as well as air with various environmental pollutants, may provoke exercise-induced asthma and should be avoided. However, when an athlete with asthma must compete in these conditions, a scarf should be worn around the face and mouth to humidify and filter inspired air.[67,68]

Patients with asthma often have difficulty in predicting their pulmonary function status and therefore should record a log of peak flow measurement, usually twice daily.[69]

In summary, for the athlete with asthma, simple precautions are best:

1. Wear scarf around face and mouth to humidify and warm inspired air.
2. Avoid competition if very cold weather is expected.
3. Keep twice-daily log of peak flow measurements.
4. Perform appropriate warm-up exercises.

Diabetes

Management of diabetes is challenging. One must deal with a complex set of relationships, eg, physician-child, physician-parent, parent-child, physician-parent-child. If diabetes is well controlled metabolically and the child is well motivated, there are usually no restrictions on physical activity, and the child can expect to compete on equal grounds with nondiabetic athletes.[70–74]

Benefits of Exercise

Exercise has proven benefits for patients with diabetes, since it affects glucose metabolism and insulin action. Insulin sensitivity is increased up to a full day after intense exercise (70%–80% of $\dot{V}O_2$ max) and several hours after moderate exercise.

Benefits of Exercise

Prolonged exercise lasting more than 60 minutes may enhance insulin sensitivity for up to 24 hours after completion of exercise.[71,72] Improved glucose transport has also been shown after physical exercise.[73] The effects of exercise on glycemic control in children and adolescents have failed to conclusively show a benefit. Studies have shown positive and negative results.[74,75]

Studies have failed to consistently show whether diabetics who partake in regular physical activity are more physically fit. Insulin works more effectively on glucose uptake when $\dot{V}O_2$ max is higher.[76] Several studies have indicated that the work capacity of diabetic adolescents did not differ from that in their healthy counterparts.[77,78] Huttunen et al[79] studied physical fitness in children and adolescents with insulin-dependent diabetes mellitus (IDDM) and found that the physical work capacity of diabetic boys was lower than that of nondiabetic boys; there was no difference between girls. It was suggested that good physical fitness in boys is associated with better metabolic control[79] (Table 14–3).

There are risks of exercise as well. Hypoglycemia resulting from hyperinsulinemia can occur if a diabetic does not reduce insulin dose before exercise. Serum glucose concentration will decrease because exercising muscle increases glucose use, and the extra insulin blocks glucose release by the liver and fatty acid from adipose tissue. Hyperglycemia occurs if a patient with poor metabolic control is deprived of insulin. With insufficient insulin levels, hepatic glucose production exceeds peripheral glucose and ketogenesis results because of increased release of lipolytic horomones.[68] Diabetic complications such as neuropathy, retinopathy, and nephropa-

TABLE 14–3. Positive Effects of Exercise on Diabetes

PROVED BENEFICIAL EFFECTS	POSSIBLE BENEFICIAL EFFECTS
Increased insulin sensitivity	Decreased fasting glucose level
Improved glucose transport	Decreased hemoglobin A1c
Decreased heart rate and blood pressure at rest	Improved lipid profile
Maintenance of lean body mass with weight reduction	Reduced coronary risk
Improved self-esteem and self-confidence	

From Bar-Or O: The young athlete with chronic disease. Clin Sports Med 14:709–726, 1995.

thy are infrequently seen in children but should be considered. Severe elevation of blood pressure has been known to theoretically increase the risk of retinal hemorrhage or renal infarction and therefore should be avoided.[80]

Recommended Sports

Young athletes with well-controlled IDDM theoretically can participate and compete on equal grounds with nondiabetic athletes. Recommended sports include those where there is constant and known energy expenditure per time, such as running, cycling, or swimming. Sports that incorporate short, high-intensity energy spurts where the energy expenditure is usually unknown, such as hockey, baseball, and football, pose a more difficult management problem. Other less recommended activities include those in which glucose monitoring and carbohydrate administration can become difficult, such as scuba diving, hang gliding, wind surfing, mountaineering, auto racing, or motor cycle racing.

Anemia

Anemia has numerous causes; however, iron deficiency is the leading cause of anemia in childhood and adolescence.[81] Athletes may have iron deficiency, but studies have failed to show whether athletes have a higher prevalence of anemia.[81] Sports anemia is a misleading term that usually describes delusional anemia. When tested, athletes often demonstrate below normal hemoglobin levels and normal iron and ferritin levels. This is usually explained by an expanded plasma volume secondary to regular aerobic exercise.[82,83] Athletes have a higher hemoglobin level per kilogram of body weight when corrected for blood volume.[84] Iron deficiency is more prevalent in athletes who participate in endurance sports, ie, distance running, swimming, cycling, cross-country skiing, than other sporting activities. Proposed causes include repeated heel strike, stool loss, sweat loss, gastrointestinal hemorrhage, and hematuria.[85]

Exercise performance can be reduced in the athlete with iron deficiency. $\dot{V}O_2$ max declines with decreases in hemoglobin concentration.[86,87] Iron supplementation improves exercise performance in the iron deficient athlete but not in the nonanemic athlete.[88–91] Endurance athletes have resorted to blood doping (ie, transfusion) to improve performance. This is controversial, however. Two studies show that blood doping can increase $\dot{V}O_2$ max,[88,92] and two others demonstrate that it decreases race time.[93,94] Recombinent human erythropoietin (rEPO) has also been used by endurance athletes to enhance performance.[95]

To obtain sufficient iron, the athlete should eat a well-balanced diet. Recommended high-iron content foods for young athletes include red meat, turkey, chicken, liver, lima beans, shellfish, and green vegetables. Red meat should be eaten twice weekly. Vitamin C also increases iron absorption; a glass of orange juice with a meal is a simple way to aid iron absorption. Coffee and tea should be discouraged, since they promote iron loss in documented deficiency. Oral elemental iron therapy should be given at a dose of 6 mg/kg/d. Iron supplementation (serum ferritin <12 μg/L) should also be provided for the nonanemic iron-deficient athlete to prevent anemia.[96,97]

Obesity

Obesity has been described as the most prevalent chronic pediatric disease.[98] The following changes have been described in children and adolescents when exercise was administered alone or in conjunction with dietary changes and behavioral modification: decrease in body weight,[99,100] increase in bone density, decrease in percent body fat,[101] and a reduction in resting blood pressure.[99,102] Psychosocial effects have also been described: an increase in the child's self–body image, self-esteem, and ability to adjust to peers.[103,104]

Only in the past decade has pediatric exercise science been strengthened by a fresh look at physical and psychological benefits and harm of exercise, training, and sports in children with chronic diseases. In a classic 1990 review article, my colleague Oded Bar-Or[98] analyzed the situation for childhood asthma, cerebral palsy, coronary risk, cystic fibrosis, diabetes mellitus, hypertension, myopathies, and obesity. Sadly he concluded that "Most of the published intervention studies are deficient on design by not including randomly assigned (or matched) controls."[98] He pointed out other constraints: the need to maintain other treatments, the progression of some disease, and the small pool of suitable subjects.

The problem of inadequate populations does not apply to childhood obesity. Unhappily, that disability has many subjects needing attention that fits the rehabilitation mode. With his associates and students, Bar-Or has focused on physical activity, adiposity, and obesity in adolescents.

Bar-Or[68,98] reported a review of the evidence that the level of physical activity or total energy expenditure affects adiposity in obese and nonobese adolescents. Many interventional studies have shown that a small (1%–3% body fat) reduction in adiposity results from physical training in the general adolescent population. Lifestyle activities (eg, walking to and from school) appear to have a more lasting effect than regimented activities (eg, calisthenics or jogging).

For obese adolescents, Bar-Or[68,98] recognizes that the low level of motivation in obese adolescents to adhere to a training program is a negative factor that must be addressed and overcome. Modification of eating patterns is recommended, as is behavior modification for both the parents and the child or adolescent (in separate groups). Epstein et al[100] reported the superiority of modified lifestyle over regimented activities.

THE FEMALE ATHLETE TRIAD

Disordered Eating

The young female athlete who is driven to excel in her sport or pressured to have a thin physique may attempt to lose weight or body fat by developing patterns of disordered eating. This may lead to menstrual dysfunction and subsequent premature osteoporosis. These three conditions, that is, disordered eating, amenorrhea, and osteoporosis form what has been termed *the female athlete triad*.[105] There is a spectrum of disordered eating behaviors that range from mild (restricting food intake only slightly or binging and purging only occasionally) to severe (restricting food intake significantly, as in anorexia nervosa, or binging and purging on a regular basis, as in bulimia nervosa).[106] Disordered eating behavior has been observed in young female athletes, and one study of 487 female elite swimmers aged 9 to 18 years revealed that 60.5% of average weight and 17.9% of underweight girls were trying to lose weight, 62% were skipping meals, and 77% were eating smaller meals to lose weight, 12.7% were vomiting, 2.5% were using laxatives, and 1.5% were using diuretics.[107]

Disordered eating is seen in athletes participating in all sports. However, some sports place athletes at higher risk for development of these abnormal behaviors. These sports are those in which subjective judging encourages lean appearance, such as gymnastics, diving, figure skating, dance, and synchronized swimming; sports that emphasize body leanness for optimal performance, such as long-distance running, swimming, and crosscountry skiing; and sports that use weight classifications, such as rowing, body building, and martial arts.[108] Disordered eating may impair athletic performance and increase risk for injury. Decreased caloric intake and fluid and electrolyte imbalance can result in decreased endurance strength reaction time, speed, and ability to concentrate. The body initially adapts to these changes, and a decrease in performance may not be seen for some time, leading athletes to falsely believe that disordered eating practices are harmless.[109]

Disordered eating can also have psychological and medical complications, including depression, fluid and electrolyte imbalance, and changes in the cardiovascular, endocrine, gastrointestinal, and thermal regulatory systems. Some of these complications are potentially fatal, and in nonathletes treated for eating disorders, the death rate has been reported as high as 18%.[110,111] Limited space available in this chapter does not allow full discussion of these changes.

Amenorrhea

Amenorrhea is classified as primary or secondary. Primary amenorrhea, or delayed menarche, is present when the subject has not begun menses by age 16 years. Secondary amenorrhea is defined as the absence of at least three to six consecutive menstrual cycles in a woman who has been menstruating. The prevalence of amenorrhea has been difficult to determine, in part because of the variability in definition. It has been reported to be between 3.4% and 66% in some segments of the athletic population, compared with 2% to 5% in the general population.[112,113] The prevalence of primary and secondary amenorrhea in the young athlete is unknown. Frisch et al[114] found that athletes who began training prior to menarche experienced delayed onset of menses and had increased incidence of amenorrhea when compared with girls who began training after menarche. She noted that each year of training prior to menarche delayed menarche by 5 months.[114] There is growing evidence to suggest that exercise-associated amenorrhea may be the result of an energy drain. Women who fail to meet their energy needs because of inadequate caloric intake and who develop low T3 (triiodothyronine) levels and stress with resulting hypercortisolism may also be associated with impairment of the hypothalamic-pituitary axis.[115,116]

Osteoporosis

Osteoporosis in the young female athlete refers to inadequate bone formation and premature bone loss, resulting in low bone mass and increased risk of fracture. Premature osteoporosis may be a result of amenorrhea and oligomenorrhea, and may be partially irreversible despite resumption of menses, estrogen replacement therapy, or calcium supplementation.[117–119] Osteoporosis can develop in the appendicular as well as the axial skeleton and increases the incidence of stress fracture.[120,121] Genetic predisposition has also been found to be a strong predictor of peak bone density.[122]

Bone Mineral Density

Bone mineral density (BMD) increases throughout adolescence; however, the amenorrheic teenager remains osteopenic in comparison with regularly menstruating controls.[123–127] Amenorrheic adolescents, both athletes and nonathletes, have been found to have lower bone mineral density than their eumenorrheic counterparts. This may be due to decreased bone accretion as well as increased bone loss.[124] Girls who have lower weight during adolescence and higher age at menarche have lower BMD when compared with their peers. Weight gain and return of menses results in increased BMD.[124,128] There is new evidence to suggest that not all groups of competitive athletes with menstrual irregularities may be at risk of osteoporosis. Slemenda et al[129] reported that high-intensity exercise over many years may increase BMD in specific skeletal sites despite amenorrhea. They report elite adolescent ice skaters have significantly higher BMD in the lower skeleton than controls do, despite menstrual dysfunction.[129] Similar findings have been reported in runners.[130]

Screening for Female Athlete Triad

The female athlete who presents to the physician with a stress fracture or menstrual irregularities should be screened. Signs of disordered eating (Table 14–4) may be recognized by parents, coaches, trainers, teammates, or school nurses and brought to the physician's attention.

TABLE 14–4. Signs of Disordered Eating

1. Repeatedly expressing concerns about being or feeling fat, even when weight is average or below average
2. Preoccupation with food, calories, and weight
3. Increasing criticism of one's body
4. Secretly eating or stealing food
5. Eating large meals, then disappearing or making trips to the bathroom
6. Excess laxative use; laxative packages in athlete's locker
7. Periods of severe caloric restriction or repeated days of fasting
8. Relentless excessive physical activity that is not part of the training regimen
9. Avoiding situations in which the athlete may be observed while eating
10. Wearing baggy or layered clothing

Disordered eating is often best treated with a multidisciplinary team approach. The physician monitors medical status and athletic participation; the nutritionist provides appropriate nutritional guidance; and the mental health professional addresses the psychological issues. Increasing caloric intake is the preferred method of treatment. Other causes of amenorrhea should be ruled out. It is helpful to monitor BMD with dual-energy x-ray absorptiometry. The need for calcium and hormone therapy can be evaluated on the basis of the results of BMD testing. Oral contraceptives are often acceptable to athletes in the adolescent age group, as many have friends who use them for menstrual dysfunction.[108,131,132]

Education about the female athlete triad is the key to prevention. Athletes, coaches, training staff, and physicians, as well as parents, need to be educated about the risks and warning signs of disordered eating, menstrual dysfunction, and bone loss. Educational material is available from the American College of Sports Medicine.

Children of all ages are subject to many of the same problems as adults are. Physical factors such as fatigue, pain, inflammation, and tissue disruption may or may not be similar in adults and children. No clear research has confirmed or denied this important puzzle.

REFERENCES

1. Chambers RB: Orthopedic injuries in athletes (ages 6 to 17). Am J Sports Med 7:195, 1979
2. Izant RJ, Hubay CA: The annual injury of fifteen million children: a limited study of childhood accidental injury and death. J Trauma 6:56, 1966
3. Lenaway DD, Ambler AG, Beaudry BE: The epidemiology of school-related injuries: new perspectives. Am J Prev Med 8:193, 1992
4. American College of Sports Medicine: Current Comment: Prevention of sports injuries of children and adolescents. Med Sci Sports Exerc 25(8 suppl):1, 1993
5. Smith AD: Sports Medicine Musculoskeletal Considerations for Children and Adolescents. In Nicholas JA, Hershman EB (eds): The Lower Extremity and Spine in Sports, 2nd Ed. Mosby, St. Louis, 1995
6. Bright RW, Burstein AH, Elmore SM: Apophyseal-plate cartilage: a biomechanical and histological analysis of failure modes. J Bone Joint Surg 56A:688, 1974

7. Bak K: Separation of the proximal tibial epiphysis in a gymnast. Acta Orthop Scand 62:293, 1991

8. Lepse PS, McArthur RE, McCullogh FL: Simultaneous bilateral evulsion fracture of the tibial tuberosity. Clin Orthop 229:232, 1988

9. Winkler AR, Barnes JC, Ogdan JA: Break-dance hip: chronic evulsion of the anterosuperior iliac spine. Pediatr Radiol 17:501, 1987

10. Bailey DA, Wedge JH, McCulloch RG, et al: Epidemiology of fractures of the distal end of the radius in children as associated with growth. J Bone Joint Surg Am 71A:1225, 1989

11. Mizuta T, Benson WM, Foster BK, et al: Statistical analysis of the incidence of physeal injuries. J Pediatr Orthop 7:518; 1987

12. Birch JG, Herring JA, Wenger DR: Surgical anatomy of selected physes. J Pediatr Orthop 4:224, 1984

13. Jowsey J: Age changes in human bone. Clin Orthop 17:210, 1960

14. Light TR, Ogden JA: The anatomy of physeal torus fractures. Clin Orthop 188:103, 1984

15. Ogden JA: The uniqueness of growing bones. In: Kin RE, Wilkins KE, Rockwood CA (eds): Fractures in Children, 3rd Ed. JB Lippincott, Philadelphia, 1991

16. Murabarnk SJ, Carroll MC: Familial osteochondritis dissecans of the knee. Clin Orthop 140:131, 1979

17. Murabarnk SJ, Carroll MC: Juvenile osteochondritis dissecans of the knee: etiology. Clin Orthop 157:200, 1981

18. Berndt AL, Harty M: Transchondral fractures (osteochrondritis dissecans of the talus). J Bone Joint Surg 41A:988, 1959

19. Bohlman HH: Acute fractures and dislocations of the cervical spine: an analysis of three hundred hospitalized patients and review of the literature. J Bone Joint Surg 61A:1119, 1979

20. Clark CA, Ogden JA: Development of the menisci of the human knee joint. J Bone Joint Surg 65B:1538, 1983

21. Abdon P, Mats B: Incidence of meniscal lesions in children: increase associated with diagnostic arthroscopy. Acta Orthop Scand 60:710, 1989

22. Steaniski CL, Harvell JC, Fu F: Observations on acute knee hemarthroses in children and adolescents. J Pediatr Orthop 13:506, 1993

23. Bailey DH, Wedge JH, McCulloch RG, et al: Epidemiology of fractures of the distal end of the radius in children as associated with growth. J Bone Joint Surg 71A:1225, 1989

24. Ekeland A, Holtmoen A, Lystad H: Lower extremity equipment-related injuries in Alpine recreational skiers. Am J Sports Med 21:201, 1993

25. Salter RB, Harris WR: Injuries involving the epiphyseal plate. J Bone Joint Surg 45A:587–622, 1963

25a. Salter RB: Textbook of Disorders and Injuries of the Musculoskeletal System, 3rd Ed. Williams & Wilkins, Baltimore, 1999, p. 505

26. Peterson HA, Burkhart SS: Compression injury of the physeal growth plate: fact or fiction? J Pediatr Orthop 1:377, 1981

27. Ogden JA: Skeletal growth mechanism injury patterns. J Pediatr Orthop 2:371, 1982

28. Bradley GW, Shives TC, Samuelson KM: Ligament injuries in the knees of children. J Bone Joint Surg 61A:588, 1979

29. Clanton TO, DeLee JC, Sanders B, Neidre A, et al: Knee ligament injuries in children. J Bone Joint Surg 61A:1195, 1979

30. Lysens RJ, Ostyn MS, Vanden Auweele Y, et al: The accident prone and overuse prone profiles of the young athlete. Am J Sports Med 17:612, 1989

31. Micheli LJ, Ireland ML: Prevention and management of calcaneal epiphysitis in children: an overuse syndrome. J Pediatr Orthop 7:34, 1987

32. Smith AD, Stroud L, McQueen C: Flexibility and anterior knee in adolescent elite figure skaters. J Pediatr Orthop 11:77, 1991

33. Orava S, Puranen J: Exertion injuries in adolescent athletes. Br J Sports Med 12:4, 1978

34. Kibler WB, Chandler TJ, Uhl T, Maddux RE: A musculoskeletal approach to the pre-participation physical examination: preventing injury and improving performance. Am J Sports Med 17:525, 1989

35. Shoen RP, Moskowitz RW, Goldberg VM: Soft Tissue Rheumatic Pain: Recognition, Management, Prevention, 2nd Ed. Lea & Febiger, Philadelphia, 1987, p. 225

36. Swenson EJ, Hough DO, McKeag DB: Patellofemoral dysfunction: how to treat, when to refer patients with problematic knees. Postgrad Med 82:125, 1987

37. Nicholas JA, Hershman EB (eds): The Lower Extremity and Spine in Sports Medicine, vol. 1. CV Mosby, St Louis, 1986, p. 1013

38. Merchant AC, Mercer RL, Jacobson RH, Cool CR: Roentgenographic analysis of patellofemoral congruence. J Bone Joint Surg 56A:1391, 1974

39. Hughston JC: Subluxation of the patella. J Bone Joint Surg 50A:1003, 1968

40. Insall J, Salvati E: Patella position in the normal knee joint. Diagn Radiol 101, 1971

41. Lancourt JE, Cristini JA: Patella alta and patella Infra. J Bone Joint Surg 57A:1112, 1975

42. Fairbanks HAT: Internal derangement of the knee in children and adolescents. Proc R Soc Med 30:427, 1937

43. Steadman JR: Nonoperative measures for patellofemoral problems. Am J Sports Med 7:374, 1979

44. DeHaven KE, Dolan WA, Mayer PJ: Chondromalacia patella in athletes: clinical presentation and conservation management. Am J Sports Med 7:5, 1979

45. DeHaven KE, Dolan WA, Mayer PJ: Chondromalacia patella and the painful knee. Am Fam Phys 21:117, 1980

46. Sandow MJ, Goodfellow JW: The natural history of anterior knee pain in adolescents. J Bone Joint Surg 67B:36, 1985

47. Bradley JD, Brandt KD, Katz BP, et al: Comparison of an anti-inflammatory dose of ibuprofen, and analgesic dose of ibuprofen, and acetaminophen in the treatment of patients with osteoarthritis of the knee. N Engl J Med 325:87, 1991

48. Grana WA, Yates C: Patellofemoral pain: a prospective study. Orthopedics 9:663, 1986

49. Kettlecamp B: Current concepts review: management of patellar malalignment. J Bone Joint Surg 63A:1344, 1981

50. Henry JH, Crosland JW: Conservative treatment of patellofemoral subluxation. Am J Sports Med 7:12, 1979

50a. Moller BN, Krebs B: Dynamic knee brace in the treatment of patellofemoral disorders. Arch Orthop Trauma Surg 104[6]:377–379, 1986

50b. Moller BN, Krebs B, Tidemand-Dal C, Aaris K: Isometric contractions in the patellofemoral pain syndrome. An electromyographic study. Arch Orthop Trauma Surg 105[1]:24–27, 1986

51. Sousa DR, Gross MT: Comparison of vastus medialis obliques: vastus lateralis muscle integrated electromyographic ratios between healthy subjects and patients with patellofemoral pain. Phys Ther 71:310, 1991

52. Caine D, Roy S, Singer KM, Broekhoff J: Stress changes of the distal radial growth plate: a radiographic survey and review of the literature. Am J Sports Med 20:290, 1992

53. Carter SR, Aldridge MJ, Fitzgerald R, Davies AM: Stress changes of the wrist in adolescent gymnasts. Br J Radiol 61:109, 1988

54. Mandelbaum BR, Bartolozzi AR, Davis CA, et al: Wrist pain syndrome in the gymnast: pathogenetic, diagnostic and therapeutic considerations. Am J Sports Med 17:305, 1989

55. Vender MI, Watson K: Acquired Madelung-like deformity in a gymnast. J Hand Surg 13:19, 1988

56. Gerber SD, Griffin PP, Simmons BP: Breakdancer's wrist: a case report. J Pediatr Orthop 6:98, 1986

57. Reider B, Yurkofsky J, Mass D: Scaphoid waist fracture in a weight lifter: a case report. Am J Sports Med 21:329, 1993

58. Troffer DS, Patton JJ, Jackson DW: Non-union of a first rib fracture in a gymnast. Am J Sports Med 19:198, 1991

59. Waninder KN, Lombardo JA: Stress fracture of index metacarpal in a tennis player. Med Sci Sports Exerc 25:S21, 1993

60. Shaffer TE: Schering symposium on sports medicine: the uniqueness of the young athlete: introductory remark. Am J Sports Med 8:370, 1980

61. Monahan T: Side-lined asthmatics get back in the game. Phys Sports Med 14:61, 1986

62. Voy RO: The US Olympic Committee experience with exercise-induced bronchospasm. Med Sci Sports Exerc 18:328, 1986

63. Fitch K, Morton AR, Blanksby BA: Effects of swimming training on children with asthma. Arch Dis Child 51:190, 1976

64. Schnall R, Ford P, Gillam I, et al: Swimming and dry land exercises in children with asthma. Aust Pediatr J 18:23, 1982

65. Szentagothai K, Gyene I, Szocska M, et al: Physical exercise program for children with bronchial asthma. Pediatr Pulmonol 3:166, 1987

66. Bundgaard A: Physical training in bronchial asthma. Scand J Sports Sci 10:97, 1989

67. American Academy of Pediatrics, Committee on Sports Medicine and Fitness: Assessing physical activity and fitness in the office setting. Pediatrics 93:686, 1994

68. Bar-Or O: The young athlete with chronic disease. Clin Sports Med. 14:709, 1995

69. Morton A, Fitch K: Asthmatic drugs and competitive sport. Sports Med 14:228, 1992

70. Dorchy H, Poortman SJ: Sport and the diabetic child. Sports Med 7:248, 1989

71. Rachterea T-L, Hespel P: Metabolic responses to exercise. Diabetes Care 15:1767, 1992

72. Sane T, Helve E, Pelkonen R, et al: The adjustment of diet and insulin dose during long term endurance exercise in type I (insulin dependent) diabetic men. Diabetologia 31:35, 1988

73. Goodyear LJ, Hirshman MF, Valyou PM, et al: Glucose transporter number, function and subcellular distribution in rat skeletal muscle after exercise training. Diabetes 41:1091, 1992

74. Campaigne BN, Gilliam TV, Spencer ML, et al: Effects of a physical activity program on metabolic control and cardiovascular fitness in children with insulin dependent diabetes mellitus. Diabetes Care 7:57, 1984

75. Larsson Y, Persson P, Sterky G, et al: Functional adaptation to rigorous training and exercise in diabetic and non-diabetic adolescents. J Appl Physiol 19:629, 1964

76. Arslanian S, Nixon PA, Becker D, et al: Impact of physical fitness and glycemic control on in

vivo insulin action in adolescents with IDDM. Diabetes Care 13:9, 1990

77. Hagan RD, Marks JF, Warren PA: Physiological responses of juvenile onset diabetic boys to muscular work. Diabetes 28:1114, 1979

78. Hebbelinck M, Loeb H, Meersseman H: Physical development and performance capacity in a group of diabetic adolescents. Acta Pediatr Belg 28:151, 1974

79. Huttenen NP, Haar ML, Kanip M, et al: Physical fitness of children and adolescents with insulin dependent diabetes mellitus. Ann Clin Res 16:1, 1984

80. Campaigne BN, Alapman RM: Exercise in the Clinical Management of Diabetes. Human Kinetics Publishers, Champaign, IL, 1994, pp. 39–46, 61–70

81. Dallman PR: Iron deficiency and relation to nutritional anemias. In: Nathan DG, Oski FA (eds): Hematology of Infants and Childhood, 3rd Ed. WB Saunders Co, Philadelphia, 1987, p. 288

82. Eichner ER: Sports anemia, iron supplements and blood doping. Med Sci Sports Exerc 24:315, 1992

83. Weight LM, Darge BL, Jacobs P: Athletes' pseudo anemia. Eur J Appl Physiol 62:358, 1991

84. Dill DB, Baraithwaite K, Adams WC, et al: Blood volume of middle distance runners: effect of 2300 m altitude comparison with non-athletes. Med Sci Sports 6:1, 1974

85. Lampe JW, Slavin JL, Apple FS: Iron status of active woman and the effect of running a marathon on bowel function and gastrointestinal blood loss. Int J Sports Med 12:173, 1991

86. Nickerson HJ, Tripp AD: Iron deficiency in adolescent cross country runners. Phys Sports Med 11:60, 1983

87. Woodson RD: Hemoglobin concentration and exercise capacity. Ann Rev Respir Dis 129:S72, 1984

88. Ekblom B, Goldbarg AN, Gullbring B: Response to exercise after blood loss and reinfusion. J Appl Physiol 33:175, 1972

89. Woodson RD, Will RE, Lenfant C: Effect of acute and established anemia on OT transport at rest, submaximal, and maximal work space. J Appl Physiol 44:36, 1978

90. Weswig PH, Winkler W: Iron supplementation and hematologic data of competitive swimmers. J Sports Med Phys Fit 14:112, 1974

91. Pate RR, Magurie M, Van Wyke J: Dietary iron supplementation in women athletes. Phys Sports Med 7:81, 1979

92. Buick FJ, Geldhill N, Froese AB, et al: Effect of enduced erythrocythemia on aerobic work capacity. J Appl Physiol 48:636, 1980

93. Brian AJ, Simon TL: The effect of red blood cell reinfusion on 10 k race time. JAMA 257:2761, 1987

94. Williams MH, Wesseldine S, Somma T, et al: The effect of induced erythrocythemia on 5 minute treadmill run time. Med Sci Sports Exerc 13:169, 1981

95. Eichner ER: Sports anemia, iron supplements, and blood doping. Med Sci Sports Exerc 24:315, 1992

96. Rowland TW: Iron deficiency in the young athlete. Pediatr Clin North Am 37:1152, 1990

97. Selby GS: When does an athlete need iron? Phys Sport Med 19:96, 1991

98. Bar-Or O: Disease specific benefits of training in the child with a chronic disease: what is the evidence? Pediatr Exerc Sci 2:299, 1990

99. Brownell KD, Kelman JH, Stunkard AJ: Treatment of obese children with and without their mothers: changes in weight and blood pressure. Pediatrics 71:515, 1983

100. Epstein LH, Wing RR, Koeske R, et al: A comparison of lifestyle change and programmed aerobic exercise on weight and fitness changes in obese children. Behav Ther 13:651, 1982

101. Moody DL, Wilmore JH, Jirandola RN, Royce JP: The effects of a jogging program on the body composition of normal and obese high school girls. Med Sci Sports 4:210, 1972

102. Rocchini AP, Katch V, Anderson J, et al: Blood pressure in obese adolescents: effects of weight loss. Pediatrics 82:16, 1988

103. Peckos PS, Spargo JA, Held FP: Program and results of a camp for obese adolescent girls. Postgrad Med 27:527, 1960

104. Stanley EJ, Jlaser HH, Elevin DG, et al: Overcoming obesity in adolescents: a description of a promising endeavor to improve management. Clin Pediatr 9:29, 1970

105. Yeager KK, Augustino R, Nattiv A, Drinkwater B: The female athlete triad: disordered eating, amenorrhea, osteoporosis. Med Sci Sports Exerc 25:775, 1993

106. Johnson MD: Disordered eating in active and athletic women. Clin Sports Med 13:355, 1994

107. Dummer GM, Rosen LW, Heusner WW, et al: Pathogenic weight control behaviours of young competitive swimmers. Phys Sports Med 15:75, 1987

108. Van de Loo DA, Johnson MD: The young female athlete. Clin Sports Med 14:687, 1995

109. Rosen LW, McKeag DB, Hough DO, et al: Pathogenic weight control behaviour in female athletes. Phys Sports Med 14:79, 1986

110. Johnson MD: Disordered eating in the active and athletic woman. Clin Sports Med 13:355, 1994

111. Ratnasuriya RH, Eisler I, Szmukler GI, et al: Anorexia nervosa: outcome and prognostic factors after 20 years. Br J Psychiatry 158:495, 1991

112. Loucks AB, Horvath SM: Athletic amenorrhea: a review. Med Sci Sports Exerc 17:56, 1985

113. Shangold M, Rebar RW, Wentz AC, et al: Evaluation and management of menstrual dysfunction in athletes. JAMA 263:1665, 1990

114. Frisch RE, Gotz-Welberg ENAV, McArthur JW, et al: Delayed menarche and amenorrhea of college athletes in relation to age of onset of training. JAMA 246:1559, 1981

115. Loucks AB, Mortola JF, Girton L, et al: Alterations in the hypothalamic pituitary, ovarian and hypothalamic pituitary, adrenal axes in athletic women. J Clin Endocrinol Metab 68:402, 1989

116. Loucks AB, Heath EN: Induction of low T_3 syndrome in exercising women occurs at a threshold of energy availability. Am J Physiol 266:R817, 1994

117. Cann CE, Martin MC, Genant HK, Jaffe RB: Decreased spinal mineral content in amenorrheic women. JAMA 251:626, 1984

118. Drinkwater BL, Bruemmer B, Chestnut CH III: Menstrual history as a determinant of current bone density in young athletes. JAMA 263:545, 1990

119. Drinkwater BL, Nilson K, Ott S, Chestnut CH III: Bone mineral density after resumption of menses in amenorrheic athletes. JAMA 256:380, 1986

120. Myburgh KH, Bachrach LK, Lewis B, et al: Low bone mineral density at axial and appendicular sites in amenorrheic athletes. Med Sci Sports Exerc 25:1197, 1993

121. Myburg KH, Hutchins J, Fataar AB, et al: Low bone density is an etiology factor for stress fractures in athletes. Ann Intern Med 113:754, 1990

122. Seeman E, Harper JL, Bauch LA: Reduced bone mass in daughters of women with osteoporosis. N Engl J Med 302:554–558, 1989

123. Bachrach LK, Guido D, Katzman D, et al: Decreased bone density in adolescent girls with anorexia nervosa. Pediatrics 86:440–447, 1990

124. Bachrach LK, Katzman DK, Litt IF, et al: Recovery from osteopenia in adolescent girls with anorexia nervosa. J Clin Endocrinol Metab 72:602–606, 1991

125. Dhuper S, Warren MP, Brooks-Gunn J, et al: Effects of hormonal status on bone density in adolescent girls. J Clin Endocrinol Metab 71:1083, 1990

126. Emans SJ, Grace E, Hoffer FA, et al: Estrogen deficiency in adolescents and young adults: impact on bone mineral content and effects of estrogen replacement therapy. Obstet Gynecol 76:585, 1990

127. White CM, Hergenoeder AC, Klish WJ: Bone mineral density in fifteen to twenty-one-year-old eumenorrheic and amenorrheic subjects. Am J Dis Child 146:31, 1992

128. Dhuper S, Warren MP, Brooks-Gunn J, et al: Effects of hormonal status on bone density in adolescent girls. J Clin Endocrinol Metab 71:1083, 1990

129. Slemenda CW, Johnston CC: High intensity activities in young women: site specific bone mass effects among female figure skaters. Bone Miner 20:125, 1993

130. Robinson T, Snow-Harter C, Gillis D, et al: Bone mineral density and menstrual cycle status in competitive female runners and gymnasts [abstract]. Med Sci Sports Exerc 25:S549, 1993

131. Emans SJ, Goldstein DP: Pediatric and adolescent gynecology. Little, Brown and Co, Boston, 1990

132. Marshall LA: Clinical evaluation of amenorrhea in active and athletic women. Clin Sports Med 13:371, 1994

NEUROMUSCULAR CONSIDERATIONS

15

Epilepsy in Sports Medicine

DEAN M. WINGERCHUK

At the beginning of spring the boy ought to be purged and his life ordered as follows: He should rise early, take a moderate walk to the gymnasium where he would meet his master of exercises, who would be charged with the details, but as a general principle the exercises would be calculated to warm up the body in order to expel excess material and should aim at strengthening the head and the cardia. (Galen: excerpt from a letter to the father of an epileptic boy)[1]

Participation in regular exercise or athletic activities improves physical and psychological well-being. This is especially important for persons with epilepsy, as they are likely to be less physically fit and more socially isolated than the general population.[2] The benefits of exercise may improve quality of life, a subject of increased attention for persons with chronic seizures.

Despite Galen's advice on the subject, epileptics are often excluded from sports for two main reasons. The first is fear that exercise will precipitate a seizure, which then may cause injury. The second is concern that repeated mild head injuries, which may occur during contact sports, will worsen epilepsy. Although certain sporting activities may justify exclusion for reasons of safety, precautionary measures are often overgeneralized. Unfortunately, the lack of objective data that address these issues led to three revisions of American Medical Association policy statements between 1968 and 1978.[3-5] This has contributed to uncertainty and inconsistency in patient counseling.

We hope that this chapter will provide a practical summary of what is known about the relationship between sports and epilepsy and assist health care professionals in patient counseling.

We begin by reviewing seizure classification because this has implications for treatment and prognosis. Next, we discuss the current understanding of the relationships between physical exercise, seizures, and injuries. We then use available data, policy statements, and opinion to formulate guidelines useful in counseling youths and adults who compete in sports. Finally, we address the special case of the endurance athlete.

SEIZURES AND EPILEPSY: DEFINITIONS, CLASSIFICATION, AND RESPONSE TO TREATMENT

A seizure is the clinical manifestation of excessive or hypersynchronous abnormal activity of neurons of the cerebral cortex.[6] Epidemiologic studies indicate that 8% to 10% of the general population will suffer at least one seizure during their lifetime.[7,8] However, the term *epilepsy* is reserved for the setting of recurrent, unprovoked seizures. Approximately 3% to 4% of the population living to age 80 develop epilepsy, amounting to more than 3 million people in Canada and the United States.

There are two main categories of seizures: partial and generalized.[9] Partial seizures have clinical or electroencephalographic (EEG) evidence of focal onset and are either simple or complex. Consciousness and awareness are preserved in simple partial seizures and their clinical manifestations depend on the area of discharge origin. For example, seizures confined to motor cortex cause contralateral motor manifestations. Similarly, simple partial seizures may be sensory or visual if those cortical areas are involved in isolation. Complex partial seizures (psychomotor seizures, temporal lobe seizures) alter awareness; clinical hallmarks include motor automatisms (such as semipurposeful fumbling of the hands or lip-smacking) and amnesia for the event. Each type of partial seizure may secondarily generalize (due to bilateral spreading of electrical discharges), resulting in a generalized tonic-clonic seizure (grand mal) with loss of consciousness and convulsive movements. Partial seizures often have an underlying structural cause, such as mesial temporal sclerosis or a neoplasm.

Generalized seizures are characterized by EEG recordings that show diffuse, bilateral electrical discharges *at onset*. There are many clinical varieties of generalized seizures, including *absence* (petit mal), *generalized tonic-clonic, astatic* (drop attacks), and *myoclonic seizures*. Generalized seizures usually alter consciousness, often have a genetic basis, and are uncommonly caused by structural lesions.

Seizure classification is essential to determine treatment and prognosis. Different antiepileptic drugs (AEDs) are used for partial and generalized seizures. Partial seizures often indicate a structural brain lesion (e.g., arteriovenous malformation or tumor) that may itself have implications for physical activity. Some patients have an identifiable *epileptic syndrome* that portends a certain prognosis. Certain epileptic syndromes (e.g., benign rolandic epilepsy; absence) affect the patient during a portion of his or her childhood or adolescence and virtually always resolve spontaneously before adulthood. Other syndromes, such as progressive myoclonic epilepsy, are associated with other neurologic abnormalities and a poor long-term prognosis. Magnetic resonance imaging (MRI) of the brain, an EEG, and other laboratory studies may be required to diagnose seizure type or epileptic syndrome.

Modern treatment of epilepsy has improved the outlook for most patients. Approximately 50% of epileptics treated with AEDs will be seizure-free and do not require any change in lifestyle. A further 20% will have infrequent seizures that usually do not limit activity. The remaining 30% of patients will have seizures frequently enough to cause significant incapacitation and lifestyle impairment. The implications for working, driving, and athletics are different for each group.

The evaluation, treatment, and counseling of epileptic patients require considerable expertise. Therefore any health care professional asked to counsel a patient with seizures regarding sporting activity should consult a neurologist skilled in the comprehensive management of these disorders.

DO EPILEPTIC PATIENTS BENEFIT FROM EXERCISE AND PARTICIPATION IN SPORTS?

Many epileptics lead sedentary lives, are less physically fit than nonepileptics, and have limited social contact. They often have diminished self-esteem and self-confidence.[10] Unwarranted restriction of activities and team sports can only worsen this perceived inequality. Regular exercise improves general physical fitness and provides psychological and social benefits. In one study, patients reported improved seizure control when they maintained a regular exercise program; however, another report showed no benefit on seizure frequency.[11,12] The next section outlines the relationships between exercise and epilepsy.

THE EVIDENCE: INTERACTIONS BETWEEN EXERCISE, SEIZURES, SEIZURE CONTROL, AND INJURY

The following questions are inevitable.

Does Exercise Precipitate Seizures in People with Epilepsy?

Several groups have addressed this question by monitoring EEG patterns in epileptic patients before, during, and immediately after exercise.[13-15] Patients with epilepsy usually had epileptiform abnormalities on EEG even when they were not experiencing a clinical seizure. This abnormal background was generally suppressed during activity. After exercise the abnormal pattern transiently worsened but remained below the preexercise level. (Clinical seizures are not mentioned in these reports.)

Clinical studies indicate that the risk of a seizure is reduced during exercise. The most common time for a group of newly exercising epileptic women to have a seizure is in the cooldown period following aerobic activity.[16] Indirect corroboration of this clinical evidence is provided by the apparent rarity of seizures triggered only by exercise.[17] In summary, the available data suggest that seizures are suppressed during aerobic exercise and are somewhat more likely to occur in the subsequent cool-down period.

The mechanism underlying the possible suppression of seizures by exercise was considered to be alteration in acid-base balance, but experiments have not convincingly shown that exercise-induced changes in blood pH would significantly affect brain function.[13] Although voluntary hyperventilation activates certain seizure types, this is physiologically quite different from increased ventilation driven by exercise. The mechanism of the effect of exercise on the seizure threshold remains unclear but is probably multifactorial and may include the effects of brain-derived β-endorphins, which have an anticonvulsant effect.[18]

Other clinical phenomena that occur during exercise may also alter seizure risk. Sustained attention and vigilance can reduce the frequency of epileptiform abnormalities on EEG, whereas fatigue and physical and psychological stress can precipitate seizures.[19,20] Competitive pressure in sports is likely to introduce all of these factors simultaneously.

Metabolic imbalances, such as electrolyte disorders, may precipitate seizures in normal people. However, these types of alterations are usually a risk only in prolonged, extreme physiologic or environmental conditions. These issues are addressed in the section concerning the endurance athlete.

Does Exercise Alter Seizure Control?

Existing studies conclude either that exercise has no measurable effect or that it improves seizure control.[12,16,21] Importantly, there are no studies that suggest that control is worsened by athletics. The available evidence (clinical opinion, small uncontrolled case series) seems to support the view that maintenance of a regular exercise program reduces seizure frequency, but more data are needed.

Does Exercise Alter Antiepileptic Drug Levels or Metabolism?

Drug dosages and schedules do not have to be modified when patients are involved in athletics or training regimens.[11,22,23] However, AED levels may be altered significantly by severe metabolic stresses, such as water intoxication (see The Endurance Athlete). In addition, close attention must be paid to potential drug interactions, including increased metabolism of AEDs in patients taking androgenic steroids or other medications that induce hepatic enzymes.[24]

Do Head Injuries Cause Seizures or Affect Seizure Control in Epileptics?

Significant head trauma greatly increases the risk of epilepsy in persons with no history of seizures. Epidemiologic studies from Rochester, Minnesota, show that severe injuries (intracranial mass lesions or unconsciousness for longer than 24 hours) increase the relative risk (RR) almost thirtyfold (absolute risk, 12%).[25] Moderate injuries (unconsciousness for 30 minutes to 24 hours or a nondepressed skull fracture) confer a risk of 2% for a few years after the event (RR − 1). Mild head trauma (amnesia or unconsciousness for less than 30 minutes), which accounts for about 80% of civilian cases, does not increase the risk of epilepsy. These data on mild injuries, which would include virtually all concussions experienced during contact sports, are only partially reassuring because they do not include persons who already have epilepsy and do not take into account repeated traumas.

Another two questions of importance to epileptics are (1) What is the effect of head trauma on preexisting epilepsy? and (2) What are the effects of repeated, mild head traumas that may occur during contact sports?

The answer to each question is unknown. Intuitively, one would expect a moderate or severe head injury to worsen seizure control in an epileptic. One experienced neurologist (15,000 patients over 34 years) reported that he had not encountered a single case of recurrent seizures related to head injury in his epileptic patients.[26] In a retrospective study of 1,000 patients with post-traumatic epilepsy,[27] 14 had preexisting epilepsy. Only one of these patients had an early seizure (a seizure within 1 week of head trauma), and the subsequent frequency pattern of seizures in all patients was the same as before the injury.[27] In a separate study, five adults with a history of remote epilepsy (no seizures for up to 14 years or seizures in infancy only) experienced early seizures after head injury. Two of the five suffered from persistent seizures thereafter.

As mentioned above, there are few studies that address the effects of multiple, mild episodes of head trauma that may occur in collision sports. For example, experiments have shown that repeatedly heading the ball in soccer does not cause brain dysfunction, although it is possible that transient, subclinical damage occurs.[28,29] However, the weight of clinical experience suggests that this is not a significant risk factor and should not preclude participation for an athlete with epilepsy (see guidelines).

Whether the epileptic brain is more susceptible to trauma remains unclear. It is likely that the cause of the epilepsy, the degree of seizure control, and the severity of the head injury play a role in determining immediate (and possibly longer-term) seizure frequency.

Do Seizures Cause Injuries?

Few studies address this question. No significant difference in number of accidents was found between children with epilepsy and those without the disorder (Fischer and Daute, referenced in van Linschoten et al).[30] Population-based studies conflict regarding whether epileptics are overrepresented in head injury victims.[31,32] A British study of epileptic inpatients documented that 2.7% of all seizures (6.1% of all seizures associated with falling) resulted in a head injury.[33] Almost all injuries were minor, requiring dressing or a few sutures. Only three intracranial hemorrhages were recorded in the series of over 27,000 seizures.

About 7% of epileptics die from accidents.[34] However, only about 5% of these deaths are attributable to seizure-related injuries, and most of these are due to bathtub drownings.[35] The relative risk of injury or drowning during swimming is increased fourfold in epileptics, but the absolute risk is small.[36,37] It is likely that improved safety would have prevented a number of the deaths reported in these studies.

These data suggest that the risk of harm from seizures is small but definite. This risk is probably modified significantly by the setting in which the patient has a seizure and by the use of appropriate safety measures, such as the buddy system for swimming.

CLINICAL DECISION-MAKING GUIDELINES

In this section we present the most common general categories of problems facing the neurologist and sport medicine physician when caring for patients with epilepsy. We begin with existing policy statements.

Advisory Group Policy Statements

In 1983 the Committee on Children with Handicaps and the Committee on Sports Medicine wrote the following:

> Proper medical management, good seizure control, and proper supervision are essential if children with epilepsy are to participate fully. . . . Common sense dictates that situations in which a seizure could cause a dangerous fall should be avoided. . . . Swimming should be supervised; no competitive underwater swimming is acceptable. Participation in contact or collision sports should be given individual consideration according to the specific problem of the athlete.[38]

In response to a letter inquiring as to whether a person with epilepsy should be allowed to train as a scuba diving instructor, the Professional Advisory Board of the Epilepsy Foundation of America stated:

> We strongly believe that persons with epilepsy whose seizures are controlled can and should lead full lives without any personal restrictions. . . . The risks for a person who has had epilepsy that is now controlled whether receiving medication or not are somewhat greater than for a person without a history of seizures. The magnitude of these risks is small but also related to the type of seizure, the duration of control, and, perhaps, the type of activity. The Epilepsy Foundation believes that it is also the right of the individual to evaluate those risks and undertake any activity for which he feels the risks are reasonable. In the case of such a person becoming a scuba diving instructor, we do not believe that such an individual who may be subject to the risks defined above should involve other persons who do not have such risk without their specific knowledge and consent.[39]

Scenario 1: Advice Regarding Athletics After a Single Seizure

Following a first-ever seizure, an attempt is made to determine whether the seizure was **pro-**

voked (i.e., caused by modifiable precipitating factors, such as electrolyte abnormalities or illicit drug use) and whether it is **symptomatic** (i.e., due to an underlying disease, such as a tumor). The first question is usually answered with a careful history and blood tests, and the latter question by brain imaging. It is imperative that all athletic and competitive physical activities be suspended until a neurologic evaluation has been completed.

If investigations define controllable factors that likely provoked the seizure (e.g., metabolic, toxic, or drug-induced seizures), prevention of further events may simply require avoidance of these precipitating factors. There is no contraindication to immediate return to athletics if this requirement is met. If neurologic investigations uncover a symptomatic cause (e.g., a tumor), the likelihood of seizure recurrence is high and further athletic endeavors should be suspended until the causative disorder is definitively treated. The decision regarding return to athletic activity depends on the nature and treatment of the primary lesion.

The most common scenario, especially in young adults, is that no precipitating cause will be found. Opinions among neurologists differ regarding the need for anticonvulsant therapy in this situation. The risk of subsequent unprovoked seizures is estimated to be 30% to 70% in the first 3 years after the initial event.[40,41] Therefore many of these young adults will soon fulfill the criteria for epilepsy. These patients should be started on an AED and monitored for as long as necessary to ensure compliance (using serum AED levels) before clearance is given to participate in sports.

Recommendations. With the above scenario—

1. Patients with a *single, unprovoked seizure of unknown cause* should be treated with an AED and cleared for athletics only when compliance is certain.

2. Following a *single provoked seizure* due to metabolic or toxic causes, we recommend that athletic activity, including contact sports (see Scenario 2), be allowed if the cause can be reliably avoided.

3. If there is a *structural cause* for seizures, we recommend AED therapy and definitive treatment of the lesion before return to athletics.

Scenario 2: Guidelines for Sports Activities in Epileptic Teenagers and Young Adults

Epileptic adolescents are rarely members of competitive individual or team sports, usually due to dissuasion or prohibition from parents or physicians. Physicians should endorse physical activity for its benefits on general health and (possibly) seizure control. However, patients and parents often inquire about taking part in specific sports or recreational activities. What information can one use to guide the adolescent or young adult who wishes to be a full participant in activities with his or her peers? We make decisions based on three essential questions, each of which is addressed below (see Table 15–1):

1. **What type(s) of seizure does the person have?** A complete clinical description of all seizures is required, including types, triggering factors, presence of an aura, diurnal pattern, seizure duration, characteristics of the postictal period, and prior injuries due to seizures.

Simple partial seizures are not a contraindication to any activities, as long as the person has not experienced secondarily generalized seizures. Complex partial seizures, which transiently impair awareness, are much more common. If an aura is not present, activities that may result in serious injury should even a transient lapse in consciousness occur must be prohibited. Although a patient may be able to recog-

---

TABLE 15–1. Considerations for Patient Counseling Regarding Sports

Epilepsy Characteristics

Seizure classification
Seizure frequency (degree of control)
Presence of aura
Accompanying disorders
Medication compliance
Prior head injuries (see section of text on concussion and sports)

Sport Characteristics

Risk of falls
Risk of drowning
Contact or noncontact sport
Individual or team sport
Endurance event
Supervision

nize a *stereotypic, invariably present* aura and extricate himself from an activity, it is not recommended that this be used to justify participation in potentially dangerous activities.

The presence of generalized tonic-clonic seizures presents the same problems as complex partial seizures without aura, except that the seizures are often longer, are associated with changes in body posture and tone, and have more prolonged postictal states. These factors probably increase the risk of injury during athletic activity and, depending upon the sport, may also place other participants at risk.

2. **How well controlled are the seizures?** The degree of seizure control is the most important factor in the need to impose restrictions. As previously mentioned, about 70% of patients treated with AEDs will become seizure-free or have only infrequent seizures. In addition, epilepsy that is under complete control for a period of 2 years carries a relapse risk that is the same as the risk of a first seizure.

Collateral history from family members is essential to establish whether control has been achieved, because subtle seizures may not be recognized by the patient. The collateral history should be obtained from someone with a primary interest in the safety of the patient rather than his or her athletic potential. Athletes may underreport seizures in order to continue competing, and well-meaning but misguided relatives or friends (including coaches) may do the same. Seizure frequency should be documented, preferably by using a diary, so that the effects of medication can be assessed accurately. In general, one needs to treat a patient with AEDs for at least 4 weeks to have confidence in the effectiveness of the drug.

There are several **modifiable factors** that can affect seizure frequency. The most important is medication compliance. Collateral history and sequential blood levels can establish this. Some epileptics are noncompliant because they view the need for medication as a stigma of epilepsy, but motivated athletes may become extremely compliant when they realize that it can make the difference in determining whether they can participate in sports. Noncompliance should raise suspicions of the patient's misreporting of seizure frequency as well. Limited experimental evidence indicates that perspiration and exercise do not significantly affect AED levels.

Patients should clearly understand that they are more susceptible to the effects of physiologic stressors than nonepileptics. Therefore identification of potential triggers is beneficial in reducing the number of seizures. These triggers include sleep deprivation, use of alcohol, and abuse of any central nervous system stimulants, illicit drugs, or performance-enhancing agents.

3. **What are the sporting activities that the person wishes to partake in?** The decision to allow an epileptic patient to participate in a sporting activity depends on which sport is desired. The most recent American Medical Association policy statement endorses the view that persons with epilepsy should be unrestricted in participating in any sport (contact or otherwise) in which the setting does not endanger the health of the person or fellow participants. Table 15–2 provides a general guide, although each case must be managed on an individual basis.

Noncontact sports that take place in a safe setting, such as golf or racquet sports, are allow-

---

TABLE 15–2. Recommendations on Specific Sports for the Epileptic Patient with Regular Seizures

Activities to Be Avoided

Scuba diving
Parachuting
High altitude climbing
Gliding
Aviation
Motor-racing
Boxing

Activities Requiring Precautions or Supervision

Water skiing
Swimming
Canoeing
Surfing (including wind surfing)
Sailing

Activities Requiring Knowledge of Seizure Type and Sports

Cycle racing
Skating
Horseback riding
Gymnastics

Adapted from van Linschoten R, Backx FJG, Mulder OGM, Meinardi H: Epilepsy and sports. Sports Med 10:9-19, 1990.

able for any epileptic. A common issue concerns participation in contact sports, such as hockey and football. In this situation, adequate seizure control is mandatory. Coaches and trainers should be made aware of the condition and be educated in appropriate first aid for seizures. As detailed above, there is no objective evidence that contact sports, even with repeated blows to the head, result in worsening of epilepsy. We recommend that epileptic persons with adequate seizure control be cleared to compete in these activities as long as their parents or guardians understand and accept the inherent risks of competition.

There are certain activities in which a seizure may not only endanger the well-being of the patient but also his teammates or co-participants. These activities include swimming, scuba diving, and sky diving. Swimmers should always use the "buddy system." In these situations, all participants must be aware of the possibility that the patient may have a seizure, accept that risk, and possess a basic knowledge of first aid with respect to seizures.

Counseling. Answers to the three questions discussed above will provide adequate information to counsel the individual patient with epilepsy regarding sports participation. Since most patients will have infrequent or no seizures and since most activities are allowable, counseling usually entails outlining potentially dangerous sports, emphasizing the avoidance of precipitating factors and the importance of maintaining medication compliance, and encouraging close physician follow-up.

Scenario 3: Discontinuing Antiepileptic Medication in the Athlete

The decision to discontinue medications in a well-controlled epileptic can be difficult . The relapse rate in adults is approximately 30% to 65% and is highest in the first 2 years after discontinuing the medication. Relapse is more common in patients who have adolescent or adult-onset epilepsy than in those with childhood epilepsy.[42–45] In general, the patient with the highest likelihood of success has a normal neurologic examination, has no history of brain disease or evidence of a structural lesion, has a normal EEG, and has been controlling his or her symptoms with a single drug for more than

2 years. For these reasons, we recommend that adolescents and young adults who are competing in sports with a potential risk of injury either do not discontinue their medications or do so gradually (over months).

Scenario 4: The Endurance Athlete

In recent years there has been a tremendous increase in the number of athletes competing in demanding endurance sports, such as marathon running, long-distance cycling, and triathlon events. The protracted physiologic stresses experienced in these events may result in metabolic abnormalities that affect seizure control. For example, hyponatremia caused by overhydration (water intoxication) during endurance events may trigger seizures in otherwise healthy people.[46] These dramatic fluid balance changes may alter AED levels, but this has not been studied in the setting of endurance sports. Hypoglycemia has been reported to cause seizures during and after marathon running.[47] Hyperthermia can also trigger seizures, and prolonged exercise in hot and humid conditions increases this risk.[48] Participants in endurance events are advised to gradually increase their levels of activity during training, remain compliant with medications, pay close attention to appropriate water and electrolyte replacement, and avoid prolonged elevations of core body temperature.

CONCLUSIONS

People with controlled epilepsy should lead an active and complete lifestyle with little or no restriction. Participation in sports improves physical and emotional health and may have a beneficial effect on seizure frequency.

There are no absolute rules concerning these issues, and we have based our guidelines upon available evidence and current clinical practice.

Ultimately, decisions should be made by the patient, optimally with informed counseling from physicians. Advances in medical and surgical treatment of epilepsy have afforded these able-bodied athletes to compete on an even playing field. Guidance from knowledgeable physicians can continue this trend.

REFERENCES

1. Temkin O: The Falling Sickness. Johns Hopkins Press, Baltimore, 1945, p. 71

2. Bjørholt PG, Nakken KO, Røhme K, Hansen H: Leisure time habits and physical fitness in adults with epilepsy. Epilepsia 21:83–87, 1990

3. The Committee on the Medical Aspects of Sports of the American Medical Association: Convulsive disorders and participation in sports and physical education. JAMA 206:1291, 1968

4. The Committee on the Medical Aspects of Sports of the American Medical Association: Epileptics and contact sports. JAMA 229:820–821, 1974

5. The Committee on the Medical Aspects of Sports of the American Medical Association: Medical Evaluation of the Athlete: A Guide. American Medical Association, Washington, DC, 1979

6. Engel J Jr: Terminology and classifications. In Engel J Jr: Seizures and Epilepsy. FA Davis, Philadelphia, pp. 3–21, 1989

7. Hauser WA, Kurland LT: The epidemiology of epilepsy in Rochester, Minnesota, 1935 through 1967. Epilepsia 16:1–66, 1975

8. Woodbury LA: Incidence and prevalence of seizure disorders including the epilepsies in the United States of America: a review and analysis of the literature. In Plan for Nationwide Action on Epilepsy, Vol. 4. Commission for the Control of Epilepsy and Its Consequences, Washington, DC, 1977. US DHEW Publ #(NIH)78-279, pp. 24–77

9. Commission on Classification and Terminology of the International League Against Epilepsy: Proposal for classification of epilepsies and epileptic syndromes. Epilepsia 26:268–278, 1985

10. Ryan R, Kempner K, Emlen AC: The stigma: epilepsy as self-concept. Epilepsia 21:433–435, 1980

11. Nakken KO, Løyning T, Taubol O: Epilepsy and physical fitness. Tidsskr Nor Laegeforen 105:1136–1138, 1985

12. Nakken KO, Bjørholt PG, Johannessen SI, et al: Effect of physical training on aerobic capacity, seizure occurrence, and serum level of antiepileptic drugs in adults with epilepsy. Epilepsia 31:88–94, 1990

13. Götze W, Kubicki S, Munter M, Teichmann J: Effect of physical exercise on seizure threshold (investigated by electroencephalographic telemetry). Dis Nerv Syst 28:664–667, 1967

14. Kuijer A: Epilepsy and exercise, encephalographical and biochemical studies. In Wada JA, Penry JK (eds): Advances in Epileptology: The Tenth Epilepsy International Symposium. Raven, New York, 1980, p. 543

15. Berney TP, Osselton JW, Kolvin I, et al: Effect of discotheque environment on epileptic children. Br Med J 282:180–182, 1981

16. Ericksen HR, Ellertsen, B, Grønningsaeter H, et al: Physical exercise in women with intractable epilepsy. Epilepsia 35:1256–1264, 1994

17. Ogunyemi AO, Gomez MR, Klass DW: Seizures induced by exercise. Neurology 38:633–634, 1988

18. Frenk H: Pro- and anticonvulsant effects of morphine and the endogenous opioids: involvement and interactions of multiple opiate and non-opiate systems. Brain Res 6:197–210, 1983

19. Miller JW, Hall CM, Holland KD, Ferrendelli JA: Identification of a median thalamic system regulating seizures and arousal. Epilepsia 30:493–500, 1989

20. Temkin NR, Davis GR: Stress as risk factors for seizures among adults with epilepsy. Epilepsia 25:450–456, 1984

21. Denio L, Drake ME, Pakalnis A: The effect of exercise on seizure frequency. J. Med 20:171–176, 1989

22. Cowart VS: Should epileptics exercise? Physician Sports Med 14:183–191, 1986

23. Latines-Bridges B, Gifford-Jorgensen RA: Exercise and sports for children with specific chronic illnesses. Nurse Practitioner 10:22–30, 1985

24. Katzung BG: Basic and Clinical Pharmacology. Lange Medical Publications, Los Altos, Calif, 1982

25. Annegers JF, Rocca WA, Hauser WA: Causes of epilepsy: contributions of the Rochester Epidemiology Project. Mayo Clin Proc 71:570–575, 1996

26. Livingston S, Berman W: Participation of epileptic patients in sports. JAMA 224:236–238, 1973

27. Jennett B: Epilepsy after Non-Missile Head Injuries, 2nd Ed. Heinemann, London, 1975

28. Tysvaer AT, Storli OV: Soccer injuries to the brain: a neurologic and electroencephalographic study of active football players. Am J Sports Med 17:573–578, 1989

29. Jordan SE, Green GA, Galanty HL, et al: Acute and chronic brain injury in United States National Team soccer players. Am J Sports Med 24:205–210, 1996

30. van Linschoten R, Backx FJG, Mulder OGM, Meinardi H: Epilepsy and sports. Sports Med 10:9–19, 1990

31. Annegers J, Grabow J, Groover R, et al: Seizures after head trauma: a population study. Neurology 30:683–689, 1980

32. Hauser W, Tabaddor K, Factor P, Finer C: Seizures and head injury in an urban community. Neurology 34:746–751, 1984

33. Russell-Jones DL, Shorvon SD: The frequency and consequences of head injury in epileptic seizures. J Neurol Neurosurg Psychiatr 52:659–662, 1989

34. Orlowski JP, Rothner FO, Lueders H: Submersion accidents in children with epilepsy. Am J Dis Child 136:777–780, 1982

35. Pearn J: Epilepsy and drowning in childhood. Br Med J 1:1510–1511, 1978

36. Hauser WA, Annegers JF, Elveback LR: Mortality in patients with epilepsy. Epilepsia 21:399–412, 1980

37. Zielinski JJ: Epilepsy and mortality rate and cause of death. Epilepsia 15:191–201, 1974

38. American Academy of Pediatrics Committee on Children with Handicaps and Committee on Sports Medicine: Sports and the child with epilepsy. Pediatrics 72:884–885, 1983

39. Dreifuss FE: Epileptics and scuba diving (Letter). JAMA 253:1877–1878, 1985

40. Hauser WA, Anderson VE, Loewenson RB, McRoberts SM: Seizure recurrence after a first unprovoked seizure. N Engl J Med 307:522–528, 1982

41. Elwes RDC, Chesterman P, Reynolds EH: Prognosis after a first untreated tonic-clonic seizure. Lancet 2:752–753, 1985

42. Callaghan N, Garrett A, Goggin T: Withdrawal of anticonvulsant drugs in patients free of seizures for two years. N Engl J Med 318:942–946, 1988

43. Overweg J, Binnie CD, Oosting J, Rowan AJ. Clinical and EEG prediction of seizure recurrence following antiepileptic drug withdrawal. Epilepsy Res 1:272–283, 1987

44. Berg AT, Shinnar S: The risk of seizure recurrence after a first unprovoked seizure: a quantitative review. Neurology 41:965–972, 1991

45. Medical Research Council Antiepileptic Drug Withdrawal Study Group: Randomized study of antiepileptic drug withdrawal in patients in remission. Lancet 337:1175–1180, 1991

46. Noakes TD, Goodwin N, Rayner BL, et al: Water intoxication: a possible complication during endurance exercise. Med Sci Sports Exerc 17:370–375, 1985

47. French JK: Hypoglycemia-induced seizures following a marathon. N Z Med J 96:407, 1983

48. Millington JT: Should epileptics scuba dive (Letter). JAMA 254:3182–3183, 1985

16

Concussion in Sports

DAVID W. DODICK

Concussion, defined as a traumatically induced alteration in mental status, not necessarily with loss of consciousness, is the most common sequela of trauma to the head during sports-related activity. Although concussive head injuries can occur in almost any form of athletic activity, they occur most frequently in contact sports, such as football, boxing, ice hockey, martial arts, or wrestling, or from high-velocity collisions or falls in basketball, soccer, gymnastics, or cycling.[1] They can also occur without a direct blow to the head when a sufficient force is applied to the brain, such as might occur with a severe whiplash type of injury.[2] The incidence of these injuries is difficult to obtain because accurate reporting by athletes, families, the medical community, and the media is inconsistent. However, it has been estimated that approximately 250,000 concussions and an average of eight deaths due to head injuries occur every year in football alone.[3] This estimate is based on a survey that found that 20% of U.S. high school football players experience one or more concussions during a single football season.[4] Although recent evidence suggests that the true incidence of concussions in varsity football may be closer to 100,000 per year,[5] the magnitude of the problem is no less staggering.

The substantial incidence of concussive head injuries in competitive sports is magnified by the fact that an athlete who has sustained one concussion is at a fourfold[4] to sixfold[6] increased risk of having a subsequent concussion. This can occur even when the concussive head injuries have been separated by months or years. Also, the ability to process new information may be reduced after a mild head injury and the

severity and duration of this functional impairment may be greater with repeated head injuries. This, of course, could lead to poor decision making in a game situation, which could decrease the athlete's ability to avoid potentially dangerous situations, further increasing the risk of repeated head injuries and the potential for long-term sequelae. This compounding risk exposes the athlete to the possibility of many head injuries over a career, the cumulative effect of which may result in persistent clinical symptoms as well as permanent cognitive and psychological sequelae.

In addition to the very real concern of permanent long-term neurologic sequelae, successive minor head injuries occurring within a short interval may indeed result in a fatal outcome called the *second impact syndrome*.[7-11] This devastating phenomenon refers to a syndrome of fatal cerebral edema that occurs in an athlete who suffers a minor head injury while still symptomatic from a previous injury. The second injury leads to autoregulatory dysfunction, cerebrovascular congestion, cerebral edema, intracranial hypertension, and fatal brain herniation.

Until recently, concussive head injuries in sports have been underrecognized and their importance minimized by physicians, coaches, trainers, and athletes themselves. The management of these athletes has been guided mainly by anecdotal experience without attention to our evolving understanding of the pathophysiology of traumatic brain injury. However, the delayed long-term consequences of concussive head injuries have recently received considerable media attention because of several high-profile athletes whose careers have been threatened or terminated as a result of repeated concussions.

PRACTICE OPTIONS

The need for a practice parameter inspired the American Academy of Neurology to develop recommendations for the management of concussion in sports based on the available scientific data and multidisciplinary expert consensus. These recommendations are considered *practice options* (Table 16–1) and are based on expert consensus and a review of the available literature from 1966 to 1996.[12] The available evidence was divided into classes I, II, and III using the definitions outlined in Table 16–1. However, because of the nature of the topic, no class I studies on this subject exist.

The development of these practice options and the recognition of their importance by the Academy have received national exposure and media attention. These practice parameters have been widely endorsed by medical specialists and national organizations. They have served to underscore the importance of close observation and assessment of the injured athlete to prevent catastrophic outcomes of acute structural brain injury, raise awareness of the phenomenon of the second impact syndrome, and highlight the potential for long-term irreversible cognitive and psychological sequelae from cumulative brain injury due to repetitive trauma. They also provide valuable guidance regarding the safety of an athlete's return to competition.

The following discussion will review the clinical features and grading system developed by a quality subcommittee of the American Academy of Neurology and currently used for concussive head injuries. An approach to the sideline evaluation and management of the injured athlete, including return-to-play recommendations, will be outlined. Finally, long-term management and retirement of the head-injured athlete will be briefly discussed, despite the absence of formal recommendations or guidelines in this area.

EVALUATION OF THE INJURED ATHLETE

Concussion

The hallmarks of cerebral concussion are confusion and amnesia. These may occur immediately after a blow to the head,[13] or they may be delayed for several minutes.[14] Confusion may be manifested as a disturbance of vigilance with marked distractibility, inability to maintain a coherent stream of thought, and an inability to perform a sequence of goal-directed movements.[15] During the acute postinjury phase, the athlete may exhibit a vacant stare, delayed verbal and motor responses, disorientation for time and place, incoordination, incoherent speech, or loss of consciousness, although the latter is *not* a requisite for the diagnosis. Symptoms that the athlete may experience and report are outlined in Table 16–2. These symptoms are divided into early and late features, although they may not occur in a typical time course in all individuals.

In a minority of athletes, some of these symptoms become persistent, resulting in what is known as the postconcussion or posttraumatic syndrome. Headaches and dizziness are the most prominent symptoms and are usually aggravated by exercise, anxiety, and stress. Fatigue, irritability, depression, impaired concentration, and

---

TABLE 16–1. Definitions

Practice Options

Standards: Generally accepted principles for patient management that reflect a high degree of certainty that is based on class I evidence; or, when circumstances preclude randomized clinical trials, overwhelming evidence of class II studies that directly address the question.

Guidelines: Recommendations for patient management that may identify a particular strategy or range of management strategies and that reflect moderate clinical certainty based on class II evidence or strong consensus of class III evidence.

Options: Other strategies for patient management for which there is unclear clinical certainty (i.e., based on inconclusive or conflicting evidence or opinion).

Class Definitions

Class I: Evidence provided by one or more well-designed randomized controlled clinical trials

Class II: Evidence provided by one or more well-designed clinical trials

Class III: Evidence provided by expert opinion, nonrandomized historical controls, case series, or case reports

TABLE 16–2. Symptoms of Concussion

Early (minutes and hours)

Headache
Dizziness or vertigo
Lack of awareness of surroundings
Nausea or vomiting

Late (days to weeks)

Persistent headache
Lightheadedness, blurred vision
Dysequilibrium
Poor concentration, short-term memory
    impairment
Easy fatigability
Irritability
Unusual sensitivity to environment (noise, light,
    children playing)
Anxiety, depression, insomnia

short-term memory are also common accompanying symptoms. There appears to be a strong correlation between the degree and extent of postconcussive symptoms and the number of previous head injuries,[16] again indicating that the cumulative effects of repeated head injuries play a significant role in the level of posttraumatic disability.

Acute Injury Management

Management of a cerebral concussion in an athlete on the sidelines should be guided by the same principles used to evaluate any patient with a traumatic brain injury irrespective of the activity. The objectives of this evaluation are to urgently identify symptoms and signs of serious intracranial pathology, such as an intracranial hemorrhage, and to prevent a catastrophic injury by allowing the athlete to prematurely return to action. Clearly, any athlete who experiences a prolonged impairment of consciousness or persistent alteration in mental status or who has abnormalities on neurologic examination requires urgent transfer to a trauma center and neurosurgical consultation.

All athletes suspected of having concussions should undergo a thorough sideline evaluation by properly trained individuals, including a mental status examination, neurologic examination, and provocative exertional maneuvers as outlined in Table 16–3. Although preliminary, this brief evaluation has been subjected to standardized study and appears to be a feasible and clinically valid approach to the sideline assessment of a head-injured athlete.[17] The decision as to if and when the athlete can return to play will depend upon the grade of the concussion

TABLE 16–3. Sideline Evaluation

Mental status testing	
Orientation	Time, person, place, and situation (opposition, game time, score, circumstances of injury)
Concentration	Serial seven's (100 − 7, 93 − 7, etc.)
	Months of year in reverse
Memory	Recall of 3 words and 3 objects at 0 and 5 minutes
	Recent newsworthy events
	Names of teams in prior contest
	Details of the contest (plays, strategy, etc.)
Neurologic examination	
Pupils	Symmetry and reaction
Coordination	Finger to nose, tandem gait
Sensation	Romberg test, finger to nose (eyes closed)
Exertional testing	40-yard sprint
	5 pushups/5 sit-ups/5 knee bends

If any symptoms appear during or after exertional testing (headache, blurred vision, dizziness, nausea, confusion, etc.), player is removed from contest.

(Table 16–4) as determined by the severity of the concussion and the duration of posttraumatic symptoms. The following discussion outlines the scheme used for grading concussions and recommendations (practice options) for acute injury management and for determining the time delay necessary before an athlete can safely return to play.

SECOND-IMPACT SYNDROME

Second-impact syndrome refers to a fatal syndrome of malignant cerebral edema and brain herniation that is thought to be the result of a second concussion occurring in an athlete who has not fully recovered from a previous concussion (athlete still symptomatic [e.g., dizziness, headache]). The second injury presumable leads

---

TABLE 16–4. Grades of Concussion

Grade I Concussion ("Dinged" or "Bell Rung")

Transient confusion
No loss of consciousness
Concussion symptoms or mental status abnormalities on examination *resolve in less than 15 minutes*

Recommendation for return to play
Return to play. However, a second grade I concussion in the same contest eliminates the player from competition immediately. May return to play in 1 week but only if asymptomatic for 1 week at rest and with exertion.

Grade II Concussion

Transient confusion
No loss of consciousness
Concussion symptoms or mental status abnormalities on examination *last more than 15 minutes*

Recommendations
Remove from contest, frequent on-site evaluations for evolving intracranial pathologic conditions with evaluation the following day by a trained examiner.
Computed tomography (CT) or magnetic resonance imaging (MRI) brain scan recommended if headache or other symptoms persist longer than 1 week. Season is terminated if an abnormality consistent with brain swelling, contusion, or other intracranial pathologic condition is present on CT or MRI.

Return to play
Return to play only after a physician has performed a neurologic examination and the athlete has remained asymptomatic at rest and with exertion for 1 week (after second grade II concussion, play suspended for minimum of 2 asymptomatic weeks).

Grade III Concussion

Any loss of consciousness, either brief (seconds) or prolonged (minutes)

Recommendations
Athlete is transported immediately to hospital emergency room by ambulance if worrisome signs are detected or still unconscious. The cervical spine should be immobilized if indicated. Athlete is admitted to hospital if any signs of pathology are detected or mental status remains impaired.
A thorough neurologic evaluation should be performed emergently with appropriate neuroimaging. Neurologic status should be assessed daily until all symptoms have stabilized or resolved.
Urgent neurosurgical evaluation is mandated when unconsciousness is prolonged, neurologic examination is abnormal, or mental status changes persist or worsen.

Return to play
Brief grade III concussion (seconds): play suspended for a minimum of 1 asymptomatic week
Prolonged grade III concussion (minutes): play suspended for a minimum of 2 asymptomatic weeks
Following second grade III concussion: play suspended for a minimum of 1 asymptomatic month
If CT or MRI indicates cerebral edema, contusion, or any trauma-related intracranial abnormality, play suspended for the remainder of the season; athlete should be discouraged from ever returning to play

to autoregulatory dysfunction, cerebrovascular congestion, brain edema, increased intracranial pressure (ICP), and, potentially, death. This phenomenon has been recognized for decades and is supported by experimental evidence[18,19] as well as numerous case reports[7-11] describing fatal outcomes, even with a trivial second head injury (e.g., tapping of helmets in a huddle) in teenage athletes as well as young adults. It is therefore widely accepted that athletes are prohibited without exception from engaging in any contact sport until all postconcussive symptoms have resolved both at rest and during provocative exertional testing (Table 16–4).

PERSISTENT NEUROPSYCHOLOGICAL SEQUELAE

It has been well documented that repeated concussive head injuries can lead to cumulative and lasting neuropsychologic and emotional deficits.[20-22] Neurobehavioral deficits (learning, memory, cognition) may be objectively identified in as many as 66% of patients after a single minor head injury as long as 3 months after the injury,[23] and significant and sustained neuropsychologic abnormalities have been demonstrated to occur after only two minor head injuries.[20] These deficits may be subtle and go unrecognized even during a comprehensive neurologic and mental status examination.

For these reasons, neuropsychological testing has been routinely used to document head injury sequelae and to provide a sensitive guide to ongoing and cumulative problems following athletic head injuries. Neuropsychometric evaluations involve a series of cognitive and behavioral problems and suggest strategies for optimizing recovery. Moreover, the results of these tests are currently being used by several authorities to assist in the decision-making process of when to allow athletes to return to competition after a concussive head injury. Resolution of the neuropsychological deficits that are felt to have arisen from the head injury is required before granting permission to return to any contact sport.

Most professional sports organizations require a baseline neuropsychometric evaluation as part of a preemployment physical. This provides a baseline assessment to which future assessments can be compared in an effort to document the presence of cognitive deficits that can be attributed to the injury. Until evidence-based criteria for retirement of a professional athlete are developed, failure to demonstrate resolution of newly acquired neuropsychological deficits should preclude high-risk sports for the athlete.

SUMMARY AND CONCLUSIONS

Concussive head injuries occur frequently in all forms of athletic endeavor, although they are more common in contact or high-velocity sports that predispose athletes to collision. Unfortunately, these sometimes subtle injuries have often gone undetected. Further, the management approach to these head-injured athletes has been haphazard and guided by anecdote and instinct rather than by neuroscience and evidence-based medicine. Although the majority of these injuries are benign, there is a potential for catastrophic outcome as well as short- and long-term neuropsychological sequelae if athletes are permitted prematurely to return to competition. This can threaten not only their future in competitive sports, but also their life.

The need therefore to develop a standardized, feasible, and valid evaluation and management approach led to the development of a **practice parameter with evidence-based practice options and recommendations** regarding appropriate timing for an athlete's return to competition. These guidelines should serve as minimum time periods, and when in doubt, the managing physician should always favor the conservative side.

Return to Play. In addition to the severity of the concussion and the duration of posttraumatic symptoms, the decision to allow an athlete to return to play should also take into account the total number of concussions sustained by the athlete, the temporal frequency of the concussions (whether they are occurring in rapid succession), the degree of impact or the severity of the injury required to give an athlete a concussion (lesser degrees of trauma with each successive head injury), the importance and complexity of the position (quarterback), and the likelihood of future head injuries, which will depend on the sport (boxing or football vs tennis or golf). Finally, not only do athletes need to be completely asymptomatic both at rest and with exertion before returning to play, but also complete resolution of documented neuropsychological deficits should be a prerequisite to returning to contact sports.

Education and Research. In the future, a continued aggressive effort to educate team trainers, physicians, and coaches about the symptoms and signs and appropriate management of cerebral concussion is needed. A standardized neuropsychologic test battery needs to be designed and tailored to detect those measures that are most sensitive to concussive head injuries. Such a test battery should be administered to all competitive athletes during the screening medical evaluation so that changes and resolution in these measurements can be accurately determined. Finally, large prospective studies are required to determine the physical, neurologic, and neuropsychological sequelae of multiple concussions. This will lead to refinement of these preliminary guidelines as well as to recommendations for retirement of competitive athletes.

REFERENCES

1. Dick RW: A summary of head and neck injuries in collegiate athletics using the NCAA Injury Surveillance System. In Hoerner EF (ed): Head and Neck Injuries in Sports. American Society for Testing and Materials, Philadelphia, 1994
2. Lindenberg R, Freytag E: Brainstem lesion characteristics of traumatic hyperextension of the head. Arch Pathol 90:509–515, 1970
3. Cantu RC: When to return to contact sports after a cerebral concussion. Sports Med Digest 10:1–2, 1988
4. Gerberich SG, Priest JD, Boen JR, et al: Concussion incidences and severity in secondary school varsity football players. Am J Public Health 73:1370–1375, 1983
5. Kelly JP, Rosenberg JH: Diagnosis and management of concussion in sports. Neurology 48:575–580, 1997
6. Zemper E: Analysis of cerebral concussion frequency with the most commonly used models of football helmets. J Athletic Training 29:44–50, 1994
7. Saunders RL, Harbaugh RE: The second impact in catastrophic contact-sports head trauma. JAMA 252:538–539, 1984
8. McQuillen JB, McQuillen EN, Morrow P: Trauma, sports, and malignant cerebral edema. Am J Forensic Med Pathol 9:12–15, 1988
9. Fekete JF: Severe brain injury and death following minor hockey accidents: the effectiveness of the "safety helmets" of amateur hockey players. Can Med Assoc J 99:1234–1239, 1968
10. Cantu RC: Second-impact syndrome. Clin Sports Med 17(1):37–44, 1998
11. Kelly JP, Nichols JS, Filley CM, et al: Concussion in sports: guidelines for the prevention of catastrophic outcome. JAMA 226:2867–2869, 1991
12. Practice Parameter: The management of concussion in sports (summary statement). Report of the Quality Standards Subcommittee. Neurology 48:581–585, 1997
13. Fisher CM: Concussion amnesia. Neurology 16:826–830, 1966
14. Yarnell PR, Lynch S: Retrograde memory immediately after concussion. Lancet 1:863–864, 1970
15. Mesulam MM: Principles of Behavioral Neurology. FA Davis, Philadelphia, 1985
16. Carlsson GS, Svardsodd K, Welm L: Long-term effects of head injury sustained during life in three male populations. J Neurosurg 67:197–205, 1987
17. McCrea M, Kelly JP, Kluge J, et al: Standardized Assessment of Concussion in football players. Neurology 48:586–588, 1997
18. Moody RA, Ruamsuke S, Mullan SF: An evaluation of decompression in experimental head injury. J Neurosurg 29:586–590, 1968
19. Langfitt TW, Weinstein JD, Kassell NF: Cerebral vasomotor paralysis produced by intracranial hypertension. Neurology 15:622–641, 1965
20. Gronwall D, Wrightson P: Cumulative effects of concussion. Lancet 2:995–997, 1975
21. Leininger BE, Gramling SE, Fannell HD, et al: Neuropsychological deficits in symptomatic minor head injury patients after concussion and mild concussion. J Neurol Neurosurg Psychiatry 53:293–296, 1990
22. Bream HT: Post concussion syndrome: a case study. Athletic Therapy Today 1(1):7–10, 1996
23. Rimel RW, Giordani B, Barth JR: Disability caused by minor head injury. Neurosurgery 9(3):221–228:1981

Neuropsychology in Sports

M. ALAN J. FINLAYSON ▪ MARK R. LOVELL

Psychology has a lengthy history in sport. Recent advances in the field of health psychology have led to increasing emphasis upon wellness models and human performance. Sport psychology has contributed to and grown with this rise in health consciousness.[1] The field of sport neuropsychology is a relative newcomer and has developed from a recognition of the significance of the consequences of brain injury for athletes.[2] This field applies knowledge regarding mild traumatic brain injury (MTBI) or concussion to sport injury.

This chapter provides a brief overview of MTBI, reviews the use of neuropsychological testing for athletes who participate in football and ice hockey, and summarizes our experiences in using neuropsychological assessment procedures to evaluate athletes following an MTBI. We specifically review the current neuropsychological testing programs within the National Hockey League (NHL) and National Football League (NFL) and discuss the extension of these programs downward to athletes at the college, high school, and junior high/middle school levels. In addition, intervention strategies for MTBI are presented.

PATHOPHYSIOLOGY OF MTBI

Detailed discussion of the pathophysiology of brain damage has been provided elsewhere.[3,4] The impact of force on delicate brain tissues accounts for the basic pathophysiology of neurotrauma. This may take the form of relatively focal damage associated with translational or sagittal forces and characterized by abrasion, coup or contracoup, and occasionally hematoma. In addition, rotational or angular forces are frequently associated with diffuse axonal injury (DAI). Diffuse injury can also occur through shearing and stretching of vessels and fibers or as consequence of ischemia, anoxia/hypoxia, and brain swelling. It is generally accepted that these processes occur on a continuum. That is, the mechanisms of brain trauma are the same for mild, moderate, and severe injury, differing only in degree. Although immediate event-specific forces are critical determinants of the subsequent course of recovery, attention is being paid to subsequent neurochemical and metabolic factors that exert their impact over time.

There is increasing evidence that neurochemical factors are critical determinants of the extent of damage in brain injury.[5] These authors (Novack, Dillon, and Jackson) articulate the disruptive effects of trauma (ischemic or anoxic) on cell metabolism and note the high frequency of ischemic damage (90%), particularly hippocampal (80%), seen in postmortem examination of brains following neurotrauma. They also point out that, even in the case of DAI, the deleterious impact of neurochemical changes may be only seen in the hours following insult. Thus consideration of the extent of damage must extend beyond only the investigation of impact-specific structural changes to also include biochemical and metabolic effects. These latter efforts may establish some hope for pharmacologic intervention to limit the effects of trauma or, perhaps, even reverse them.

Recent evidence has come forth to identify the critical factor in the brain's postconcussion vulnerability. Hovda[6] described a series of investigations that led him to conclude that metabolic dysfunction was key to both the production and maintenance of this vulnerability. He postulates that, with brain injury, there is an increased demand for glucose by the brain coupled with a yet to be explained reduction in cerebral blood flow that hampers the delivery of glucose to the brain tissue. Thus the resulting pathophysiology is a function of the brain's inability to restore chemical and ionic equilibrium.

SECOND-IMPACT SYNDROME

Second impact syndrome (SIS) can arise for an individual when a second brain injury is sustained while the person is still symptomatic from a first brain injury.[7-9] The incidence of this syndrome is relatively low, and it is usually confined to the pediatric or adolescent population. However, it has gained prominence because of its often fatal but preventable occurrence. The interested reader is referred to Cantu's recent chapter[9] for a more detailed discussion of this topic. However, its occurrence highlights the need for adequate evaluation of concussion and its course in children and young adults.

The typical course is that the individual sustains MTBI with associated postconcussion symptoms. A problem arises when the person returns to the playing field or active competition before these problems have resolved. A second, often trivial, insult can lead to a rapid neurologic crisis and death. It is thought that the second trauma precipitates irregularities in, or loss of, the regulation of the blood supply to the brain, which subsequently results in a sudden and dramatic increase in intracranial pressure with dire consequences. Because of the often fatal consequences of this syndrome, many clinicians are adamant that individuals should not engage in contact sports while symptomatic from previous brain injury. In fact, it is an often-stated view that further delay of return to play following attainment of asymptomatic status is justified because of this high risk. (See also Chapter 16.)

INCIDENCE

Several reviews of data regarding head injury associated with sports have appeared recently.[10,11] Clarke and Jordan[10] have raised several methodologic concerns that serve as cautions in the study of sport-related injury. For example, sufficient data must be available to permit adequate evaluation. Injury rate alone is seen as insufficient, and health burden can only be determined by viewing the rate in the context of the number of participants actually at risk. Further, the subtleties of calculating athletic exposure must be considered in the accurate determination of injury risk and injury rate. Finally, they note that classification issues and diagnostic accuracy and clarity can be particularly problematic in neurotrauma.

Davis and McKelvey[11] reported that *football* accounts for more than 250,000 brain injuries annually in the United States, not including injuries that may not have been reported because of the athlete's reluctance to report the injury. In *horseback riding* they report that brain injury accounts for more than 60% of riding deaths and more than 17% of all riding-related injuries. These authors report that brain injury is present in 87% of *professional boxers,* an alarmingly high prevalence. In sports such as *skiing, hockey,* or *skating,* brain injury accounts for 46% of all injuries sustained. In **soccer,** 5% of players are estimated to have received brain injury. Recent data[12] have shown that long-term neuropsychological deficits are associated with professional soccer play and may well be attributable to heading and its frequency.

In a review of boxing-related fatalities from January 1918 to January 1997, Ryan[13] reported that, on average, nine fatalities occurred per year. However, he described a lack of data regarding details that might permit more adequate documentation of less catastrophic consequences of injury to the brain in boxing. In summarizing earlier studies, Ryan concluded that the presence and extent of neurologic problems in boxers appeared to relate to the number and frequency of bouts fought. These studies included examination of boxers and neuropathologic postmortem examination of brains. Jordan[14] identified the need to move beyond fatality rate alone. He argued that persistent and prolonged neurologic consequences are rare at the amateur level; however, he cited several studies documenting the incidence and prevalence of acute concussion symptoms in professional boxers. Jordan also differentiated acute injury effects from the chronic effects associated with parameters that, in essence, reflect the consequences of increased exposure and the cumulative effects of repeated injury.

Thus traumatic brain injury associated with sports participation is a major public health concern. Thurman, Branche, and Sniezek[15] have estimated that approximately 300,000 sports-related traumatic brain injuries occur annually. As the authors point out, not only does frequency of injury contribute to the severity of the problem but also the general youthfulness of the injured athlete coupled with the long-term consequences of the cumulative effect of repeated injury. To manage this problem, the authors propose problem identification, including risk factors, along with the development and implementation of intervention programs with appropriate evaluation. To accomplish such a task requires extensive data from large populations. A minimum of 1.5 million athletes participate in organized football or ice hockey on an annual basis, and it is estimated that up to 20% of these athletes experience traumatic brain injury annually while participating in these sports.[16] Growing concerns about permanent brain injury as a result of multiple MTBIs have led to stepped-up efforts to more effectively evaluate the injured athlete and have resulted in the creation of large-scale evaluation programs within both the NFL and the NHL. As part of these efforts, specific neuropsychological examination has been incorporated in order to provide reliable and valid data regarding the neurobehavioral consequences of MTBI.

TIMELINE FOR EVALUATION OF THE ATHLETE

Initial Assessment

The evaluation of the athlete with a concussion begins on the playing field, and the first assessment of the athlete's status is usually completed by the team physician or athletic trainer. This evaluation should involve an assessment of the player's orientation to place, game, and details of the contest. The athlete's recall of events preceding the collision (retrograde amnesia) should also be evaluated. The ability to learn and retain new information (anterograde amnesia) should also be tested via a brief sideline memory test. The player should be asked to repeat three to five words until he or she can do so consistently. The player should be checked for recall of this list within 5 minutes. Brief tests of at-

tentional capacity, such as recitation of digits in backward order or backward recitation of months of the year, are also useful.

Finally, the player should be observed for emerging postconcussive symptoms, such as headache, nausea, imbalance, or on-field confusion.[17] On-field assessment of the athlete has recently been standardized to allow a more systematic evaluation of MTBI after it has occurred.[18] However, this very brief evaluation is not a substitute for more formal neuropsychological testing and should not serve as the primary basis for making decisions regarding return to the field or ice.

Formal Evaluation

The formal neuropsychological evaluation of the athlete should take place within 24 hours of the suspected MTBI, whenever possible. Many athletes who have experienced only very mild concussions may appear to be symptom free by this time, but we suggest a neuropsychological assessment to evaluate more subtle aspects of cognitive functioning. If the athlete displays any cognitive deficits on testing or continues to exhibit postconcussive symptoms, a detailed follow up neuropsychological evaluation is recommended approximately 5 days later. We have found that this time interval represents both a useful and a practical follow-up interval and allows for a reassessment of the athlete before the next scheduled game, which, in the case of football, usually takes place on the following Saturday or Sunday.

NEUROPSYCHOLOGICAL TESTING IN FOOTBALL: HISTORICAL ROOTS

Although many of the risks associated with collision sports have been discussed in the scientific literature for decades, the systematic study of MTBI in athletics has been a recent phenomenon. To date, only a few studies have been published that have formally used neuropsychological testing in North American football. Although a number of projects are currently underway at both the college and professional level, only a few completed studies of athletes have used neuropsychological testing.

Historically, the first major study of concussion in football athletes involved the cooperative efforts of the University of Virginia, the Ivy League schools, and the University of Pittsburgh. This study was directed by Dr. Jeffrey Barth at the University of Virginia in the early 1980s and involved more than 2,300 athletes.[19,20] These athletes were given a baseline evaluation before the beginning of the season, and repeat testing was completed if the player experienced an MTBI during the season. Follow-up testing was conducted 24 hours after an MTBI, again at 5 days and 10 days, and after the season. This study revealed subtle and rapidly resolving difficulties in cognitive functioning on tests sensitive to information-processing speed, compared to a control group. Along similar lines, Lovell and his colleagues[21] conducted a study of high school students who underwent neuropsychological testing both before and after experiencing a concussion. Players' test performances were compared to their preseason baseline testing, and mild changes in cognitive functioning were evident 24 hours after injury, but the athletes' performance had improved substantially 72 hours after the concussion.

Based on the need for more sensitive MTBI evaluation procedures in professional football players, a neuropsychological evaluation program was instituted in 1993 with the Pittsburgh Steelers.[22] This represented the first clinically oriented project structured to assist team medical personnel in making return-to-play decisions following a suspected MTBI. This approach involved the formal evaluation of each player before the beginning of the season to provide a basis for comparison in the event of an MTBI during the season. Testing was then repeated within 24 hours after a suspected MTBI and again before the return of the athlete to playing (approximately 5 days after injury). Preseason, baseline evaluation of the athletes is conducted for several reasons. First, individual players vary with regard to their level of performance on tests of memory, attention/concentration, mental processing speed, and motor speed. Second, some players perform poorly on the more demanding tests because of preinjury learning disabilities, attention deficit disorder, or other factors, such as test-taking anxiety. In addition, the player's concussion history may affect performance on subsequent neuropsychological evaluations.

As seen in Table 17–1, the NFL test battery was constructed to evaluate multiple aspects of cognitive functioning but is heavily oriented toward the evaluation of attentional processes, visual scanning, and information processing, although the test battery also evaluates verbal memory, upper extremity motor speed, coordination, and speech fluency. The tests that made up the battery were administered using standardized instructions to avoid variation in test results across testing sessions and across teams. This test battery has gained wide acceptance within the NFL and is now part of a league-supported program that involves over half the teams in the league.

RECENT STUDIES AT THE AMATEUR LEVEL

In addition to the use of neuropsychological testing in the NFL, several other large-scale projects are currently underway at the college level that have continued to demonstrate the usefulness of neuropsychological testing in documenting the effects of concussion.[28] For instance, a multisite study is currently underway at Michigan State University, the University of Florida, and the University of Pittsburgh (M. Collins, personal communication, 1998). This study has resulted in the preseason baseline evaluation of more than 250 football athletes to date and is beginning to yield important information regarding the reliability and validity of neuropsychological testing procedures across different institutions and across multiple testings. In addition to the multisite study cited above, a multisport project that includes football players is being completed at Pennsylvania State University under the direction of Dr. Ruben Echemendia (personal communication, 1998). This study has involved the evaluation of both male and female athletes from other sports in addition to football players and will yield important data regarding the incidence of concussion in other contact sports, such as basketball and ice hockey. This study is also unique in that it includes athletes from noncontact sports, such as baseball and tennis, as control subjects. Although these more recent studies have not yet published their results, they provide excellent models for the study of amateur athletes and should yield important information within the next several years.

TABLE 17–1. NFL Neuropsychological Test Battery

TEST	ABILITY EVALUATED
Orientation Questions	Retrograde and anterograde amnesia, orientation to place and time
Hopkins Verbal Learning Test (HVLT)[24]	Memory for words (verbal memory)
Brief Visuospatial Memory Test—Revised (BVMT-R)[25]	Visual memory
Trail Making Test[26]	Visual scanning, mental flexibility
Controlled Oral Word Fluency[27]	Word fluency, word retrieval
WAIS-III Symbol Search[23]	Visual scanning, visual search
WAIS-III Digit Symbol[23]	Visual scanning, information processing
WAIS-III Digit Span[23]	Attention span
Post-Concussion Symptom Inventory[22]	MTBI symptoms
Delayed recall from HVLT	Delayed memory for words
Delayed recall from BVMT-R	Delayed memory for designs

This table lists the neuropsychological tests that were originally used by the Pittsburgh Steelers and a number of other NFL teams. This test battery has recently been revised with the addition of several tests from the *Wechsler Adult Intelligence Scale-III (Symbol Search, Digit Symbol,* and *Digit Span).*[23] The *Hopkins Verbal Learning Test (HVLT)*[24] consists of a 12-word list that is presented to the athlete on three consecutive trials. The athlete is checked for recall after each presentation and again following a 20-minute delay period. The *Brief Visuospatial Memory Test-Revised (BVMT-R)*[25] evaluates visual memory and involves the presentation of six abstract spatial designs on three consecutive trials. Similar to the *HVLT,* the athlete's recall following each trial and his or her delayed recall are evaluated. Both the *HVLT* and the *BVMT-R* have multiple equivalent forms that minimize practice effects and make them ideal for use with athletes who are likely to undergo evaluation on multiple occasions throughout the course of their careers. The *Trail Making Test*[26] consists of two parts and requires the athlete to use spatial scanning and mental flexibility skills. The *Controlled Oral Word Association Test*[27] requires the athlete to recall as many words as possible that begin with a given letter of the alphabet within a 60-second period. This is completed for three separate letters and provides a measure of verbal fluency. In addition to the neuropsychological tests mentioned above, it is important to monitor the athlete's symptoms. The *Post-Concussion Symptom Inventory* has recently been developed and is currently being used by the NFL.[22]

NEUROPSYCHOLOGICAL TESTING IN ICE HOCKEY

Similar to the sport of football, ice hockey is a collision sport that can and does result in MTBIs. Recent interest in studying MTBI in hockey players has developed as the result of several converging forces. First, heightened media exposure has led to a general awareness of the potential danger of MTBI in hockey. Second, the large-scale neuropsychologic testing project underway in the NFL has demonstrated the feasibility and utility of conducting neuropsychological testing in large groups of athletes. This section details some current research underway in the sport of ice hockey, but first some unique aspects of ice hockey with regard to MTBI are reviewed.

Although athletes who participate in the sports of football and ice hockey share many characteristics, there are differences between hockey and other sports, such as football, that are worthy of mention. For example, the speed at which the athletes typically skate is quite fast and rules of the game result in continuation of high-speed play, with minimal stoppage of play for substitutions. This results in players being at near peak physical performance during their shift. This increases the speed at which the game is played and therefore increases the potential for high-velocity collisions on the ice. In addition, maneuverability on skates is poorer in certain situations, which may result in difficulty in avoiding high-speed collisions on the ice. Finally, the boards in hockey represent a potential source of injury that does not exist in football or other sports played in an open field.

A Model for Use of Neuropsychological Assessment Procedures in Ice Hockey

A number of factors must be taken into consideration when establishing a clinical evaluation program for college level or professional level hockey players. In particular, the benefit of baseline testing and the need for brief but sensitive test procedures are as important in working with hockey players as they are with football players. The need to perform baseline evaluations of more than 20 athletes, often within a 24-hour period, creates a definite challenge to the neuropsychologist. This is particularly important at the professional and college levels, where the athletes have multiple demands on their time that may include practice, team meetings, classes, and often demanding travel schedules.

Although the time pressures in working with large groups of athletes are similar with both football and hockey players, several factors make evaluation of the hockey athlete particularly challenging. First, multiple languages are spoken within the professional hockey ranks (e.g., French, English, Russian, Czechoslovakian, Swedish, Finnish, German). Although examination of each athlete in his or her native language may appear to be the most effective way of evaluating the athlete both at baseline and following an MTBI, this is highly impractical and would require that multilingual neuropsychologists be readily available in all NHL cities. For this reason, it is far more practical to use test procedures that are not heavily language dependent. The assessment of players in their native tongue would also impede league or sportwide efforts to study performance on standardized tests because of limitations in translating languages directly. Another more realistic alternative is for the neuropsychologist to rely more heavily on measures that do not require a high degree of comfort with one language, such as English. Such an approach should focus on information-processing speed or psychomotor functioning, which are known to be affected by MTBI.

In addition, the logistics of a typical hockey schedule differ significantly from football. In professional football, games are typically played on weekends and the teams return home, often immediately after the game. This allows for the neuropsychological assessment of athletes with concussions in the home city within 24 to 48 hours of injury. However, in the professional hockey ranks, teams often embark on long (2- to 3-week) road trips and frequently receive medical treatment outside their home city. Therefore any leaguewide program aimed at the systematic evaluation of MTBI needs to be structured so that athletes can be assured that they

will have access to neuropsychological testing, regardless of where a game is being played. This requires cooperation at the conference or league level.

Selection of a Neuropsychological Test Battery for Ice Hockey

As noted earlier in this chapter, the application of neuropsychological assessment strategies to ice hockey provides specific challenges. As is the case with football the need for brevity must be balanced against the need to sample functioning across multiple cognitive domains. The test battery should be constructed to evaluate the athlete's functioning in the areas of attentional processes, information-processing speed, fluency, and memory. Although numerous tests can provide information regarding the athlete's ability to function in these domains, procedures should also be selected that have multiple equivalent forms or that have been thoroughly researched with regard to the expected practice effects. Although much more research needs to be completed that investigates the use of specific neuropsychological tests with athletes, a test battery developed for use with ice hockey has been suggested by the NHL/NHLPA Neuropsychological Advisory Board members. This group is composed of Drs. Mark Lovell, Alan Finlayson, Ruben Echemendia, William Barr, and Elizabeth Parker. The test battery can be administered in approximately 30 minutes and samples multiple cognitive domains. In keeping with our previous experience with amateur and professional football, we suggest preseason baseline testing, follow-up testing within 24 to 48 hours of a suspected MTBI, and a 5-day follow-up evaluation. Our suggested test battery is detailed in Table 17–2.

INTERVENTION

Intervention strategies following MTBI are generally aimed at the elimination or reduction of the constellation of symptoms that have come to represent the postconcussion syndrome.[32] Pharmacologic and other medical intervention is beyond the scope of this chapter. Summaries of such interventions can be found elsewhere.[33,34] Although most interventions follow a more gen-

TABLE 17-2. NHL/NHLPA Neuropsychological Test Battery*

TEST	ABILITY EVALUATED
Orientation Questions	Retrograde and anterograde amnesia, orientation to place and time
Hopkins Verbal Learning Test (HVLT)[24]*	Word learning
Color Trail Making[30]	Visual scanning, mental flexibility
Controlled Oral Word Association Test[27]*	Word fluency, word retrieval
Ruff Figural Fluency Test[29]	Design fluency
Penn State Symbol Cancellation Test (R. Echemendia, personal communication, 1998)	Visual scanning, attention
Symbol Digit Modalities[31]	Visual scanning, immediate memory
Post-Concussion Symptom Inventory[22]	Postconcussive symptoms
Delayed recall from HVLT	Delayed recall for words

The *Hopkins Verbal Learning Test*[24] was discussed in Table 17–1. The *Ruff's Figure Fluency* test[29] is a relatively new test that requires the athlete to rapidly draw a series of unique designs while under time pressure. Although use of this test has yet to be formally evaluated with athletes, its nonverbal nature may be ideal for use with athletes for whom English is a second language. The *Color Trail Making* test[30] was developed to provide a culture-fair alternative to the widely used *Trail Making Test.*[26] The *Symbol Digit Modalities Test*[31] measures mental processing speed. *The Penn State Cancellation Test* (R. Echemendia, personal communication, 1998) is a test that measures visual scanning and attentional processes and requires the athlete to cross out symbols that are embedded within an array of other symbols. In addition to the neuropsychological tests listed above, the neuropsychologist should carefully evaluate noncognitive symptoms of MTBI. The *Post-Concussion Symptom Inventory* scale[22] described elsewhere in this text has been found to be useful in this regard. Finally, the athlete should be checked for orientation to year, month, date of the month, and day of the week and should also be questioned regarding his or her last memory before the hit (*retrograde amnesia*) and first memory following the hit (*anterograde amnesia*).
*Suggested for English-speaking athletes only.

eral strategy, some authors have focused on sleep disturbance and pain in MTBI.

Richter, Cowan, and Kaschalk[35] have argued for caution when attributing ongoing neurocognitive difficulties to cerebral pathology in cases of MTBI with accompanying sleep disturbances. They proposed a treatment protocol for MTBI that includes the following:

1. Patient and family education
2. Treatment of sleep disorder
3. Treatment of associated psychological disturbance in posttraumatic stress symptoms
4. Restoration of normal mobilization

Emphasis is placed on education and issues ranging from medication to concepts of illness behavior with the goal of self-control and self-management of symptoms. In the presence of sleep disorder, discussion focuses on sleep hygiene procedures and, in more complicated cases, appropriate investigations and judicious use of medication. Cognitive behavioral techniques, including education, desensitization, and psychological activation, are recommended to reduce psychological factors arising from injury. Finally, the authors encouraged physical activation in a graduated fashion. These techniques are combined in a holistic manner to reestablish self-control and mastery in the individual client. It is their belief that such a treatment protocol can avoid the iatrogenic harm associated with exclusively diagnostic or passive approaches to management. They echoed the point made previously[36] that chronic pain is a frequent co-morbidity with MTBI. In fact, according to Uomoto and Esselman,[36] headache is more frequently associated with MTBI than other severity levels. They also note that other pain (ie, neck, shoulder, back) persists to a greater degree in this group.

Pryse-Phillips and colleagues[37] proposed guidelines for management of migraine headache using nonpharmacologic interventions. Their extensive review highlighted the paucity of studies that meet the methodologic standards expected in clinical trials. They found that, in general, nonpharmacologic management resulted in a reduction in frequency or severity of headache in approximately 30% to 45% of subjects. However, methodologic problems were such that the question of placebo effect could not be adequately addressed. Interestingly, they emphasized the importance of patient education and the role that avoidance of migraine trigger factors can play in minimizing the clinical problem. Nevertheless, they did recommend that nonpharmacologic therapies had a role in the clinical management of migraine headache.

Perhaps not surprisingly, many of the recommendations for psychological intervention following MTBI are consistent with the treatment survey results of Mittenberg and Burton.[38] Their survey of clinicians dealing with individuals with postconcussion syndrome revealed that education, reassurance, psychological support, cognitive reattribution of symptoms, and gradual reactivation were associated with a better treatment outcome. Mittenberg and his colleagues have incorporated these principles into a treatment manual for therapists[39] and a similar handbook for patients.[40]

The importance of adequate education cannot be underestimated. Minderhoud, Boelens, Huizenga, and Saan[41] documented a marked reduction in postconcussional sequelae following a program of information and encouragement. However, care must be taken in providing such information and patient education must be more than mere diagnostic labeling. Such a practice has been shown to actually contribute to the problem that the intervention was designed to reduce.[42]

Clearly, brief psychological intervention based on the cognitive-behavioral model can successfully reduce the number of reported symptoms and shorten the duration of such symptoms in individuals with postconcussion syndrome.[43] This work has been extended further by Paniac,[44] who reported on his own efforts at early intervention following MTBI. He found that one session of appropriate information and education was just as effective (as measured by reduction in subjective symptoms in the treatment groups) as a multidisciplinary assessment and treatment program.

Prevention

Any discussion of treatment strategies must recognize the adage that an ounce of prevention is worth a pound of treatment. In athletic pursuits, prevention can occur on many levels. For example, the development of equipment standards can range from a consideration of personal protective devices, such as helmet type, to environmental considerations, such as the nature of the playing surface. Standards alone, however, will not prevent injury, and adherence to standards by manufacturers and facility owners and compliance by players are essential. In addition, rules of play or conduct along with appropriate enforcement can serve to reduce injury in the athlete. Other variables, such as long distance travel and frequency of contests, may also contribute to injury risk, but their impact has yet to be studied. Prevention measures must not be arbitrary, and the impact of any changes needs to be carefully evaluated for injury reduction. For example, Clarke and Jordan[10] cite data showing the reduction in brain injury following the development of uniform standards for football helmets. They further cite the success in reducing fatal cerebral and spinal injuries following the rule change with respect to head-first tackling and blocking. Unfortunately, few sports have yet developed sufficient data collection methods to permit the necessary evaluations.

SUMMARY

This chapter has reviewed the potential uses of neuropsychological testing to document neurocognitive changes associated with MTBI in athletes and to aid in charting recovery and evaluating intervention. We have specifically focused on the approach that is currently used by both the NFL and the NHL and by a number of college teams. Although research is currently in its initial stages, neuropsychological assessment programs should yield important new information in the months and years to come.

REFERENCES

1. Van Raalte JL, Brewer BW (eds): Exploring Sport and Exercise Psychology. American Psychological Association, Washington, DC, 1996
2. Matser EJT: Sports neuropsychology. In Jordan BD (ed): Sports Neurology, 2nd Ed. Lippincott-Raven Publishers, Philadelphia, 1998, pp 15–27
3. Povlishock JT, Valadka AB: Pathobiology of traumatic brain injury. In Finlayson MAJ, Garner SH (eds): Brain Injury Rehabilitation: Clinical Considerations. Williams & Wilkins, Baltimore, 1994, pp 11–33
4. Alexander MP: Mild traumatic brain injury: pathophysiology, natural history, and clinical management. Neurology 45:1253–1260, 1995

5. Novack TA, Dillon MC, Jackson WT: Neurochemical mechanisms in brain injury and treatment: a review. J Clin Exp Neuropsychol 18:685–706, 1996

6. Hovda DA: The neurobiology of cerebral concussion: Why is the brain so vulnerable after a concussion? Paper presented at Sports Related Concussion and Nervous System Injuries, Lake Buena Vista, March 1998.

7. Schneider RC: Head and Neck Injuries in Football. Williams & Wilkins, Baltimore, 1973

8. Saunders RL, Harbaugh RE: Second impact in catastrophic contact sports head trauma. JAMA 538–539, 52, 1984

9. Cantu RC: Second-impact syndrome. In Cantu RC (ed): Clinics in Sports Medicine: Neurologic Athletic Head and Neck Injuries. WB Saunders Co., Toronto, 1998, pp 37–44

10. Clarke KS, Jordan BD: Sports neuroepidemiology. In Jordan BD (ed): Sports Neurology, 2nd Ed. Lippincott-Raven Publishers, Philadelphia, 1998

11. Davis TM, McKelvey MK: Medico-legal aspects of athletic head injury. In Cantu RC (ed): Clinics in Sports Medicine: Neurologic Athletic Head and Neck Injuries. WB Saunders Co., Toronto, 1998, pp 71–82

12. Matser EJT, Dessels AGH, Jordan BD, et al: Chronic traumatic brain injury in professional soccer players. Neurology, 51:791–796, 1998

13. Ryan AJ: Intracranial injuries resulting from boxing. In Cantu RC (ed): Clinics in Sports Medicine: Neurologic Athletic Head and Neck Injuries. WB Saunders Co., Toronto, 1998, pp 155–168

14. Jordan BD: Boxing. In Jordan BD (ed): Sports Neurology, 2nd Ed. Lippincott-Raven Publishers, Philadelphia, 1998, pp 351–366

15. Thurman DJ, Branche CN, Sniezek JE: The epidemiology of sports-related traumatic brain injuries in the United States: recent developments. J Head Trauma Rehabil 13 (2):1–8, 1998

16. Gerberich SG, Priest JD, Boen JR, et al: Concussion incidences and severity in secondary school varsity football players. Am J Public Health 73 (12):1370–1375, 1983

17. Kelly JP, Rosenberg JH: Diagnosis and management of MTBI in sports. Neurology 48:575–580, 1997

18. McCrea M, Kelly JP, Kluge J, et al: Standardized assessment of MTBI in football players. Neurology 48:586–588, 1997

19. Barth J, Alves W, Ryan T, et al: Mild head injury in sports: neuropsychological sequelae and recovery of function. In Levin H, Eisenberg H, Benton A (eds): Mild Head Injury. Oxford University Press, New York, 1989, pp 257–275

20. Macciocchi S, Barth JT, Alves W, et al: Neuropsychological functioning and recovery after mild head injury in collegiate athletes. Neurosurgery 39(3):510–514, 1996

21. Lovell M, Maroon J, Haag B: Cognitive functioning in high school football players. A paper presented at the annual convention of the International Neuropsychological Society. Vancouver, 1989

22. Lovell MR: Evaluation of the professional athlete. In Bailes JE, Lovell MR, Maroon JC (eds): Sports-Related Concussion. Quality Medical Publishers, St Louis, 1998

23. Wechsler D: Wechsler Adult Intelligence Scale—III. The Psychological Corporation, San Antonio, 1997

24. Brandt J: The Hopkins Verbal Learning Test: development of a new memory test with six equivalent forms. Clin Neuropsychologist 5:125–142, 1991

25. Benedict RHB: Brief Visuospatial Memory Test—Revised. Psychological Assessment Resources, Odessa, Fla, 1997

26. Reitan R: Validity of the trail making test as an indicator of organic brain damage. Percept Mot Skills 8:271–276, 1958

27. Benton A, Hamsher K: Multilingual Aphasia Examination. University of Iowa Press, Iowa City, 1978

28. Lovell M, Collins M: Neuropsychological assessment of the college football player. J Head Trauma Rehabil 13(2):9–26, 1998

29. Ruff R: Ruff Figural Fluency Test. Psychological Assessment Resources, Odessa, Fla, 1988

30. D'Elia L, Satz P: The Color Trail Making Test. Psychological Assessment Resources, Odessa, Fla, 1989

31. Smith A: Symbol Digit Modalities Test Manual. Western Psychological Services, Los Angeles, 1982

32. Kay T: Neuropsychological treatment of mild traumatic brain injury. J Head Trauma Rehabil 8(3):74–85, 1993

33. Zazler MD: Neuromedical diagnosis in management of post concussive disorders. In Horn LJ, Zazler ND (eds): Medical Rehabilitation of Traumatic Brain Injury. Hanley and Belfus, Philadelphia, 1996, pp 133–170

34. Horn LJ: Post concussive headaches. In Malanga GA (ed): Spine: State of the Art Reviews, 12:377–393, 1998

35. Richter KJ, Cowan DM, Kaschalk SM: A protocol for managing pain, sleep disorder, and associated psychological sequelae of presumed mild head injury. J Head Trauma Rehabil 10:7–15, 1995

36. Uomoto JM, Esselman BC: Traumatic brain injury and chronic pain: differential types and rates by head injury severity. Arch Phys Med Rehabil 74:61–64, 1993

37. Pryse-Phillips WEN, Boddick DW, Edmeads JG, et al: Guidelines for the non-pharmacologic management of migraine in clinical practice. Can Med Assoc J 159:47–54, 1998

38. Mittenberg W, Burton DE: A survey of treatments for post concussion syndrome. Brain Injury 8: 429–437, 1994

39. Ferguson RJ, Mittenberg W: Cognitive-behavioural treatment of post concussion syndrome: a therapist's manual. In Van Hasselt V, Hersen M (eds): Sourcebook of Psychological Treatment Manuals for Adult Disorders. Plenum Press, New York, 1995, pp 615–655

40. Mittenberg W, Zielinski R, Fichera S: Recovery from mild head injury: a treatment manual for patients. Psychother Private Practice 12:37–52, 1993

41. Minderhoud JM, Boelens MEN, Huizenga J, Saan RG: Treatment of minor head injuries. Clin Neurol Neurosurg Psychiatry 82:127–140, 1980

42. Haynes RB, Sackett DL, Taylor DW, et al: Increased absenteeism at work after detection and labeling of hypertensive patients. N Engl J Med 229:741–744, 1978

43. Mittenberg W, Tremont G, Zielinski R, et al: Cognitive-behavioural intervention of post concussion syndrome. Arch Clin Neuropsychol 11:139–145, 1996

44. Paniac C: Informed treatment. Recovery 9:22–24, 1998

18

Exercise in Neuromuscular Conditions

GUNNAR GRIMBY

GENERAL ASPECTS

Usually neuromuscular disorders are defined as diseases or injuries in the peripheral motor neuron. In this presentation, however, disorders mainly located in the upper motor neurons also are included, such as spinal cord injury and stroke. The exercise problems in upper motor neuron lesions will, however, only be considered from the muscular performance point of view, not including, for example, aspects on perception or cognition.

When evaluating the use of exercise in various neuromuscular conditions the following principal questions should first be answered.

Questions

- Are there neuropathic or myopathic muscular changes?
- In *neuropathy,* to what degree has the loss of motor units been compensated by reinnervation and muscle fiber hypertrophy? What is the resulting muscular performance capacity?
- In *myopathy,* which muscular structures are damaged and what might the reaction be at overload? Is there a progressive or relatively stable condition? Is the myopathy in a relatively early or late stage? Will there also be cardiopathic changes?
- Is the *neural control* altered, and will there be changes in muscular tone and stiffness? What secondary effects on muscle structure and function might be caused by an altered innervation and neural control?
- Will factors of importance for muscle endurance be affected, and should muscle fatigue be specially considered?

- Is the cardiorespiratory performance affected? Which etiologic factors can be identified? To what extent will cardiorespiratory capacity limit the ability for muscular exercise?

USE AND MISUSE OF EXERCISE

Before use and misuse of exercise in various conditions, including some exercise guidelines, are discussed, *general aspects* will be given with respect to the above mentioned questions.

Exercise can be divided into resistance and endurance programs. Endurance can emphasize local muscle endurance or whole body endurance.

Resistance Training

In resistance training it is generally accepted that the initial effects of a training program usually are in the improvement of neural activation.[1] Different approaches to study changes in neural activation are used. With the superimposed single twitch technique the question is whether all motor units are activated. With tetanic muscle stimulation, the effect of maximal neural activation may be simulated. The use of electromyographic (EMG) recordings together with strength measurements has some methodologic problems at repeated recordings on different occasions. Nevertheless, the increase in maximal EMG without an increase in the ratio between EMG and muscle force would indicate an increased neural activation without muscle hypertrophy.

After a certain period in normal subjects (presumably a couple of weeks), the resistance training will stimulate and result in muscle fiber hypertrophy with an increased muscle volume. Differences here may be seen among different fiber types and also depending on the pattern of the resistance exercise with respect to intensity, speed of movement, number of repetitions, etc. The training effects are rather task specific, which must be taken into consideration in designing training programs.

In patients with disorders of the peripheral motor neuron, lack of optimal neural activation might occur and can be analyzed with any of the approaches mentioned above. There might, however, already be an overuse of practically all motor units in certain daily activities, and then increased neural activation with training in those activities would not be expected. Because the stimulus for increase of the contractile proteins and muscle fiber hypertrophy is increased muscle tension due to the resistance load, the questions in myopathies are whether there is any capacity to react positively to the increased load or if that will have negative effects with damage of muscle fiber elements. In neuropathy, on the other hand, there is a large potential for muscle fiber hypertrophy, if not already reached spontaneously, as can be seen in postpolio muscles.[2,3]

In disorders of the upper motor neuron, the basic dysfunction is failure of neural motor control, resulting in, for example, altered antagonist activation and co-contraction. There may also develop some muscle weakness, but more rarely a major reduction of muscle volume occurs. In impaired motor control, there will also be changes in muscle tone resulting in an increased muscle stiffness. Exercise programs must emphasize the effect of various activities and posture on muscle tone and if possible reduce counteracting antagonist and co-contraction activity. Exercise programs should also aim to improve the motor control, for example, by motor learning principles. Increase in muscle tone and stiffness will, however, not only have negative effects, as will be discussed more specifically. With slight changes in motor control, resistance training may have effects not too different from in normal subjects.

Endurance Training

Endurance training will have both central and peripheral effects. Central effects are reduction of heart rate and ventilation, increased stroke volume of the heart at a certain submaximal workload, and also reduction in arterial blood pressure. Peripheral effects are increased capillarization, increase in oxidative muscle enzymes, and other metabolic changes. Changes in the muscular reaction to exercise will have an effect on the central cardiorespiratory control mechanisms. It is now well documented that part of the adaptation to an increased exercise performance is limited to exercise with the specific trained muscle groups (eg, with one-legged training studies). This has some application in training with hemisymptoms, the muscle adaptation being different in the extremities of the two sides. There is reason to believe that the adaptation and level of training are suboptimal in the muscles and in the cardiorespiratory system in many conditions with neuromuscular disorders. There is, however, limited information in the literature. In some disorders there are specific limitations in the cardiorespiratory function, as in stroke patients with an additional coronary heart disease,[4] in spinal cord injury, poliomyelitis, and other neuropathies affecting respiratory muscles, and in muscle dystrophy with respiratory muscle weakness. This must naturally be considered when evaluating cardiorespiratory performance and endurance.

The possibility to use peripheral training principle[5] with endurance training of several separate muscle groups to get the peripheral adaptation to endurance exercise has been applied in different clinical situations, as in patients with cardiac failure.[6] This principle could be used also in neuromuscular conditions with central factors limiting cardiorespiratory performance. Another way to get peripheral muscle adaptation and with some general benefit for the cardiorespiratory performance is the use of functional electrical stimulation (FES) of paretic muscles, as in subjects after spinal cord injury.[7]

MYOPATHIES

Most studies of exercise has been made in boys with Duchenne muscular dystrophy and in adults with myotonic dystrophy. There is a concern of overload because the cytoskeleton in the muscle cell has a limited tolerance to an increased load and might be further damaged. There are, however, reports of increased strength in boys 5 to 11 years old with Duchenne muscular dystrophy using a submaximal isokinetic training program.[8] From uncontrolled studies in Duchenne (subjects 5 to 10 years old), limb-girdle (subjects 8 to 39 years), and facioscapular (subjects 22 to 45 years) muscular dystrophy, Vignos and Watkins[9] concluded that exercise programs do *not* result in overwork weakness when properly supervised but may increase muscle strength. Other more recent studies about resistance training in adults with slowly progressive disorders[10–12] have indicated beneficial effects, but control groups are lacking or the opposite extremity has been used as a control. In a randomized control study[13] of 33 adult subjects with myotonic dystrophy training three times per week for 24 weeks with weights adapted to their force, the trained group of subjects showed neither positive nor negative average effects of the training program, evaluating strength as well as performance in various activities. However, there were indications that the stronger subjects—those with less muscle damage—could show some trainability, which also is in agreement with the findings of Milner-Brown and Miller.[10] In a study by McCartney et al.[14] of various disorders using superimposed single twitch technique, it was demonstrated that the increase in muscle strength could be the result of neural factors.

Electrical stimulation has been used to strengthen muscles in muscular dystrophy. At a frequency of 5 to 10 Hz for 1 hour three times daily for 7 to 11 weeks, stimulation of the tibialis anterior muscle in boys 5 to 12 years gave a significant increase in maximal voluntary contraction, whereas the contralateral unstimulated leg showed no significant change.[15] Interestingly, the effect of electrical stimulation did not appear until after 6 weeks of stimulation, indicating muscular contribution to the increased muscle strength. A possible explanation given was that growth of regenerating fibers became more rapid. In a study of adults 17 to 62 years of age with progressive muscular dystrophies, electrical stimulation with 30 Hz during 2 to 14 months combined with voluntary contractions could increase knee extensor but not anterior tibialis strength. The contralateral unstimulated knee extensor muscles showed considerably less increase. The stimulation was initially 30 minutes on alternate days and was then increased to 2 hours per day, 5 days per week.

In a recent report on resistance training in five patients with sporadic inclusion body myositis,[16] the repetition maximum as a measure of muscle strength increased after 12 weeks by 25% to 120% but was not seen in isometric muscle strength measurements. Repeated muscle biopsies did not reveal changes in the number and degree of degenerating fibers or inflammation. There was no evidence of immunocytotoxic exacerbation. This first study in a small number of patients points to the use of resistance exercise also in inflammatory myopathies, at least in less affected muscles. It is possible that such muscles experience some degree of disuse since other muscles are more affected and limit the activity level of the person. Strength training could then delay the progression of muscle weakness and atrophy in certain muscle groups when applied in the early stage of the disease.

Taken together, there might be some trainability for resistance exercise in myopathies, at least in younger patients or with light to moderate muscle deterioration. *Neural factors* are likely to be mainly responsible for the effect of training, which points to the specificity for trained type of exercise and may, for example, explain part of the lack of measured effects by Lindeman et al.[13] Overworked weakness is not recorded in well-monitored programs.

The importance of objective muscle strength measurements should be stressed. Manual muscle testing is *not* sufficient; hand-held myometers or dynamometers should be used, as should continuous recording of training load. In addition to any specific resistance training program, functional daily activities should be encouraged.

Respiratory muscles might also be trained with the same limitations as above for skeletal muscles. There are reports of increased respiratory muscle strength after inspiratory resistive training[17] and also of increased endurance of ventilation.[18] In more recent studies, Wanke et al.[19] and Vilozni et al.[20] demonstrated that inspiratory muscle training could improve inspiratory muscle strength and endurance after just 1 month of training in the early stage of Duchenne muscular dystrophy. However, the risk of causing respiratory muscle fatigue by training programs has been pointed out,[21] and it is necessary to be cautious with respiratory muscle training, probably still more so than with skeletal muscles.

There are few reports on the feasibility and effect on endurance training programs in muscular dystrophy. Reduced aerobic work performance is found, related not only directly to the reduced muscle mass but also to the relatively sedentary life-style due to gradual loss of muscle strength. Wright et al[22] recently reported the effect of a walking program 15 to 30 minutes 3 to 4 days per week at 50% to 60% of the heart rate reserve of the subjects, thus a low-intensity training program. Seven of the eleven subjects, with a mean age of 37 years and slowly progressive neuromuscular disease, had myotonic dystrophy and one had limb girdle dystrophy (LGS); the remaining three had hereditary motor and sensory neuropathy (HMSN). There was a significant reduction in the heart rate at submaximal workload, but the increase in peak power output and maximal oxygen uptake was insignificant. It was concluded that a low-intensity type of training is well tolerated and may increase physical capacity in this type of subject with the exception of the subject with LGS, who also was the weakest and had a problem keeping his target heart rate at training.

NEUROPATHIES

Poliomyelitis

Studies in subjects with poliomyelitis sequelae have provided further insight into the adaptive processes in the skeletal muscle. The relatively high intensity load during repeated short daily activities, such as rising from a chair or climbing stairs, can lead to muscle fiber hypertrophy, as already pointed out. In general it seems that the adaptation to force development has a priority compared to the adaptation to endurance.[23] Because of increased interest in the late polio symptoms, such as those seen in postpolio syndrome,[24] some studies have analyzed the adaptation to exercise. Both resistance training and endurance training have been studied.

Resistance Training

Resistance training can have an effect on both neural and muscular factors. Einarson[25] was able to demonstrate in 12 postpolio subjects that a combined program of isokinetic and isometric training of the knee extensors three times per week for 6 weeks could increase the strength in the order of 17% and with no change in the untrained knee flexors. The subjects had grade 3+ or more on the manual muscle testing scale before training. Although muscle fiber areas increased in most subjects, there was no significant change in the group of subjects, indicating that the main training effect was caused by the neural factors. The training effect was partly maintained 6 to 12 months afterward. There was no evidence of histopathologic changes with exercise indicating no negative effects of the training program.

Fillyaw and colleagues[26] studied a long-term nonfatiguing resistance exercise program with weights according to the 10 RM (repetition maximum) principle (every other day for 1 to 2 years) in 17 subjects with postpolio syndrome. They found an average increase of 8.4% in strength in the trained knee extensor and arm flexor muscles; 10 RM increased an average of 78%.

Agre and co-workers[27,28] also reported increased strength from nonfatiguing exercise without adverse effects. In their first study[27] on 12 subjects in a supervised home program, weights were used for knee extensor training. Although the dynamometric measured strength did not increase significantly, the average amount of weight that the subjects could lift increased by over 60%. There was no change in the serum concentration of creatine kinase or the amount of jitter and blocking in the EMG. Also, the second report[28] on seven postpolio subjects with both dynamometer and weight training showed no adverse effects and an increase in isometric and isokinetic strength by 36% and 15%, respectively, and of the maximum weight by 47%. Also, the endurance measured as the time the subjects could hold 40% of maximal voluntary contraction increased after training.

Spector and co-workers[29] showed also that a supervised resistance training program could be conducted without serologic and histologic evidence of muscular damage. In six subjects with postpolio muscular atrophy, training increased strength in knee extensors by 41% and 61% and in elbow extensors by 54% and 71% in two types of dynamic tests. There was no change in muscle cross-sectional area as measured by magnetic resonance imaging. Up to 20% improvement was maintained after cessation of training.

To sum up, in postpolio subjects with a remaining muscle strength above what is needed to counteract the gravity effect on the extremity, a well-supervised nonfatiguing resistance training program can be used without adverse effects and with usually a substantial increase in strength, probably mainly caused by improved neural activation of the muscle. Muscles with a demonstrated overuse in daily activities,[30] such as walking, seen in tibialis anterior muscle, have not been studied with respect to additional training.

Endurance Training

Evidence in the literature is less clear on endurance training, and this topic has several aspects to take into account, namely, the various limiting factors for exercise in the cardiorespiratory system, in muscles, or in joints. From the cardiorespiratory standpoint, postpolio subjects are usually deconditioned.[31,32] Jones and colleagues[33] reported in a controlled study an increase in aerobic power by 15% after a 16-week, thrice weekly aerobic exercise program, in 16 training subjects, but there was no change in the control group of 21 subjects. Subjectively the exercising subjects noted a decrease in fatigue during their daily activities.

A 6-month, twice weekly combined endurance and strength training program in groups studied by Ernstoff et al.[34] increased peak exercise performance on an exercise ergometer, reduced heart rate (6 bpm) at 70 W, and increased maximal heart rate (12 bpm). Muscle strength increased in some muscle groups. Except for one subject, there were no adverse effects. That one subject, who deteriorated in function, had a very unusual fiber composition (recorded in several muscle groups) with a high proportion of type II fibers and also marked fatigue both at testing and at training. The subject still wanted to participate and demonstrated during the subsequent half year, with reduced activity, a return to pretraining strength values and less fatigue. This case demonstrates the necessity to carefully monitor training programs.[35]

Also, the movement energetics can be improved by aerobic training, as shown by Dean and Ross,[36] without improved cardiorespiratory conditioning. The importance of distributing exercise and rest intervals to avoid fatigue in polio muscles, which may recover slower than normal muscles, has been stressed by several authors, such as Agre and Rodriquez.[37]

No studies have been performed on flexibility exercises, since joint contractures may impair the ability to function. Avoidance of pain is also necessary in the training programs, and pain has recently been demonstrated to be more prominent in moderately weak extremities in relatively active individuals than in those with greater weakness.[38] This indicates the need to give advice to monitor the exercise patterns with respect to intensity and distribution of activity and rest periods, particularly in relatively mobile individuals. The role of exercise in persons with postpolio syndrome has been summarized by Agre.[39] Pool training often can be recommended and may reduce pain and modify activity pattern.

Respiratory Training

Respiratory muscle training has only been sparsely studied in subjects after polio, and respiratory limitation to exercise is rather uncommon, since those individuals also are limited by their extremity muscle weakness.

Peripheral Neuropathies

Patients with hereditary motor and sensory neuropathy (HMSN) were studied by Lindeman et al,[13] who conducted a 24-week home training program three times per week in 13 patients using 13 other patients as randomized controls. Weight training was used initially at 60% of 1 RM, and in a later part of the training up to 80% of 1 RM and different lower leg muscles were trained. Isokinetic knee extension strength increased by 14% and flexion strength by 13%. The time for comfortably walking 6 meters decreased. The study gave no indication whether the increase in strength was due to neural or muscular factors.

Home exercise training program effects have also been reported in patients with chronic peripheral neuropathy, an immune-mediated peripheral nerve root disorder with symmetric motor and sensory involvement of both proximal and distal muscles.[40] An exercise program of strengthening various muscle groups with Thera-Band and cycling or walking for 10 to 20 minutes was used daily. Training took place in 14 subjects during 6 weeks with 14 subjects randomized to a control group. Manual muscle testing was used, and the results were expressed in an averaged muscle score (AMS). AMS increased in the training group compared with the control group. The training group also increased in the physical limitation scale of the instrument SF-36. Positive effects from low-intensity (50% to 60% of heart rate reserve) training by walking were described in subjects with HMSN studied together with subjects with muscular dystrophy[22] (see discussion of myopathies).

In *Guillain-Barré syndrome* (GBS), the manifestations are heterogeneous and the outcome differs, as described in a large-scale prospective study.[41] The effect of training will depend on the remaining muscular impairment, but training effects similar to those in other neuropathic conditions would be expected. Pitetti et al[42] described positive effects of endurance training in a case study.

MYASTHENIA GRAVIS

Myasthenia gravis is characterized clinically by muscular weakness and fatigability caused by a decrease in the amount of acetylcholine at the neuromuscular junction. The exact etiology is unknown, but it is probably linked to an autoimmune disorder. The weakness increases with exercise, which is used for testing. Light activities of short duration can be without problems, whereas patients may have difficulty performing prolonged moderate activities. The feasibility and effects of physical training can therefore be questioned. However, Lohi and co-workers[43] demonstrated in 11 patients with mild or moderate myasthenia gravis that a resistance training program of 27 to 30 sessions gave a 23% increase of maximal voluntary force of the knee extensors. There was no significant change on the untrained control side. No change was noted in the fatigue test with repetitive maximal isometric muscle contractions. The patients did not experience any subjective discomfort or any adverse effect of the training. Thus physical training could be carried out safely in patients with mild myasthenia gravis.

SPINAL CORD INJURY

In patients with paresis or paralysis below the injury level and normal innervated muscles above this level, the effect of training differs depending on which muscles are involved. For the paretic muscles, effects of resistance training would be similar to those in the neuropathies discussed above. In normal innervated muscles there is a great need for strengthening training to allow for as much independence in transfer and locomotion as possible. Effects on strength and endurance have also been demonstrated in several reports with an adaptation similar to well-trained normal subjects, for example, an increased level of oxidative enzymes, increased capillarization, and even an increased proportion of type I fibers[44] in the anterior portion of the deltoid muscle in trained wheelchair users. The training program should follow similar lines as in able-bodied subjects.

For the cardiorespiratory adaptation, however, the autonomic nervous system will have a role that can be altered in this patient group. The heart rate increase by exercise will be reduced in tetraplegic subjects[45] because of the lack of sympathetic drive in the cervical spine lesion. In subjects with lower spinal cord lesion and paraplegia, an exaggerated heart rate response might be found because of several factors, such as hemodynamic dysregulation imposed by the lower extremity immobilization and the vasomotor dysfunction. The reduced venous return may contribute to an elevated heart rate response to exercise.

Functional Electrical Stimulation

An approach to training that has received interest during recent years is the use of FES. By using multichannel FES–assisted ambulation, Jacobs et al[7] showed after 32 sessions during 11 weeks a significant increase also in peak power output, peak oxygen uptake, and peak values to fatigue at arm ergometry. The submaximal heart rate levels were also lower after training. Thus this training resulted in task-nonspecific training adaptation with an improved cardiovascular adaptation. Such a training approach may benefit subjects' participation in efforts demanding upper body activities.

Studies on the adaptation of the paretic muscles with neuromuscular electrical stimulation at leg bicycle exercise have also been performed. A 10% increase in peak oxygen uptake at leg exercise was noted by Hooker et al[46] in eight males with spinal cord lesions. In the trained muscles, changes were seen after 6 and 12 months in the myosin heavy chain (MHC) distribution, with a dominance of MHC IIA, as in the more oxidative and fatigue-resistant muscle fibers, instead of equal amounts of MHC IIA and MHC IIB.[47] This finding shows also that the paralyzed muscles can adapt with training.

Because many of the subjects with spinal cord lesions are in the younger age-groups there is a relatively widespread interest to participate in various sport activities. Present knowledge about optimal training procedures and adaptive mechanisms for physical training is limited but still gives valuable basic information. Further studies also directly related to various sport activities are needed with measurement of energy expenditures, mechanical efficiency at wheelchair propulsion, and thermoregulation, which might be impaired.

STROKE

The effect of stroke on exercise performance depends on several factors: the degree of deterioration of motor control, increased motor tone, deconditioning, and the effect of any cardiovascular disorders.[4] There is also still controversy concerning the feasibility and benefit of resistance exercise in stroke patients. All these aspects cannot be dealt with here, and this review will mainly concentrate on the effect of resistance and endurance training programs in patients with a moderate loss of ability in locomotor activities and who are or will be walkers. Recent approaches in walking training will also be discussed.

Deficits in muscular strength are among the most common impairments following stroke. Although a number of authorities have suggested that it is not appropriate to measure muscle strength and that, at the least, such measurements are difficult to interpret, there are a number of recent reports on muscle strength[48] and also on the effects of resistance training in stroke patients. Decreased strength has been demonstrated not only on the side contralateral

to the brain lesion but also on the ipsilateral side. Patients with hemiparesis not only may have difficulty in generating the force but also a reduced ability to generate the force within a certain time frame. The stroke patient, however, does not seem to have a greater rate of decline in force across increasing velocities than normal subjects have.[48]

Several factors are involved in the reduction in muscle strength in stroke patients.[49] A decreased number of functional motor units after stroke has been demonstrated by McComas et al.[50] There may be changes in the recruitment order of motor units and in the motor unit firing rate. A concomitant activation of the antagonist muscles will result in a net reduction of the produced torque.[51] However, spasticity of the antagonists does not seem to have a major role in limiting the force production of the agonist muscles,[52] but if limitation does occur, it is more by passive mechanical properties of the antagonist muscles. An increased muscle stiffness in the agonists can, however, have a positive effect on the development of force in a fast eccentric-concentric muscle activation, such as in running or jumping, and contribute to a larger than normal increase of the concentric force after an eccentric activation.[53]

Muscle atrophy may develop but has been described differently with respect to fiber types, probably because of different samples of patients and different timing after onset of stroke. Edström[54] and, recently, Hachisuka et al[55] reported that there can be a dominance of type II atrophy, which is assumed partly to be due to disuse, and that unknown central trophic factors also are suggested.

The question is then to what extent the reduction in muscle fiber size and muscle strength after stroke is reversible by training. In a recent study by Miller and Light,[56] graded resistive exercise gave similar effects in the paretic and the nonparetic side on different performance variables. Thus this type of exercise did not have detrimental effects in the paretic muscles. Reports have started to appear on an increase in strength after resistance training in stroke patients.[57] Eccentric knee extensor training was found to have some advantages compared with only concentric training in the study by Engardt et al,[57] which reported increased restraint of the antagonist muscles.

There are also reasons to assume that a reduced endurance may develop in stroke patients. Reduced oxidative capacity of the paretic muscles has been demonstrated.[58] In the only randomized study yet, 10 weeks of modified bicycle ergometer training improved maximal oxygen uptake by 14%, which is similar to what is expected in healthy older persons.[59] Interestingly, the maximal work performance increased more, which suggested that there was also an improvement of mechanical efficiency at least in the trained type of exercise. An improved mechanical efficiency, as indicated by reduced energy expenditure at a fixed submaximal workload after low-intensity treadmill aerobic training, was demonstrated after a 6-month program in stroke patients (mean age 67 years; on average 3 years since stroke). The subjects also performed the submaximal workload with a lower heart rate and respiratory exchange ratio. This suggests that task-oriented aerobic exercise may improve functional mobility and the cardiovascular fitness profile in this population.

Further resistance and endurance training studies are needed, particularly in the later period of rehabilitation and after the ordinary rehabilitation programs are finished.

A training approach that has received considerable interest in recent years is the use of partial body support for initiating the walking training. It could also be useful in later stages in stroke patients with low walking performance. The concept is based on the assumption that by walking with body weight support, spinal reflexes may be used in the training and that the stabilization of the body will enhance the walking pattern. In a single case design, Hesse et al[60] could demonstrate improvements in gait ability and walking velocity with partial body support training, and results were positive in a controlled study by Visitin et al.[61] The clinical usefulness of this addition to traditional walking training remains, however, to be further studied.

PRACTICAL COMMENTS

In the choice of exercise programs there are several aspects to consider.

Aim of the Program

- Is the main aim to increase strength or endurance or a combination?

- Does endurance involve cardiovascular fitness or local muscle endurance or both?
- Can different components of the program compromise each other?
- Are there limiting factors besides the impaired neuromuscular function?
- What are the overall aims with respect to improvement of ability in daily activities?

A recent report on muscle dysfunction in relation to physical disabilities in the elderly population by Dutta et al[62] focused on different aspects of ability in performance that also are relevant for younger individuals with chronic disabilities.

Ability to Perform a Normal Daily Workload of Activities. Not only the necessary muscle strength to perform the different daily activities has to be taken into account, but also the performance speed and the time the person can perform the individual activities. Thus training must also include activities during natural functional circumstances.

Ability to Do High-Demand Tasks of Normal Daily Life Quickly and Without Advance Notice ("Emergency" Tasks). High-demand tasks include abruptly stopping at a crosswalk, avoiding persons in a crowded area, and rising from a ground position (voluntarily or after a fall). This requires training of fast and appropriate muscle activation and indicates specific training for certain situations.

Ability to Engage in Physical Activities Sufficient to Maintain Cardiovascular Fitness. To this should also be added "and to support body weight control." Muscle dysfunction that restricts the ability to perform moderate activities, such as walking (or comparable energy expenditure in wheelchair driving), could have significant negative health effects, such as weight gain and increased risk for the "metabolic" syndrome (increased insulin resistance, diabetes, hypertension) in addition to reduced cardiovascular fitness. It is important to understand the limiting factors for various activities to design suitable exercise programs and instruction for habitual daily activities.

Maintenance of Normal Biomechanics of Motion. Alterations in biomechanics of motion could increase energy expenditure and contribute to physical disabilities, such as osteoarthrosis and back pain. These could be precipitated or aggravated by the altered biomechanics of motion. It is important in the design of a training program to choose activities that do not further impair the biomechanical disorders and also, if necessary, arrange so that unstable joints are stabilized with orthoses and proper shoes are worn.

Choice of Intensity and Timing

The first questions to be asked are as follows:

- *On the muscular level.* Is it a myopathic or neurogenic condition? Are there specific fatigue problems, such as impaired neuromuscular transmission or muscle metabolic failure?
- *On the "central" level.* Is there a deteriorated motor control? Are there changes in the afferent signals from proprioceptors, vision, or hearing, or is there an impaired perception of those signals? Will this lead to balance problems or specific learning problems for different motor tasks? Are there cardiovascular limiting factors to be taken into account?

Myopathic Conditions

High resistance training should be avoided because it can lead to overload and further deterioration of muscle function. Submaximal training, especially in early clinical stages, could be beneficial and probably act through a better neural muscle activation and maintenance of endurance. Training is better with relatively short and not too fatiguing sessions repeated more often. This will increase the possibility to monitor and avoid unwanted side effects. It is important to find general exercises that can maintain cardiovascular fitness within the ability level of the person, such as cycling, wheelchair driving, pool exercises, and swimming.

Neuropathic Conditions

The risk for overload is less. The choice of training intensities depends to a large extent on the amount of neurogenic changes, utilization of compensatory mechanisms, reinnervation, and muscle fiber hypertrophy. Experience from analyses of muscle function and training experiences in postpolio individuals gives some guidelines.

If there is only a minor neuropathic change with good compensation and preserved or only slightly reduced muscle function, training should be performed as in normal individuals. High resistance training programs can be used also as general fitness programs.

With moderately reduced muscle function and when different muscle groups show different degrees of deterioration, programs have to be more individualized. Short periods of high resistance training may be used, if properly supervised. However, the training should start on a submaximal level and an improved neural activation might be achieved in addition to better fatigue resistance.

Training of local muscle endurance as well as of cardiovascular fitness should be included. Exercises should be chosen that are not limited by low function in certain muscle groups. Pool exercises, swimming, and bicycling have been successful exercises.

It is important to allow proper rest intervals, because the recovery after a fatiguing session might be prolonged. Repeated measurements of muscle function should be used to monitor the program. If signs of overload occur, the intensity should be reduced and usually the function recovers soon.

In persons with marked deterioration of muscle function in general or in specific key muscle groups, training programs to improve strength may not be feasible or may even be deleterious. In contrast, the exercise programs should emphasize learning to achieve energy-saving patterns of activity, an appropriate balance between activity and rest, and also maintenance of muscle endurance and if possible cardiovascular fitness.

Also, if cardiac or respiratory function is limited, this has to specifically be taken into account in the choice of the training program.

Altered Motor Control

- The effect of altered motor control should be evaluated. Is there an increased motor tone and muscle stiffness?
- Will certain types of physical activities enhance or even reduce muscle tone? Is there

evidence of co-contraction of synergists or antagonists, and what are the functional consequences of such an activity?

- Physical training may have to be modified.

However, recent studies support that resistance training can be performed and will have positive functional effects in patients with partial recovery of motor function and that it may reduce disuse muscle atrophy. Endurance may also be reduced by lack of activity, and endurance training should be encouraged in mobile stroke patients.

Group training and participation in regular training programs can be encouraged in persons with moderate motor deficits.

In patients with spinal cord lesions, functional electrical stimulation of paretic muscles seems to be useful in addition to the voluntary training of nonparetic muscles.

REFERENCES

1. Sale OG: Neural adaptation to resistance training. Med Sci Sports Exerc 20:S135–S145, 1988
2. Grimby G, Einarsson G, Hedberg M, Aniansson A: Muscle adaptive changes in postpolio subjects. Scand J Rehabil Med 21:19–26, 1989
3. Borg K, Borg J, Edström L, Grimby L: Effects of excessive use of remaining muscle fibers in prior polio and LV lesion. Muscle Nerve 11:1219–1230, 1988
4. Roth EJ: Heart disease in patients with stroke: incidence, impact, and implications for rehabilitation. Arch Phys Med Rehabil 74:752–760, 1993
5. Gaffney FA, Grimby G, Danneskiold-Samsöe B, Halskov O: Adaptation to peripheral muscle training. Scand J Rehabil Med 13:11–16, 1981
6. Cider Å, Tygesson H, Hedberg M, et al: Peripheral muscle training in patients with clinical signs of heart failure. Scand J Rehabil Med 29:121–127, 1997
7. Jacobs PL, Nash MS, Klose KJ, et al: Evaluation of a training program for persons with SCI paraplegia using the Parastep 1 ambulation system: part 2. Effects on physiological responses to peak arm ergometry. Arch Phys Rehabil Med 78:794–798, 1997
8. de Lateur BJ, Giaconi RM: Effect on maximal strength of submaximal exercise in Duchenne muscular dystrophy. Am J Phys Med 58:26–36, 1976
9. Vignos PJ, Watkins MP: The effect of exercise in muscular dystrophy. JAMA 197:843–848, 1966
10. Milner-Brown HS, Miller RG: Muscle strengthening through electric stimulation combined with low-resistance weights in patients with neuromuscular disorders. Arch Phys Med Rehabil 69:14–19, 1988
11. Aitkens SG, McCrory MA, Kilmer DD, Bernauer EM: Moderate resistance exercise program: its effect in slowly progressive neuromuscular disease. Arch Phys Med Rehabil 74:711–715, 1993
12. Kilmer DD, McCrory MA, Wright BS, et al: The effect of a high resistance exercise program in slowly progressive neuromuscular disease. Arch Phys Med Rehabil 75:560–563, 1994
13. Lindeman E, Lefflers P, Spaans F, et al: Strength training in patients with myotonic dystrophy and hereditary motor and sensory neuropathy: a randomized clinical trial. Arch Phys Med Rehabil 76:612–620, 1995
14. McCartney N, Moroz D, Garner SH, McComas AJ: The effects of strength training in patients with selected neuromuscular disorders. Med Sci Sports Exerc 20:362–368, 1988
15. Scott OM, Vrbova G, Hyde SA, Dubowitz V: Responses of muscles with Duchenne muscular dystrophia to chronic electrical stimulation. J Neurol Neurosurg Psychiatry 49:1427–1434, 1986
16. Spector SA, Lemmer JT, Koffman BM, et al: Safety and efficacy of strength training in patients with sporadic inclusion body myositis. Muscle Nerve 20:1242–1248, 1997
17. DiMarco AF, Kelling J, Sajovic M, et al: The effects of inspiratory resistive training on respiratory muscle functions in patients with muscular dystrophy. Muscle Nerve 8:284–290, 1985
18. Estrup C, Lyager S, Naera N, Olsen C: Effect of respiratory muscle training in patients with neuromuscular diseases and normals. Respiration 50:36–43, 1986
19. Wanke T, Toifl K, Merkle M, et al: Inspiratory muscle training in patients with Duchenne muscular dystrophy. Chest 105:475–482, 1994
20. Vilozni D, Bar-Yishay E, Gur I, et al: Computerized respiratory muscle training in children with Duchenne muscular dystrophy. Neuromuscul Disord 4:249–255, 1994
21. Smith PEM, Coakley JH, Edwards RHT: Respiratory muscle training in Duchenne muscular dystrophy. Muscle Nerve 11:784–785, 1988
22. Wright NC, Kilmer DD, McCrory MA, et al: Aerobic walking in slowly progressive neuromuscular disease: effect of a 12-week program. Arch Phys Med Rehabil 77:64–69, 1996
23. Tollbäck A: Neuromuscular compensation and adaptation to loss of lower motoneurones in man. Studies in prior-polio subjects. Karolinska Institute, Stockholm, Doctoral thesis, 1995
24. Halstead LS, Rossi CD: Post-polio syndrome: clinical experience with 132 consecutive outpa-

tients. In Halstead LS, Wiechers DO (eds): Research and clinical aspects of the late effects of poliomyelitis. Birth Defects 23(4):13–16, 1987

25. Einarson G: Muscle conditioning in late poliomyelitis. Arch Phys Med Rehabil 72:11–14, 1991

26. Fillyaw MJ, Badger GD, Goodwin GD, et al: The effects of long-term non-fatiguing resistance exercise in subjects with post-polio syndrome. Orthopedics 14:1253–1256, 1991

27. Agre JC, Rodriquez AA, Franke TM, et al: Low-intensity, alternative day exercise improves muscle performance without apparent adverse effect in postpolio patients. Am J Phys Med Rehabil 75:50–58, 1996

28. Agre JC, Rodriquez AA, Franke TM: Strength, endurance, and work capacity after muscle strengthening exercise in postpolio subjects. Arch Phys Med Rehabil 78:681–686, 1997

29. Spector SA, Gordon PG, Feuerstein IM, et al: Strength gains without muscle injury after strength training in patients with post polio muscular atrophy. Muscle Nerve 19:1282–1290, 1996

30. Grimby L, Tollbäck A, Müller U, Larsson L: Fatigue of chronically overused motor units in prior polio patients. Muscle Nerve 19:728–737, 1996

31. Owen RR, Jones D: Polio residual clinic: conditioning exercise program. Orthopedics 8:882–883, 1985

32. Stanghelle JK, Festvåg L, Aksnes AK: Pulmonary function and symptom limited exercise stress testing in subjects with late sequelae of poliomyelitis. Scand J Rehabil Med 25:125–129, 1993

33. Jones DR, Speier J, Canine K, et al: Cardiorespiratory responses to aerobic training by patients with postpoliomyelitis sequelae. JAMA 261:3255–3258, 1989

34. Ernstoff B, Wetterqvist H, Kvist H, Grimby G: Endurance training effect on individuals with postpoliomyelitis. Arch Phys Med Rehabil 77:843–848, 1996

35. Grimby G, Einarsson G: Post-polio management. Crit Rev Phys Rehabil Med 2:189–200, 1991

36. Dean E, Ross J: Effect of modified aerobic training on movement energetics in polio survivors. Orthopedics 14:1243–1246, 1991

37. Agre JC, Rodriquez AA: Intermittent isometric activity: its effect on muscle fatigue in post polio subjects. Arch Phys Med Rehabil 72:971–975, 1991

38. Willén C, Grimby G: Pain, physical activity and disability in individuals with late effects of polio. Arch Phys Med Rehabil 79:915–919, 1998

39. Agre JC: The role of exercise in the patient with post-polio syndrome. Ann N Y Acad Sci 753:921–934, 1995

40. Ruthland JL, Shields RK: The effects of a home exercise program on impairment and health-related quality of life in persons with chronic peripheral neuropathies. Phys Ther 77:1026–1039, 1997

41. Beghi E, Bono A, Bogliun G: The prognosis and main prognostic indicators of Guillain-Barré syndrome. A multicentre prospective study of 297 patients. Brain 119:2053–2061, 1996

42. Pitetti KH, Barrett PJ, Abbas D: Endurance exercise training in Guillain-Barré syndrome. Arch Phys Med Rehabil 74:761–765, 1993

43. Lohi EL, Lindberg C, Andersen O: Physical training effects in myasthenia gravis. Arch Phys Med Rehabil 74:1178–1180, 1993

44. Schantz P, Sjöberg B, Widebeck A-M, Ekblom B: Skeletal muscle of trained and untrained paraplegics and tetraplegics. Acta Physiol Scand 161:31–39, 1997

45. Hjeltnes N: Cardiorespiratory capacity in tetra- and paraplegia shortly after injury. Scand J Rehabil Med 18:65–70, 1986

46. Hooker SP, Scremin AM, Mutton DL, et al: Peak and submaximal physiologic responses following electrical stimulation leg cycle ergometer training. J Rehabil Res Dev 32:361–366, 1995

47. Mohr T, Andersen JL, Biering-Sörensen F, et al: Long term adaptation to electrically induced cycle training in severe spinal cord injured individuals. Spinal Cord 35:1–16, 1997

48. Bohannon RW: Measurement and nature of muscle strength in patients after stroke. J Neuro Rehab 11:115–125, 1997

49. Bourbonnais D, Noven SV: Weakness in patients with hemiparesis. Am J Occup Ther 43:313–319, 1989

50. McComas AJ, Sica REP, Upton ARM, Aquilera N: Functional changes in motoneurones of hemiparetic patients. J Neurol Neurosurg Psychiatry 40:183–193, 1973

51. Knutsson E, Mårtensson A: Dynamic motor capacity in spastic paresis and its relation to prime mover dysfunction, spastic reflexes and antagonist co-contraction. Scand J Rehabil Med 12:93–106, 1980

52. Gowland C, de Bruin H, Basmajian JV, et al: Agonist and antagonist activity during voluntary upper-limb movement in patients with stroke. Phys Ther 72:624–633, 1992

53. Svantesson U, Stibrant Sunnerhagen K: Stretch-shortening cycle in patients with upper motor neuron lesions due to stroke. Eur J Appl Physiol 75:312–318, 1997

54. Edström L: Selective changes in the sizes of red and white muscle fibers in upper motor lesions and Parkinsonism. J Neurol Sci 11:537–550, 1970

55. Hachisuka K, Umezu Y, Ogata H: Disuse muscle atrophy of lower limbs in hemiplegic patients. Arch Phys Med Rehabil 78:13–18, 1997

56. Miller GJT, Light KE: Strength training in spastic hemiparesis: should it be avoided? J Neuro Rehabil 9:17–28, 1997

57. Engardt M, Knutsson E, Jonsson M, Sternhag M: Dynamic muscle strength training in stroke patients: effects on knee extension torque, electromyographic activity, and motor function. Arch Phys Med Rehabil 26:419–425, 1995

58. Saltin B, Landin S: Work capacity, muscle strength and SDH activity in both legs of hemiparetic patients and patients with Parkinson's disease. Scand J Clin Lab Invest 35:531–538, 1975

59. Macko RF, DeSouza CA, Tretter LD, et al: Treadmill aerobic exercise training reduces energy expenditure and cardiovascular demands of hemiparetic gait in chronic stroke patients. A preliminary report. Stroke 28:326–330, 1997

60. Hesse S, Bertelt C, Jahnke MT, et al: Treadmill training with partial body weight support compared with physiotherapy in nonambulatory hemiparetic patients. Stroke 26:976–981, 1995

61. Visintin M, Barbeau H, Korner-Bitensky N, Mayo NE: A new approach to retrain gait in stroke patients through body weight support and treadmill stimulation. Stroke 29:1122–1128, 1998

62. Dutta C, Hadley EC, Lexell J: Sarcopenia and physical performance in old age: overview. Muscle Nerve Suppl 5:S1–S9, 1997

REGIONAL CONSIDERATIONS

19

Rehabilitation of the Shoulder

KAARE KOLSTAD ■ TIMOTHY F. TYLER ■ STEPHEN J. NICHOLAS

The shoulder plays an essential role in all sports. It has obvious importance to the athlete involved in baseball, tennis, swimming, and other overhead sports as well as contact sports. However, it is equally important in sports that require balance such as ice skating, horseback riding, and skiing.

The shoulder joint is responsible for supporting and positioning the arm and hand in space. It does this through a series of coordinated musculoskeletal links moving proximal to distal. To effectively understand and treat shoulder injuries, it is important to realize that the shoulder is not simply one joint but an alliance of four joints whose movement involves many muscles. Fifteen muscles provide scapular motion; nine muscles provide glenohumeral motion; and six muscles support the scapula on the thorax.[1] It is this shoulder complex that must be treated in its entirety when an injury occurs.

The peer-reviewed published literature on rehabilitation of the shoulder offers little reproducible data because most studies lack randomized trials. In fact, most of the reported data have come from case series without controls. Nonetheless, rehabilitation of the shoulder from sports injuries has progressed significantly over the past two decades. Much of the advancement has come from a better understanding of shoulder function. The genesis of this understanding stems from basic and clinical research involving functional anatomy, biomechanics, kinesiology, and physiology in both normal and pathologic shoulders. Increased comprehension of the shoulder complex has led to improved treatments. The aim of this chapter is to summarize the current understanding of the shoulder and present rehabilitation guidelines and protocols designed to preserve and restore normal shoulder function. Randomized trials will be included when available to better explain the efficacy of various shoulder rehabilitation modalities.

FUNCTIONAL ANATOMY AND BIOMECHANICS

The shoulder complex differs from other joints of the body because of its multiple articulations, large range of motion, and its inherent instability at the glenohumeral joint. The shoulder complex is a fine balancing act between mobility and stability. Joint stability is maintained by both static and dynamic factors.

Joints and Static Stabilizers

The shoulder complex is made up of four joints, the sternoclavicular (SC), the acromioclavicular (AC), the scapulothoracic, and the glenohumeral (GH). The SC joint is the only bony attachment of the entire upper limb to the axial skeleton. It is a synovial joint between the medial end of the clavicle and the notch of the sternum. The ligaments that support this joint are important in supporting the weight of the shoulder and arm at rest.[2] This joint allows much of the scapular motion, such as elevation, depression, protraction, and retraction that occurs with arm movement.[3] At the SC joint, 35 degrees of upward motion, 35 degrees of anteroposterior motion, and 45 to 50 degrees of axial rotation occur.[4] Because the joint is fortified with such strong ligaments, the clavicle will usually break before the joint is disrupted.

The AC joint is formed by the lateral end of the clavicle and the acromion process of the scapula. The AC joint is stabilized by several ligaments. This joint is important in providing additional range of motion to the scapula during arm elevation. It allows physiologic winging of the scapula, abduction and adduction of the scapula, and tilting of the inferior angle of the scapula away from the chest wall.[3] This joint is commonly injured in sports activities. Different degrees of sprains occur at this joint. When the ligaments are completely torn, it is referred to as an AC separation. It is important that this joint remain mobile for proper shoulder function.

The scapulothoracic joint is not a true joint but the movement of the scapula on the posterior thoracic rib cage. The scapula remains largely suspended by muscular action on the posterior thoracic rib cage and forms the base of support for arm movement by positioning its lateral apex, the glenoid process, with the humeral head. The maintenance of these muscles is critical for joint stability and can be positively affected with proper physical therapy protocols.

The glenohumeral joint, which is commonly referred to as the shoulder joint, is a synovial joint between the head of the humerus and the glenoid cavity of the scapula. The ball is maintained in the socket by several mechanisms. First, the socket is deepened by a cartilaginous sleeve called the labrum. When this structure is injured during a dislocation, it is referred to as a Bankart lesion and often needs to be repaired with surgery. A capsular sleeve encompasses the joint and provides a checkrein at the extremes of motion. The capsular sleeve has various thickenings that form a dynamic ligament complex that is crucial to providing resistance to GH joint subluxation at the extremes of motion.[5–7] The rotator cuff muscles, which will be discussed more thoroughly later, help steer the humeral head in the center of the glenoid and provide compression across the joint.[8] The rotator cuff is important in both stability and impingement. The rotator cuff muscles also insert into the capsule tissue providing a means to increase the stiffness and the torsional rigidity of these static stabilizers.[7] A negative pressure is maintained in the joint, which has been found to be important in resisting inferior subluxation of the GH joint when the arm is at the side of the body.[9,10] There are also external mechanisms to the GH joint, such as proper scapular function, which are critical to both joint stability and the avoidance of subacromial impingement and internal impingement. It is interesting to note that the bulk effect of the primary movers such as the deltoid, pectoralis major, and latissimus dorsi muscles has not been shown to contribute to joint stability.[11]

Muscles

The specific coordination of the muscles that support the shoulder complex is paramount to the intricate interrelationship between function and stability. The dynamic stabilizers are comprised of three muscle groups: the scapular muscles, which attach the axial skeleton to the scapula, the rotator cuff muscles, which attach the scapula to the humerus, and the primary movers, which attach the axial skeleton and the scapula to the humerus. The individual muscles in each group will be described below.[12]

Six muscles directly suspend the scapula from the axial skeleton and position it properly. The serratus anterior originates from the first eight ribs and inserts on the medial border and the inferior angle of the scapula. Its role is to stabilize the scapula during arm elevation by pulling the scapula against the chest wall, providing a base of support and preventing excessive winging. However, it is also involved as part of a coordinated team of muscles that position the glenoid in space beneath the humeral head. In this manner it contributes to sliding the scapula forward on the rib cage, known as protraction or abduction of the scapula. Boxers protract their scapula when punching and tend to have well-developed serratus anteriors. Scapular rotation is paramount for overhead activities.

EMG studies done on pitchers during throwing demonstrated that the anterior serratus muscle is highly active in the late cocking, acceleration, and follow-through phases of pitching.[13] In another EMG study by Glousman et al[14] on recurrent shoulder instability, athletes demonstrated diminished activity in the serratus anterior throughout all phases of throwing but especially in the acceleration and the follow-through phases.

There are two rhomboid muscles. The rhomboid minor originates from the spinous process of the seventh cervical and first thoracic vertebrae and inserts on the medial border of the scapula near the base of the scapular spine. The rhomboid major originates from the spinous processes of the second through fifth thoracic vertebrae and inserts into the medial border of the scapula inferior to the rhomboid minor. These muscles are involved with retraction of the scapula also known as adduction of the scapula. Kibler noted that if the scapula is not properly retracted during overhead motion, undue stress could be placed on the anterior structures of the glenohumeral joint.[15] In an EMG study by Jobe et al,[16,17] the rhomboids were found to be highly active during the acceleration and deceleration phases of pitching. In the acceleration phase these muscles contract eccentrically, holding the scapula back by stabilizing its medial border. In the deceleration phase they would also be contracting eccentrically, stopping the scapula from pulling off the chest wall anteriorly. Although these muscles are small, it is evident that they are important in overhead activities.

The upper trapezius and levator scapulae will be considered together because of their similar function. The upper trapezius originates from the superior nuchal line coming from the external occipital protuberance of the skull and the seventh cervical vertebra and inserts on the distal third of the clavicle and the acromion process of the scapula. The levator scapulae originates from the transverse processes of cervical vertebrae 1 through 4 and inserts on the superior angle of the scapula and the medial border adjacent to the base of the scapular spine. In a person standing with the arms at the sides little muscle activity has been recorded with an electromyogram in either the trapezius or levator scapulae.[18] However, the upper trapezius and levator scapula are critical to upward rotation of the scapula, which is needed for arm movement over the head. If these muscles are not functioning properly, the scapula will not elevate with the arm, and subacromial impingement will result.

The pectoralis minor originates from the second through sixth ribs and inserts onto the medial side of the coracoid process of the scapula. It protracts the scapula when it is retracted and pulls the lateral angle downward or rotates the scapula downward if the scapula is rotated upward.[4]

The second group of muscles, which are important for dynamic shoulder stabilization, make up the rotator cuff. Although the rotator cuff is composed of four different muscles, it often functions as one synergistic unit that is extremely important in generating joint compressive forces. The rotator cuff has been shown to play an important role in the pathogenesis of recurrent instability of the shoulder by many authors.[14,17,19-24]

The subscapularis muscle originates from the costal surface of the scapula and inserts into the lesser tuberosity of the humerus. By itself it acts as an internal rotator of the humerus. It has been shown to become attenuated with recurrent dislocations.[21] Others have noted the ability to diminish the incidence of recurring instability with a rehabilitation program that strengthens the rotator cuff, especially the subscapularis.[19] Glousman et al have shown significant misfiring of the subscapularis in the late cocking and follow-through phases of pitching.[14]

The supraspinatus muscle originates from the fossa supraspinata and passes laterally under the coracoacromial arch to attach to the greater tuberosity of the humerus. As it passes under the coracoacromial arch, the tendon and synovium can become pinched, leading to inflammation and pain. In the athlete this condition usually results from poor arthrokinematics secondary to instability and muscle weakness and imbalance. This condition is referred to as impingement syndrome. By itself the supraspinatus is an elevator of the humerus.

The infraspinatus and the teres minor are considered together because they are the primary external rotators of the arm. The infraspinatus muscle originates from the fossa infraspinata and travels laterally to insert on the posterior aspect of the greater tuberosity of the humerus. The teres minor muscle originates from the central third of the lateral border of the scapula below the scapular neck to pass behind the long head of the triceps and insert onto the inferoposterior aspect of the greater tuberosity of the humerus. The teres minor and triceps have been shown to be important as a restraining mechanism to anterior dislocation.[21] Both muscles also have been shown to be important decelerators during pitching with the teres minor showing the highest level of activity during this phase of throwing.[13]

Finally, although the biceps is not part of the rotator cuff, its long head originates on the superior glenoid tubercle and passes directly between the subscapularis and the supraspinatus on its way to inserting on the tuberosity of the radius. It can function as a humeral head depressor when the arm is in external rotation.[25,26] It also has been shown to contribute significantly to anterior and posterior stability.[27]

The third and last group of muscles that make up the shoulder complex are the primary movers. This group is made up of the deltoid, latissimus dorsi, pectoralis major, and the teres major. The largest and most important muscle of the glenohumeral muscles is the deltoid muscle. It originates from the lateral third of the clavicle, the acromion, and the spine of the scapula and inserts into the deltoid tuberosity along the anterolateral aspect of the proximal humerus. The deltoid functions as three separate muscles, anterior, middle, and posterior, depending on the plane of motion. Unlike the anterior and posterior deltoid with their parallel fibers, the middle section is multipennate muscle and subsequently the most powerful part of the deltoid. The middle deltoid is actively involved in all motions involving the elevation of the shoulder.[28] The anterior deltoid along with the middle section is active in forward elevation of the arm in the scapular plane. Because the scapular plane is the most functional plane of motion for the shoulder in everyday activities, Neer described this as the most important part of the deltoid.[29] When the arm is elevated in the coronal plane, abduction, the middle and posterior sections of the deltoid are most active. On EMG studies during pitching, all portions of the deltoid were active in early cocking and deceleration phases with minimal activity during the other phases with the exception of the acceleration phase, which showed a high level of activity in the posterior deltoid.[13] Interestingly enough no deltoid deficit was noted in an EMG study looking at the muscles of the shoulder complex during throwing activities in those individuals with glenohumeral instability.[14]

The teres major muscle originates from the lower third of the lateral border of the scapula and passes around the anterior aspect of the humerus and in front of the long head of the triceps to insert onto the crest of the lesser tubercle. When not resisting force, the teres major is quiescent in normal activities of the shoulder.[30] One study found that it was only active when it was needed to maintain a static position to resistance.[3] Against force it internally rotates, adducts, and extends the arm.[31]

Two muscles in the shoulder complex, the latissimus dorsi and the pectoralis major, originate on the axial skeleton and insert on the humerus. They cross two joints, the scapulothoracic and the glenohumeral. The latissimus dorsi originates from the spinous processes of the lower six thoracic vertebrae, all of the lumbar vertebrae, part of the sacrum, the posterior crest of the ilium, and the lower three ribs and inserts on the crest of the lesser tubercle. It functions to extend, adduct, and internally rotate the arm.[32] It can also indirectly rotate the scapula downward by the pull of the humerus. It has been shown to be important in torque development during throwing activities and as an important muscle in the deceleration phase of pitching.[33] The pectoralis major originates from the medial third of the clavicle, the manubrium and body of the sternum, and the cartilages of the first six ribs and inserts on the lower portion of the greater tuberosity. The major function is internal rotation and adduction. It indirectly functions as a depressor of the lateral angle of the scapula, and the clavicular head is a weak flexor of the arm.[32] This muscle was most active during late cocking and acceleration phases of pitching.[13] Both the pectoralis major and the latissimus dorsi augment the energy that is transferred from the trunk to the arm. These two muscles were the only ones to demonstrate a positive correlation with peak torque developed during isokinetic testing and throwing speed.[34]

Dynamic Stabilizers and Force Couples

In the preceding pages the muscles that make up the shoulder complex were described but not how they act to stablize it. As a group, the muscles of the shoulder function as accelerators, decelerators, and stabilizers. The eccentric action of muscle on the shoulder complex is especially important. Eccentric action of these muscles helps to decelerate joint motion and absorb energy, thereby placing fewer demands on the ligamentous restraints.[31] The eccentric action of muscle is more suitable as a joint stablizer than concentric action is because the force generated with an eccentric contraction increases with negative velocity as compared to a concentric contraction, whose force decreases with increasing velocity. The net effect is that functionally stretching muscle (eccentric contraction) at a given velocity can generate a much higher force than the same muscle that is shortening (concentric contraction) at the same velocity.[31] In addition, the energy cost per unit of velocity under identical forces is much less when a muscle is lengthened compared to when it is shortened at the same velocity. Therefore, eccentric muscle contractions are much better suited for the repetitive endurance activities involving the shoulder and must be emphasized in the rehabilitation of the shoulder.

The torque and stiffness of a joint are controlled by muscles that produce opposing forces to one another.[30] When both the agonist and antagonist muscles are activated across a joint, the stiffness of the joint and therefore the stability of the joint will increase, but the torque generated will be low. If the antagonist muscle is inhibited, however, the stiffness of the joint will be low, but the torque produced will be high. The coactivation of muscles across a joint to protect it is one of the principal reasons for using closed chain exercises in the early rehabilitation period of an injured joint. The question that must be addressed for the glenohumeral joint, which unlike other joints has minimal static contraints, is how it maintains stiffness or joint compression without compromising its ability to generate the high torque forces seen in the overhead athlete. The demands of the shoulder are met by the primary torque-producing muscles (ie, deltoid, pectoralis major, and latissimus dorsi) with the synergistic action of the rotator cuff muscles and long head of the biceps providing joint compression. The larger primary movers like the deltoid have long lever arms, which make them good torque producers, whereas the rotator cuff muscles attach close to the axis of rotation, making them more suitable for joint compression. In fact, the compressive forces of the rotator cuff along with an intact glenoid and labrum have been shown to approximate the motion of a ball and socket joint.[35–37] In other words the head of the humerus is maintained in the center of the glenoid throughout the full range of motion of the shoulder.

To better understand the dynamic stability of the shoulder, the concept of a force couple must be grasped. A force couple involves two groups of muscles working together to produce a motion. There are three basic types of force couples: one involves the coordinated activity of synergists, the second involves a coordinated coactivation of an agonist muscle and antagonist muscle that pull in opposite directions to impose rotation about an axis, and the third involves coordinated activation of an agonist muscle with simultaneous inhibition of its antagonist muscle.[3,15] The primary example of a synergistic force couple occurs in the GH joint between the deltoid and the rotator cuff. As abduction begins with the arm at the side, the pull of the deltoid is directed vertically, creating a shear force at the GH joint. This shear force is countered by the depressive forces placed on the humeral head by the synergistic activity of three of the rotator cuff muscles: the infraspinatus, the teres minor, and the subscapularis. These muscles lie beneath the center of rotation and thereby can have a depressive effect on the humeral head. In addition, the fourth rotator cuff muscle, the supraspinatus, which is nearly perpendicular to the GH joint, can impart a compressive force across the joint when its action is combined with that of the other rotator cuff muscles. This coordinated synergism results in a stable joint fulcrum whereby the humeral head is maintained and compressed in the center of the glenoid. When this mechanism is not functioning properly, instability or impingement or both can result. Examples of coordinated coactivation of agonist and antagonist muscles would be the upper trapezius and levator scapulae working with the lower trapezius and serratus anterior muscles to control scapular rotation. Examples of the coordinated activation-inhibition of antagonistic muscle groups would include the trapezius and rhomboids working with the serratus anterior to protract and retract the scapula in order to follow arm movements, and the pectoralis–latissimus dorsi–subscapularis working with the posterior deltoid–infraspinatus–teres minor to create glenohumeral internal and external rotation. These force couples often are disrupted with injury or surgery and must be properly reestablished if the shoulder is going to recover properly.

The six muscles that support the scapula must fire in a coordinated sequence to provide a normal functioning shoulder. This is analogous to the musicians in a symphony each performing a given movement to produce the final sound of the composition. If one of the musicians is not playing properly or in the right sequence, the outcome will be flawed. The same is true of scapular movement in relationship to the shoulder complex. The muscles that support the scapula are responsible for three major functions. First they provide a stable base or platform by positioning and holding the glenoid in the proper orientation so that the glenohumeral joint can properly function. Without this proper base of operation the scapula would slide from side to side, making the glenohumeral joint unstable. For example, if it slid too far laterally, the glenoid would become antetilted, placing excessive stress on the anterior structures of the glenohumeral joint.[38] In fact, many overhead athletes tend to have excessive joint laxity at the glenohumeral joint that remains stable because of the healthy and well-coordinated function of the supporting scapula musculature. Second, these muscles dynamically position the glenoid with the humeral head so that efficient glenohumeral movement can occur through the action of the shoulder muscles. Remember that the deltoid and the rotator cuff muscles originate on the scapula. Therefore, it is this positioning of the scapula in the proper relationship to the arm that allows the proper length-tension relationships to be maintained among the glenohumeral muscles. Finally, the periscapular muscles can fix the scapula to the thoracic rib cage, providing a base of support from which muscles that originate on the scapula, such as the rotator cuff, can function properly.

Kinesiology

The shoulder is the most mobile joint in the body. This mobility of the shoulder is possible for several reasons. First, the relatively large ball of the humeral head in comparison to the small glenoid socket gives little bony support to the joint. Only one third of the humeral head is in contact with the glenoid at any one time. Second, the ample volume of the shoulder capsule allows a large amount of joint laxity. Finally, the scapula is highly mobile because of the limited constraint by the clavicle.[15] Between the glenohumeral and scapulothoracic joints there can be 0 to 180 degrees of arm elevation, with 120 degrees occurring at the glenohumeral joint and 60 degrees occurring at the scapulothoracic joint.

This coordinated movement between the humerus and scapula, called the scapulohumeral rhythm by Codman, is critical for arm elevation. The classic teaching of a 2:1 ratio for glenohumeral to scapulothoracic joint motion was identified by Lockhart and later confirmed in the classic work by Inman, Saunders, and Abbott.[3] They found this ratio to be consistent from 30 to 170 degrees of motion in the coronal plane. This was an average, however. Over the first 30 degrees of abduction the movement of the scapula was inconsistent, moving medial, lateral, or not at all. Because of this inconsistency, they termed this the *setting phase*. Poppen and Walker demonstrated that there is a 4:1 glenohumeral to scapulothoracic ratio of motion in the first 25 degrees of arm elevation, which changes to a 5:4 ratio from 25 to 180 degrees.[22]

In another study, Freedman and Munro, who were the first to look at glenohumeral and scapulothoracic motion in the scapular plane, found an approximate ratio of 3:2 from 0 to 90 degrees, 5:4 from 90 to 135 degrees, and greater than 5:2 from 135 to 170 degrees.[39] Furthermore, other authors have shown a large degree of individual variation in the first 30 degrees of elevation, which is greatly affected when resistance is applied to the arm.[39] The scapula not only abducts (upward rotation) but also rotates forward (winging) with arm elevation. The scapula must move with the humeral head to position the glenoid under the head of the humerus, providing a stable base of support.

Rowe, in a great analogy, compared it to a seal balancing a ball on its nose. To obtain full abduction of the arm, external rotation is required. Maximum elevation occurred at 35 degrees of external rotation. This allows clearance of the greater tuberosity under the acromion.[40] Morrey et al also demonstrated that the external rotation loosens the inferior glenohumeral ligament, thereby enabling full elevation of the arm.[4] Maximum glenohumeral elevation in full internal rotation is limited to 115 degrees. The shoulders' excessive laxity and complex anatomy allows a great range of motion, more than in any other joint. Consequently it is prone to soft tissue injury resulting in instability.

The shoulder complex also possesses the subacromial space, which acts in some ways as a second joint cavity to the humeral head, predisposing it to the stress of repetitive loading and potential development of impingement sequelae.[41] When the posterior capsule becomes tight, limiting internal rotation of the shoulder, the head actually rises with arm elevation. This occurs because the glenohumeral joint no longer acts as a ball and socket and hinges on the tight posterior capsule, predisposing it to subacromial impingement. That is why gaining full symmetric internal rotation of the shoulder is so important.

Body Linkage

The shoulder works as part of a complex musculoskeletal linkage. When a pitcher is throwing, the force generated to accelerate a ball starts from the legs and feet pushing off the ground and is propagated up through the pelvis, spine, and into the shoulder complex and down the arm. This is all accomplished by a linkage system made up of multiple joints and overlapping muscle attachments. For example, when the pitcher throws, the shoulder is incapable of generating and producing the forces needed to throw a 90-mile-per-hour fastball by itself. The spine and trunk muscles transfer the ground reaction forces up from the lower extremities into the upper extremity. The anteroposterior directed ground reaction force is funneled into the rotational force of the shoulder.[42] This force transfer is also helped with some of the prime movers such as the pectoralis major and the latissimus dorsi. When the spine is not working properly, it can put undue stress on the shoulder, leading to injury. In fact, the mass of the trunk contributes more than 50% of the kinetic energy and velocity to the pitched ball. This is illustrated quite nicely by the water polo player who can only generate 50% of the ball's velocity without his feet on the ground.[42]

The health of the shoulder depends upon this linkage system. If lateral trunk flexion, a major source of abduction force upon the shoulder, is lost, more reliance will be placed on the shoulder musculature as energy generators. This can lead to early fatigue and injury. A force transfer occurs during the late cocking and acceleration phases of throwing. The trunk acts as a rigid cylinder via muscle tension provided by the thoracolumbar fascia. As the shoulder and arm rapidly accelerate, the trunk decelerates.

Inefficient force transfer sets the shoulder up for injury. For example, if the trunk opens up prematurely while the arm is cocked, the anterior glenohumeral joint will experience tensile overload after many cycles of this pathologic throwing motion. The spine also acts to attenuate the forces across the shoulder during the deceleration and follow-through phases of throwing. It does this by reacquiring energy from the shoulder by trunk lateral bending and forward rotation, thereby dissipating the distraction forces on the shoulder.

Therefore it is critical during rehabilitation of the shoulder to consider the whole kinematic chain looking at strength imbalances, inflexibilities, fatigued body components, instability, and improper sequencing. It must be remembered that the shoulder is linked to the spine and trunk as well as the elbow, forearm, and wrist.[43] If the shoulder rehabilitation program is to succeed, it must incorporate these additional regions.

AN EVIDENCE-BASED ALGORITHM FOR SHOULDER REHABILITATION

Treatment of pain or dysfunction at the shoulder is complex. The pain or dysfunction can be caused by macrotrauma, such as dislocation or surgery, or by microtrauma, such as subtle instability that presents as impingement.[44] In both cases, healing and rehabilitation occur in an overlapping series of four stages: inflammation, proliferation, remodeling, and maturation.

After an injury or a surgical procedure, rehabilitation can address certain areas that are identified as abnormal in relation to the uninvolved extremity. Rehabilitation cannot restore a labrum that has been torn or remove a bone spur located in the subacromial space. Rehabilitation can, however, relieve pain and restore mobility, stability, and function to the injured shoulder.[41,45] All injuries to the athlete's shoulder require rehabilitation to restore the full range of motion and strengthen the shoulder throughout the range before the athlete returns to the playing field.[46]

Shoulder Injury and Repair

Once the shoulder has been injured or has undergone surgery, it must have time to heal.

This is a morphologically complex process. The clinician may evaluate the patient at any one of the four stages of healing. It is important to note that age, tissue quality, nutritional status, degree of injury, mechanical stress, and other factors all influence the healing process.

The initial response, the inflammation stage, begins with the cell's release of histamine, a potent vasodilator. At this point, endothelial buds start to proliferate into the wounded area, and monocytes and macrophages appear. Biochemical changes, including increased water content in the injured tissue, take place. This stage reaches its maximum synthesis in 5 days. Rest at the injured site is essential for healing to occur. Uncontrolled movement during this stage can destroy this fragile clot and healing cell matrix. Goals during this stage are to decrease discomfort and inflammation. Controlling the amount of trauma and bleeding in the injured area can decrease hypoxic injury and edema formation. Minimizing this sequela can result in earlier mobility and accelerate the recovery process.[47]

The second stage, the proliferation phase, is characterized by rapid cellular activity. If the surgery or injury is to a ligamentous tissue, a specific process takes place: immature collagen framework is laid down; elastin production begins; and the water weight is decreased. The healing ligament begins to form unorganized collagen cross-link profiles that seem to increase the tensile strength of the matrix.[48] Formal rehabilitation usually begins at some point during this stage. It is now that proximal and distal strengthening, restoration of mobility in areas away from the injured site, and aerobic training may begin. The maintenance of strength and vital capacity can provide valuable physiologic and psychological benefits to the injured athlete.

The third stage, remodeling of the tissues, usually begins 6 weeks after the injury. During this stage, collagen turnover is restored to near normal levels. As the tissue matures, the cellular profile of the injured area undergoes a realignment of connective tissue in line with the tension encountered.[49] Tissues are highly susceptible to stress during this period. The muscles surrounding the injury will provide protection and help minimize the stress on the healing tissue, which is paramount in expediting recovery. Restoration of the full range of motion and increased

strength are primary goals during this stage of healing.

The final stage, maturation, continues slowly in the months and year to come. During this period the tissue regains its normal appearance. The collagen fibers are continually being organized in a dynamic process in response to the load and direction of force that they encounter. Although factors involved in the ongoing maturation are not well understood, it is clear that immobilization is detrimental to the rehabilitation process and to the overall tensile strength of the tissue.[48] Total restoration of mobility and stability will allow patients to function fully and should be the climax of this final stage of healing. Regaining proprioception and sports-specific training should be emphasized during this stage.

THE EXERCISE PRESCRIPTION

Phase I: Modalities

In the early phases of rehabilitation shortly after an acute injury or surgery, local modalities can provide comfort to the painful shoulder. Nonsteroidal antiinflammatory drugs (NSAIDs) can diminish pain and inflammation in the early stages of an injury. They work by inhibiting the formation of prostaglandins. Prostaglandins can sensitize nerve endings and dilate blood vessels, leading to increased pain and swelling.

In one review article, in which 11 known double-blinded, randomized, and placebo-controlled studies were cited, eight were helped.[50] In Shelbourne's study involving postoperative anterior cruciate ligament reconstruction patients, preemptive analgesia using NSAIDs at the start, during, and after surgery met with a great deal of success.[51] In the study, NSAIDs significantly lowered the patients' need for narcotic medication and gave them pain-free motion earlier in their postoperative course than would otherwise have been expected. NSAIDs produce mild side effects, such as stomach upset, in a large percentage of patients, but these are usually short term and not dangerous. They do, however, produce serious and potentially harmful side effects in a small percentage of patients. To help avoid these problems, NSAIDs should be given for only short periods, ranging from 10 to 14 days, and taken with meals and should not be prescribed for patients with a history of ulcers or NSAID sensitivity. If there should be stomach pain or signs of gastrointestinal bleeding, the medicine needs to be stopped immediately, and if symptoms dictate, the patient should be seen by a physician urgently.

Cryotherapy is the use of cold modalities. There are many forms of cryotherapy, such as ice packs, ice massage, chemical sprays, and cold compression devices. When one is treating the shoulder, it is important to identify the goal or structures the cryotherapy is directed toward. Cryotherapy has the physiologic effect of vasoconstriction, which decreases swelling and inflammation by reducing blood flow.[43] Although cryotherapy may reduce shoulder joint effusion, there is evidence that cryotherapy to the shoulder joint is unable to reach the glenohumeral joint or subacromial space as measured by indwelling temperature probes.[52] However, the previous study did not examine the patients' perception of pain. Cryotherapy has been shown to be an effective analgesic.[53] Cold modalities slow nerve conduction velocity and may activate the gate theory of pain relief. Speer et al[53] were able to show that cryotherapy could provide perceived pain relief following arthroscopic shoulder surgery. Following a cryotherapy treatment session, pain and superficial inflammation are reduced. We use the shoulder cryocuff to reduce posttherapy pain and inflammation (Fig. 19–1).

Low frequency transcutaneous electrical nerve stimulation (TENS) is another noninvasive method of providing pain relief. Morgan et al[54] found TENS to be an effective means of pain alleviation in patients with adhesive capsulitis who are undergoing arthrography. In a prospective randomized study the researchers concurred that TENS was an effective therapeutic alternative to medication for shoulder pain relief. In this study the diagnoses of the cause of shoulder pain were multiple.[55] Successful pain relief has been documented in up to 60% to 70% of patients using this modality.[43]

Heat can be a useful modality in reducing spasm and promoting healing of the shoulder.[43] Heating tissue has been shown to be an effective means of assisting in the stretching of the shoulder. Heating the tissue prior to stretching increases the viscoelastic properties of the shoulder. Our preferred method of heating the shoulder is to have the patient seated with the arm on a table with moist heat in the axilla

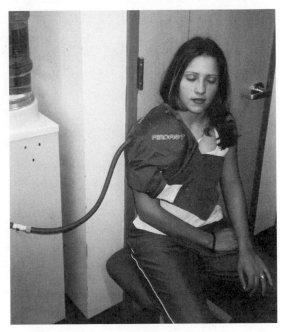

FIGURE 19–1. A patient with cryocuff on her shoulder following a rehabilitation session.

and over the shoulder (Fig. 19–2). Heat reduces muscle spasms and increases metabolism and blood flow by stimulating vasodilation of the blood vessels supplying this tissue. Heat reduces muscle spasm, speeds healing of nonacute muscular contusions, relieves pain, and decreases connective tissue stiffness. Heat is not indicated in the presence of a joint effusion, acute injuries, or a compromised sensorium.

Ultrasound heats deep tissues and may provide pain relief. Ultrasound is the use of sound waves to achieve a thermal or nonthermal effect. Depth of penetration is determined by the frequency used. This technique can be extremely beneficial for heating the shoulder joint capsule and increasing circulation to the tendinous portion of the rotator cuff. Good results were achieved with patients who received ultrasound treatment for subacromial bursitis. These same results, however, were found in a group of patients who received diathermy, another means of deep heating.[56] In contrast, Downing and Weinstein's prospective randomized double-blind study found ultrasound added no additional benefit to therapeutic exercise in the treatment of the shoulder.[57] Nykanen supported these findings in a group of painful shoulders treated with pulsed ultrasound.[58] At our institute

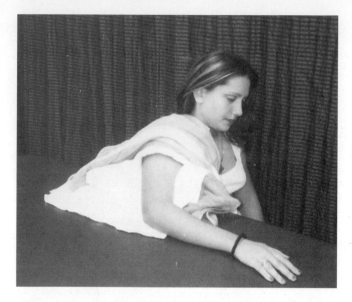

FIGURE 19–2. The application of moist heat directed to the glenohumeral joint.

ultrasound is not the modality of choice for global heating of shoulder structures and may be more appropriate for localized deep heating.

Phonophoresis is an effective method of delivering topical medication through the skin to an area through the use of ultrasound.[33] Cortisone has been shown to reduce inflammation. Although phonophoresis is commonly used on shoulder tendonitis, its efficacy has not been specifically tested. In a double-blind study using phonophoresis, Griffin et al demonstrated on a multitude of diagnoses that 68% of patients who received cortisone cream did better than patients who got the placebo cream.[59] Only 45% of the cases involved the shoulder. If this technique is chosen, depth of penetration may be enhanced by massaging the cortisone to the area first and then applying moist heat to enhance permeability.[60] It has been our experience that 5 to 10 treatments are sufficient to determine if this modality will be beneficial.

Passive range of motion and grade I and II mobilizations can be offered early in treatment to reduce pain and discomfort.[61,62] This is dependent on the injury or surgery. Lastayo et al[63] revealed that both manual and mechanical continuous passive range of motion was safe and produced the same outcome following repair of the rotator cuff. The patients in this study initiated passive pendulum exercises three to four times per day starting the day after surgery.

Phase 2: The Linkage to the Shoulder

Whatever the shoulder diagnosis, the importance of its linkage to the torso cannot be underestimated. Rehabilitation of the shoulder starts proximal to the glenohumeral joint. Proper arthrokinematics of the sternoclavicular, acromioclavicular, and scapulothoracic joints needs to be reestablished if hypomobility exists.[64–66] In the case of hypermobility, stability needs to be restored. This goal can be obtained through rehabilitation with improvement of muscular stability or through surgical intervention.

Hypomobility of the sternoclavicular joint can be mobilized posterior to increase retraction or anterior to increase protraction (Fig. 19–3). This mobility is essential after the first 30 degrees of clavicular elevation when the costoclavicular ligament becomes taut and the clavicle rotates to allow full active range of motion of the shoulder.[65,66] Minimal accessory joint motion is essential at the acromioclavicular joint. An effective method of achieving an anterior glide of the acromioclavicular joint is mobilization with the patient in the sitting position. One hand stabilizes the scapula while the other provides an anterior force on the posterior acromion (Fig. 19–4). Even though passive scapulothoracic hypomobility is rare, mobility needs to be achieved for full shoulder range of motion to take place. The scapula can be mobilized in

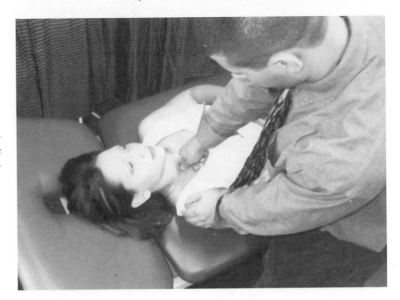

FIGURE 19–3. The clinical position to deliver a posterior glide force to mobilize the sternoclavicular joint.

the sidelying position with the patient facing the therapist. In this position a clinician can make a transition from passive range of motion to providing isometric manual resistance to elevation-depression and protraction-retraction (Fig. 19–5).

Once this milestone of mobility has been restored to these proximal joints, scapular strengthening and reestablishment of glenohumeral joint mobility can begin. Six primary scapular muscles provide the force couples that move

the scapula in a synchronous fashion. These muscles include the serratus anterior, trapezius (upper, middle, lower), rhomboid major and minor, levator scapular, and pectoralis minor.[16] Scapular stabilization exercises should be directed toward strengthening muscles that have atrophied or lost endurance. Conversely, it may be necessary to train a patient to inhibit scapular stabilizer activity so that normal force couple activity may transpire.

When training the scapular stabilizers, one must take into consideration that these muscles do not generate a large amount of torque. Correspondingly, these muscles need to have a high level of endurance to provide necessary force couples to maintain the position of the glenoid fossa for proper arthrokinematics. In fact, cadaver studies have demonstrated the stabilizing nature of the trapezius muscle, showing a larger proportion of slow twitch fibers in all portions of the muscle.[67] McQuade and Smidt[68] have confirmed that scapulothoracic motion increases with fatigue of the scapular stabilizers during scaption, (ie, glenohumeral flexion in the scapular plane). The possible relative immobilization of the shoulder may add to the needed emphasis of scapula strengthening, since immobilization has been shown to selectively atrophy type I motor units. Scientific data suggest that in shoulder fatigue, scapular motion increases, altering scapulohumeral rhythm. It seems that the fatigued scapular stabilizers are unable to provide proximal stability for distal mobility of the humerus.[69]

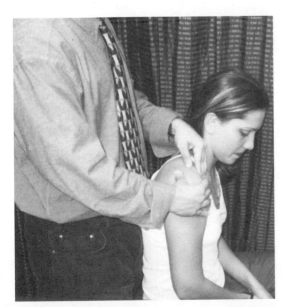

FIGURE 19–4. A method of achieving anterior glide of the acromioclavicular joint.

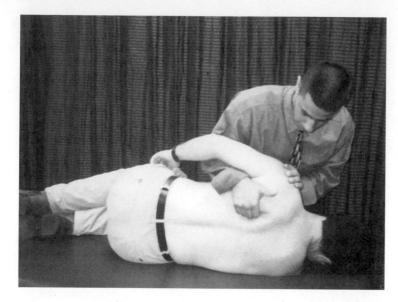

FIGURE 19–5. An effective position for manual therapy of the scapulothoracic joint. In this position the clinician can mobilize the scapula or provide resistance to the motions of the scapula.

At our institution we have seen several patients with shoulder instability secondary to scapular winging, providing another piece of evidence supporting the importance of scapular musculature in shoulder stability. The global evidence provides crucial support for initiating a strengthening and endurance program for the periscapular muscles. Therefore, at our institute we train all scapular stabilizers by performing three to five sets of exercises to their fatigue.

To have normal scapulohumeral rhythm, dynamic stability of this joint needs to be restored. Many authors have examined the EMG activity during shoulder-strengthening exercises, but when choosing the appropriate exercise the clinician must keep the activity pain free and protect the injury or surgical repair.[70–74] An EMG study of 16 shoulder exercises was performed by Moseley et al[74] to determine optimal motor recruitment of scapular muscles. Maximum activation of the rhomboids and middle trapezius was achieved with a rowing exercise. The serratus anterior muscle was significantly activated with a push-up with a plus. The seated press-up exercise fired the pectoralis minor and some latissimus dorsi muscle fibers. Scaption strongly emphasized the upper and lower trapezius and levator scapula. Further research is needed to determine the role of the scapula in shoulder pathology.

The only two upward and outward rotators of the scapula are the serratus anterior and the lower trapezius. These vital muscles need endurance to maintain the force couple with the powerful upper trapezius muscles. Some clinicians feel it may be the strong influence of the upper trapezius and relative inactivity of the lower trapezius that promote abnormal biomechanics.[75] When performing exercises in the sitting or standing position, patients may influence the firing of the lower trapezius by pressing their sternum forward while retracting the scapulae slightly[50] (Figs. 19–6 and 19–7). Currently we are working on EMG evidence to support this hypothesis. On the basis of clinical observation, upper trapezius atrophy and weakness are not commonly seen in shoulder pathology unless there is neurologic involvement. Therefore, upper trapezius strengthening is not commonly prescribed at our clinic. The milestone of achieving scapular stability and normal scapulohumeral rhythm should be met before strengthening above 90 degrees of abduction begins.

Strengthening of muscles distal to the injury or repair should be incorporated at this time. Specifically, the biceps should be strengthened even when not involved because it has been found to be a depressor and stabilizer of the humeral head.[25,26]

In addition, spinal and abdominal muscles need to provide a solid base of support so that the origins (the spine) of the scapular stabilizers remain fixed during distal movement. Moreover, it has been documented that during throwing more than 50% of the kinetic energy is generated in the trunk, torso, and lower extremities.[34,76]

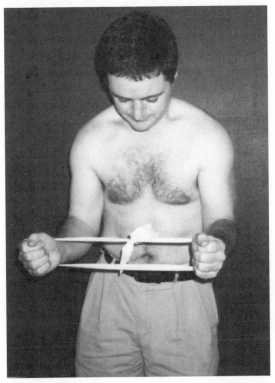

FIGURE 19–6. A posture of a forward head and rounded shoulders will put the scapular stabilizers in a stretched position. This position may put these muscles at a mechanical disadvantage.

Phase 3

As a result of shoulder pain, hypomobility of the glenohumeral joint often accompanies the diagnosis. Normal arthrokinematics are restored through joint mobilization and stretching of the glenohumeral joint capsule and the surrounding tissues.[77] Accessory joint motion is essential for normal roll and glide, which is necessary for full range of motion. Active range of motion of the shoulder has been correlated to patients' ability to perform activities of daily living.[78] Pain free submaximal isometric strengthening of the rotator cuff muscles may begin despite the lack of normal glenohumeral arthrokinematics, which should be restored, however, before isotonic strengthening is initiated.

The restoration of accessory glenohumeral joint motion is achieved through joint mobilization. Anterior glide of the humeral head can be performed with a common exercise called pendulums or Codman's exercise. Anterior glide is an involuntary accessory motion that is essen-

tial for external rotation. Humeral head inferior glide is needed to prevent impingement of structures between the greater tubercle and the acromion during shoulder flexion. Long axis distraction of the arm can provide a gentle inferior glide (Fig. 19–8). More force can be applied in this plane with the patient supine and the shoulder at 90 degrees of abduction. The clinician should be able to palpate for gapping under the acromion (Fig. 19–9). The final accessory joint motion is glenohumeral posterior glide, which is needed for osteokinematic internal rotation and flexion.[77] A technique for mobilizing the humeral head posteriorly is to place the patient supine, grasp the arm at the epicondyles, and place the free hand under the glenohumeral joint. Providing a posterior force at the elbow through the axis of the humerus will stretch the posterior capsule. Active assistive and passive range of motion will help maintain the restored accessory joint range of motion. Using kinematic analysis and EMG, McCann et al[72] demonstrated that passive range of motion exercises involve

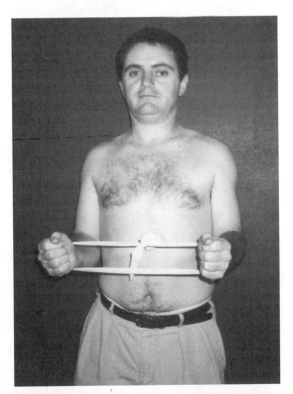

FIGURE 19–7. A postural position with the chest up and shoulders retracted back slightly may facilitate lower trapezius and shoulder retractor muscle activity.

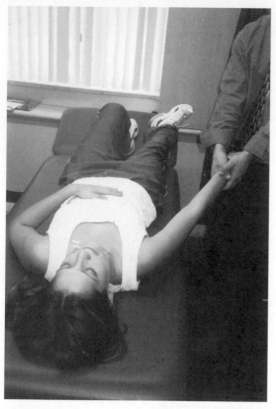

FIGURE 19–8. A caudal force is given to provide a long axis distraction.

minimal EMG activity and can be initiated early in rehabilitation. Once the milestone of normal glenohumeral osteokinematics is achieved and the patient has passive flexion and abduction to

90 degrees, strengthening may begin in the plane of the scapula to 90 degrees of elevation.[46] Stretching may also be phased in at this point.

Flexibility of the shoulder is a component of mobility that allows the patient to place the hand in the correct position. Stretching should be implemented only when side-to-side differences are identified and should not be done indiscriminately.[79] In fact, hypomobility in a patient with anterior subluxation may be a protective mechanism. Antithetically, Harryman et al state that oblique glenohumeral translations are not the result of ligamentous insufficiency or laxity; instead they result when the capsule is asymmetrically tight.[80] A tight posterior capsule is thought to cause anterosuperior migration of the humeral head with forward elevation of the shoulder, possibly contributing to impingement. In addition, posterior capsule tightness has been linked clinically to a loss of internal rotation range of motion.[81] Tyler et al[81] have developed a new valid and reliable method of measuring posterior capsule tightness (Fig. 19–10). An effective method of stretching this area is to stabilize the patient's scapula at the inferior angle manually while the patient provides a cross chest adduction force (Fig. 19–11). The inferior capsule is stretched with the arm overhead and the elbow in full flexion. A passive stretch is given by placing the opposite hand on the involved elbow and providing overpressure.

Stretching to regain mobility can be advanced through active assistive range of motion by hav-

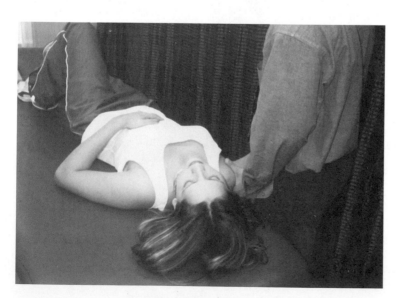

FIGURE 19–9. The position for inferior glide of the glenohumeral joint.

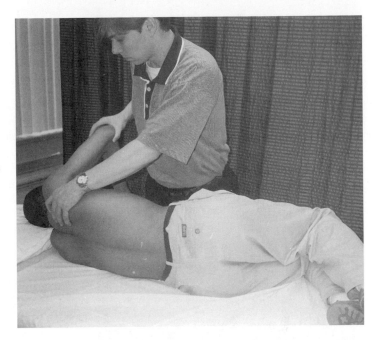

FIGURE 19-10. A clinical position to evaluate posterior capsule tightness.

ing the uninvolved upper extremity help with the use of pulleys and cane stretches. All of these are isotonic rotator cuff strengthening exercises.[73,82] Much as they do for the scapular muscles, the force couples of the subscapularis, infraspinatus, and teres minor provide dynamic stability to centralize the humeral head. Rhythmic stabilization exercises are ideal for rotator cuff awareness and stabilization (Fig. 19-12). Kelly et al[71] established the optimal position for maximum activation of selected shoulder muscles in healthy individuals. The infraspinatus and posterior deltoid were most active when contracted isometrically in a position of 90 degrees of abduction and 45 degrees of internal rotation. These researchers, however, did not explore the muscle activity in the plane of the scapula. The same rationale employed for scaption is used when one is initiating isotonic external rotator cuff strengthening.[37] External rotation performed in the scapular plane with a freeweight while the patient is in a sidelying position is an effective method of starting isotonic strengthening. Townsend et al[83] confirmed

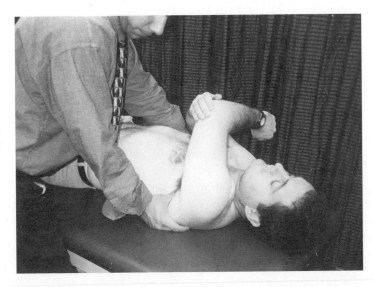

FIGURE 19-11. Manual stabilization is needed at the inferior angle of the scapula to effectively stretch the posterior capsule.

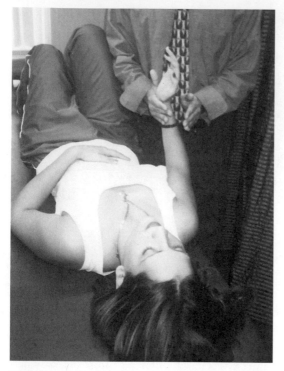

FIGURE 19-12. The internal and external rotators are activated alternately to perform rhythmic stabilization.

this by using EMG during 17 shoulder exercises and found external rotation with the patient in the sidelying position to be the best exercise, activating 80% to 88% of the infraspinatus and teres minor. Blackburn et al[84] found these muscles to be maximally active on EMG with the patient prone and the elbow and shoulder at 90 degrees of flexion and abduction. Using elastic resistance in the standing position can provide a foundation for a home exercise program. Hintermeister et al[85] examined the EMG activity and applied a load during shoulder rehabilitation exercises. The results showed a peak load for all exercises ranging from 21 to 54 N. This study justifies the use of elastic resistance for low initial loading of rotator cuff muscles for postinjury and postoperative patients. It also provides the shoulder muscles with an eccentric exercise component that is inherent in training with elastic resistance.

A continuum of positioning for external rotator strengthening should be implemented to protect and provide a mechanical advantage to the shoulder. The progression should start at 0 degrees abduction and progress to the scapular plane followed by 90 degrees abduction.[86]

Phase 4

Once scapular and humeral head stabilizer strength milestones have been reached (which varies for each patient and is dependent on age and size), patients may begin more aggressive strengthening away from the plane of the scapula. The rationale for setting a strength goal is based on the findings of McQuade and Smidt.[68] These researchers demonstrated that as the resistance increased during elevation in the scapular plane, the ratio of scapulohumeral rhythm increased from 2:1 to 4.5:1, glenohumeral to scapular motion. Conversely, as the arm was elevated through passive range of motion, the scapulohumeral rhythm decreased. Therefore, strengthening is directed toward maintaining the strength of the stabilizers and increasing strength of the prime movers away from the plane of the scapula. This is more demanding on the joint capsule and requires more rotator cuff strength. However, there is no scientific evidence to determine when it is appropriate to start strengthening away from the scapular plane. Strengthening throughout the full range of motion is a goal during this phase.

Strengthening the rotator cuff will permit a progression of isotonic strength training away from the scapular plane and into more demanding planes. Straight planes that isolate weak muscles should continue to be implemented. Combined movement patterns are used to establish muscle timing and improve proprioception and kinesthesia awareness. Proprioceptive neuromuscular facilitation (PNF) is a specific pattern of treatment techniques originally described for use in neurologic patients. These techniques have since been integrated into the orthopedic population. Specifically, upper extremity patterns can help activate the shoulder rotators while they are performing functional movements.[46] A drawback to PNF training, however, is that the amount of resistance and the clinician's ability to consistently grade the amount of resistance make PNF training impractical in the orthopedic setting.[86] PNF may be time consuming in some clinics. Other methods of resistance such as cable column resistance, elastic tubing, freeweight, and isokinetics may be more suitable. Improvement in rotator cuff strength will foster progression to strengthening in a position of 90 degrees of shoulder abduction and 90 degrees of elbow flexion. Resistance may begin with freeweights in the prone and supine positions progressing to elastic resistance in the standing position. At this time submaximal isokinetic exercising can be implemented with a slow progression toward maximal activity.

Training position is an integral factor in isokinetic exercises. It is suggested that isokinetic rotator cuff strengthening begin in the plane of the scapula. This position allows for unrestricted arthrokinematics.[40] A therapeutic rational can be made for a continuum of positioning for isokinetic strengthening of the internal and external rotators. Isokinetic strengthening would begin in the plane of the scapula, then progress to 45 degrees of shoulder abduction. A position of 90 degrees abduction should be reserved for advanced training. In this position, increased rotator cuff strength is needed to help provide stability when capsular stress is at a maximum and geometric joint stability is at a minimum.[37] The efficacy of these different isokinetic positions is separate and distinct for the internal and external rotators.[87] Isokinetic testing between the scapular plane and the frontal plane has revealed increased strength values in the scapular plane for the external rotators but not for the internal rotators.[88] Soderberg and Blaschek[89] found the strongest isokinetic position for the internal rotators to be at 0 to 20 degrees of shoulder abduction. In postsurgical patients the recovery of isokinetic strength has been correlated to the size of repaired rotator cuff tears and require 1 year to return to normal strength.[82]

Providing isokinetics is expensive and space consuming; therefore other means of advanced strengthening may be implemented. Closed kinetic chain exercise used with plyometric exercise can be an excellent method of training. The advantages and benefits of closed kinetic chain and plyometric training have been established in the lower extremity.[90] The current trend in rehabilitation is to incorporate these types of training in upper extremity rehabilitation. Closed kinetic chain exercise is a concept more accepted in shoulder rehabilitation.[91] Proprioceptive input, diagonal movement patterns, proximal stability, and co-contraction were found to be safe exercises early in rehabilitation, recording minimal muscular activity.[72] Regaining full external rotation range of motion can be difficult at times. It is necessary to stretch and evaluate the external rotation motion at 0, 45, and 90 degrees abduction. Different portions of the capsule and its ligamentous attachments are stretched at different degrees of abduction.[6,92] Internal rotation range of motion may also be evaluated and stretched in the same manner.

A primary goal later in this phase of treatment includes restoring dynamic stability to the glenohumeral joint. Scaption is usually the precursor to other isotonic exercises. Flexion 30 to 45 degrees anterior to the frontal plane provides a sound rationale for initiating isotonic strengthening. Scaption promotes a higher degree of congruence between the humeral head and the glenoid fossa, providing a solid fulcrum for the humerus to pivot off of. This congruence provides maximal synovial joint contact promoting joint nutrition.[22,93] Furthermore there is less twisting of the joint capsule in the scapular plane, and rotator cuff stresses are minimized.[40] In addition, this position furnishes an optimal length-tension relationship for the supraspinatus and deltoid muscles and provides an excellent mechanical advantage for producing torque.[94] Last, strengthening in the scapular plane places the glenohumeral joint in a position of functional movement.[86] Scaption is effective and safe for strengthening the supraspinatus. Numerous studies have examined selective activation of the supraspinatus muscle and found no one position selectively isolates the supraspinatus.[84,95–97] Scaption should start with no resistance and increased repetitions. This recommendation is based on the study by McQuade and Smidt,[68] who found an increase in scapular stabilizer muscle activity with increased resistance during scaption. The arc of motion of isotonic strengthening may need to be modified at first. Later, progression to greater arcs should be permitted but limited to only 90 degrees to prevent impingement.

Although isometric strengthening of the internal and external rotators may have begun early on, a position of minimal stress should be used to protect the injury or repair when one is initiating upper extremity closed kinetic chain exercises. Wall push-ups progressing to push-ups on unsteady surfaces are commonly used.

An EMG analysis of the scapular stabilizers during this progression revealed increased level of activity in the serratus anterior and upper trapezius but not the lower trapezius.[98]

The use of plyometrics in the upper extremity involves the application of a distal load on the upper extremity. This requires agonist and antagonist muscles to control the deceleration of a force. This places the viscoelastic components of the agonist into a shortened position. The preparation for motion reversal in the shoulder provides the potential to increase force generation during the concentric contraction. The type of pathology will dictate whether these modes of training are appropriate.[46,90] Cordasco et al[99] have examined the EMG analysis of the shoulder during plyometrics. The results found this technique to be a protective method of strengthening that is functional. However, these were healthy subjects using two hands during the exercises. A progression of plyometrics may include single arm throwbacks with a medicine ball standing a foot away from the wall. The patient would continue to throw moving farther distances away from the wall. However, there is no evidence to support the functional carry over from isokinetic or plyometric strength training.[100]

CONCLUSION

The exercise prescription is a continuum of rehabilitation phases based on scientific rationale, each ending by achieving a milestone before progressing forward. However, none of these milestones are set in stone, nor is every exercise distinct to that phase. The goals and milestones will need to be modified based on the performer, pathology, and performance demands. No exercise prescription should be viewed as a rigid protocol to follow word for word but as a guideline for which we base the specific rehabilitation process.

REFERENCES

1. Griffin KM, Bonci C, Solane B: Prevention and rehabilitation of shoulder injuries in throwing athletes. In Nicholas JA, Hershman EB (eds): The Upper Extremity in Sport Medicine. Mosby, St Louis, 1995
2. Kent BE: Functional anatomy of the shoulder complex. Phys Ther 51:867–888, 1971
3. Inman VT, Saunders JB, Abbott LC: Observation on the function of the shoulder joint. Am J Bone Joint Surg 1A:1–30, 1944
4. Morrey BF, Itoi E, An K: Biomechanics of the shoulder. In Rockwood CA, Matsen FA (eds): The Shoulder. W.B. Saunders, Philadelphia, 1998
5. Ferrari DA: Capsular ligaments of the shoulder. Anatomical and functional study of the anterior superior capsule. Am J Sports Med 18:20–24, 1990
6. O'Brien SJ, Neves MC, Arnoczky SP, et al: The anatomy and histology of the inferior glenohumeral ligament complex of the shoulder. Am J Sports Med 18:449–456, 1990
7. Warner JJP, Caborn DNM, Berger R, et al: Dynamic capsuloligamentous anatomy of the glenohumeral joint. J Shoulder Elbow Surg 2:115–133, 1993
8. Warner JJP, Flatow EL: Anatomy and biomechanics. In Bigliani LU (ed): The Unstable Shoulder. AAOS, Rosemont, IL, 1996
9. Kunmar VP, Balasubramianiam P: The role of atmospheric pressure in stabilising the shoulder: an experimental study. J Bone Joint Surg 67B:719–721, 1985
10. Warner JJP, Deng X, Warren RF, et al: Superoinferior translation in the intact and vented glenohumeral joint. J Shoulder Elbow Surg 2:99–105, 1993
11. Motzkin NE, Itoi E, Morrey BF, An K: Contribution of passive bulk tissues and deltoid to static inferior glenohumeral stability. J Shoulder Elbow Surg 3:313–319, 1994
12. Hollinghead WH, Rosse C: Textbook of Anatomy. Harper & Row, Philadelphia, 1985
13. DiGiovine NM, Jobe F, Pink M, Perry J: An electromyographic analysis of the upper extremity in pitching. J Shoulder Elbow Surg 1:15–26, 1992
14. Glousman R, Jobe F, Tibone J, et al: Dynamic electromyographic analysis of the throwing shoulder with glenohumeral instability. J Bone Joint Surg 70:220–226, 1988
15. Kibler WB: Orthopaedic knowledge update shoulder and elbow. In Norris TR (ed): Rehabilitation of the Shoulder. AAOS, Chicago, 1997, pp 289–298
16. Gowan ID, Jobe F, Tibone J, et al: A comparative electromyographic analysis of the shoulder during pitching. Am J Sports Med 15:586–590, 1987
17. Jobe F, Moynes DR, Tibone J, Perry J: An EMG analysis of the shoulder in pitching. A second report. Am J Sports Med 12:218–220, 1984
18. Paine RM, Voight M: The role of the scapula. J Orthop Sports Phys Ther 18:386–391, 1993

19. Aronen JG, Regan K: Decreasing the incidence of recurrence of first time anterior shoulder dislocation with rehabilitation. Am J Sports Med 12:283, 1984

20. Basmajian JV, Bazant FJ: Factors preventing downward dislocation of the abducted shoulder joint. J Bone Joint Surg 41A:1182, 1959

21. Cain PR, Mutschler TA, Fu FH, Lee SK: Anterior stability of the glenohumeral joint: a dynamic model. Am J Sports Med 15:144, 1987

22. Poppen NK, Walker PS: Normal and abnormal motion of the shoulder. Bone Joint Surg 58A:195–201, 1976

23. Saha AK: Dynamic stability of the glenohumeral joint. Acta Orthop 42:491–505, 1971

24. Symeonides PP: The significance of the subscapularis muscle in the pathogenesis of recurrent anterior dislocation of the shoulder. J Bone Joint Surg 54B:476, 1972

25. Kumar VP, Satku K, Balasubramaniam P: The role of the long head of biceps brachii in the stabilization of the head of the humerus. Clin Orthop 244:172–175, 1989

26. Rodosky MW, Harner CD, Fu FH: The role of the long head of the biceps muscle and superior glenoid labrum in anterior stability of the shoulder. Am J Sports Med 1:121–130, 1994

27. Itoi E, Motzkin NE, Morrey BF: The stabilizing function of the long head of the biceps with the arm in the hanging position. Orthop Trans 16:775, 1992

28. Perry J: Muscle control of the shoulder. In Rowe CR (ed): The Shoulder. Churchill Livingstone, New York, 1988

29. Neer CS: Shoulder Reconstruction. W.B. Saunders, Philadelphia, 1990

30. Basmajian JV, Deluca CJ: Muscles Alive: Their Functions Revealed by Electromyography, 5th Ed. Williams & Wilkins, Baltimore, 1985, pp 223–289

31. Speer KP, Garrett WE: Musclar control of motion and stability about the pectoral girdle. In Matsen FA, Fu FH, Hawkins RJ (eds): The Shoulder: A Balance of Mobility and Stability. AAOS, Rosemont, IL, 1993

32. Jobe CM: Gross anatomy of the shoulder. In Rockwood CA, Matsen FA (eds): The Shoulder. W.B. Saunders, Philadelphia, 1998

33. Davick JP, Martin RK, Albright JP: Distribution and deposition of tritiated cortisol using phonophoresis. Phys Ther 68:1672–1675, 1988

34. Bartlett LR, Storey MD, Simons BD: Measurement of upper extremity torque production and its relationship to throwing speed in the competitive athlete. Am J Sports Med 17:89–91, 1989

35. Howell S, Kraft T: The role of supraspinatus and infraspinatus muscles in glenohumeral kine-matics of anterior shoulder instability. Clin Orthop 263:128–134, 1991

36. Howell S, Galinat BJ: The glenoid-labral socket: a constrained articular surface. Clin Orthop 243:122–125, 1989

37. Howell SM, Galinat BJ, Renzi AJ, Marone PJ: Normal and abnormal mechanics of the glenohumeral joint in the horizontal plane. J Bone Joint Surg 70A:227–232, 1988

38. Kibler WB: Role of the scapula in the overhead throwing motion. Contemp Orthop 22:525–532, 1991

39. Freedman L, Munro RR: Abduction of the arm in the scapular plane: scapular and glenohumeral movements. A roentgenographic study. J Bone Joint Surg 48A:1503–1510, 1966

40. Johnston TB: The movements of the shoulder-joint: a plea for the use of the 'plane of the scapula' as the plane of reference for movements occurring at the humero-scapular joint. Br J Surg 25:252–260, 1937

41. Neer CS: Impingement lesions. Clinical Orthop 173:70–77, 1983

42. Weinstein SM: The role of the spine in the throwing athlete. AAOSM, Vancouver, 1998

43. Krumholz AL, Gelfand B, O'Connor PA: Therapeutic modalities. In Nicholas JA, Hershman EB (eds): The Lower Extremity and Spine in Sports Medicine, 2nd Ed. Mosby, St. Louis, 1995, Vol 1, pp. 207–234

44. Parker RD, Seitz WH: Shoulder impingement/instability overlap syndrome. J South Orthop Assoc 6(3):197–203, 1997

45. Frieman BG, Albert TJ, Fenlin JM: Rotator cuff disease: a review of diagnosis, pathophysiology and current trends in treatment. Arch Phys Med Rehabil 75:604–609, 1994

46. Kibler WB: Shoulder rehabilitation: principles and practice. Med Sci Sports Exerc 4:S40-S50, 1998

47. Knight K: The effects of hypothermia on inflammation and swelling. Athletic Training 11:7–10, 1976

48. Woo SL-Y, Inoue M, McGurk-Burleson E, Gomez MA: Treatment of the medial collateral ligament injury. II. Structure and function of canine knees in response to differing treatment regimens. Am J Sports Med 15:22, 1987

49. Dahners LE: Ligament contraction: a correlation with cellularity and action staining. Trans Orthop Res Soc 11:56, 1986

50. Weiler JM: Medical modifiers of sports injury: the use of nonsteroidal anti-inflammatory drugs (NSAID's) in sports soft tissue injury in tendinitis. I: Basic concepts. Clin Sports Med 11(3):625–644, 1992

51. Shelbourne D, Liotta FJ, Goodloe SL: Preemptive pain management program for anterior cruciate ligament reconstruction. Am J Knee Surg 11(2):116–119, 1998

52. Levy AS, Kelly B, Lintner S, Speer K: Penetration of cryotherapy in treatment after shoulder arthroscopy. Arthroscopy 13:461–464, 1997

53. Speer KP, Cavanaugh JT, Warren RF, et al: A role for hydrotherapy in shoulder rehabilitation. Am J Sports Med 21:850–853, 1993

54. Morgan B, Jones A, Mulcahy K, et al: Transcutaneous electric nerve stimulation (TENS) during distension shoulder arthrography: a controlled trial. Pain 64:265–267, 1995

55. Herrera-Lasso I, Mobarak L, Fernandez-Dominguez L, et al: Comparative effectiveness of packages of treatment including ultrasound or transcutaneous electrical nerve stimulation in painful shoulder syndrome. Physiotherapy 79:251–254, 1993

56. Lehmann JF, Erickson DJ, Martin GM, et al: Comparison of ultrasonic and microwave diathermy in the physical treatment of periarthritis of the shoulder. Arch Phys Med Rehabil 35:627–634, 1954

57. Downing DS, Weinstein A: Ultrasound therapy of subacromial bursitis: a double blind trial. Phys Ther 66:194–199, 1986

58. Nykanen M: Pulsed ultrasound treatment of the painful shoulder: a randomized, double-blind, placebo-controlled study. Scand J Rehabil Med 27:105–108, 1995

59. Griffin JE, Echternach JL, Price RE, et al: Patients treated with ultrasonic driven hydrocortisone and with ultrasound alone. Phys Ther 47:594–601, 1967

60. Cameron MH, Monroe LG: Relative transmission of ultrasound by media customarily used for phonophoresis. Phys Ther 72:142–148, 1992

61. Maitland G: Peripheral Manipulation. Butterworth, London, 1977

62. Kisner C, Colby LA: Peripheral joint mobilization. In Therapeutic Exercise Foundation and Techniques, 2nd Ed. F.A. Davis, Philadelphia, 1990

63. Lastayo PC, Wright T, Jaffe R, Hartzel J: Continuous passive motion after repair of the rotator cuff. J Bone Joint Surg 80A:1002–1011, 1998

64. Kamkar A, Irrgang JJ, Whitney SL: Nonoperative management of secondary impingement syndrome. J Orthop Sports Phys Ther 17:212–224, 1993

65. Peat M: Functional anatomy of the shoulder complex. Phys Ther 66:1855–1865, 1986

66. Schenkman M, Rugo de Cartaya V: Kinesiology of the shoulder complex. J Orthop Sports Phys Ther 8:438–450, 1987

67. Lindman R, Eriksson A, Thornell LE: Fiber type composition of the human male trapezius muscle: enzyme-histo-chemical characteristics. Am J Anat 189:236–244, 1990

68. McQuade KJ, Smidt GL: Dynamic scapulohumeral rhythm: the effects of external resistance during elevation of the arm in the scapular plane. J Orthop Sports Phys Med 27:125–133, 1998

69. McQuade KJ, Dawson J, Smidt GL: Scapulothoracic muscle fatigue associated with alterations in scapulohumeral rhythm kinematics during maximum resistive shoulder elevation. J Orthop Sports Phys Ther 28:74–80, 1998

70. Ballantyne B, O'Hare S, Paschall J, et al: Electromyographic activity of selected shoulder muscles in commonly used therapeutic exercises. Phys Ther 73:668–682, 1993

71. Kelly B, Kadrmas W, Kirkendall D, Speer K: Optimal normalization tests for shoulder muscle activation: an electromyographic study. J Orthop Res 14:647–653, 1996

72. McCann P, Wootten M, Kadaba M, Bigliani L: A kinematic and electromyographic study of shoulder rehabilitation exercises. Clin Orthop 288:179–188, 1993

73. McMahon PJ, Jobe FW, Pink MM, et al: Comparative electromyographic analysis of shoulder muscles during planar motions: anterior glenohumeral instability versus normal. J Shoulder Elbow Surg 2:118–123, 1996

74. Moseley JB, Jobe FW, Pink M, et al: ECG analysis of scapular muscles during a shoulder rehabilitation program. Am J Sports Med 20:128–134, 1994

75. McConnell J: The McConnell approach to the problem shoulder. (Course notes.) Lenox Hill Hospital, New York, October 17–18, 1997

76. Toyoshima S, Hoshikawa T, Miyashita M, Oguri T: Contribution of the body parts to throwing performance. In Nelson RC, Morehouse CA (eds): Biomechanics IV. University Park Press, Baltimore, pp. 169–174, 1974

77. Mulligan E: Conservative management of shoulder impingement syndrome. Athletic Training 23:348–353, 1988

78. Triffitt PD: The relationship between motion of the shoulder and the stated ability to perform activities of daily living. J Bone Joint Surg 80A:41–46, 1998

79. Litchfield R, Hawkins R, Dillman C, et al: Rehabilitation of the overhead athlete. J Orthop Sports Phys Ther 18:433–441, 1993

80. Harryman DT, Sidles JA, Clark JM, et al: Translation of the humeral head on the glenoid with passive glenohumeral motion. J Bone Joint Surg 72A:1334–1343, 1990

81. Tyler TF, Roy T, Nicholas SJ, Gleim GW: Reliability and validity of a new method of measuring posterior shoulder tightness. J Orthop Sports Phys Ther 29(5):262–269, 1999

82. Rokito AS, Zuckerman JD, Gallagher MA, Cuomo F: Strength after surgical repair of the rotator cuff. J Shoulder Elbow Surg 1:12–17, 1996

83. Townsend H, Jobe F, Pink M, Perry J: Electromyographic analysis of the glenohumeral muscles during a baseball rehabilitation program. Am J Sports Med 19:264–272, 1991

84. Blackburn TA, McLeod WD, White B, Wofford L: EMG analysis of posterior rotator cuff exercises. Athletic Training 25:40–45, 1990

85. Hintermeister RA, Lange GW, Schultheis JM, et al: Electromyographic activity and applied load during shoulder rehabilitation exercises using elastic resistance. Am J Sports Med 2:210–220, 1998

86. Wilk KE, Arrigo C: Current concepts in the rehabilitation of the athletic shoulder. J Orthop Sports Phys Ther 18:365–378, 1993

87. Walmsley RP, Szybbo C: A comparative study of the torque generated by the shoulder internal and external rotators in different positions and at varying speeds. J Orthop Sports Phys Ther 9:217, 1987

88. Greenfield BH, Donatelli R, Wooden MJ, Wilkes J: Isokinetic evaluation of shoulder rotational strength between the plane of scapula and the frontal plane. Am J Sports Med 18:124–128, 1990

89. Soderberg GJ, Blaschek MJ: Shoulder internal and external rotation peak torque production through a velocity spectrum in differing positions. J Orthop Sports Phys Ther 8:518, 1987

90. Komi P, Bosco C: Utilization of stored elastic energy in leg extensor muscles by men and women. Med Sci Sports 10:261, 1978

91. Wilk KE, Voight ML, Keirns MA, et al: Stretch-shortening drills for the upper extremities: theory and clinical application. J Orthop Sports Phys Ther 17:225–239, 1993

92. Turkel SJ, Panio MW, Marshall JL, et al: Stabilizing mechanisms preventing anterior dislocation of the glenohumeral joint. J Bone Joint Surg 63A:1208–1217, 1981

93. Saha AK: Mechanism of shoulder movements and a plea for the recognition of "zero position" of glenohumeral joint. Clin Orthop 173:3–10, 1983

94. Lucas DB: Biomechanics of the shoulder joint. Arch Surg 107:425–432, 1973

95. Malanga GA, Jenp YN, Growney ES, An KN: EMG analysis of shoulder positioning in testing and strengthening the supraspinatus. Med Sci Sports Exerc 6:661–664, 1996

96. Jobe F, Moynes DR: Delineation of diagnostic criteria and a rehabilitation program for rotator cuff injuries. Am J Sports Med 10:336–339, 1982

97. Rowlands LK, Wertsch JJ, Primack SJ, et al: Kinesiology of the empty can test. Am J Phys Med 74:302–304, 1995

98. Lear LJ, Gross MT: An electromyographical analysis of the scapular stabilizing synergists during a push-up progression. J Orthop Sports Phys Ther 28(3):146–156, 1998

99. Cordasco FA, Wolfe IN, Wootten ME, Bigliani LU: An electromyographic analysis of the shoulder during a medicine ball rehabilitation program. Am J Sports Med 3:386–392, 1996

100. Heiderscheit BC, McLean KP, Davies GJ: The effects of isokinetic vs. plyometric training on the shoulder internal rotators. J Orthop Sports Phys Ther 23:125–133, 1996

SUGGESTED READINGS

Bonci CM, Hensal FJ, Torg JS: A preliminary study on the measurement of static and dynamic motion at the glenohumeral joint. Am J Sports Med 14.12–17, 1986

Boublik M, Hawkins R: Clinical examination of the shoulder complex. J Orthop Sports Phys Ther 18:379–385, 1993

Clark J, Sidles JA, Matsen FA: The relationship of the glenohumeral joint capsule to the rotator cuff. Clin Orthop 254:29–34, 1990

Clark JM, Harryman DT: Tendons, ligaments, and capsule of the rotator cuff. J Bone Joint Surg 5:713–725, 1992

Conroy DE, Hayes KW: The effect of joint mobilization as a component of comprehensive treatment for primary shoulder impingement syndrome. J Orthop Sports Phys Ther 28:3–14, 1998

Dillman C, Fleisig G, Andrews J: Biomechanics of pitching with emphasis upon shoulder kinematics. J Orthop Sports Phys Ther 18:402–408, 1993

Gleim GW, McHugh M: Flexibility and its effects on sports injury and performance. Sports Med 5:289–299, 1997

Haggmark T, Eriksson E, Jansson E: Muscle fiber type changes in human skeletal muscle after injuries and immobilization. Orthopedics (9):181, 1986

Hama H, Morinaga T, Suzuki K, et al: The infraspinatus test: an early diagnostic sign of muscle weakness during external rotation of the shoulder in athletes. J Shoulder Elbow Surg 2:257–259, 1993

Hawkins RJ, Kennedy JC: Impingement syndrome in athletes. Am J Sports Med 8:151–158, 1980

Helmig P, Sojbjerg JO, Kjaefsgaard-Andersen P, et al: Distal humeral migration as a component of multidirectional shoulder instability. Clin Orthop 252:139–143, 1990

Helmig P, Sojbjerg JO, Sneppen O, et al: Glenohumeral movement patterns after puncture of the joint capsule: an experimental study. J Shoulder Elbow Surg 2:209–215, 1993

Hutton RS: Neuromuscular basis of stretching exercises. In Paavo KV (ed): Strength and Power in Sport. The Encyclopaedia of Sports Medicine and IOC Medical Commission Publication. Blackwell Scientific Publications, Oxford, 1991, pp 29–38

Itoi E, Motzkin NE, Morrey BF, et al: Contribution of axial arm rotation to humeral head translation. Am J Sports Med 22:499–503, 1994

Itoi E, Tabata S: Conservative treatment of rotator cuff tears. Clin Orthop 275:165–173, 1992

Jobe F, Pink M: Classification and treatment of shoulder dysfunction in the overhead athlete. J Orthop Sports Phys Ther 18:427–432, 1993

Johansen RL, Callis M, Potts J, Shall L: A modified internal rotation technique for overhand and throwing athletes. J Orthop Sports Phys Ther 21:216–219, 1995

Kronberg M, Nemeth G, Brostrom L: Muscle activity and coordination in the normal shoulder. Clin Orthop 257:76–85, 1990

Lippitt SB, Harris SL, Harryman DT, et al: In vivo quantification of the laxity of normal and unstable glenohumeral joints. J Shoulder Elbow Surg 3:215–223, 1994

Lundin P, Berg W: A review of plyometric training. National Strength Conditioning Assoc J 13:22–30, 1991

Meister K, Andrews JR: Classification and treatment of rotator cuff injuries in the overhand athlete. J Orthop Sports Phys Ther 18:413–421, 1998

Neer CS: The shoulder in sports. Orthop Clinics North Am 8:583–591, 1997

Nicholas JA, et al: The importance of a simplified classification of motion in sports in relation to performance. Orthop Clin North Am 8:499, 1977

Paavo KV: Stretch-shortening cycle. In Paavo KV (ed): Strength and Power in Sport. The Encyclopaedia of Sports Medicine and IOC Medical Commission Publication. Blackwell Scientific Publications, Oxford, 1991, pp 169–179.

Pagnani MJ, Warren RF: Stabilizers of the glenohumeral joint. J Shoulder Elbow Surg 3:173–190, 1994

Peacock EE: Wound Repair, 3rd Ed. WB Saunders, Philadelphia, 1984

Pearl ML, Perry J, Torburn L, Lawerence HG: An electromyographic analysis of the shoulder during cones and planes of arm motion. Clin Orthop 284:116–127, 1992

Richards DB, Kibler WB: Sports-related shoulder rehabilitation: an overview of concepts. J Musculoskeletal Med 14:44–63, 1997

Saha AK: Dynamic stability of the glenohumeral joint. Acta Orthop Scand 42:491–505, 1971

Shankwiler JA, Burkhead WZ: Diagnosis, evaluation, and conservative treatment of impingement syndrome. Operative Tech Sports Med 2:89–97, 1994

Sobel JS, Kremer I, Winters JC, et al: The influence of the mobility in the cervicothoracic spine and the upper ribs (shoulder girdle) on the mobility of the scapulohumeral joint. J Manipulative Physiol Ther 7:469–474, 1996

Tata GE, Ng L, Kramer JF: Shoulder antagonistic strength ratios during concentric and eccentric muscle actions in the scapular plane. J Orthop Sports Phys Ther 18:654–660, 1993

Thompson WO, Debski RE, Boardman ND, et al: A biomechanical analysis of rotator cuff deficiency in a cadaveric model. Am J Sports Med 24:286–292, 1996

Thorsteinsson G, Stonnington HH, Stillwell GK, et al: The placebo effect of transcutaneous electrical stimulation. Pain 5:31–41, 1978

Torstensen TA, Meen HD, Stiris M: The effect of medical exercise therapy on a patient with chronic supraspinatus tendinitis. Diagnostic ultrasound-tissue regeneration: a case study. J Orthop Sports Phys Ther 20:319–327, 1994

Voight ML, Hardin JA, Blackburn TA, et al: The effects of muscle fatigue on and the relationship of arm dominance to shoulder proprioception. J Orthop Sports Phys Ther 6:348–352, 1996

Warner JJP, Micheli LJ, Arslanian LE, et al: Scapulothoracic motion in normal shoulders and shoulders with glenohumeral instability and impingement syndrome: a study using Moire topographic analysis. Clin Orthop 285:191–199, 1992

Yamshon LJ, Bierman W: Kinesiologic electromyography. Arch Phys Med 647–651, 1948

20

Sports Injuries of the Wrist and Hand

JOHN V. BASMAJIAN ■ DINESH A. KUMBHARE

Rehabilitation of hand and wrist problems in athletes and sportspersons of all kinds and of all ages has been handicapped, even in modern times, by confusion over causes and their diagnostic criteria, intensity of acute treatments (including surgery), and postacute care. This chapter casts a critical eye on the existing evidence in the literature and attempts to weigh the importance of what is largely based on the long experience of respected clinicians. Our review found no study that approaches the gold standard. The wrist and hand constitute an uncharted territory.

Many books are devoted to the exhaustive treatment of the musculoskeletal and neurologic problems of the upper limb, including the wrist and hand, but few, if any, deal with the decision-making process and evidence-based practice in rehabilitation problems of the wrist and hand. This chapter does not review the literature. Rather, we will choose the significant conditions of the wrist and hand that may be experienced by amateur sportspersons and professional athletes in their sporting activities.

Athletes are susceptible to the same neuropathies seen in nonathletes, and most sports nerve injuries are not unique to sports; thus the general concepts of neurapraxia, axonotmesis, and neurotmesis, and the anatomy, healing, and functioning of the nerves are similar between athletes and nonathletes. However, there are some distinctions between athletes and non-athletes:

1. Athletes' propensity to push their bodies to their absolute limit, working with their bodies in extreme positions and being subjected to severe and repetitive trauma

2. Ongoing participation in sports despite pain or clear evidence of tissue damage
3. The intense desire to return to sporting activity at nearly any cost

CARPAL TUNNEL SYNDROME

Carpal tunnel syndrome (CTS) is defined as entrapment of the median nerve within the carpal tunnel. There is a distinction between median nerve injury and the nonspecific signs and symptoms of carpal tunnel syndrome. True CTS can be defined as objective confirmation of median nerve injury; therefore by definition CTS is a clinical diagnosis. Symptoms of CTS include numbness and tingling in the median nerve distribution of the thumb, index finger, middle finger, and radial half of the ring finger; numbness in the entire hand (autonomic disturbance associated with CTS); nocturnal aggravation of hand symptoms; pain in the wrist at night that can be shaken out; pain in the wrist after frequent use of wrists and hands; dropping or difficulty holding items; and pain referred more proximally in the upper limb.[1-3]

In the literature, signs associated with CTS vary greatly. The problems with this literature include the following:

- Only subjective data were used to diagnose CTS in many studies.
- Provocative maneuvers were described and performed inconsistently.
- There were significant technical limitations for the signs. A list of signs with sensitivities and specificities of published studies can be found in Table 20–1.

TABLE 20–1. Sensitivity and Specificity of Carpal Tunnel Syndrome Signs

CONDUCTION SIGN	SENSITIVITY (%)	SPECIFICITY (%)	SAMPLE SIZE	NERVE STUDIES*
Hoffmann-Tinel[74]				
Phalen[75]	73	Not reported	654	None
Seror[76]	63	55	100	Good
Posch, Marcotte[32]	9	Not reported	1201	None
Szabo et al[77]	61	Not reported	23	Good
Golding et al[78]	26	80	39	Poor
Durkan[79]	56	80	36	Poor
DeKrom et al[15]	25	59	44	Good
Hennessey, Kuhlman[3]	23	87	228	Good
Phalen				
Phalen[75]	73	Not reported	654	None
Posch, Marcotte[32]	10	Not reported	1201	None
Szabo et al[77]	70	Not reported	23	Good
Golding et al[78]	10	86	39	Poor
Durkan[79]	70	84	36	Poor
DeKrom et al[15]	48	55	44	Good
Hennessey, Kuhlman[3]	51	76	228	Good
Reverse Phalen				
Werner et al[19]	55	100	50	Good
LeBan et al[80]				
LaBan et al[80]	90	100	20	Good
Square Wrist				
Gordon et al[81]	74	76	80	Good
Hennessey, Kuhlman[3]	69	73	228	Good
Thenar Weakness				
DeKrom et al[15]	39	80	44	Good
Hennessey, Kuhlman[3]	66	66	228	Good
Thenar Atrophy				
Phalen[75]	44	Not reported	654	None
DeKrom et al[15]	16	94	44	Good
Golding et al[78]	3	100	39	Poor
Two-Point Discrimination				
Szabo[77]	22	Not reported	23	Good
Spindler, Dellon[82]	64	Not reported	74	Good
Gellman et al[83]	33	Not reported	67	Poor
Hypesthesia				
Phalen[75]	79	Not reported	654	None
Golding et al[78]	15	93	39	Poor
DeKrom et al[15]	39	59	44	Good
Hennessey, Kuhlman[3]	51	85	228	Good
Carpal Compression				
Durkan[79]	87	90	36	Poor
DeKrom et al[15]	5	94	44	Good
Hennessey, Kuhlman[3]	28	74	228	Good

TABLE 20–1. Sensitivity and Specificity of Carpal Tunnel Syndrome Signs *Continued*

CONDUCTION SIGN	SENSITIVITY (%)	SPECIFICITY (%)	SAMPLE SIZE	NERVE STUDIES*
Tourniquet				
Gellman et al[83]	65	60	67	Poor

*Good, Standard electrodiagnostic techniques performed and referenced. The study is reproducible. *Poor*, Electrodiagnostic techniques not described or inadequately described. The study is not reproducible.

Incidence

Nordstrom and colleagues[4] studied the incidence of diagnosed CTS in Wisconsin and Minnesota. They conducted a prospective study to ascertain all cases of incident disease during a 2-year period. Newly diagnosed, probable, or definite CTS ($N = 309$) occurred at a rate of 3.46 cases per 1,000 person-years (95% confidence interval = $3.07 - 3.84$).[4] They believed this to accurately reflect the incidence of diagnosed CTS in a general population. Little is known about the incidence of CTS in the athletic population. Krivickas and Wilbourn reported peripheral nerve injuries in 169 athletes with 190 sports injuries to nerve fibers.[5] They reported 80% of the injuries occurred in the upper extremity; the most common injuries were burners ($N = 38$) and cervical radiculopathies ($N = 18$), followed by median ($N = 28$), axillary ($N = 22$), ulnar ($N = 19$), suprascapular ($N = 14$), and peroneal ($N = 11$) mononeuropathies. This is the largest reported case series of sports-related nerve injuries to date. Athletes participated in 27 sports, but over one third of injuries were sustained playing football. A similar incidence for injuries was also described by Feinberg et al in 1997.[6]

Epidemiology

Not much information on CTS in the athletic population is available. It has been extensively studied in the occupational literature and will not be reviewed in this chapter. An excellent reference appears in *Physical Medicine & Rehabilitation Clinics of North America* (August 1997), and the reader is directed to this extensive reference for more information. CTS, as stated earlier, has nonspecific signs and symptoms. Most epidemiologic studies performed on CTS have included abnormalities of the median nerve since this is objective and precise, and the signs and symptoms associated with CTS are nonspecific. The Industrial Injuries Committee of the American Society for Surgery of the Hand, after reviewing more than 2,000 articles, recently concluded that "no causal relationship is established between work activities and any median nerve injury."[7] Median nerve slowing is more common in women than in men. Men accounted for 22% of those with CTS in a benchmark study performed at the Mayo Clinic from 1961 to 1980.[8]

Familial Occurrence

Certain familial medical conditions, such as amyloidosis, mucopolysaccharidosis, mucolipidosis, and polyneuropathy, may affect the median nerve at the carpal tunnel. Also, a relationship between Dupuytren's contracture (thickened palmar tissue) and CTS has been found with trisomy of chromosome 8 in five of nine patients with Dupuytren's contracture and in five patients with CTS. A thickened carpal ligament may be the cause of symptoms.[9] The familial occurrence of median nerve slowing or CTS is reported among several ethnic and nationality groups.[10]

Aging

The aging process may be a factor in the development of median nerve injury. The Mayo Clinic[11] found a significant co-variance between age and all median sensory conductions in 330 healthy subjects. Letz and Gerr[12] studied 4,462 army personnel and found a 0.127 m/sec/yr slowing of median sensory conduction and a 0.108 m/sec/yr change in median motor latency ($P < .0001$). Stetson and colleagues[13] in 1992 reported similar findings.

Several studies linking obesity, shorter height, or weight gain to CTS report a co-variance or direct relationship between increased BMI (body mass index) and median slowing in the carpal tunnel.[12,14–19]

Johnson Wrist Ratio

The Johnson wrist ratio is the wrist depth divided by the width. Ernest W. Johnson observed that women most likely to develop symptoms of CTS during pregnancy were those with "squarish" wrists. That is to say, those with a higher wrist ratio.[20] The positive co-variance between the wrist ratio and median nerve slowing is not yet clearly explained. Square-wristed individuals may have thicker carpal ligaments or a smaller carpal tunnel cross-sectional area, or there may be other characteristics affecting median nerve function that have yet to be worked out.[21]

Medical Conditions

Many medical conditions are associated with symptoms of CTS. However, establishing a causal relationship between these conditions and median nerve injury is difficult. This is because multiple medical conditions may co-exist and personal factors such as age, BMI, and wrist ratio must also be considered. Medical conditions showing such an association include diabetes, thyroid disorders, rheumatoid arthritis, abnormalities of growth hormone, dialysis, space-occupying lesions, and anomalous muscles. A complete review of these conditions is beyond the scope of the present chapter.

Pathophysiology

Most clinicians agree that CTS should be thought of as a repetitive strain disorder. In a susceptible individual the stress results in edema and increased pressure within the carpal tunnel. Factors that lead to irritation and sometimes deterioration of the median nerve as it traverses the tunnel include repetitive stress, pressure, edema, and any characteristics of the individual, as previously described. Pressure of the tunnel was studied by a number of researchers, including Gelberman and colleagues[22] and Mubarak and colleagues.[23] Mubarak et al inserted a Wick catheter into the carpal tunnel and measured pressures of 12 controls and of patients with CTS. In the experimental group, at neutral wrist angle, the mean pressure was measured at 32 mm Hg, an average of 94 mm Hg in flexion and an average of 110 mm Hg in extension. In the controls the average pressure at neutral wrist angle was 2.5 mm Hg, at maximum flexion it was 31 mm Hg, and at maximum extension it was 30 mm Hg.[23] Such data are supported by other researchers.[24,25]

Lundberg et al[26] studied 16 healthy volunteers to examine the relationship between increased carpal tunnel pressure and the development of CTS. Intracanal pressures were measured using wrist catheter monitoring, and external compression at the wrist was applied to achieve intratunnel pressures of 90 mm, 60 mm, and 30 mm Hg. Nerve conduction studies of motor and sensory components of the median nerve were checked at baseline and every 5 minutes during the period of compression. Results of this important study demonstrate mild hand paresthesias at 30 mm Hg within 10 to 15 minutes of the onset of compression, and with compression at 60 or 90 mm Hg a rapid complete sensory conduction block occurred followed by a motor block for 10 to 30 minutes. This pivotal study establishes a correlation between increased carpal tunnel pressure and localized nerve dysfunction.

TREATMENT OF CARPAL TUNNEL SYNDROME

Splinting

Immobilization through splinting has been employed to reduce time spent at extreme wrist angles. Splints can be used for both nighttime and daytime, leaving the hands relatively free to perform daytime activities. Kruger et al[27] studied 105 patients with CTS with positive electromyograms (EMGs). Patients were placed in neutral angle splints for 17 months. Sixty-seven percent of these patients reported relief. All patients demonstrated improved sensory distal latencies, but those reporting subjective relief of symptoms showed improvement in both sensory and motor distal latency.

Antiinflammatory Medications

The efficacy for the use of nonsteroidal antiinflammatory drugs (NSAIDs) alone is not well documented for the treatment of CTS.[28] Steroids have shown some positive effects for the treatment of CTS. Harskovitz and colleagues[29] treated patients with CTS with 20 mg of prednisone daily for 1 week, followed by 10 mg daily for the second week. Symptoms improved initially quite rapidly, but their effect waned over 8 weeks after discontinuation of therapy. Therefore it is thought that this treatment in isolation is probably not effective.

Steroid Injections

Steroid injections have been widely used as a conservative treatment for CTS. This treatment was thought to offer the benefits of reducing the edema and therefore the pressure within the carpal tunnel, thereby providing symptom relief. Several authors, however, have suggested the possibility of median nerve damage as a significant side effect of such injections.[30-32] Overall success rates of steroid injections have varied in the literature from 60% to 90%.[28] These early studies, however, provided limited information regarding improvement and focused on short-term follow-up only. Giannini et al[33] injected 31 hands of 21 CTS patients with 40 mg of triamcinolone. At 6-month follow-up, 35% of the hands had complete relief, and 58% had partial relief. Sensory nerve conduction studies improved in 74% and motor nerve conduction in 65%. Girlander et al[34] studied 53 wrists in 32 patients with CTS in whom 15 mg of methylprednisolone or normal saline was injected. The follow-up was every 2 months for 2 years. At 6 months 50% of the patients had worsened symptomatology, and at 2-year follow-up only 8% of the wrists remained "completely cured."

The following studies have looked at splinting combined with steroid injections. Gelberman et al[35] stated that symptom resolution occurred in 39% of patients. Weiss et al[36] completed a prospective blinded study of 76 wrists in 56 patients; all were treated with 6 mg of betamethasone and placed in a neutral angle splint for 4 weeks. Final follow-up was at an average of 11 months. At 1 month the symptom "cure" rate was 50%, but this deteriorated to 13% at 11 months. Kaplan et al[37] studied 263 hands in 260 patients with CTS. All patients received a splint and either nonsteroidal antiinflammatory medication, oral steroids, or a steroid injection into the carpal tunnel. Six-month follow-up was carried out. Factors identified that correlated with poor outcome included age less than 50 years, duration of symptoms of longer than 10 months, constant paresthesias, stenosing flexor tenosynovitis, and positive Phalen's test in less than 30 seconds. When none of these factors were present the authors reported two thirds of their cases had a cure at 14-month follow-up. When one factor was present, 40.4% were cured, and when two factors were present, 16.7% were cured; when three factors were present, 6.8% were cured at the 1-month follow-up. Other factors identified as poor prognostic indicators have included increased body mass, specific wrist dimensions, and occupational factors such as ongoing workmen's compensation cases, use of laboratory tools, and repetitive hand motions.[38]

Vitamin B₆

Vitamin B$_6$ (pyridoxine) has been used for the treatment of CTS because it has gained some anecdotal popularity secondary to its ability to affect the pain threshold. Stransky et al,[39] using a randomized, double-blinded, placebo-controlled trial, studied the effects of vitamin B$_6$ on patients with CTS. The experimental group received 200 mg of vitamin B$_6$ daily. At 10-week follow-up there was no change in symptoms or electrodiagnostic studies. Wu et al[40] showed similar findings when vitamin B$_6$ supplements were compared with splinting, steroid injections, and a combination of steroids and splinting.

Surgery

The definitive treatment after failed conservative therapy for CTS is surgery. Carpal tunnel surgery can be performed using open or endoscopic techniques. The endoscopic technique has the following advantages: less tissue trauma, less postoperative pain, faster recovery, and smaller scars. Also, patients do not have to stay in the hospital for very long with the endoscopic approach. The consensus of one study[41] was that patients who were treated using the endoscopic method appeared to return to work sooner than patients treated with the open approach. This was regardless of workers' compensation status.

There are also reports of higher grip and pinch strength obtained earlier in the recovery period for the endoscopic method. Complications of surgery range from chronic pain to neurapraxia and infection or nerve transection. Complication rates as low as 0.5% to as high as 7% have been reported.[41]

A PROPOSED MEDICAL TREATMENT STRATEGY

This treatment strategy for CTS is proposed based on the best available evidence in the literature and the experience of the authors.

1. You must definitively diagnose CTS and rule out any other entities that may contribute to the patient's symptoms. This is usually possible with a thorough history, physical examination, and electrodiagnostic studies. Should an alternative diagnosis arise, treat as appropriate.
2. *Appropriate ergonomics*: correct positioning of the hands should be maximized to reduce the time spent in extremes of flexion and extension.
3. Recommend a reduction in the amount of repetitive work, if possible. Routine breaks should also be taken if possible.
4. Arrange a general fitness program with weight reduction and cardiovascular fitness.
5. Provide splinting with the wrist in neutral position. Such a splint should be worn for 2 to 3 weeks, and then the patient should be reassessed.
6. In conjunction with wrist splinting, an anti-inflammatory dose of NSAIDs should be prescribed, with the patient warned of possible side effects.
7. If the patient remains symptomatic, consider the risks and benefits of a corticosteroid injection and proceed with the injection with the patient's informed consent. The volume injected would be minimized as much as possible by using as concentrated a preparation of corticosteroids as possible. This should minimize neural trauma.
8. If there is no response to the above treatments, then you should refer the patient for consideration of surgical release of the median nerve at the carpal tunnel.

Differential Diagnosis

It is essential to exclude conditions that can mimic CTS. This can be accomplished through EMG nerve conduction studies. A patient may present with symptoms that mimic CTS, but another diagnosis may result from performing EMG nerve conduction studies, for example, proximal median neuropathy with entrapment of the median nerve (at the pronator teres muscle or at the ligament of Struthers). These patients would have low-amplitude compound muscle and sensory nerve action potentials of the median nerve and slowing of conduction velocity in the forearm. Such patients would be carefully studied using needle EMG, because this important test will likely lead to the correct diagnosis.[42]

The needle EMG also assists in diagnosing cervical radiculopathy and brachial plexus lesions. A combination of cervical radiculopathy and CTS—the so-called double crush syndrome—first was reported by Upton and McComas in 1973[43] and is now becoming more widely accepted. A proposed mechanism for this syndrome is that a proximal lesion (e.g., at a cervical root) makes the distal nerve more susceptible to entrapment at normal entrapment sites, such as the carpal tunnel.[44]

Cervical radiculopathy, especially in a C6 territory, may present clinically with symptoms very similar to CTS, and it can be difficult on history and physical examination alone to make the distinction between C6 radiculopathy and CTS. Needle EMG evidence of cervical radiculopathy can assist in making this diagnosis.[45] Cervical radiculopathy has been found to coexist with CTS in 6% to 14% of patients.[46,47]

Gnatz[48] analyzed 1,070 consecutive electrodiagnostic studies. The incidence of cervical radiculopathy, CTS, and a combination of the two diagnoses was calculated, revealing 15% as CTS, 3.9% as cervical radiculopathy (all levels), and 1.1% as a combination of CTS and cervical radiculopathy (double crush syndrome).

Patients may meet the electrodiagnostic criteria for CTS but fail to respond appropriately to treatment; this may occur if patients have concomitant CTS and cervical radiculopathy. Eason and colleagues[49] have demonstrated that patients who have concomitant CTS and cervical radiculopathy have worse outcomes after carpal tunnel release than those with CTS alone.

The patient with **concomitant polyneuropathy and CTS** also poses a challenging problem. Polyneuropathy may predispose the peripheral nerves to entrapment neuropathy.[48] In such challenging patients the electromyographer will likely be faced with prolonged distal latencies of all or most peripheral nerves, and he or she should look for latency differences between the median and other peripheral nerves. Electrodiagnostically it is also important to thoroughly evaluate for peripheral neuropathy, including needle EMG of distal and proximal muscles to determine the extent of axonal loss. This assists in establishing a diagnosis, as well as in the process of prognostication.

Finally, **brachial plexus lesions and syringomyelia** can present with symptoms that may mimic CTS, and a significant number of patients with posttraumatic and congenital syringomyelia may have peripheral nerve entrapments as well.[50] Electrodiagnostically, one must rely on nerve conduction studies combined with F waves and needle EMG to define the extent of the pathology.[48]

Thoracic outlet syndrome is a clinical entity in which patients present with moderate to severe pain, paresthesias, weakness, and varying degrees of dysfunction of the arm and hand. This condition usually afflicts young to middle-aged healthy active adults with an aching pain that typically begins in the back of the shoulder and spreads to involve the medial aspect of the arm and forearm and into the ring and little fingers. The pain is exacerbated by arm elevation or by carrying objects such as grocery bags or luggage. These activities also stimulate numbness, tingling, progressive weakness, and even swelling, coolness, and discoloration of the fingers.

There are two different forms of neurogenic thoracic outlet syndrome. The classic or undisputed form of neurogenic thoracic outlet syndrome is usually caused by a congenital band from a bone anomaly (cervical rib or long C7 transverse process seen on x-ray). There are abnormal nerve conduction studies, and needle examination reveals axonal damage in a C8–T1 distribution.[51] These patients usually have neurologic findings, either in a C8–T1 distribution or the ulnar distribution, and have atrophy of the intrinsic muscles of the hand. Surgery has been found to assist the majority of these types of patients.[52,53]

The **"disputed" type of neurogenic thoracic outlet syndrome** is more common; it presents with pain as the primary complaint, accompanied by paresthesias, weakness, and dysfunction of the hand, again most frequently in the ulnar nerve distribution. This group of patients, however, does not have any muscle wasting or electrodiagnostic abnormalities. Conservative treatment is usually advocated for these patients, including physical therapy, various medications, injections, biofeedback, psychotherapy, and restricted use of the limb.[54]

Bony and soft tissue congenital anomalies in the neck and thoracic outlet region are common and are thought to predispose a large part of the general population to develop neurovascular symptoms that affect the upper extremity. Firsov[55] reported that cervical ribs were found in 0.27% of the population and 77% occurred in women. These soft tissue anomalies may remain symptomatically dormant until some activity or event causes muscle spasm or hypertrophy as a result of occupational arm position. Examples are hairdressing, athletic activities such as weightlifting, or trauma to the cervical region that results in long-term muscle contraction. Machleder and colleagues[56] demonstrated histochemical changes of scalene muscle fibers before and after neck trauma. They found an abundance of myosin isoform variation type 2 fibers, which are thought to cause tetanic contraction of muscles after trauma to the cervical muscles.[56] Sanders and colleagues[57] found similar changes in scalene muscles and reported that there were double the number of connective tissue cells following neck injury. The degree of compression is thought to vary with the type, tension, rigidity of the anomalous structures, severity of the trauma or strain involved, and age, gender, occupation, and general activities of the patient.[54]

The **vascular thoracic outlet syndrome** is due to arterial insufficiency from subclavian artery compression, varying from aneurysm to emboli or vessel occlusion. This can result in intermittent coolness, fatigue, advanced ischemia, and even gangrene, depending on the severity of the vascular compromise. Venous symptoms have also been reported and can vary from mild intermittent swelling and duskiness of the arm from subclavian vein compression, to constant severe edema, pain, deep discoloration, and pulmonary emboli (35%) from vein damage and thrombosis.[54]

The Elevated Arm Stress Test (EAST). The most consistent clinical test for thoracic outlet syndrome has been the EAST, originally described by Roos.[58] Both arms are held in the "surrender" position, and opening and closing of the hands precipitate the patient's usual symptoms within 3 minutes in practically all cases of neurogenic, arterial, and venous thoracic outlet syndrome. It is described by Roos as a quick, noninvasive, painless, and free test that can be performed by anybody anywhere. Roos also stated that the EAST is quite specific for thoracic outlet syndrome and does not reproduce the symptoms of a cervical disc, spondylosis, or cubital tunnel or carpal tunnel syndromes.[58] The light exercise of the hands in the 90 degree abduction, external rotation shoulder position is believed to cause maximum functional compression of the brachial plexus and subclavian vessels by narrowing the costoclavicular space and tightening the cervical muscles.

The EAST, however, remains controversial since Wilbourn demonstrated that there was a high incidence of positive results in normal persons and 92% positive results in patients with CTS.[59] Barsotti and Chiaroni[60] demonstrated similar findings in 150 normal persons at 2 minutes into the EAST. Therefore the specificity and sensitivity of this test are in question.

• • •

Although electrodiagnostic studies are excellent laboratory procedures for diagnosing true neurogenic thoracic outlet syndrome, they are not helpful for diagnosing disputed neurogenic thoracic outlet syndrome because they are invariably normal.[59]

Pathogenesis of neurogenic outlet syndrome remains controversial, and thus a number of theories have been advanced. Table 20–2, adapted from Wilbourn,[59] gives some of these theories. Many theories combine two or more of the listed factors and attempt to provide some unification by suggesting that there are predisposing causes, for example, fibrous bands combined with an inciting cause, such as trauma.

TABLE 20–2. Some Theories Regarding Pathogenesis of Disputed Neurogenic Thoracic Outlet Syndrome

Congenital Anomalies

Cervical ribs abnormal. First thoracic ribs, fibrous bands, scalene muscle insertional abnormalities, abnormal descent of scapula.

Postural Factors

Disuse atrophy, muscle balance, secondary muscle shortening, compensatory muscle overuse, forward displacement of shoulder.

Trauma Sequelae

Brachial plexus scarring with or without plexus elements bound to other structures and inability to move sufficiently. Hemorrhage into and subsequent fibrosis contractures and shortening of anomalous bands or scalene muscles; change in muscle fiber type in scalene muscles.

Adapted from Wilbourn A: Thoracic outlet syndrome is over-diagnosed. Muscle Nerve 22:130–136, 1999. Reprinted by permission of John Wiley & Sons, Inc.

"STINGERS" OR "BURNERS"

Stingers are a common problem encountered by the sports physician. Signs and symptoms include unilateral shoulder or upper extremity pain with burning dysesthesias, accompanied by arm weakness immediately following contact. The distribution usually follows the C5–6 nerve root or the upper trunk or both. The dysesthesias occur along the lateral aspect of the arm, radiating into the thumb and index finger with weakness typically found in the deltoid, biceps, and supraspinatus and infraspinatus muscles. These problems rarely last longer than approximately 1 minute or so; however, prolonged and even permanent injuries have been reported in the literature.[61]

The incidence of stingers is unknown, since most go unreported. In one survey,[61] only 30% of all stingers were reported to the team. The authors of this survey suggested that as many as 65% of all football players may experience the problem at some time during their playing careers. Meyer et al[62] reported that among U.S. football players 30% of all defensive ends and linebackers had stingers that caused lost time from practice or play during a season.

The mechanism of injury is controversial and likely multifactorial. The various proposed mechanisms include the following:

1. Direct trauma and compression of the fixed brachial plexus in the area of Erb's point
2. Traction injury to the brachial plexus and/ or nerve roots when the head is forced into lateral rotation and the shoulder is forcefully depressed away from the head and neck
3. Nerve root compression with cervical hyperextension and lateral flexion impinging the nerves on the side of the lateral flexion, similar to the Spurling maneuver[61–63]

Cervical spinal canal stenosis may increase the risk of stingers. Meyer and colleagues[62] examined this by finding a high correlation between a low Torg ratio and the risk of sustaining stingers in three groups of U.S. football players: (1) stingers with lost time, (2) neck pain with lost time, and (3) asymptomatic group with no lost time. The Torg ratio is the anteroposterior width of the spinal canal divided by the anteroposterior width of the vertebral body. A measurement of less than 0.8 suggests, but does not diagnose, significant spinal stenosis.

A low Torg ratio has been implicated in patients who have repeated burners and is associated with an increased risk of transient quadriparesis or spinal cord injury.[64] This important paper proposes the following criteria for "spear tackler's spine":

1. Developmental narrowing (stenosis) of the cervical canal (Torg ratio less than 0.8)
2. Persistent straightening or reversal of normal cervical lordotic curve on erect lateral x-ray
3. Concomitant preexisting posttraumatic x-ray abnormalities of the cervical spine, for example, congenital fusion, disc herniation or bulge, compression fractures, or ligamentous laxity
4. Documentation of having employed spear tackling techniques (axial loading)

Torg et al[64] found that 4 out of 15 athletes in their series developed spinal cord injury, and therefore they suggest that athletes with spear tackler's spine be excluded from participation in high-risk sports that expose their cervical spine to axial loading.

Electrodiagnostic abnormalities in stingers are numerous and nonspecific. Most patients have EMG abnormalities in the anterior myotomes only, and a minority demonstrate involvement of the dorsal rami. The most common location of abnormalities is the upper trunk or a C5–6 distribution or both. The typical neurogenic changes of positive sharp waves, fibrillation potentials, and abnormalities of motor unit potentials can be found. The exact incidence of such abnormalities is, at this time, unknown.[63,65,66] Wilbourn[67] reported low sensory nerve action potentials in the lateral antebrachial cutaneous nerve and median nerve recorded from the thumb. Markey et al[63] reported delayed nerve conduction latencies most commonly in the axillary and musculocutaneous nerves of the upper extremity. In 1988, Bergfeld and colleagues[68] reported that EMG abnormalities were present in up to 80% of patients after a 5-year follow-up.

No randomized clinical trials on treatment of stingers were found in the literature. Experienced clinicians[61,63] have used total contact neck, shoulder, chest orthoses as cervical collars and Cabway collars in addition to neck rolls and exercises. Proper coaching techniques are also probably quite important.

Repeated stingers may be a reason to justify restriction of participation in sports, especially if there are persistent signs and symptoms. Most clinicians recommend using clinical criteria for when the athlete can return to play. Athletes with no residual symptoms, no weakness, and good range of motion can usually return to play safely. The role of EMG in decision making for return to sport is limited, and we do not believe that the EMG criteria should supersede the clinical evaluation. This is supported by Bergfeld et al,[68] and athletes with abnormal spontaneous activity should be closely monitored. However, these abnormalities alone should not preclude return to play.[69]

The presentations of most peripheral nerve injuries in athletes are similar to those in the normal population. There are abnormalities on electrodiagnostic testing despite "normal" participation in sports activities. Therefore caution should be exercised when interpreting these electrodiagnostic "abnormalities." The return to sport is a clinical decision not based on any one diagnostic test.

TENDONITIS OF WRIST AND HAND

Among adults, tendonitis and tenosynovitis of the digital flexors can occur equally often in those who play or do not play sports. Both primary care and rehabilitation appear to be similar for everyone. In early rehabilitation (as in emergency care) two classes of treatment are widely employed: (1) oral or injectable drugs and (2) braces for the wrist, hand, and digits; commercial or custom-made splints; and compressive bandaging.

Although both patients and physicians appear to feel instant relief from both approaches, no evidence exists (or appears to be sought) to test the efficacy of these specific maneuvers. The modern trust in pharmacy and the ancient trust in the curative influence of rest overcome (almost) everyone's skepticism. Also, no one has come up with a truly better, more specific attack.

Oral Analgesics and Antiinflammatory Agents

Relief of pain is usually a major requirement, and the spectrum of oral agents for pain, from aspirin to codeine, is broad. However, no specific scientific studies exist of their effects on wrist and hand pain in athletes with tendon problems. The ultimate judge of efficacy is the patient, and the degree of return to attempted activity is usually a personal issue. For better or worse, many athletes still subscribe to the dubious theory of "no pain—no gain," but no clear general law regarding athletes' return to activity has emerged from substantive research.

Oral anti-inflammatory agents for tendonitis and tenosynovitis of the hand fall into two categories: (1) nonsteroidal (e.g., indomethacin, phenylbutazone, sulindac) and (2) corticosteroids (e.g., dexamethasone, prednisone, triamcinolone). Here, as elsewhere in this chapter, the *art* of medicine overwhelms the *science,* and the careful judgment of a well-trained physician appears to be the athlete's best hope for recovery of wrist and hand function. Over-the-counter medications, now becoming more and more potent, may cause overwhelmingly more egregious side effects; trainers and therapists should be cautious rather than casual about them.

Injection of Corticosteroids

Although basic research studies provide strong evidence that glucosteroids have a clear-cut local effect on synovial tissues, it should be noted that injected cortisone and hydrocortisone clear rapidly from joint cavities (and presumably from tendon sheaths) and are dissipated in 60 to 70 minutes.[70] Longer-acting drugs (e.g., triamcinolone hexacetonide) are favored for long-term synovial inflammation in arthritis.[71] They may be more suitable for direct injection into hand tendon sheaths. The rare cases of serious damage to tendons must be kept in mind.[72] Again, we must rely on the *art* not the science of individual physicians.

Hand and Finger Splints

As in the acute phase of treating painful hands, a wide variety of commercial splints and elastic gloves are available. Little or no evidence exists that these provide reparative function, but athletes and nonathletes feel that their protective influence warrants their costs. A good case could be made on general principles for avoiding rigid immobilization, but no scientific clinical studies are available.

SPRAINS/STRAINS AND BONY INJURIES

Participation in violent competitive sports guarantees a crop of limb injuries; the wrist and hand are not immune. Probably the most common disabling conditions result from repeated overuse (see following discussion), but acute episodes of trauma can cause sprains/strains and bony injuries. Generally, the acute care for these conditions is well established, with the direct application of cold and pressure being almost a religious exercise. The rationale is based on both (1) common sense and experience and (2) reliance on the relevant basic sciences. However, clinical sciences say very little either in support or in rejection of this common practice.

The aftermath of sprains, strains, and bony injuries of the hand in the competitive athlete often reveals a determination to get back into the fray. In spite of a local problem that is painful and constitutes a handicap to performance (e.g., the damaged throwing hand of a quarterback or the catching hands of a receiver), athletes often make decisions that aggravate their condition. The healing power of time—with or without enforced rest—is not given a fair chance by many athletes. (Generally, women athletes are more logical.) The thoughtful clinician may need to be forceful to prevent further injury, but again, no clear scientific evidence exists for this cautious approach, only common sense.

Bony injuries are generally the province of surgeons who may or may not count on rehabilitation personnel for follow-up. In any case, critical decisions regarding the steps toward a return to full sports activities are clearly the responsibility of the surgeon. Of course, managers, trainers, and the athlete will place pressure on clinicians, but bony injuries probably heal no faster in athletes than in others. Again, the time factor is an important part of the equation.

The widespread use of splints and bandages has little or no scientific evidence, but they appear to provide emotional support more than any physical support. Probably no serious harm is done.

Severe wrist injuries of athletes deserve a special mention regarding the transition from surgical to rehabilitation care. These include, for example, ulnar collateral ligament injury (skier's thumb), de Quervain's tenosynovitis, triangular fibrocartilage injury, tendonitis of flexor carpi ulnaris and radialis, scaphoid fracture, and baseball finger.

After rigid nonremovable devices are removed, rehabilitation teams prefer removable splints to permit range-of-motion and strengthening exercises. Experience appears to be universal that these are essential for recovery and to avoid limitation of normal movements. Therapists are cautious to avoid overstretching stiff joints and muscles and often use heat application to the parts being stretched. Why? Common sense and experience. Generally, strengthening exercises move from (1) passive to (2) isometric to (3) isotonic to (4) isokinetic for the same reasons. Apparently, no one has tried the opposite order of (4) to (1). Perhaps it would be better, but we may never know.

OTHER OVERUSE INJURIES

In the modern age of computer usage, office workers probably experience more overuse injuries of the wrist and hand than athletes. Repetitive compression of an athlete's ulnar nerve with ensuing local inflammation where the nerve enters its tunnel against and beyond the hook of the hamate—ulnar tunnel syndrome—is common among several groups, including cyclists (handlebar palsy). Ulnar tunnel syndrome is also seen among baseball catchers, handball players, and hockey goalies.[73] Surgery is uncommon, but rehabilitation requires the suspension of the activities and postures of the wrist that aggravate the symptoms.

Similarly, digital nerve repetitive compression and injury (e.g., bowler's thumb) can be treated with conservative care. Trigger digits, in which stenosing tenosynovitis causes snapping of the digits, are common in sports that require repetitive forceful gripping of handles (e.g., gymnasts, golfers, weightlifters); they may be treated conservatively. However, surgical release—a relatively minor operation with the patient under local anesthetic—may require subsequent minimal rehabilitation exercises with or without supervision of a therapist or trainer.

In summary, conservative care (rest, altered hand usage, analgesics, and sometimes corticosteroids) is the usual approach that appears quite adequate for overuse symptoms. However, there is no clinical scientific demonstration of the efficacy of the wide variations used in retraining the athlete's hand and performance for the sport that caused the problem.

REFERENCES

1. Caccia MR, Galimberti V, Valla PL, et al: Peripheral autonomic involvement in carpal tunnel syndrome. Acta Neurol Scand 88:47–50, 1993
2. Hennessey WJ, Johnson EW: Carpal tunnel syndrome. In Johnson EW, Peas WS (eds): Practical Electromyography, 3rd Ed. Williams & Wilkins, Baltimore, 1996, pp 195–216
3. Hennessey WJ, Kuhlman KA: The anatomy, symptoms, and signs of carpal tunnel syndrome. Phys Med Rehabil Clin North Am 8(3):439–457, 1997
4. Nordstrom DL, DeStefano F, Vierkant RA, Laybe PM: Incidence of diagnosed carpal tunnel syndrome in a general population. Epidemiology 9(3):342–345, 1998
5. Krivickas LS, Wilbourn AJ: Sports and peripheral nerve injuries: report of 190 injuries evaluated in a single electromyography laboratory. Muscle Nerve 21(8):1092–1094, 1998
6. Feinberg JH, Nadler SF, Krivickas LS: Peripheral nerve injuries in the athlete. Sports Med 24(6):385–408, 1997
7. Vender MI, Kasdan ML, Truppa KL: Upper extremity disorders: a literature review to determine

work relatedness. J Hand Surg [Am] 20:534–541, 1995

8. Stevens JC, Beard CM, O'Fallon WM, et al: Conditions associated with carpal tunnel syndrome. Mayo Clin Proc 67:541–546, 1992

9. Bonnici AV, Birjandi F, Spencer JD, et al: Chromosomal abnormalities in Dupuytren's contracture and carpal tunnel syndrome. J Hand Surg [Br] 17:349–355, 1992

10. Radecki P: The familial occurrence of carpal tunnel syndrome. Muscle Nerve 17:325–330, 1994

11. Dyck PJ, Litchy WJ, Lehman KA, et al: Variables influencing neuropathic end points: The Rochester Diabetic Neuropathy Study of Healthy Subjects. Neurology 45:1115–1121, 1995

12. Letz R, Gerr F: Co-variants of human peripheral nerve function: I. Nerve conduction velocity and amplitude. Neurotoxicol Teratol 16:95–104, 1994

13. Stetson DS, Albers JW, Silverstein BA, et al: Effects of age, sex, and anthropol metric factors on nerve conduction measures. Muscle Nerve 15:1095–1104, 1992

14. Czeuz KA, Thomas JE, Lambert EH, et al: Long term results of operation for carpal tunnel syndrome. Mayo Clin Proc 41:232–241, 1966

15. De Krom MCTFM, Kester ADM, Knipschild PG, et al: Risk factors for carpal tunnel syndrome. Am J Epidemiol 132:1102–1110, 1990

16. Nathan PA, Keniston RC: Carpal tunnel syndrome and its relation to general physical condition. Occupational diseases of the hand. Hand Clin 9:253–261, 1993

17. Radecki P: Variability in the median and ulnar nerve latencies: implications for diagnosing entrapment. J Occup Environ Med 37:1293–1299, 1995

18. Vessey MP, Villard-Mclntosh L, Weates D: Epidemiology of carpal tunnel syndrome in women of child bearing age: findings in a large cohort study. Int J Epidemiol 19:655–659, 1990

19. Werner RA, Alders JW, Franzblau A, et al: The relationship between body mass index and the diagnosis of carpal tunnel syndrome. Muscle Nerve 17:632–636, 1994

20. Johnson EW, Jatens T, Poindexter D, et al: Wrist dimensions: correlation with median sensory latencies. Arch Phys Med Rehabil 64:556–557, 1983

21. Radecki P: Carpal tunnel syndrome: effects of personal factors and associated medical conditions. Phys Med Rehabil North Am 8(3):419–436, 1997

22. Gelberman HR, Hergenroeder PT, Hargens AR, et al: The carpal tunnel syndrome: a study of carpal canal pressures. J Bone Joint Surg Am 63:380–384, 1981

23. Mubarak JS, et al: The Wick catheter technique for measurement of intramuscular pressure: new research and clinical tool. J Bone Joint Surg Am 58:1016–1020, 1976

24. Rempel D, Manojlovic R, Levinsohn OG: The effect of wearing a flexible wrist splint on carpal tunnel pressure during repetitive hand activity. J Hand Surg [Am] 19(1):106–110, 1994

25. Cobb TK, An KN, Cooney WA: Effect of lumbrical muscle incursion within the carpal tunnel on carpal tunnel pressure: a cadavaric study. J Hand Surg [Am] 20(2):186–192, 1995

26. Lundberg G, Gelbarman RH: Metal median nerve compression in the carpal tunnel: functional response to experimentally induced controlled pressures. J Hand Surg [Am] 7:252–259, 1982

27. Kruger VL, Kraft GH, Deitz TC, et al: Carpal tunnel syndrome: objective measures and splint use. Arch Phys Med Rehabil 72:517–520, 1991

28. Burke DT: Conservative management of carpal tunnel syndrome. Phys Med Rehabil Clin North Am 8(3):513–528, 1997

29. Harskovitz S, Berger AR, Lipton RB: Low dose, short term oral prednisone in the treatment of carpal syndrome. Neurology 45:1923–1925, 1995

30. Laskey ME, Segal R: Median nerve injury from local steroid injection in carpal tunnel syndrome. Neurosurgery 26:512–515, 1990

31. Minamikama Y, Peimer CA, Kambee K, et al: Tenosynovial injection for carpal tunnel syndrome. J Hand Surg [Am] 17:178–181, 1992

32. Posch JL, Marcotte DR: Carpal tunnel syndrome: an analysis of 1201 cases. Orthop Rev 5:25–35, 1976

33. Giannini F, Passero S, Cioni R, et al: Electrophysiologic evaluation of local steroid injection in carpal tunnel syndrome. Arch Phys Med Rehabil 72:738–742, 1991

34. Girlander P, Dattola R, Venuto C, et al: Local steroid injection in idiopathic carpal tunnel syndrome: short and long term efficacy. J Neurol 240:187–190, 1993

35. Gelberman HR, Aronson D, Weisman MH: Carpal tunnel syndrome: results of a prospective trial of steroid injection and splinting. J Bone Joint Surg Am 62:1181–1184, 1980

36. Weiss AP, Sachar K, Gendreau M: Conservative management of carpal tunnel syndrome: a reexamination of steroid injection and splinting. J Hand Surg [Am] 19:410–415, 1996

37. Kaplan SJ, Glickel S, Eaton RG: Predictive factors in the non-surgical treatment of carpal tunnel syndrome. J Hand Surg [Br] 15:106–108, 1990

38. Burke DT: Conservative management of carpal tunnel syndrome. Phys Med Rehabil Clin North Am 8(3):513–528, 1997

39. Stransky M, Rubin A, Lava NS, et al: Treatment of carpal tunnel syndrome with vitamin B$_6$: a double blinded study. South Med J 82:841–842, 1987

40. Wu SF, Chan RC, Hsu TC: Diagnostic evaluation of conservative treatment in carpal tunnel syndrome. Chin Med J 48:125–130, 1991

41. Armstrong MB, Villaobos RE: Surgical treatment of carpal tunnel syndrome. Phys Med Rehabil Clin North Am 8(3):529–539, 1997

42. Gross BT, Jones HR: Proximal median neuropathies: electromyographic and clinical correlation. Muscle Nerve 15:390–395, 1992

43. Upton AR, McComas AJ: The double crush in nerve entrapment syndromes. Lancet 2:359–362, 1973

44. Dellon AL, MacKinnon SE: Chronic nerve compression model for the double crush hypothesis. Ann Plast Surg 26:259–264, 1991

45. Eisen A: Electrodiagnosis of radiculopathy. Neurol Clin 3:495–510, 1985

46. Cassvan A, Rosenberg A, Rivera LF: Ulnar nerve involvement in carpal tunnel syndrome. Arch Phys Med Rehabil 67:290–292, 1986

47. Kuntzer T: Carpal tunnel syndrome in 100 patients: sensitivity, specificity of multi-neurophysiological procedures and estimation of axonal loss of motor, sensory and sympathetic nerve fibers. J Neurol Sci 127:221–229, 1994

48. Gnatz SM: The role of needle electromyography in the evaluation of patients with carpal tunnel syndrome: needle EMG is important. Muscle Nerve 22(2):282–283, 1999

49. Eason SY, Belsole RJ, Greene TL: Carpal tunnel release: analysis of suboptimal results. J Hand Surg [Br] 10:365–369, 1985

50. Dyro FM, Rossier AB: Electrodiagnostic abnormalities in 15 patients with post-traumatic syringomyelia: pre and post-operative studies. Paraplegia 23:233–242, 1985

51. Wilbourn AJ: Thoracic outlet syndrome surgery causing severe brachial plexopathy. Muscle Nerve 9:632–634, 1986

52. Gilliat RW, Lequesne PM, Logue V, Sumner A: Wasting of the hand associated with a cervical rib or band. J Neurol Neurosurg Psychiatry 33:615–624, 1970

53. Kelly TR: Thoracic outlet syndrome: current concepts of treatment. Ann Surg 190:657–662, 1979

54. Roos DB: Thoracic outlet syndrome is under diagnosed. Muscle Nerve 22(1):127–129, 1999

55. Firsov GI: Cervical ribs and their differentiation from underdeveloped first ribs. Arkh Anat Gistol Embriol 67:101–103, 1974

56. Machleder HI, Moll F, Verity A: The anterior scalene muscle in thoracic outlet syndrome: histochemical and morphometric studies. Arch Surg 121:1141–1144, 1986

57. Sanders RJ, Jackson CGR, Baushero N, Pearce WH: Scalene muscle abnormalities in traumatic thoracic outlet syndrome. Am J Surg 159:231–236, 1990

58. Roos DB: Congenital anomalies associated with thoracic outlet syndrome: anatomy, symptoms, diagnosis and treatment. Am J Surg 132:771–778, 1976

59. Wilbourn AJ: Thoracic outlet syndrome is over-diagnosed. Muscle Nerve 22(1):130–136, 1999

60. Barsotti J, Chiaroni P: Thoracic outlet syndrome: diagnosis by Roos' test. Presse Med 13:1335, 1984

61. Sallis RE, Jones K, Knopp W: Burners: offensive strategy for an under-reported injury. Phys Sports Med 20(11):47–55, 1992

62. Meyer SA, Schulte KR, Kallaghan JJ, et al: Cervical spinal stenosis and stingers in collegiate football players. Am J Sports Med 22(2):158–166, 1994

63. Markey KL, Dibenedetto M, Curl WW: Upper trunk brachial plexopathy: the stinger syndrome. Am J Sports Med 21(5):650–655, 1993

64. Torg JS, Sennett B, Pavlov H, et al: Spear tacklers spine: an entity precluding participation in tackle football and collision activities that expose the cervical spine to axial energy inputs. Am J Sports Med 21(5):640–649, 1993

65. Hershman EB: Brachial plexus injuries. Clin Sports Med 9:311–329, 1990

66. Poindexter DP, Johnson EW: Football shoulder and neck injury: a study of the "stinger." Arch Phys Med Rehabil 65:601–602, 1994

67. Wilbourn AJ: Electrodiagnostic testing of neurological injuries in athletes. Clin Sports Med 9(2):229–245, 1990

68. Bergfeld JA, Hershman EB, Wilbourn AJ: Brachial plexus injury in sports: a five year followup. Orthop Trans 12:743–744, 1988

69. Andary MT: Electrodiagnoses in upper extremity sports injuries. 1995 AAEM Course F: Sports and Occupational Disorder—the role of electrodiagnosis, pp 21–27

70. Gray RG, Gottlieb NL: Intra-articular corticosteroids: an updated assessment. Clin Orthop (177):235–263, 1983

71. Goss JA, Adams RF: Local injection of corticosteroids in rheumatic diseases. J Musculoskeletal Med 10:92, 1993

72. Leadbetter WB: Anti-inflammatory therapy in sports injury: the role of non-steroidal drugs and corticosteroid injection. Clin Sports Med 14:353–410, 1995

73. Plancher KD, Peterson RK, Steichen JB: Compressive neuropathies and tendinopathies in the athletic elbow and wrist. Clin Sports Med 15:331–371, 1996

74. Wilkins RH, Brody IA: Neurological classics: Tinel's sign and Hoffmann's sign. Arch Neurol 24:573–575, 1971

75. Phalen GS: The carpal tunnel syndrome: seventeen years' experience in diagnosis and treatment of 654 hands. J Bone Joint Surg Am 48:211–228, 1966

76. Seror P: Tinel's sign in the diagnosis of carpal tunnel syndrome. J Hand Surg [Am] 12:364–365, 1987

77. Szabo RM, Gelberman RH, Dimick MP: Sensibility testing in patients with carpal tunnel syndrome. J Bone Joint Surg Am 66:60–64, 1984

78. Golding DN, Rose DM, Selvarajah K: Clinical tests for carpal tunnel syndrome: an evaluation. Br J Rheumatol 25:388–390, 1986

79. Durkan JA: A new diagnostic test for carpal tunnel syndrome. J Bone Joint Surg Am 73:535–538, 1991

80. LaBan MM, Friedman NA, Zemenick GA: "Tethered" median nerve stress test in chronic carpal tunnel syndrome. Arch Phys Med Rehabil 67:803–804, 1986

81. Gordon C, Bowyer BL, Johnson EW: Electrodiagnostic characteristics of acute carpal tunnel syndrome. Arch Phys Med Rehabil 68:545–548, 1987

82. Spindler HA, Dellon AL: Nerve conduction studies and sensibility testing in carpal tunnel syndrome. J Hand Surg [Am] 7:260–263, 1982

83. Gellman RW, Gelberman RH, Tan MA, et al: Carpal tunnel syndrome: an evaluation of the provocative diagnostic tests. J Bone Joint Surg Am 68:735–737, 1986

Acute Lower Back Pain: Concise Review of Nonsurgical Treatments

DINESH A. KUMBHARE ▪ JOHN V. BASMAJIAN

Low back pain (LBP) is experienced by most people at some time in their lives; it is estimated that general yearly prevalence in the United States is between 15% and 20%.[1] Many therapeutic interventions are available for the treatment of acute LBP. The effectiveness of most of these interventions, however, has not yet been demonstrated beyond doubt.[2] The current interest in evidence-based medicine has led to an extensive increase in publications. This chapter discusses the commonly used nonsurgical treatments of acute nonspecific LBP and reviews the levels of evidence available. To assist the clinician in making diagnostic and treatment decisions, algorithms based on efficacious treatments are presented in Table 21–1 and Appendix A.

LBP is a symptom not a diagnosis, and a precise pathoanatomic or pathophysiologic diagnosis is usually elusive. Thus perhaps 95% of patients are labeled "mechanical" LBP, a nonspecific entity. Local inflammation and muscle tension may have important etiologic roles. An expert panel has concluded that for most patients with LBP an unambiguous diagnosis is impossible because of the poor associations between symptoms, pathology, and image findings.[3] There is controversy regarding the validity of many common diagnoses. Some experienced clinicians believe that skeletal muscle spasm does not exist,[4] and there is good evidence that muscle tenderness is not reproducible by physicians.[5] There is substantial controversy about the definitions of segmental instability, sacroiliac strain, and facet joint syndrome.[6]

It is important to distinguish between acute and chronic back pain because the prognosis and response to therapy differ substantially. The prognosis of acute LBP is excellent, with 60% to 80% of patients improving within 2 weeks of onset. In patients with chronic pain the overall prognosis is bleaker. Further, it is widely accepted that for patients with chronic pain nonorganic factors complicate responses to treatment.

Below is a concise review of the available literature. For more detailed information the reader is referred to the numerous review and original articles referenced.

BED REST

Bed rest has been a common treatment modality for acute LBP until recently, when several trials have shown harmful effects. Wiesel et al[7] studied 80 army combat trainees with acute nonradiating LBP and normal neurologic straight leg raising tests and radiologic examination. They were admitted to the hospital and randomly assigned to bed rest or an ambulatory group. Both groups received acetaminophen, one tablet twice daily. The study was discontinued after 14 days even if the patients continued to experience pain. The bed rest group returned to full activity significantly earlier than the ambulatory group ($P < .001$). The bed rest group also had significantly less pain ($P < .005$). The major drawback to this study was that the outcome assessments were not blinded and the pain reporting was on an arbitrary scale. There are also questions about the generalizability of this study since the combat trainees were forced to undergo a specific treatment.

TABLE 21–1. Initial Assessment of Acute Low Back Symptoms

Low Back Pain Red Flags

Cancer or infection
   Age >50 years (also consider abdominal aortic
     aneurysm) or <20 years
   History of cancer
   Unexplained weight loss
   Failure to improve with 4–6 weeks of
     conservative therapy
   Unrelenting night pain
   Intravenous drug use
   Fever >38°C
   Immune suppression
   Recent bacterial infection
Cauda equina syndrome or rapidly progressive
   neurologic deficit
   Loss of bowel or bladder function
   Saddle anesthesia
   Leg weakness
   Progressive neurologic deficit in lower extremity
History of recent (significant) trauma

Gilbert et al[8] conducted a randomized trial of 252 patients with acute LBP with and without radiating pain into the legs and no neurologic, significant spinal or pelvic pathology. The patients were randomized to one of four treatment groups: (1) bed rest for at least 4 days; (2) bed rest, physiotherapy, and education; (3) physiotherapy and education; or (4) control group with analgesics only. The patients were observed for 3 to 44 days. At the end of the trial there were no significant differences among the groups on the main outcome measures of activity discomfort scale and mean recovery period. However, the bed rest group experienced a significant but small increase of restrictions of daily activities ($P < .034$). This group also took longer to achieve a normal level of activities and consumed more analgesics.

Deyo et al[9] studied the effects of 2 and 7 days of bed rest involving 203 patients with mechanical LBP without neurologic deficits. Seventy-eight percent had acute pain, defined as symptoms lasting less than 30 days. Patients were randomly assigned to 2 days or 7 days of bed rest. All patients received recommendations for local heat applications, exercise, and weight loss. At 3-week follow-up there was no significant difference between the two groups on all out-

come measures: functional status, perceptions, symptoms, signs, and use of services except for the 2-day group, which missed significantly less time off work ($P = .01$). There were some major flaws with this landmark study: The time that the 7-day group actually rested in bed was an average of 3.9 days. This study does not address the issue of bed rest or no bed rest. Also, there was poor patient recruitment and follow-up. Only 203 of the 450 eligible patients were randomized to treatment groups, and 189 and 179 patients were available at 3-week and 3-month follow-up periods. No explanation is provided for this.

Malmivaara et al[10] studied three groups: (1) bed rest for 2 days, (2) mobilization exercise, and (3) continuation of ordinary activities as tolerated (control group); 186 patients with acute or acute on chronic LBP without neurologic deficit or sciatic syndrome were randomly assigned to the three groups. Sciatic syndrome was defined as at least one neurologic deficit or a positive Lasègue sign at 60 degrees or less. The following outcomes were assessed at 3 and 12 weeks: return to work, straight leg raising, lumbar flexion, and Oswestry back disability index. After 3 and 12 weeks, the patients in the control group had better recovery than those prescribed either bed rest or exercises. There were statistically significant differences favoring the control group in the duration of pain, pain intensity, lumbar flexion, ability to work measured subjectively, Oswestry back disability index, and number of days absent from work. Recovery was slowest among patients assigned to bed rest. The overall costs of care differed significantly among the three groups, with care for the group continuing with normal activities costing less than the other groups. There was 89% follow-up at 3 weeks and 87% follow-up at 12 weeks. The study design did not allow for complete blinding of treatments, but a placebo effect seemed an unlikely explanation for the success of the control treatment. The authors concluded that avoidance of bed rest and continuing with ordinary activities as tolerated provided the most rapid recovery in patients with acute LBP without neurologic deficits.

These studies suggest that avoiding bed rest and maintaining ordinary activity as tolerated lead to the most rapid recovery (level 1 evidence). Widespread use of this strategy is expected to result in substantial savings to the health care system. Even though these studies were not performed in the sports medicine population, the same principles would apply since the treatments of soft tissue injuries should be the same in this group. The literature search conducted did not reveal any studies of acute nonspecific LBP in athletes of sufficient quality to include in this review.

DRUG THERAPIES

There are numerous problems with the existing literature on drug therapy for soft tissue injuries.[6] One of the greatest deficits in the existing literature is the failure to provide an adequate description of patients and outcomes.[11] Reporting of relevant outcomes is also problematic. Usually, only patient symptom relief, spinal range of motion, or changes in muscle activity are recorded, but this says nothing about a patient's daily functioning. Efforts to describe or control for co-interventions, group contamination, and patient compliance are often omitted from published reports.[6]

Appropriate research design is important in all therapeutic research, but the opportunity to be misled is especially high in studies of LBP. In part this is because of the highly favorable natural history of LBP. Many studies have shown that 80% or more of patients with LBP will show substantial recovery within a few weeks,[12–16] it is likely that improvement will be seen after any therapy, even if it is ineffective. This represents the natural history of this condition. Another problem is the placebo effect, which can be enormous among patients treated with painful conditions. Placebo responses follow the typical patterns of pharmacologic response seen with active drugs, for example, dose response and duration of effect.[17] Also, the reader is referred to Chapter 11 on complementary therapies for a more thorough discussion on the nonspecific (placebo) effects. Another potential problem is the statistical concept of regression toward the mean. This suggests that patients whose conditions are at an extreme level at the beginning of the study will tend toward a more average level (because of random variability) by the end of the study. This concept usually applies because patients generally seek medical attention when their symptoms are most extreme.

Analgesics

Six randomized controlled trials (RCTs) (Table 21–2) were identified, but using the criteria set out in Table 21–3,[2] only one was considered to be of high methodologic quality.[18] Based on this information there is level 2 evidence that analgesics are not more effective than nonsteroidal anti-inflammatory drugs (NSAIDs) and no evidence (level 4) that analgesics are more effective than electroacupuncture or ultrasound for acute LBP.[2]

Nonsteroidal Anti-Inflammatory Drugs (NSAIDs)

Of 19 RCTs identified (Table 21–4), 10 were considered high quality[18–27] and 9 of low quality.[7,28–35] Based on this information there is level 1 evidence that NSAIDs are more effective than a placebo in patients with uncomplicated acute LBP but not in acute sciatica. There is level 1 evidence that NSAIDs are *not more effective* than analgesics. Also, numerous trials demonstrate that the various types of NSAIDs are equally effective for acute LBP.

When prescribing NSAIDs one should keep in mind their potential side effects, such as dyspepsia, gastric erosion, ulceration and bleeding, interference with control of hypertension, and cardiac failure.[36] Another important side effect is deterioration in renal function. These effects are usually attributable to the inhibition of prostaglandin synthesis. These potential risks should be weighed against any therapeutic benefits before prescribing NSAIDs.

In recent years ketorolac has been introduced as an injectable NSAID and ketoprofen has become available as a cream. Although these have become popular treatments acutely, a recent study suggests that they are no more effective than oral ibuprofen.[37]

Muscle Relaxants

Muscle relaxant drugs are widely used for the treatment of acute LBP, although their use is somewhat controversial.[6] This is because it is uncertain whether these drugs offer any additional benefit over analgesics or NSAIDs. Given this starting point, eight high-quality RCTs[38–45] and five low-quality RCTs[46–50] were identified

TABLE 21–2. Details of Randomized Controlled Trials on the Effectiveness of Analgesics for Acute Low Back Pain

REFERENCE	ANALGESICS DOSE/ FREQUENCY/DURATION (NO. OF PATIENTS)	REFERENCE TREATMENT(S) (NO. OF PATIENTS)	RESULTS
Videman et al[18]	(1) Meptazinol 200 mg qid/ 3 wk (35)	(R) Diflunisal 250 mg qid/4 wk (35)	Mean change in degree of pain (100 mm VAS) at 3 wk: (1) 45 vs (R) 40; similar improvement regarding capacity for daily tasks (data in graphs); no significant differences; side effects similar; (1) 19 vs (R) 23 patients
Wiesel et al[7]	(11) Acetaminophen (dosage not given) bid/2 wk (?) (12) Codeine 60 mg qid/2 wk (?) (13) Oxycodone + aspirin 1 tab qid/2 wk (?)		Mean (SD) number of days before return to full activity: (11) 5.6 (0.6), (12) 5.2 (0.6), (13) 5.6 (0.7); no significant differences; no data on side effects given
Brown et al[50]	(1) Acetaminophen 300 mg + codeine two 50 mg caps initially; then one cap q4h/15 d (21)	(R) Diflunisal (caps) initial dose 1000 mg, 500 mg q12/15 d (19)	Pain assessment by patient and investigator on 3-point ordinal scale shows similar improvement curves (data in graphs); number of patients rating drugs as excellent or very good: (1) 9 vs (R); no significant differences; more side effects in (1) 10 than in (R) 3
Evans et al[31]	(11) Dextropropoxyphene 32.5 mg + two paracetamol 325 mg caps qid/1 wk (30 c.o.) (12) Paracetamol two 500 mg caps qid/1 wk (30 c.o.)	(R1) Aspirin three 300 mg caps qid/1 wk (30 c.o.) (R2) Indomethacin 50 mg tid/1 wk (30 c.o.) (R3) Mefenamic acid two 250 mg caps tid/1 wk (30 c.o.) (R4) Phenylbutazone 100 mg tid/1 wk (30 c.o.)	Mean daily pain index during intervention period (4-point ordinal scale): (11) 1.7, (12) 1.7, (R1) 1.4, (R2) 1.5, (R3) 1.4, (R4) 1.4; (R3) significantly different from (11) and (12); (R1) significantly different from (11); more side effects in (R1) 20, (R2) 19, and (11) 19 than in (R3) 12, (12) 13, and (R4) 4
Hackett et al[65]	(1) Paracetamol 2 tabs q4h (?)	(R) Electroacupuncture 2 treatments in 4 d (?)	Pain scores (VAS) pretreatment and after 1, 2, and 6 wk: (1) 54.5, 23.4, 22, 13.7 vs (R) 52.7, 23.2 18.3, 3.3; (R) significantly less pain after 6 wk.
Nwuga et al[86]	(1) Analgesics (unspecified) (?)	(R1) Ultrasound (?) (R2) Placebo ultrasound (?)	Proportion of patients pain free after 4 wk: (1) 6.8%, (R1) 40.7%, (R2) 12%; (R1) significantly more improved than (1)

bid, twice per day; tid, three times per day; qid, four times per day; tabl, tablet; cap(s) capsules; ?, number of patients not given; ADL, activities of daily living; VAS, visual analogue scale.

that studied the effectiveness of muscle relaxants (Table 21–5). Based on this information one may conclude that muscle relaxant drugs reduce pain intensity. Unfortunately no comment can be made regarding their effects on muscle spasm. Trials comparing the various muscle relaxants reported no differences with regard to their effects on pain intensity. Therefore there is level 1 evidence that muscle relaxants are more effective than placebo in reducing pain for acute LBP. There is also level 1 evidence that different types of muscle relaxants are equally effective for acute LBP.

Epidural Steroid Injection

The rationale for epidural injection of local anesthetic with corticosteroids is to reduce inflammation and swelling of affected lumbar roots, which in turn are thought to reduce pain and other symptoms of radiculopathy. Five trials are available that study epidural steroid injection.

Dilke et al[51] reported a double-blind RCT that involved 100 consecutive patients with a clinical diagnosis of lumbar radiculopathy of 1 week to 2 years' duration. The experimental group received an epidural injection of 80 mg of methylprednisolone in 10 ml of normal saline, and the control group received a superficial injection of 1 ml of normal saline. All patients underwent graded rehabilitation with hydrotherapy and exercise. The experimental group had better pain relief ($P < .01$) and a higher rate of return to work at 3 months ($P < .01$).

Sonek et al[52] studied a group of 51 patients with lumbar radiculopathy of between 12 days and 36 weeks' duration confirmed by myelography. Patients were randomly assigned to two treatment groups. The treatments included epi-

TABLE 21–3. Criteria List for the Methodologic Assessment of Randomized Controlled Trials of Therapeutic Interventions for Low Back Pain

Study Population

A   Homogeneity
B   Comparability of relevant baseline characteristics
C   Randomized procedure adequate
D   Dropouts described for each study group separately
E   <20% loss to follow-up
    <10% loss to follow-up
F   >50 subjects in the smallest group
    >100 subjects in the smallest group

Interventions

G   Interventions standardized and described
H   Pragmatic study/control group adequate*
I   Co-interventions avoided
J   Placebo controlled

Effect

K   Patients blinded[†]
L   Outcome measures relevant
M   Blinded outcome assessment
N   Follow-up period adequate

Data Presentation and Analysis

O   Intention-to-treat analysis
P   Frequencies of most important outcomes presented for each treatment group

Only Trials of Drug Therapy

Q   Compliance measured and satisfactory in all study groups

From van Tulder MW, Koes BW, Bouter LM: Conservative treatment of acute and chronic nonspecific low back pain. Spine 22(18):2128–2156, 1997.

*Criterion H was defined as "pragmatic study" for RCTs of drug therapies for which a placebo treatment was feasible; criterion H was defined as "control group adequate" for RCTs of the other therapeutic interventions.

[†]Criterion K was not assessed for trials on the efficacy of bed rest.

dural injection of 80 mg of methylprednisolone in 2 ml of normal saline. Outcome assessment was blinded. There was no significant difference between the groups in regard to pain relief or percentage of patients ultimately requiring surgical intervention.

Cuckler et al[53] treated 73 patients with lumbar radiculopathy that was radiologically proven to be due to either a herniated disc or spinal stenosis. The treatment group received epidural injection of 80 mg of methylprednisolone and procaine. The control group received procaine and sterile saline. At the 24-hour mark, 41.6% +/− 6.2% in the steroid-treated group and 43.6% +/− 6.6% in the control group experienced 75% or more relief of their symptoms. The differences were not statistically significant, and at 20 months there was no significant difference between the groups.

Ridley et al[54] studied 39 patients with clinical signs and symptoms consistent with lumbosacral nerve root compression. The duration of their symptoms was not specified. The treatment arm of the trial received epidural injection of 80 mg of methylprednisolone in 10 ml of saline, and the control arm received 2 ml of normal saline into the interspinous ligaments. At the end of 1 and 2 weeks the treatment arm experienced significantly more pain relief compared to the placebo group. However, after 24 weeks 35% of the patients who had experienced pain relief with active treatment relapsed.

Bush and Hillier[55] studied 23 patients with symptoms and signs of lumbar root compression with a duration of approximately 1 to 13 months. The experimental group received 80 mg of triamcinolone mixed with 25 ml of normal saline. The control arm received 0.5% procaine hydrochloride with 25 ml of normal saline. At the 4-week follow-up mark the active treatment group had significantly less pain ($P = .02$), "improved life-style" ($P = .02$), and improved straight leg raising ($P = .01$). At the 1-year follow-up these differences in pain and lifestyle improvement were no longer significant.

Based on these trials it is apparent that there is limited evidence on the effectiveness of epidural steroid injection for acute LBP with nerve root pain and radicular neurologic deficits (level 3). The results of these trials are difficult to generalize because of the different injection techniques and patient populations with varying durations of pain and diagnoses. It is believed that epidural steroid injections may be helpful in short-term relief of discomfort in patients with lumbar radiculopathy when other treatment methods have failed or surgery is not a desired option. Agency for Health Care Policy and Research (AHCPR)

TABLE 21–4. Details of Randomized Controlled Trials on the Effectiveness of NSAIDs for Acute Low Back Pain

REFERENCE	NSAIDs DOSE/FREQUENCY/DURATION (NO. OF PATENTS)	REFERENCE TREATMENT(S) (NO. OF PATIENTS)	RESULTS
Hosie[23]	(11) Ibuprofen caps 400 mg tid + placebo foam tid/14 d (147) (12) Felbinac (foam 3%) tid + placebo caps tid/14 d (140)		Patients (%) reporting no pain or mild pain after 1 and 2 wk: (11) 84, 92, (12) 76, 88; wk (11) significant differences; number of side effects: (11) 22, (12) 26
Amlie et al[19]	(1) Piroxicam 20 mg cap bid first 2 d, one daily next 5–7d (140)	(R) Placebo caps (142)	(1) More pain relief (VAS) than (R) after 3 d; after 7 d no significant differences; side effects similar: (1) 13%, (R) 17%
Goldie[22]	(1) Indomethacin 25 mg cap tid for course of 50 caps (25)	(R) Placebo caps (25)	Number of patients with complete relief of pain after 7 and 14 d: (1) 7, 14, (R) 9, 16; no significant differences; side effects similar: (1) 8, (R) 5
Weber et al[27]	(1) Piroxicam 20 mg cap bid first 2 d; 20 mg/d next 12 d/14 d (120)	(R) Placebo caps (94)	Reduction of pain in back and leg measured by VAS after 4 wk the same in the two groups (data graphs); no significant differences; more side effects in (1) 22 than in (R)
Bakshi et al[20]	(11) Diclofenac resinate 75 mg cap bid/14 d (66) (12) Piroxicam 20 mg cap bid/2 d + once daily for 12 d (66)		Mean pain intensity scores at rest (VAS) before and after treatment: (11) 70.0, 22.7, (12) 67.1, 21.0; efficacy excellent or good according to patients: (11) 81.8%, (12) 87.7%; no differences; side effects similar: (11) 17, (12) 15
Blazek et al[21]	(11) Diclofenac 25 mg cap qid/4 d and tid next 8 d (14) (12) Briarison 300 mg cap qid/4 d and tid next 8 d (14)		Average improvement on 5-point ordinal scale (0 = no response, 4 = very good response) during and after the intervention period of 12 d according to physician and patient: (11) 2.6, 2.8, (12) 2.8, 3; no significant differences in recovery rate; side effects: mild side effects in 3 patients in each group
Szpalski and Hayez[26]	(1) Tenoxicam 20 mg IM on day 1 +20 mg cap/d for day 2–14 (+7 d bed rest) (37)	(R) Placebo injection + placebo caps (36)	Mean pain intensity (VAS) on day 1, 8, and 14: (1) 7.4, 1.9, 0.6, (R) 7.1, 2.8, 0.8; (1) significantly better on day 8; side effects 1 patient in group (1)
Lacey et al[24]	(1) Piroxicam 10 mg cap qid/2 d and bid next 12 d (168)	(R) Placebo caps (169)	Patients (%) improved after 1 wk only in subgroups with initial moderate or severe pain: (1) 82%, 149%, (R) 53%, 38%; no difference for subgroup with mild initial pain; results after 2 wk not reported, and no data presented on side effects for subgroup with back pain
Videman et al[18]	(1) Diflunisal 250 mg cap qid/ 3 wk (35)	(R) Meptazinol 200 mg cap qid/ 3 wk (35)	Mean change in pain (100 mm VAS) at 3 wk: (1) 45, (R) 40, similar improvement regarding capacity for daily tasks (data in graphs); no significant differences; side effects similar: (1) 19, (R) 23 patients
Sweetman et al[25]	(1) Mefenamic acid 500 mg bid + placebo bid (40) and paracetamol 450 mg two caps tid + placebo bid (42)	(R1) Chlormezanone 100 mg (R2) Ethoheptazine 75 mg and meprobamate 150 mg and aspirin 250 mg two caps + placebo tid (40)	Number of patients reporting no pain after 1 and 7 d: (1) 7, 21, (R1) 12, 23, (R2) 10, 20; number of patients with adverse events: (1) 9, (R1) 10, (R2) 16
Orava[32]	(11) Diflunisal 500 mg cap bid (66) (12) Indomethacin 50 mg cap tid (67)		Percent of patients assessing therapy as good or excellent after 3 and 7 d: (11) 45%, 64%, (12) 45%, 64%; no significant differences; more side effects in (12) 31% than in (11) 18%
Wiesel et al[7]	(11) Aspirin 625 mg cap qid/2 wk (12) Phenylbutazone 100 mg cap qid (first 5 d); no further information	(R) Acetaminophen (dosage not given) bid/2 wk (?)	Mean number of days before return to full activity: (11) 5.7, (12) 6.5, (R) 5.7; no significant differences; no data on side effects given

TABLE 21–4. Details of Randomized Controlled Trials on the Effectiveness of NSAIDs for Acute Low Back Pain *Continued*

REFERENCE	NSAIDs DOSE/FREQUENCY/DURATION (NO. OF PATENTS)	REFERENCE TREATMENT(S) (NO. OF PATIENTS)	RESULTS
Agrifoglio et al[29]	(11) Aceclofenac 150 mg IM bid/2 d + 100 mg tab bid/5 d (50) (12) Diclofenac 75 mg IM bid/2 d + 50 mg tab tid/5 d (50)		No significant difference in pain intensity (VAS) before and after treatment (data in graph); percentage of patients not limited in functional impairment after treatment: (11) 65.9%, (12) 40.5%; significant; overall assessment of efficacy good/very good: (11) 85%, (12) 76%; significant side effects: (11), (12) 8
Weber and Aasand[35]	(1) Phenylbutazone two 200 mg caps tid/3 d (29); 1 cap bid next 2 d (28)	(R) Placebo caps	Number of patients reporting definite positive effect after intervention period (1) 14, (R) 8; no sgnificant differences; no side effects reported by the patients
Waterworth and Hunter[34]	(1) Diflunisal two 500 mg caps immediately; 500 mg bid/10 d (36)	(R1) Physiotherapy: local heat, ultrasound, and exercises, five 45-min session wkly (R2) Spinal manipulation or McKenzie therapy or both, five 45-min sessions wkly (38)	Mean change in pain intensity on 4-point scale after 4 and 12 d: (1) −0.9, −1.7, (R1) −0.9, −1.6, (R2) −1.1, −1.7; no significant differences in pain and mobility
Brown et al[30]	(1) Diflunisal two 500 mg caps initial dose; 500 mg q12h/15 d (19)	(R) Acetaminophen 300 mg with codeine 50 mg/2 caps initially; then 1 cap q4h/15 d (21)	Pain assessment by patient and investigator on 3-point ordinal scale shows similar improvement curves (data in graphs); number of patients rating drugs as excellent or very good: (1) 9, (R) 9; no signihcant differences; side effects: more side effects in (R) 10 than (1) 3
Evans et al[31]	(11) Aspirin three 300 mg caps qid/1 wk (30) (12) lndomethacin 50 mg tid/1 wk (30) (13) Mefenamic acid two 250 mg caps/d/1 wk (30)	(R1) Dextropropoxyphene 32.5 mg + paracetamol 325 mg caps in 2 caps qid/1 wk (30) (R2) Paracetamol two 500 mg caps tid/1 wk (30) (R4) Phenylbutazone 100 mg cap qid/1 wk (30)	Mean daily pain index during intervention period (on 4-point ordinal scale): (11) 1.4, (12) 1.5, (13) 1.4; (R1) 1.7, (R2) 1.7, (R4) 1.4; (13) significantly different from (R1 and R2); (11) significantly different from (R1); side effects: more side effects in (11) 20, (12) 19, (R1) 19 than in (13) 12, (R2) 13, (R4) 4
Aghababian et al[28]	(11) Diflunisal two 500 mg caps initially; 500 mg q8–12h/2 wk (16) (12) Naproxen two 250 mg caps lnitially; 250 mg q6–8h/2 wk (17)		Percent of patients reporting no pain (4-point ordinal scale) after 2 wk: (11) 81%, (12) 41%; no significance tests reported; no adverse experiences reported by the patients
Postacchini et al[33]	(1) Diclofenac 'full dosage'/10–14 d (34)	(R1) Chiropractic manipulation (35) (R2) Physiotherapy (31) (R3) Bed rest (29) (R4) Placebo (antiedema gel) (30)	Mean improvement on combined pain, disability, and spinal mobility score (5–32) after 3 wk, 2 and 6 mo: (1) 3.0, 10.7, 14.0, (R1) 7.5, 9.7, 12.3, (R2) 5, 8.4, 7.3, (R4) 1.8, 7.3, 11.0; (R1) significantly better than others after 3 wk; no other differences; no data on side effects reported

bid, twice per day; tid, three times per day; qid, four times per day; tabl, tablet; caps, capsules; ?, number of patients not given; ADL, activities of daily living; VAS, visual analogue scale.

guidelines from 1994 suggest for acute radicular pain epidural injections may provide a method of avoiding surgery and should be used after conservative treatments fail. The guidelines stress that limited research is currently available. Please remember that epidural injections are not benign since common side effects include allergic/anaphylactic reactions, spinal headache, and epidural hematoma or abscess.

Facet Injections

Facet joint injections with local anesthetics or corticosteroids or both may be used in the

TABLE 21–5. Details of Randomized Controlled Trials on the Effectiveness of Muscle Relaxants for Acute Low Back Pain

REFERENCE	MUSCLE RELAXANTS DOSE/ FREQUENCY/DURATION (NO. OF PATIENTS)	REFERENCE TREATMENT(S) (NO. OF PATIENTS)	RESULTS
Berry and Hutchinson[39]	(1) Tizanidine 4 mg + ibuprofen 400 mg tid/ 7 d (51)	(R) Placebo + ibuprofen 400 mg tid/7 d (54)	Mean changes (SD) in pain score (VAS 100 min) after 3 d: (1) pain at night 32.8 (20), pain at rest 25.3 (18), and pain walking 25.4 (23) vs (R) 34.6 (22), 24.9 (16), and 22.6 (13); after 7 d (1) 39.5 (32), 43.3 (29), and 34.1 (36) vs (R) 39.8 (33), 32.9 (33), and 32.8 (30); percentage of patients improved after 3 d (1) 76% vs (R) 67%, and after 7 d (1) 85% vs (R) 81%; no significant differences; (1) significantly more central nervous system side effects; (R) significantly more gastrointestinal side effects; significantly fewer patients had moderate or severe pain at rest or pain at night in (1) than in (R)
Baratta[38]	(1) Cyclobenzaprine 10 mg tid–qid/ 10 d (58)	(R) Placebo tid–qid/10 d (59)	Mean decrease in pain (10-point scale) from day 1 to 9: (1) −0.8 to −5.5 vs (R) −0.3 to −4.0; (1) significantly better; moderate to marked global improvement: (1) 71% vs (R) 25%, significant; significantly more central nervous system side effects in (1)
Casale[41]	(1) Dantrolene sodium 25 mg 1 cap/d/4 d (10)	(R) Placebo 1 cap/d/4 d (10)	Pain during maximal voluntary movement (VAS) decrease significantly more in (1) than in (R); muscle spasm significantly more improved in (1) 85% than in (R) 30%
Boyles et al[40]	(11) Carisoprodol 350 mg qid/8 d (36)	(12) Diazepam 5 mg qid/8 d (35)	Patient's assessment of muscle tension, stiffness, and overall relief significantly more improved in (11) than in (12) after 6 and 7 d; no significant difference in pain; physician's assessment of overall improvement and muscle spasm: significantly better in (11) than in (12) after 7 d, but not after 3 d; data in graphs
Hindle[43]	(1) Carisoprodol 350 mg qid/4 d (16)	(R1) Placebo qid/4 d (16) (R2) Butabarbital 5 mg qid/4 d (16)	Pain score (VAS 0–100) at baseline and after 2 and 4 d (1) 86, 33, and 15.5, (R1) 65.5, 58.5, and 64, (R2) 75.2, 58.7, and 49.1; (1) significantly more improved; ADL significantly more improved in (1) than in (R1) and (R2), but not muscle spasm
Middleton[44]	(11) Methocarbamol 400 mg + acetylsalicylic acid two 325 mg tabl qid/7 d (55)	(12) Chlormezanone 100 mg + paracetamol 450 mg in 2 tabl tid/7 d (52)	Percentage of patients with moderate to severe pain on day 1 and day 7 in (11) 87% vs (12) 85% and 52%; percentage of patients with overall improvement after treatment: (11) 66% vs (12) 61%; not significant; significantly more side effects in (12) than (11)
Dapas et al[42]	(1) Baclofen one or two 10 mg tabl tid–qid/ 10 d (100)	(R) Placebo 2 tabl qid/10 d (100)	For patients with severe symptoms at baseline: (1) significantly more improved at day 10 in pain, patient's opinion, ADL muscle spasm, and spinal mobility; significantly more side effects in (1)
Rollings et al[45]	(11) Carisoprodol 350 mg qid/7 d (28)	(12) Cyclobenzaprine HCl 10 mg qid/7 d (30)	No statistically significant differences between (11) and (12) on pain, muscle stiffness and tension, ADL, and overall relief; data in graphs
Berry and Hutchnson[46]	(1) Tizanidine 4 mg tid/ 7 d (59)	(R) Placebo tid/7d (53)	Mean (SD) pain score (VAS 100 mm) at baseline and after 3 and 7 days: pain at night (1) 32.5 (51), 32.3 (39), and 20.6 (15) vs (R) 33.1 (52), 28.8 (38), and 20.8 (18); pain at rest (1) 29.4 (51), 29.6 (39), and 23.2 (19) vs (R) 26.9 (51), 27.9 (34), and 22.9 (19); pain on movement (1) 30.0 (55), 30.4 (46), and 22.9 (18) vs (R) 27.8 (49), 25.6 (36), and 23.1 (18); no differences between (1) and (R); overall improvement after 3 and 7 d: (1) 17% and 84% of patients and (R) 8% and 82% of patients; not significant; side effects in (1) 41% and (R) 21%; (1) significantly more central nervous system side effects, (R) significantly more gastrointestinal side effects
Gold[48]	(1) Orphenadrine citrate 100 mg bid/7 d (20)	(R1) Placebo bid/7 d (20) (R2) Phenobarbital 32 mg bid/7 d (20)	Number of patients improved after 2 d: (1) 7, (R1) 0, (R2) 3; (1) significantly more improved than (R1); number of patients with reduced pain after 2 d: (1) 9, (R1) 4, (R2) 3; (1) significantly more reduced than (R1) and (R2); number of patients with side effects: (1) 5, (R1) 1, (R2) 2

TABLE 21–5. Details of Randomized Controlled Trials on the Effectiveness of Muscle Relaxants for Acute Low Back Pain *Continued*

REFERENCE	MUSCLE RELAXANTS DOSE/ FREQUENCY/DURATION (NO. OF PATIENTS)	REFERENCE TREATMENT(S) (NO. OF PATIENTS)	RESULTS
Sweetman et al[25]	(1) Chlormezanone 100 mg + paracetamol two 450 mg caps tid/7 d (42)	(R1) Mefenamic acid 500 mg tid/ 7 d (40) (R2) Ethoheptazine 75 mg + meprobamate 150 mg + aspirin two 250 mg tabl tid/7 d (40)	Number of patients with overall improvement after 7 d: (1) 24, (R1) 24, (R2) 22; not significant; number of patients reporting side effects on day 7: (1) 5, (R1) 5, (R2) 13; significant
Borenstein et al[47]	(1) Cyclobenzaprine 10 mg tid + naproxen 500 mg initially; then 250 mg qid/14 d (20)	(R) Naproxen 500 mg initially; 250 mg qid/14 d (20)	Treatment outcome significantly better on muscle spasm and tenderness in (1) than in (R); no significant differences on pain and functional capacity; significantly more side effects in (1) than in (R)
Hingorani[49]	(1) Diazepam 10 mg IM × 4/24 h + 2 mg PO qid/5 d + aspirin 10 g tid/5 d (25)	(R) Placebo four IM injections/ 24 h + PO qid/5 d + aspirin 10 g tid/5 d (25)	Number of patients improved: (1) 19 vs (R) 18; side effects: drowsiness in 7 patients (1) vs 3 in (R)
Tervo et al[50]	(1) Orphenadrine 60 mg in 2 ml IM + orphenadrine citrate 35 mg PO + paracetamol two 450 mg tabl tid/8 d (25)	(R) Placebo saline injection 2 ml + paracetamol two 450 mg tabl PO tid/8 d (25)	No significant differences in subjective impression of improvement, muscle spasm, and spinal flexion; walking and sitting ability significantly more improved in (1) than in (R); side effects in (1) 2 patients and (R) 1 patient

treatment of patients thought to have "facet syndrome." Facet syndrome is an ill-defined clinical entity that includes patients who have primarily LBP that is aggravated by extension of the spine without neurologic signs or sciatica. Facet joint injections are usually used in the treatment of chronic LBP (more than 3 months' duration). Four trials are available in the literature studying facet joint injections in patients who had chronic LBP: Jackson,[56] Lilius et al,[57] Carette et al,[58] and Nash.[59] Thorough review of the literature did not reveal any adequate studies assessing the efficacy of facet joint injections in acute LBP. These four trials reviewed facet joint injections in chronic LBP and found that neither use of steroid, saline, or local anesthetic nor the location of injection (i.e., intraarticular, pericapsular, or nerve block) made any significant difference in outcome. Based on this limited information facet joint injection cannot be recommended for the treatment of acute or chronic LBP.

Trigger Point Injections

This technique involves injection of local anesthetic with or without corticosteroid into painful soft tissues of the back, such as muscles or ligaments, to attempt to relieve discomfort.

Review of the literature revealed the following best studies.

Frost et al[60] compared trigger point injection of 0.5% carbocaine or normal saline in 53 patients who had acute neck, shoulder, and low back pain. All patients received three injections at intervals of 2 to 3 days. No subgroup analysis for patients who had back pain was provided. After the first injection the normal saline group had significantly more pain relief ($P \leq .05$), but after the second and third injections there was no significant difference between groups.

Garvey et al[62] studied 63 patients with acute back pain who received one of four treatments:

1. Trigger point injection with 1% lidocaine
2. Trigger point injection with lidocaine and steroid
3. Dry needling of trigger
4. Ethyl chloride spray (spray and stretch technique)

In addition to these treatments all patients received 4 weeks of anti-inflammatory medications and activity restriction before entry into the trial. At the end of the 2-week follow-up there was no significant difference in pain perception among groups receiving medication and those receiving needling or ethyl chloride spray ($P < .093$).

Collee et al[62] compared the analgesic effects of injection with 5 ml of 0.5% lidocaine and 5 ml of normal saline in 41 patients with iliac crest pain syndrome. These patients were divided into two groups: rheumatology clinic and general practice patients. The rheumatology patients had more chronic symptoms. The visual analog scale was used to attempt to quantify pain. No significant difference was found between groups at the 10-minute and day-7 marks. However, at the day-14 mark the lidocaine group had a significantly lower pain score. Subgroup analysis of the rheumatology clinic group of patients in the treatment arm showed that they experienced more pain relief. In the general practice patients, with a shorter duration of pain, there was no significant difference in pain relief between the two treatments.

Ongley et al[63] studied 81 patients with chronic LBP of more than 1 year's duration randomized to two treatments. The experimental group was treated with a sclerosing solution that contained 25% dextrose and glycerine in 2.5% phenol, and the control group received normal saline. At the 1-, 3-, and 6-month marks the treatment group showed a reduction in pain and disability ($P < .01$ to .04).

Based on these trials there is poor evidence available in the literature for recommending trigger point injections in the treatment of patients who have acute LBP.

Oral Steroids

Corticosteroids given orally have been used in the past for the treatment of acute lower back discomfort, especially for patients with radicular symptoms. Very limited information is available for this treatment in the existing literature.

Haimovic and Beresford[64] reported a prospective double-blind trial comparing oral dexamethasone with placebo. They used a 7-day course of oral dexamethasone starting with 64 mg in a sliding scale to 8 mg. Thirty-three patients with acute LBP and monoradiculopathy were entered into the study, and all patients were kept on bed rest for 7 days and given narcotic and nonnarcotic analgesics. At the time this trial was taking place, bed rest was believed to have a beneficial effect. They were evaluated after 7 days and at the 1- and 4-year marks regarding intensity of pain. Unfortunately, only

27 patients (82%) were available for a followup. Dexamethasone was not found to be better than placebo in the short or long term. Therefore based on this limited information, oral steroids cannot be recommended for the treatment of patients with acute LBP, especially considering the potential for serious side effects.

TRANSCUTANEOUS ELECTRICAL NERVE STIMULATION

Transcutaneous electrical nerve stimulation (TENS) has been widely used for the treatment of both acute and chronic pain. There is scant literature available studying the effects of TENS in acute LBP.

Hackett et al[65] compared the treatment effects of electroacupuncture with acetaminophen and placebo. Electroacupuncture is pulsed electrical stimulation with surface electrodes. Thirty-seven patients with acute LBP of less than 3 days' duration were randomly assigned to one of two treatment groups: (1) electroacupuncture and placebo tablets or (2) placebo electroacupuncture and acetaminophen at the end of 1 and 2 weeks. There was no significant difference between the groups, but at the 6-week mark the electroacupunture group had significantly less pain.

Hermann et al[66] studied the effects of codatron TENS on 58 injured workers with acute LBP of 3 to 10 weeks' duration. The patients were randomly assigned to one of two treatment groups: (1) active codatron TENS and exercise or (2) placebo codatron TENS and exercise. The exercise program lasted for 4 weeks. There was a significant reduction of pain in each treatment group when compared to baseline values, but there was no significant difference in percentage return to work between the groups.

Three other trials (Fox and Melzack,[67] Lehman et al,[68] Deyo et al[69]) studied the effects of TENS in patients with chronic LBP. Since they do not directly evaluate acute LBP they will not be reviewed here in detail. Generally no clinically or statistically significant differences were found between groups.

In summary, of the five clinical trials available for review, only two studied acute LBP and did not find significant differences between TENS and placebo. The three trials looking at chronic LBP also did not find any significant improvement with TENS. Therefore based on this information TENS cannot be recommended for patients with acute or chronic LBP.

EXERCISE THERAPIES

Various types of exercise regimens are frequently recommended for the treatment of acute LBP. Specific exercise programs are expected to achieve specific treatment goals, such as improved spinal mobility, strengthening of paraspinal and abdominal muscles, or improved overall strength and endurance and cardiovascular conditioning.

Lindstrom and Zachrisson[70] studied 62 patients with acute LBP of no more than 1 month's duration. The patients were randomized into three treatment groups: (1) conventional treatment (i.e., hot packs, massage, mobilization and strengthening exercise), (2) alternative treatment (i.e. intermittent pelvic traction and isometric exercise of abdominal and hip extensor muscles), and (3) control group (i.e., hot packs and rest). All patients received 10 treatments during 1 month, and assessments were performed by a physician blinded to treatment group. Patients receiving the alternative treatment arm reported a slight improvement with respect to pain.

Coxhead et al[71] reported a multicenter randomized trial of 292 patients with LBP and sciatica with an average duration of 14.3 weeks. A factorial design was used, and patients were assigned into one of the following four treatment groups: (1) traction, (2) exercise at physiotherapist's discretion, (3) manipulation, or (4) corset. At the end of 4 weeks, 78% of all patients improved irrespective of the treatment arm that they were assigned to. There were no statistically significant differences among groups.

Davies et al[72] studied 43 patients with LBP of 3 weeks to 6 months' duration. Patients were treated with either extension or isometric flexion exercise and short-wave diathermy. All patients had reduced pain and increased spinal mobility, and the time to return to work and sport was similar in each group.

Evans[73] evaluated the effects of the Kendall flexion exercise routine in 242 patients with acute LBP with or without radiation into the legs. The duration of pain for patients was less than 30 days, and patients were randomized to

one of four treatment groups: (1) flexion exercise, education, and bed rest for 4 days; (2) flexion exercise and education; (3) bed rest only; or (4) control group with analgesics only. All patients were instructed on a 20-minute exercise program to be performed daily for 2 months or longer if necessary. Follow-up was at 6 weeks, 12 weeks, and 1 year. There were no significant differences among the groups with respect to self-reported levels of pain or activity restriction.

Stankovic and Johnell[74] compared the effects of Mackenzie extension exercises with a mini-back school in a group of 100 patients with acute LBP with or without radiation into the legs. Most patients had pain for less than 1 week; some had pain for up to 4 weeks. Follow-up was at the 3-week and 1-year marks. Patients treated with the Mackenzie extension exercise protocol returned to work earlier ($P < .001$), had fewer recurrences ($P < .001$), reported lower pain levels ($P < .001$), and had improved spinal mobility ($P < .001$).

Linstrom et al[75] reported a randomized trial involving 103 Swedish auto workers who had subacute, nonspecific mechanical LBP of approximately 6 weeks' duration. The subjects received either a graded activity program or traditional therapy. The graded activity program consisted of a functional capacity assessment, a workplace visit, attendance in back school, and individualized, submaximal, gradually increasing exercises using operant conditioning principles. Patients in the traditional therapy arm received rest, analgesics, and traditional physiotherapy. Patients were observed for 3 years. At the 1-year mark the rate of return to work was significantly faster for the graded activity program ($P = .03$), and at the 2-year mark the average duration of sick leave was significantly less in the graded activity program group ($P = .05$).

Faas et al[76] studied 473 patients with acute LBP with or without radiation into the upper leg. The patients had pain for less than 3 weeks. They were randomized into one of three groups: (1) exercise therapy, which included 20 minutes of exercise twice weekly for 5 weeks; (2) usual care, which consisted of analgesics and information about back pain (ie, the importance of heat and physical activity); or (3) placebo therapy, which consisted of ultrasound therapy performed by a physiotherapist twice weekly for 5 weeks. There were no differences among groups in regard to functional health status or pain recurrence at the 1-year follow-up mark.

Gundewall et al[77] evaluated the effects of a supervised exercise program and prevention of LBP in a group of 60 nursing personnel. The subjects were randomized to receive either a supervised exercise program during work six times per month for 13 months or no intervention. The exercise program consisted of isometric and dynamic exercises to strengthen back extensor muscles. The group of patients receiving this exercise program experienced fewer recurrences in low back pain: 4% compared with 38% for the control group; fewer days of lost time from work; and a lower average duration of back pain symptoms.

Malmivaara et al[10] studied the effects of extension exercises, 2 days of bed rest, and "ordinary activity." Fifty-two patients received the extension exercise treatment, and 67 patients were entered into the other two treatment arms. Twelve weeks of follow-up was provided, and this trial revealed that ordinary activity was better than doing either extension exercises or remaining in bed for 2 days with respect to pain "disability" and the amount of sick leave.

Based on the available literature there is no evidence to suggest that an exercise program provides any significant benefit in patients who have had acute LBP (less than 4 weeks in duration). There is some evidence, however, to suggest that an exercise program can limit recurrences and duration of symptoms in future episodes of back pain. Similar conclusions have been reached in recent reviews by Faas[78] and Van Tulder et al.[2] It is becoming more clear that nonspecific exercise programs are probably not beneficial.[79] Which specific exercise is helpful is still unclear—strength vs endurance training, flexion vs extension and cardiovascular fitness (re)training.[82] There is strong evidence that exercise therapy is not more effective than other conservative treatments, including no intervention, for acute LBP (level 1 evidence).

PHYSICAL MODALITIES

Physical modalities have been used for centuries for symptomatic relief of pain. The evidence of their effectiveness in the treatment of acute LBP is at the present controversial. Given below are the best articles in the literature after extensive review.

Waterworth et al[80] reported an RCT comparing diflunisal for 10 days with physiotherapy that consisted of short-wave diathermy for 15 to 20 minutes, ultrasound for 5 to 10 minutes, flexion-extension exercises 5 days per week for 45-minute sessions, and manipulation by a physiotherapist. One hundred and four patients with acute LBP with or without radiation into the leg of less than 1 month's duration were randomized into three groups. The following outcome variables were recorded after 10 to 12 days of treatment: pain, return to work, and spinal movement. At the end of the trial most patients improved and returned to work, but there were no statistically significant differences among the groups. The major problem with this study is that it is difficult to separate the effects of the modalities from the other aspects of physical therapy. Also, the outcome assessment was not blinded.

Postacchini et al[33] studied the effects of manipulation, physiotherapy (massage), infrared daily for 2 to 3 weeks, drug therapy (Diaclofinac), placebo (antiedema gel), bed rest (20 to 24 hours for 4 to 6 days and 15 to 20 hours for 2 days), and attendance in back school (four 1-hour sessions and exercise daily). One hundred and fifty-nine patients with acute LBP with or without radiation into the legs of less than 4 weeks' duration were entered. The following outcome measurements were recorded: the patient's self-report of pain, restriction of activities of daily living, spinal mobility, muscle strength, degree of positivity of straight leg raising, and local tenderness at the 2- and 6-month follow-up. There were no statistically significant differences among the groups.

Gibson et al[81] reported an RCT involving 109 patients with LBP of between 2 and 12 months' duration who were assigned to osteopathic manipulation, short-wave diathermy, or detuned short-wave diathermy. The short-wave diathermy treatments were given three times per week, and osteopathic treatment was once per week for 4 weeks. Outcome assessments were pain, spinal mobility, local tenderness, and return to work status. The patients were observed at 2, 4, and 12 weeks. Gibson et al found that there was immediate improvement in more than one half the patients across treatment groups, and improvement was maintained at the 12-week follow-up. However, there were no significant differences among the treatment groups.

Recommendations

On the basis of the limited information available in the existing literature, it is apparent that modalities were not more efficacious than placebo. However, the literature does not provide information in regard to which modalities work best, when and how they should be applied, and whether they work equally well on "mechanical" LBP as on LBP with neurologic signs and symptoms. Considerably more research is required to answer these clinically relevant questions.

CORSETS AND ORTHOSES

The effectiveness of an orthosis may result from restriction in intersegmental motion, reduction of interdiscal pressure, and unloading of the spinal column in general. The landmark study in this area was carried out by Nachemson et al.[82] The intradiscal and intraabdominal pressures as well as myoelectrical activities of abdominal and paraspinal muscles were examined in four able-bodied volunteers wearing three different types of orthoses (corset, Rainey, and Boston extension brace). The subjects were asked to carry out six different tasks wearing each of the braces. All the braces were found to unload the spine and reduce interdiscal pressure and myoelectrical activity in two thirds of the tasks. However, none of the orthoses raised intraabdominal pressure significantly, and no one was superior in mechanical effectiveness.

Cockshead et al[71] compared the treatment effects of lumbar corsets for 292 patients with acute and chronic LBP with an average duration of 14.3 weeks. Lumbar corsets were no more efficacious than traction, manipulation, exercise, or a combination of these.

Million et al[83] assessed the ability of lumbar corsets with or without rigid support to reduce back discomfort. A randomized trial involving 19 patients with chronic back pain of at least 6 months' duration was carried out. Rigid corsets were found to be superior in relieving discomfort.

Walsh and Schwartz[84] studied the effectiveness of lumbar corsets in preventing back injury and time lost from work in a group of 90 male warehouse workers. These workers did not have any LBP and were not receiving any treatment for back injury. The workers were randomly assigned to the following three groups: no intervention (control), 1-hour session on back pain prevention and body mechanics, and education and wearing lumbosacral corsets during work hours. At the 6-month follow-up the group with education and wearing the orthoses showed substantially less time lost even though there was no change in abdominal strength, productivity, or accident rate.

Reddel et al[85] evaluated a weightlifting belt in the prevention of back injury in 642 airline baggage handlers. At the 8-month follow-up 58% of the workers who were issued belts stopped using them and there was no significant difference between treatment groups regarding back injury rate, loss or restricted workdays, and workers' compensation rates.

Recommendations

Corset and lumbar braces have been found to reduce intradiscal pressure and restrict lumbar spinal movement as well as reduce myoelectrical activity in healthy individuals. However, there is no evidence that this translates into improved pain or functional abilities and there is conflicting evidence regarding the effectiveness of corsets or belts in the prevention or reduction of impact of back pain in workers who perform frequent lifting tasks. There were no studies identified that examined the athletic population and the use of corsets or lumbar braces.

REFERENCES

1. Anderson GBJ: The epidemiology of spinal disorders. In Frymoyer JW (ed): The Adult Spine: Principles and Practice. Raven Press, Philadelphia, 1991, p 107
2. van Tulder MW, Koes BW, Bouter LM: Conservative treatment of acute and chronic nonspecific low back pain. Spine 22(18):2128–2156, 1997
3. White AA, Gordon SL: Synopsis: workshop on idiopathic low back pain. Spine 7:141–149, 1982
4. Johnson EW: The myth of skeletal muscle spasm. Am J Phys Med Rehabil 68:1, 1989
5. Waddell G, Main CJ, Morris EW, et al: Normality and reliability in the clinical assessment of backache. BMJ 284:1519–1523, 1982

6. Deyo RA: Drug therapy for back pain. Which drugs help which patients? Spine 21(24):2840–2849, 1996

7. Wiesel SW, Cuckler JM, DeLuca F, et al.: Acute low back pain: an objective analysis of conservative therapy. Spine 5:324–330, 1980

8. Gilbert JR, Taylor DW, Hildebrand A, et al: Clinical trial of common treatments for low back pain in family practice. BMJ 291:791, 1985

9. Deyo R, Diehl AK, Rosenthal M, et al: How many days of bed rest for acute low back pain? A randomized clinical trial. N Engl J Med 315:1064, 1986

10. Malmivaara A, Hakkinen U, Aro T, et al: The treatment of acute low back pain—bed rest, exercise or ordinary activity. N Engl J Med 332:351, 1995

11. Deyo RA: Conservative therapy for low back pain. Distinguishing useful from useless therapy. JAMA 250:1057–1062, 1983

12. Chavannes AW, Gubbels J, Post D, et al: Acute low back pain: patients' perception of pain four weeks after initial diagnosis and treatment in general practice. J R Coll Gen Pract 36:271–273, 1986

13. Dillane JB, Fry J, Kalton G: Acute low back syndrome—a study from general practice. BMJ 2:82–84, 1966

14. Frymoyer JW: Back pain and sciatica. N Engl J Med 318:291–300, 1988

15. Roland M, Morris R: A study of the natural history of back pain, part II: development of guidelines for trials of treatment in primary care. Spine 8:145–150, 1983

16. Spitzer WO, LeBlanc FE, Dupuis M, et al: Scientific approach to the assessment and management of activity related spinal disorders. A monograph for clinicians. Report of the Quebec Task Force on Spinal Disorders. Spine 12(Suppl), 1987

17. Turner JA, Deyo RA, Loeser JD, et al: The importance of the placebo effects in pain treatment and research. JAMA 271:1609–1614, 1994

18. Videman T, Heikkila J, Partanen T: Double blind parallel study of meptazinol versus diflunisal in the treatment of lumbago. Curr Med Res Opin 9:246–252, 1984

19. Amlie E, Weber H, Holme I: Treatment of acute low back pain with piroxicam: results of a double-blind placebo controlled trial. Spine 12:473–476, 1987

20. Bakshi R, Thumb N, Broll H, et al: Treatment of acute lumbosacral back pain with diclofenac resinate: results of a double-blind comparative trial versus piroxicam. Drug Investigation 8:288–294, 1994

21. Blazek M, Keszthelyi B, Varhelyi M, Korosi O: Comparative study of Blarison and Voltaren in acute lumbar pain and lumbo-ischialgia. Ther Hung 34:163–166, 1986

22. Goldie I: A clinical trial with indomethacin (indomee) in low back pain and sciatica. Acta Orthop Scand 39:117–128, 1968

23. Hosie GAC: The topical NSAID, felbinac, versus oral ibuprofen: a comparison of efficacy in the treatment of acute low back injury. Br J Clin Res 4:5–17, 1993

24. Lacey PH, Dodd GD, Shannon DJ: A double-blind placebo controlled study of piroxicam in the management of acute musculoskeletal disorders. Eur J Rheumatol Inflamm 7:95–104, 1984

25. Sweetman BJ, Baig A, Parsons DL: Mefenamic acid, chlormazanone-paracetamol, ethoptazine-aspirin-meprobamate: a comparative study in low back pain. Br J Clin Pract 41:619–624, 1987

26. Szpalski M, Hayez JP: Objective functional assessment of the efficacy of tenoxicam in the treatment of acute low back pain. A double-blind placebo-controlled study. Br J Rheumatol 33:74–78, 1994

27. Weber H, Holme I, Amlie E: The natural course of acute sciatica with nerve root symptoms in a double-blind placebo controlled trial evaluating the effect of piroxicam. Spine 18:1433–1438, 1993

28. Aghababian RV, Volturo GA, Heifetz IN: Comparison of diflunisal and naproxen in the management of acute low back strain. Clin Ther 9(Suppl C):47–51, 1986

29. Agrifoglio E, Benvenuti M, Gatto P, et al: Aceclofenac: a new NSAID in the treatment of acute lumbago. Multicentre single blind study vs diclofenac. Acta Therapeutica 20:33–43, 1994

30. Brown FL, Bodison S, Dixon J, et al: Comparison of diflunisal and acetaminophen with codeine in the treatment of initial or recurrent acute low back pain. Clin Ther 9(Suppl C):52–58, 1986

31. Evans DP, Burke MS, Newcombe RG: Medicines of choice in low back pain. Curr Med Res Opin 6:540–547, 1980

32. Orava S: Medical treatment of acute low back pain. Diflunisal compared to indomethacin in acute lumbago. Int J Clin Res 6(1):45–51, 1986

33. Postacchini F, Facchini M, Palmieri P: Efficacy of various forms of conservative treatment in low back pain: a comparative study. Neuro Orthop 6:28–35, 1988

34. Waterworth RF, Hunter IA: An open study of diflunisal, conservative and manipulative therapy in the management of acute mechanical low back pain. N Z Med J 98:372–375, 1985

35. Weber H, Aasand G: The effect of phenylbutazone on patients with acute lumbago-sciatica: a double blind trial. J Oslo City Hospital 30:69–72, 1980

36. Basmajian JV, Banerjee SN: Clinical Decision Making in Rehabilitation: Efficacy and Outcomes. Churchill Livingstone, New York, 1996, p 70

37. Turturro MA, Paris PM, Seaberg DC: Intramuscular ketorolac versus oral ibuprofen in acute musculoskeletal pain. Ann Emerg Med 26:117–120, 1995

38. Baratta RR: A double blind study of cyclobenzaprine and placebo in the treatment of acute musculoskeletal conditions of the low back. Curr Ther Res 32:646–652, 1982

39. Berry H, Hutchinson DR: Tizanidine and ibuprofen in acute low back pain: results of a double-blind multicentre study in general practice. J Int Med Res 16:83–91, 1988

40. Boyles WF, Glassman JM, Soyka JP: Management of acute musculoskeletal conditions: thoracolumbar strain or sprain. A double-blind evaluation comparing the efficacy and safety of carisoprodol with diazepam. Today's Therapeutic Trends 1:1–16, 1983

41. Casale R: Acute low back pain: symptomatic treatment with a muscle relaxant drug. Clin J Pain 4:81–88, 1988

42. Dapas F, Hartman SF, Martinez L, et al: Baclofen for the treatment of acute low back syndrome: a double-blind comparison with placebo. Spine 10:345–349, 1985

43. Hindle TH: Comparison of carisoprodol, butabarbital and placebo in treatment of the low back syndrome. Calif Med 117:7–11, 1972

44. Middleton RSW: A comparison of two analgesic muscle relaxant combinations in acute back pain. Br J Clin Prac 38:107–109, 1984

45. Rollings HE, Glassman JM, Soyka JP: Management of acute musculoskeletal conditions— thoracolumbar strain or sprain: a double blind evaluation comparing the efficacy and safety of carisoprodol with cyclobenzaprine hydrochloride. Curr Ther Res 34:917–928, 1983

46. Berry H, Hutchinson DR: A multicentre placebo-controlled study in general practice to evaluate the efficacy and safety of tizanidine in acute low-back pain. J Int Med Res 16:75–82, 1988

47. Borenstein DG, Lacks S, Wiesel SW: Cyclobenzaprine and naproxen versus naproxen alone in the treatment of acute low back pain and muscle spasm. Clin Ther 12:125–131, 1990

48. Gold RH: Orphenadrine citrate: sedative or muscle relaxant? Clin Ther 1:451–453, 1978

49. Hingorani K: Diazepam in backache: a double-blind controlled trial. Ann Phys Med 8:303–306, 1965

50. Tervo T, Petaja L, Lepisto P: A controlled clinical trial of a muscle relaxant analgesic combination in the treatment of acute lumbago. Br J Clin Pract 30:62–64, 1976

51. Dilke TFW, Burry HE, Grahame R, et al: Extradural corticosteroid injection in management of lumbar root compression. BMJ 16:635, 1973

52. Sonek W, Weber H, Jorgensen: Double-blind evaluation of extradural prednisolone for herniated lumbar disc. Acta Orthop Scand 48:635, 1977

53. Cuckler JM, Bernini PA, Wiesel SW, et al: The use of epidural steroids in the treatment of lumbar radicular pain. J Bone Joint Surg Am 67:63, 1985

54. Ridley MG, Kingley GH, Gibson T, et al: Outpatient lumbar epidural corticosteroid injection in the management of sciatica. Br J Rheumatol 27:295, 1988

55. Bush K, Hillier S: Controlled study of caudal epidural injections of triamcinolone plus procaine for the management of intractable sciatica. Spine 16:5(27), 1991

56. Jackson R: The facet syndrome—myth or reality? Clin Orthop 279:110, 1992

57. Lilius G, Laasonen EM, Myelynen P, et al: Lumbar facet joint syndrome J Bone Joint Surg Br 71:681, 1989

58. Carette S, Marcoux S, Pruchon R, et al: In controlled trial of corticosteroid injections into facet joints for chronic low back. N Engl J Med 325:1002, 1991

59. Nash TP: Facet joints—intra-articular steroid or nerve block. Pain Clin 3:77, 1990

60. Frost FA, Jessen B, Siggaard-Anderson J: A controlled double blind comparison of mepivacaine injection vs. saline injection of myofascial pain. Lancet 8:499, 1980

61. Garvey T, Marks MR, Weisel SW: A prospective randomized double blind evaluation of trigger point injection therapy for low back pain. Spine 14:962, 1989

62. Collee G, Dijkmans BA, Vandenbroucke JP, Cats A: Iliac crest pain syndrome in low back pain. A double blind, randomized study of local injection therapy. J Rheumatol 18:1060, 1991

63. Ongley M, Klein RG, Dorman TA, et al: A new approach to the treatment of chronic low back pain. Lancet 18:143, 1987

64. Haimovic I, Beresford HR: Dexamethasone is not superior to placebo for treating lumbosacral radicular pain. Neurology 36:1593, 1986

65. Hackett GI, Seddon D, Karminski D: Electroacupuncture compared with paracetamol for acute low back pain. Practitioner 232:163, 1988

66. Hermann E, Williams R, Stratford P, et al: A randomized trial of transcutaneous electrical nerve stimulation (codatron) to determine its benefits in a rehabilitation program for acute occupational low back pain. Spine 19:561, 1994

67. Fox EJ, Melzack R: Transcutaneous electric stimulation and acupuncture: comparison of treatment for low back pain. Pain 2:141, 1976

68. Lehman TR, Russell DW, Spratt KR, et al: Efficacy of electroacupuncture and TENS in rehabilitation of chronic low back pain patients. Pain 26:277, 1986

69. Deyo RA, Walsh NE, Martin DC, et al: A controlled trial of transcutaneous electrical stimulation (TENS) and exercise for chronic low back pain. N Engl J Med 322:1627, 1990

70. Lindstrom A, Zachrisson M: Physical therapy on low back pain and sciatica and attempt at evaluation. Scand J Rehabil Med 2:37, 1970

71. Coxhead CE, Meade TW, Inskip H, et al: Multicentral trial of physiotherapy in the management of sciatic symptoms. Lancet 8229:1065, 1981

72. Davies JE, Gibson T, Tester L: The value of exercises in the treatment of low back pain. Rheumatol Rehabil 18:243, 1979

73. Evans C: A randomized control trial of flexion exercises, education and bed rest for patients with acute low back pain. Physiother Can 39:96, 1987

74. Stankovic R, Johnell D: Conservative treatment of acute low back pain. A prospective randomized trial: Mackenzie method of treatment verses patient education in "Mini-back school." Spine 15:120, 1990

75. Linstrom I, Ohlund C, Eek C: The effect of graded activity on patients with sub-acute low back pain: a randomized perspective clinical study with an operant conditioning behavioural approach. Phys Ther 72:279, 1992

76. Faas A, Chavannes AW, Van Eijk JT, et al: A randomized placebo controlled trial of exercise therapy in patients with acute low back pain. Spine 18:1388, 1993

77. Gundewall B, Lilijearrist M, Hansson T, et al: Primary prevention of back symptoms and absence from work: a prospective randomized study among hospital employees. Spine 18:587, 1993

78. Faas A: Exercises: which ones are worth trying for which patients and when? Spine 21:2874–2879, 1996

79. Herring S: The role of exercise for the prevention of low back pain. AAPM&R Annual Assembly, 1998, p 259

80. Waterworth RF, Hunter IA: An open study of Difluzinal, conservative and manipulative therapy in the management of acute mechanical low back pain. N Z MED J 98:372, 1985

81. Gibson T, Grahame R, Harkness G, et al: Controlled comparison of short wave diathermy treatments with osteopathic treatment in non-specific low back pain. Lancet 1:1258, 1985

82. Nachemson A, Schultz A, Andersson G: Mechanical effectiveness studies of lumbar spine orthosis. Scand J Rehabil Med 9:139, 1983

83. Million R, Haavik NK, Jayson MIV, et al: Evaluation of low back pain and assessment of lumbar corsets with and without back supports. Ann Rheum Dis 40:494, 1981

84. Walsh NE, Schwartz RK: The influence of profilactic orthosis on abdominal strength and low back injury in the work place. Am J Phys Med Rehabil 69:245, 1990

85. Reddel CR, Cogleton JJ, Huchingson RD, et al: An evaluation of a weight lifting belt and back injury prevention training class for airline baggage handlers. Appl Ergonomics 23:319, 1992

86. Nwuga VCB: Ultrasound treatment of back pain resulting from prolapsed intervertebral disc. Arch Phys Med Rehabil 64:88, 1983

Algorithms for Acute Back Pain

A.1. Acute Low Back Pain Pathway

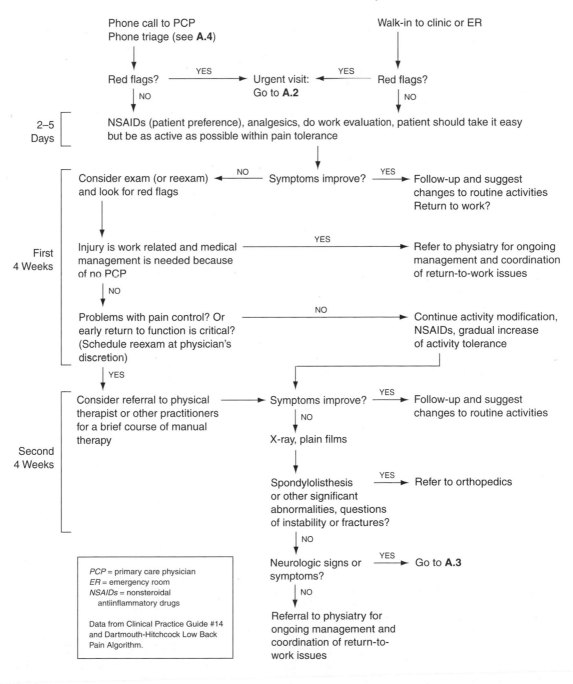

PCP = primary care physician
ER = emergency room
NSAIDs = nonsteroidal
  antiinflammatory drugs

Data from Clinical Practice Guide #14
and Dartmouth-Hitchcock Low Back
Pain Algorithm.

A.2. Initial Evaluation of Acute Low Back Pain

Patients with <3 months of activity intolerance due to LBP or back-related leg symptoms

Perform fused medical history and physical examination
Search for red flags
Examination includes neurologic screening and straight leg raising test

Any red flags? ———————————— YES

NO

In the absence of red flags, diagnostic testing is not clinically helpful in the first 4 weeks of symptoms

Red flags for spine fracture

Red flags for cancer or infection

Red flags for cauda equina syndrome or rapidly progressing neurologic deficit

Plain x-ray of lumbosacral spine; if after 10 days fracture still suspected or multiple sites of pain, consider bone and consultation before defining anatomy with CT

CBC, ESR, U/A; if still suspicious, consider consultation or seek further evidence with bone scan, x-ray, or other laboratory tests; negative x-ray alone does not rule out disease; if positive, define anatomy with MRI

Immediate consultation for emergency studies and definitive care

Evidence of serious disease?

NO

Return to pathway ←——— NO ——— Evidence of nonspinal medical problems causing referred back complaints? ——— YES ——→ Arrange appropriate treatment or consultation

Exit algorithm

CT = computed tomography
MRI = magnetic resonance imaging
CBC = complete blood count
ESR = electro skin resistance
U/A = urinalysis

Data from Clinical Practice Guide #14 and Dartmouth-Hitchcock Low Back Pain Algorithm.

A.3. Management Protocol for Neurologic Signs or Symptoms Still Evident After 4 Weeks

Patients with neurologic signs evident after 4 weeks of routine treatment

↓

Consider or discuss further imaging with neurosurgical or orthopedic consultant
Increase analgesics
Restrict activity

↓

Imaging modalities show significant disk ⎯⎯ YES ⎯⎯→ Refer to orthopedics or neurosurgery

↓ NO   ↓ NO

Consider referral to physiatry for ongoing ←⎯⎯ NO ⎯⎯ Surgical candidate?
management and coordination of return-
to-work issues   ↓ YES

                                               Surgery

Data from Clinical Practice Guide #14 and Dartmouth-Hitchcock Low Back Pain Algorithm.

A.4. Phone Triage

Patient name:_____ Interviewer:_____
Phone number:_____
Patient calls with complaint of low back pain:

HOW AND WHEN DID IT START?
_____ Major trauma (MVA, fall from height)?
_____ Work related?

→ YES → Yes—same day visit

WHAT ARE YOUR SYMPTOMS?
_____ Weakness of lower extremities?
_____ Numbness of lower extremities or buttocks (saddle distribution)?
_____ Urinary symptoms such as dysuria, urinary retention, nocturia, incontinence?
_____ Any constitutional symptoms such as fever, chills?
_____ Abdominal, pelvic, groin pain?
_____ Unable to find comfortable position?

YES → Yes to any of these—same day visit

NO ↓

_____ Age over 50 years (with new back pain)?
_____ Any history of cancer?
_____ Any recent bacterial infection (especially UTI)?
_____ Immunosuppression (steroids, transplants, or HIV)?
_____ Weight loss?

YES → Yes to any of these—visit 1–2 days

NO ↓

_____ 1. Any medication allergies? YES:_____
_____ 2. Any problems with medications such as ibuprofen (Advil, Motrin), Aleve, or aspirin?
_____ 3. Any history of ulcers or bleeding problems?
_____ 4. Do you take blood thinners such as warfarin sodium (Coumadin)?
_____ 5. Any chance of pregnancy?

YES → Yes to medication allergy for NSAIDs or to nos. 2–5

NO ↓

3 day's modification of activities (avoid activities that make pain worse). ASA, ibuprofen, or Tylenol. DOSE:_____

YES ↓

3 day's modification of activities (avoid activities that make pain worse). ES Tylenol; send information.

If you are not improving after 3 days, call your primary provider or come to the walk-in clinic.

Follow-up phone call in 4 days →
- Worse → Offer appointment in 1–2 days
- No better → Offer appointment in 2–3 days
- Improved

MVA = motor vehicle accident
UTI = urinary tract infection
HIV = human immunodeficiency virus
NSAIDs = nonsteroidal antiinflammatory drugs
ASA = acetylsalicylic acid

Hip and Knee Injuries

ROBERT W. JACKSON ■ SANDER KOËTER

Sports usually involve the younger, more physically active people of society. However, we are also witnessing a trend toward a healthier, stronger, and more physical population that, in spite of advancing age, tends to participate in sporting activities throughout a longer period of their lifetime. As a result, we are seeing an increasing number of sport injuries in the older age-group.

There are two basic types of sports injuries. The first type is due to a significant single episode of trauma, producing disruption of soft tissues or bony structures, and the second is due to repetitive minor traumatic insults that can cumulatively produce damage that eventually requires treatment. The former is more common in contact sports. The latter, which might also be grouped as *overuse injuries,* tend to be caused by minor biomechanical imbalances. For example, muscle imbalance between the agonist and antagonist muscles has been reported in tennis players, water polo players, pitchers, and runners, and a slightly malaligned varus or valgus knee usually shows signs of degeneration by the fifth decade of life.[1]

A swift return to sports is vital for the true athlete because physical inactivity reduces functional capacity. This is due not only to changes in muscle function but also to cardiorespiratory changes or loss of conditioning.

The clinical decisions physicians are faced with can best be approached in phases. Treatment options should be supported if possible by level 1 scientific evidence, but unfortunately many orthopaedic treatment options lack this evidence, and the treatment offered is based on experience or prior teaching. Moreover, any surgical treatment is very much operator dependent, and the results can be markedly influenced by the degree of skill possessed by the surgeon. Randomized trials are virtually nonexistent, and level 1 or even level 2 evidence is almost impossible to obtain. However, irrespective of the strength of evidence, any treatment must have a strong biologic basis.[2]

KNEE LIGAMENT INJURIES

Medial Collateral Ligament

In contact sports, the most commonly injured ligament is the medial collateral ligament. This can be either a sprain or a rupture, and it normally results from a blow to the outer aspect of the knee when the patient's weight is on that leg. For example, collateral ligament injuries are common in the contact sports of football and soccer but less common in ice hockey, where the sliding skate often allows the striking force to be dissipated. The presenting symptoms of medial collateral ligament injury are pain and often instability. A good history, outlining the details of the injury, is essential to analyze the severity of the injury. Details must be elicited, such as the direction of the injuring force, whether weight was being borne on the knee at impact, in what part of the knee were the initial symptoms felt, could the joint be moved immediately after the injury, could the patients stand or walk, was there a feeling of instability, and finally how rapidly did swelling occur. Slow swelling over 24 hours, for example, suggests an inflammatory response to a lesser injury, possibly extraarticular, whereas rapid swelling within 1 to 3 hours suggests a more serious injury with active bleeding inside the joint capsule due to rupture of a vascular structure, such as an anterior cruciate ligament tear or a peripheral tear of a meniscus.

Physical examination must include the application of a valgus stress to the knee, both in full extension and in slight flexion. When tested in full extension, the superficial fibers of the medial structures are tested for stability. In slight flexion the deep fibers of the medial collateral ligament are assessed. Laxity is compared with the opposite and uninjured knee and is usually graded I to III. A grade I lesion demonstrates slight opening of the medial joint line and is usually considered as a sprain of the ligament. Grade II is a moderate opening of 2 to 5 mm and represents a more severe sprain or partial tear. Grade III lesions are generally considered to be complete ruptures of the ligament. Local tenderness, either above or below the joint line, and swelling, due to either a hemarthrosis or a blood-stained synovial effusion, are also common findings after a few hours. It should be noted, however, that grade III lesions, which involve a significant rupture of the capsule as well as the medial ligament, may sometimes present with little or no swelling in the joint, since the hemorrhage and the inflammatory effusion can leak out through the torn capsule and track down in the soft tissues of the lower leg. Patients with grade III lesions can disguise the severity of the injury by walking into the office or the emergency room holding the knee stiff through strong quadriceps action. Although they have pain, paradoxically, it is usually not so severe as that of grades I and II lesions because the joint is decompressed when blood and synovial fluid leak out of the joint. Consequently the seriousness of the injury may be missed by the casual examiner. History and physical findings are, once again, two of the most important aspects of examination.

Stress x-rays are sometimes indicated, but a truly definitive evaluation involves an arthroscopic examination with the patient under anesthesia. With such an examination the true extent and severity of the medial ligament injury can be immediately established, and any other unsuspected pathology is revealed.

If the examiner is sure that he or she is dealing with an *isolated* sprain or rupture of the medial collateral ligament, no matter what the degree of laxity, most authors advocate nonoperative treatment with more than 85% good to excellent results.[3-5] However, if other signs of laxity are present, such as excessive anterior drawer or posterior drawer, it becomes a combined injury and is usually treated by the appropriate operative procedure.

Nonoperative treatment generally consists of a temporary period of immobilization using a posterior knee immobilizer or cast for relief of symptoms. This allows the patient to continue to be active, using crutches for balance and ambulation. Full weight bearing is allowed if the varus-valgus instability is controlled by the splint. Weight-bearing activity maintains some physiologic function in the limb, allowing the ankle and hip joints to continue to move, and permits the muscle action of the calf to serve as a venous pump. It also maintains some tone in those muscles. After an initial period of relative rest and protection (usually 7 to 10 days), early protected mobilization (EPM), avoiding valgus stress, is begun. This consists of active exercises for quadriceps, terminal resistance exercises, and hamstring exercises to enhance the earliest return to function. Because soft tissue healing time is approximately 3 to 4 weeks, at that point it is reasonable to allow the individual to go without external support. However, valgus angulation, rotation, and exposure to any extraneous forces should still be avoided at this stage. Return to activity at approximately 6 weeks, with protective bracing or strapping, may be considered.[6]

One should be sure, however, before embarking on a nonoperative course as outlined above that there are no associated intraarticular injuries, such as a meniscus rupture or chondral lesion. Therefore in the initial assessment of the injury, the treating surgeon may opt to do an examination with the patient under anesthesia, followed by an arthroscopic evaluation to identify and treat, in the initial stages, any meniscal tear or chondral loose body. One word of caution: if early arthroscopic evaluation of an injured knee is carried out, large amounts of irrigating fluid must be avoided, because a rent in the capsule can allow the fluid to escape into the calf, and if undetected, the escaping liters of saline can compromise the venous return of the limb.

Operative repair of the medial collateral ligament is infrequently indicated and is usually considered for the severe grade III lesions. Early protected mobilization and rehabilitation are once again essential after the initial healing phase is completed.[7]

Lateral Collateral Ligament

A similar treatment regimen for the injured lateral collateral ligament should be carried out. The lateral collateral ligament is injured with a varus strain and is not infrequently associated with a peroneal nerve injury. If the amount of varus stress applied to the knee is sufficient to rupture the collateral ligament, it is quite probable that the peroneal nerve has also been placed under considerable stretch.[8] The classic finding of a nerve lesion is inability to dorsiflex the foot or great toe along with numbness of the lateral aspect of the lower leg and foot. Usually this is a neurapraxia and recovers with time. Also be aware that the posterolateral corner and the posterior cruciate ligament are frequently injured with a varus type of stress.

To rule out or to establish a posterior cruciate injury or damage to the posterolateral corner of the joint, two physical tests are extremely important: (1) a greater than 2+ anterior drawer sign with a tibia in internal rotation and (2) a positive varus stress with the knee in full extension. Both these indicate a degree of posterior cruciate ligament insufficiency or rupture of the posterolateral ligament complex. If the knee demonstrates a positive adduction stress test in full extension, without concomitant rotation of the tibia, it is probably an isolated lateral collateral ligament injury.

After full evaluation of the situation, an isolated lateral collateral lesion is probably best treated by nonoperative measures. If there is associated posterolateral damage, however, it is generally agreed that operative repair of the posterolateral corner of the joint will produce a better end result.[9]

Anterior Cruciate Ligament

Anterior cruciate ligament injuries have been the focus of much orthopaedic attention over the past few years. It is now generally recognized that anterior cruciate ligaments can be torn by endogenous as well as exogenous forces. Exogenous forces, such as those that produce the classic O'Donoghue triad (anterior cruciate ligament plus medial cruciate ligament plus medial meniscal tears), are common in contact sports. Endogenous or self-inflicted forces occur when an athlete who is running hard decelerates to change direction or to stop suddenly, or alternatively, a skier who is falling backward tries to regain his or her balance through sudden quadriceps contraction.[10] In these situations there is a strong contraction of the quadriceps and the tibia is pulled forward (or conversely, the femur is pushed backward) by the contracting extensor mechanism to such an extent that the major restraining ligament, the anterior cruciate, can be ruptured in isolation. This can be either a partial tear, meaning a few fibers are torn (usually the posterolateral component), or a total tear, meaning the entire ligament is ripped from its origin on the femur or is torn in the midsubstance of the ligament. The common history is one where the athlete experiences a "pop" in the knee associated with pain. Rapid swelling almost always occurs because of bleeding within the joint. If the tear is unrecognized, the symptoms subside within 2 or 3 weeks, associated with the resorption of blood from the joint, and the athlete soon regains a full range of motion. The untreated patient then goes back to sporting activities and finds that on attempting to stop, to change direction, or to land from a jump, the knee gives way, since it no longer has the restraint of the anterior cruciate ligament.

Physical examination should reveal the extent of the pathology, but sometimes this is difficult in the acute stage because of pain and hemarthrosis within the joint. However, in the chronic stages or even in the subacute phase, both a positive Lachman test and a positive anterior drawer test should be identified. When there is a complete ligament rupture, the pivot shift test is always positive, as are the drawer and Lachman tests. In the case of a partial posterolateral band rupture, the pivot shift test is positive and the Lachman test is positive. However, because the anteromedial band is still intact, it will become taut in flexion and consequently produce a negative drawer test.[11] The examiner should be aware that a positive Lachman test always suggests either a partial or complete tear of the anterior cruciate ligament and is therefore the most sensitive test.

Associated injuries often include a torn meniscus or articular cartilage damage. Retrospective studies have shown that the untreated anterior cruciate is associated with a steadily increasing incidence of meniscal lesions and articular cartilage pathology over subsequent years. It is also believed that an untreated anterior cruciate ligament rupture will eventually lead to arthritic change in the joint. It has been shown by kinematic studies that even during the simple activity of walking, the cruciate-deficient knee translates 4 to 8 mm forward with each step during the unweighted swing phase of gait. At heel strike, the knee locks back into a normal gait pattern.[12] This slipping or sliding action, plus the occasional acute episode of giving way, can cause serious disruption of normal knee joint function and lead to posttraumatic arthritis some 10 to 30 years later.

There are virtually no reliable, accurate, prospective long-term natural history studies of diagnosed, but untreated, anterior cruciate ligament tears. In our experience, however, an arthroscopic diagnosis of anterior cruciate ligament damage was made in 65 patients from 1965 to 1972, and no treatment was offered for the torn anterior cruciate ligament. In fact, there was no reasonable alternative or operative treatment available at that time.[13] These patients were observed 6 years later, and somewhat surprisingly, those who had *isolated* lesions had been able to cope fairly well in terms of long-term function. However, those patients with *associated* injuries, such as a torn capsule or torn meniscus, had fared poorly. Those in both groups who gave up sports tended to do reasonably well. However, all those with combined lesions reported severe instabilities that affected the activities of daily living and had experienced several subsequent operations to treat additional tears of menisci or to attempt stabilization.

Now, with greater awareness and with the easy availability of magnetic resonance imaging (MRI), the diagnosis of a torn anterior cruciate ligament is made more frequently.

Increased awareness and better diagnosis have led to the present trend toward early operative intervention in the treatment of most anterior cruciate ligament lesions. The rationale for surgery is twofold: (1) to prevent further destruction of the joint and (2) to allow continued and safe participation in recreational and sporting activities. The advent of arthroscopy and the increased awareness of physicians that even endogenous forces can produce a rupture of the cruciate have facilitated this marked increase in the number of cases being treated by surgical means.

Arthroscopic-assisted anterior cruciate ligament reconstruction has become the standard of care. One of the most common techniques used to replace the ruptured anterior cruciate involves using a portion of patellar tendon, with a bone plug at each end, taken from the patella and the tibial tuberosity. The bone plugs are anchored in suitably created tunnels in the femur and the tibia, which creates an isometric replacement for the anterior cruciate ligament. An alternative technique uses semitendinosis tendon, usually folded double, or even quadrupled to increase the initial strength, and also anchored in bony tunnels. Other replacement materials include quadriceps tendon and allografts, either fresh or frozen, from cadavers. All these replacement tissues seem to produce reasonable results, and no matter what technique is used, the best results are virtually normal knees after an 8- to 12-month period of bony consolidation and revascularization of the grafted material.

A brief flirtation with synthetic ligaments was halted in the United States because of secondary problems due to the materials and their methods of implantation. However, this area of treatment should probably be reexplored. In this era of biomaterials research, an appropriately strong and biologically inert synthetic ligament should be eventually identified, and methods of insertion and fixation should be developed to allow an easier repair of the damaged anterior cruciate. Thus stability could be achieved without sacrifice of normal anatomical structures and without exposing the patient to the potential dangers of allograft material.

A major advance in the treatment of anterior cruciate ligaments has been in the rehabilitation of these injuries.[14] Surgical treatment is now commonly performed approximately 3 weeks following injury, which allows the patient to regain motion and some quadriceps strength and function before he or she is subjected to further trauma through surgery. Early postoperative mobilization is also necessary to avoid arthrofibrosis and to avoid further wasting of the quadriceps muscle bulk.[15]

Rehabilitation is generally conducted in three phases. Phase I, the healing phase, allows fixation of the reconstructed cruciate ligament through healing in the bone tunnels. Phase II concentrates on mobilization of the joint and strengthening of the adjacent musculature. Phase III involves the return to normal activity with protective bracing and appropriate education of the patient so that he or she avoids sudden stops or landings on the previously damaged limb, plus regaining musculature strength, increasing reaction time, and developing endurance. Full rehabilitation normally takes a minimum of 6 months. Full revascularization of the reconstructed ligament probably takes 1 year or more to be achieved.[16] The surgically treated anterior cruciate ligament with appropriate rehabilitation, barring complications, should lead to a virtually normal knee 1 year following the injury.

Complications, however, can and do occur.[17] Ligaments may loosen or tear. The surgery may be incorrectly performed, resulting in a nonisometric placement of the reconstruction, thus limiting range of motion and creating secondary problems. Arthrofibrosis or scarring within the joint may also limit range of motion. Problems may occur from the donor sites of the patellar tendon, such as patella tendonitis, rupture of the patella tendon, or fracture of the patella, and finally, a too early return to function may result in a repeat rupture of the reconstructed ligament. All these problems can be managed but usually require further surgical treatment.

On the basis of the evidence to date therefore, surgical reconstruction of the torn anterior cruciate ligament is the recommended treatment at a *grade C level*.

Posterior Cruciate Ligament

Injury to the posterior cruciate ligament occurs much less frequently than injury to the anterior cruciate ligament and comprises approximately 3% of all knee ligament injuries.[18] A severe hyperextension injury of the knee or a blow to the anterior aspect of the bent knee, causing forced posterior translation of the tibia on the femur, is the common reason. The latter mechanism can occur when a hockey player, sliding on ice, strikes a rigid goal post at the tibial tuberosity level. A similar injury can occur by falling on the bent knee with the foot plantar flexed, allowing direct ground contact on the tibial tuberosity. A direct blow to the front of the extended knee, such as a football block or tackle, can cause a hyperextension rupture of the posterior cruciate ligament and the posterior capsule.

Physical examination will show a posterior drawer sign or posterior sag of the tibia on the femur. If the posterior translation is subtle, it can often be appreciated by the examiner by running the finger or thumb down the medial side of the joint. Normally, one encounters the edge of the tibial plateau. If the tibia is subluxed posteriorly there is no plateau edge to be felt. A heightened awareness because of the history of the injury can also help the examiner to determine whether the anteroposterior laxity is due to a posterior translation or an anterior translation. Also, if anteroposterior instability (Lachman test) is present and one cannot determine whether or not this is due to anterior or posterior cruciate instability, the examiner should test for the pivot shift. If the pivot shift test is negative, then it is definitely a posterior cruciate ligament injury—because an intact anterior cruciate ligament will prevent a pivot shift. The use of MRI is also helpful in establishing the correct diagnosis, since the posterior cruciate ligament is usually well demarcated.

Posterior cruciate ligament lesions can be usefully classified into three types: (1) complete ruptures with or without avulsion of the bony insertion at the back of the tibia; (2) partial, isolated rupture of some fibers or bands of the posterior cruciate ligament; and (3) major posterior dislocations of the knee associated with multiple other injuries to the joint, such as meniscal tears or posterolateral complex disruption. Like the anterior cruciate ligament, the natural history of the untreated posterior cruciate ligament injury has not been well defined by any prospective study. Many authors[19,20] feel that this lesion does not usually lead to significant further problems within the joint. Others have shown that further problems can occur with wear on the patella and in the medial compartment of the joint.[21]

The isolated posterior cruciate ligament lesion, whether partial or complete, is usually treated nonoperatively,[20] although arthroscopic techniques in recent years have been developed to allow for the early reconstruction of the complete rupture of the posterior cruciate.[18]

Nonoperative treatment generally consists of relative rest and temporary immobilization to allow soft tissue healing to occur. The knee is usually immobilized in a comfortable degree of flexion (45 to 50 degrees) to avoid distraction of the capsule and soft tissues at the back of the joint. However, early rehabilitation must be done to avoid a subsequent flexion contracture due to healing in the flexed position. Somewhere between the second and third weeks the knee should be actively extended to the fully straight position.

Because the quadriceps mechanism and the posterior cruciate work together to stabilize the knee, one common sequela of posterior cruciate ligament rupture is chondromalacia of the patella. This is believed to be the result of the quadriceps working extra hard to stabilize the joint, thus creating increased pressure on the patellofemoral compartment. Medial compartment degenerative arthritis is also commonly seen because of the frequently associated posterolateral rotary instability from the stretched posterolateral capsular and ligamentous structures. This allows for a rotational movement to occur around the medial compartment, leading to tibial plateau damage and often associated changes on the femoral condyle.

Decision making regarding treatment must be based on both the extent of the pathology and the wishes of the patient.[22] The young patient may be more anxious to continue in sporting activities than the middle-aged patient and may therefore warrant a more aggressive approach to treatment. It is our experience that there is no really good functional brace that would assist the patient with an unstable posterior cruciate lesion to participate further in sports.

MENISCAL LESIONS

The torn meniscus is a common knee injury in sport. With the advent of arthroscopy, diagnosis and treatment of this pathology have become much more sophisticated.[23] The site and the type of tear should be diagnosed before any decision regarding treatment. Lesions that are in the outer third of the meniscus, especially in the younger age-group, have the potential to heal if stabilized.[24] It is important therefore to consider repair of a damaged meniscus if the lesion is in the "red," or vascular, area of the meniscus. This can be done with sutures (passing them from inside out or from outside in) or by various darts, arrows, or staples that hold the mobile inner fragment back to the periphery and its anatomical position. Lesions in the inner two thirds of the meniscus are considered to be in the avascular, or "white," region of the meniscus. With no significant blood supply, these tend not to heal and are generally excised under arthroscopic control. In the future, some of these lesions may be preserved by new techniques involving photodynamic welding of collagenous tissues.[25]

Physical examination may reveal a popping or catching sensation (ie, the classic McMurray test), local joint line tenderness, swelling, and a decreased range of motion. MRI may be helpful in questionable cases. However, the diagnosis can always be confirmed by arthroscopy, and at the same time, appropriate treatment can be established. Small lesions are usually resected. Larger lesions may be sutured if there is a possible opportunity for them to heal. Statistics over the years have shown that a total meniscectomy, or removal of the entire meniscus, almost invariably leads to osteoarthritic change within 10 to 15 years. Retention of the meniscal rim and removal of only the mobile inner fragment of meniscus have markedly changed that statistic.[26] Although partial meniscectomy may also lead to degenerative problems in the future,[27] the appropriate treatment at this time is to remove any unstable meniscal fragments that do not have the opportunity to heal. In the older age-group, we are beginning to see more degenerative meniscal tears involving the posterior horn of the meniscus. Again, resection is the treatment of choice.[28] Early rehabilitation involves range-of-motion exercises, strengthening exercises for quadriceps and hamstring, and exercises designed to steadily increase the endurance and reaction time of the musculature.[29,30]

CHONDRAL LESIONS

Blunt trauma or shear forces of significant magnitude can produce partial- or full-thickness lesions of the articular cartilage of a knee joint. Many studies in the past have shown that partial-thickness lesions never heal. However, full-thickness lesions that expose the underlying subchondral bone do have the propensity to heal with a fibrocartilaginous response. One classification described four types of traumatic lesions[31]:

- Type I: a linear split in the articular surface believed to be due to shear stress
- Type II: a stellate type of fracture, usually partial thickness, thought to be due to a direct contact of significant force in a focal area
- Type III: a flap of articular cartilage probably produced by a combination of shear and direct contact forces
- Type IV: a full-thickness "divot" or loss of articular cartilage also due to combinations of shear and contact forces with the resultant exposure of subchondral bone

There is no available treatment for types I and II. Type III lesions can be helped by excision of the flap at arthroscopic surgery, thus preventing the further propagation or separation of the cartilage from the underlying bone surface. Type IV lesions are generally treated by efforts to replace the cartilage by grafting or to stimulate the repair by fibrocartilage. The use of osteochondral plugs grafted from a non-weight-bearing area of the joint to the defect area is currently popular.[32] The implantation of cultured chondrocytes beneath a retaining periosteal patch is also a source of much research.[33] Most of these repair efforts are still in the experimental stage, but scientific data are being gathered to document an improvement in eventual function following such treatment.[34]

Osteochondritis Dissecans

Osteochondritis dissecans is usually seen in juvenile patients and may be due to trauma, or in the youngest patients it may be an ossification defect. Treatment, if the fragment is separating from the underlying femoral condyle, is directed toward stabilizing the fragment and improving the blood supply from the condyle to the fragment by drilling the area. In some instances removal and grafting of the involved area are necessary.[35]

Posttraumatic Degenerative Arthritis

Posttraumatic degenerative arthritis in the senior or mature athlete is seen as fibrillated articular cartilage surfaces and is often accompanied by a complex tear of the meniscus. Evidence has been gathered to support a treatment plan that involves the judicious excision of the damaged meniscus and the shaving or irrigation of the fibrillated articular cartilage surfaces at arthroscopy. This type of treatment can produce a temporary symptomatic improvement that may last months or years but does not return the knee to its preinjury status.[36]

In the very late stages, when all the damaged cartilage is worn away, eburnated bone surfaces are seen, and a varus or valgus deformity is present, which creates an increasing biomechanical imbalance. In severe cases, surgical restoration of the alignment is the only treatment option and is achieved by osteotomy, unicompartmental arthroplasty, or total joint arthroplasty.[37]

SOFT TISSUE INJURIES

Although often considered minor injuries, muscular strains and sprains are the leading cause of time lost from athletics as a result of injury. Trainers, coaches, and physicians other than orthopaedic surgeons are usually called on to manage these injuries and therefore need to be aware of proper methods of diagnosis and treatment.[38]

Hamstring Injuries

Injuries to the hamstring muscles are often slow to heal, and reinjury often occurs following a too early return to activity. It is probable that many recurrent injuries to the hamstring musculotendinous unit are the result of inadequate rehabilitation following the initial injury. The severity of hamstring injuries is usually of first or second degree, but occasionally third-degree injuries (complete rupture of the musculotendinous unit) do occur. Most hamstring strain injuries are produced by sudden acceleration while running or sprinting. Etiologic factors include poor flexibility, inadequate muscle strength or muscle endurance, dyssynergic muscle contraction during running, insufficient warm-up and stretching before exercise, awkward running style, and as mentioned, a too early return to activity before rehabilitation is complete. Treatment for hamstring injuries includes rest and immobilization immediately following injury and then a gradually increasing program of mobilization, stretching, strengthening, and activity. Permission to return to athletic competition should be withheld until full rehabilitation has been achieved, which usually means a complete return of muscle strength, endurance, and flexibility, in addition to a return of coordination and athletic agility. The athlete who tries to play himself or herself back into condition is asking for trouble. Failure to achieve full rehabilitation will only predispose the athlete to recurrent injury.[39] Proximal hamstring sprain, which can cause chronic pain over the area of the ischial tuberosity with radiation down the thigh, may benefit from surgical division of hamstring insertion at the ischial tuberosity.[40]

Tendinitis

Tendinitis is a frequent affliction of the patellar tendon or the quadriceps tendon at their respective insertions on the distal and proximal poles of the patella. Patellar tendinitis is more common in young athletes who engage in jumping sports, such as basketball or volleyball, and has been called "jumper's knee." The less common quadriceps tendinitis is usually found in athletes in their forties. Careful clinical examination reveals sharp localized pain and tenderness at the insertion points of the affected tendon, with an increase in pain produced by any activities that load the extensor mechanism. Thickening of the tendon and hyperechoic zones corresponding to fibrous scar and intratendinous calcification have been detected by ultrasonography.[41] MRI, however, is now the investigation of choice in doubtful cases, providing excellent topographic anatomy of the lesion in both the coronal and sagittal planes. Increased signal intensity in the substance of the tendon is seen along with an increased thickness of the tendon.[42]

Conservative management of tendinitis includes eccentric exercises, imposing increasing stresses on the patellar tendon in order to gradually increase its strength, combined with stretching to increase the length of the muscle-tendon

unit.[43] Surgical treatment may sometimes be necessary when conservative regimens have failed.[44] Some authors advocate surgical resection of the degenerative tissue in the tendon and drilling or excising the lower pole of the patella. Others believe impingement by the lower pole of the patella on underlying soft tissues is the causative factor in development of patellar tendinitis, and satisfactory results have been reported with arthroscopic resection of the lower pole of the patella, with no attempt at dissection of the granuloma in the tendon itself.[45] Return to sports is allowed 3 to 4 months after open surgery and earlier following arthroscopic procedure.

Chronic muscle and tendon injuries to the groin are common sports injuries. Adductor longus tendinitis and rectus femoris tendinitis by far are the most common causes of groin pain, although prostatitis and hernias should be considered in the differential diagnosis. The recommended treatment is a well-planned and gradually increased rehabilitation program during the initial stages. Surgery, for example, tenotomy of the adductor longus, has given satisfactory results in many athletes when nonsurgical treatment has failed.[46]

Bursitis

Bursitis most commonly affects the prepatellar bursae in the athletic population, particularly those sustaining a direct injury to the kneecap, as might occur during the take down maneuver in wrestling.[47] Semimembranosus-tibial collateral (SMTCL) bursitis can clinically mimic an internal derangement of the knee, typically causing pain more superior and posterior to that of the fairly common pes anserinus bursitis. MRI is useful in diagnosing SMTCL bursitis and avoiding unnecessary knee arthroscopy.[48] Treatment with rest, ice, elevation, and anti-inflammatory medication usually relieves the symptoms. However, some chronic cases require surgical excision if the chronically inflamed bursa tends to recur.

Peripatellar Pain

Peripatellar pain can occur without anatomic malalignment, history of trauma, patellar instability, or clinical evidence of patellofemoral crepitus. Frequently, the patient's pain occurs when sitting for prolonged periods of time with the knee flexed, such as when watching a sporting event. These individuals may demonstrate lateral retinacular and iliotibial band tightness. This condition, termed *patellofemoral syndrome* or *anterior knee pain syndrome,* is usually treated conservatively, with 60% to 80% satisfactory results. An exercise program performed twice daily should include iliotibial band stretching, hamstring stretching, gastrocnemius stretching, progressive resistance straight leg raising, and hip adduction strengthening.[49]

Chondromalacia Patellae

Chondromalacia of the patella should be a term reserved for the true pathologic entity of breakdown of the articular surface of the patella. Although many etiologic factors have been identified with chondromalacia patellae, those that are related to sporting injuries can usually be classified in one of three categories: (1) direct trauma, (2) recurrent subluxation, and (3) traumatic dislocation.[50]

The first category is seen in athletes who sustain direct trauma to the anterior aspect of the knee. These individuals usually have a normally aligned extensor mechanism. Direct trauma, such as smashing into the boards in hockey, can damage the articular cartilage and cause breakdown, fibrillation, fragmentation, and eventually eburnation in its end stages.[51,52]

The second group are those with slightly malaligned extensor mechanisms, as evidenced by a high Q angle or a congenital bony abnormality in terms of shape of the patella or the trochlea of the femur. In this group, repetitive motions, such as running and jumping, cause the patella to sublux to the lateral side with every extensor movement. With time, this repetitive and cumulative injury to the articular cartilage causes breakdown and the resultant symptoms of anterior knee pain due to chondromalacia patellae.[53]

The third category, that of traumatic dislocation, can occur in either the aligned or the malaligned extensor mechanism and usually results from an external force being applied to the knee. In the dislocating process, the articular cartilage is severely damaged and subsequently goes on to chondromalacia.

Chondromalacia patellae is diagnosed primarily from the history with supportive evidence being gained by physical examination, showing either the malaligned extensor mechanism or pain on compression of the patella and on direct palpation of the inferior surface of the patella.[54] X-rays of the knee should always include a tangential view of the patellofemoral articulation, showing the relationship between the patella and the underlying trochlea. It is postulated that the anterior knee pain that the individual experiences comes from the transmission of force directly to the subchondral cancellous bone of the patella, as the contact forces are no longer buffered or neutralized by the damaged articular cartilage. The subchondral bone, which previously was protected from such forces, develops stress fractures in many of the cancellous trabeculae. The stress fractures eventually heal, which is evidenced by progressive thickening of the subchondral bone on x-ray examination. Eventually the patella is able to withstand the compressive stresses of extending the knee as in running and jumping, and thus the symptoms finally abate. In most instances, therefore, nonsurgical management is advised. However, if a 6-month supervised course of nonsurgical management that includes relative rest, aspirin or other nonsteroidal anti-inflammatories (to minimize symptoms), and stretching and strengthening exercises for the extensor mechanism fails to relieve the symptoms, one should consider some form of surgical treatment.

In the direct trauma group, arthroscopic surgery performing an excisional debridement of the fragmenting articular cartilage area has been proven to be quite effective. If the patient has a degree of extensor malalignment, arthroscopic surgical debridement of the patella plus a lateral release to allow a change in the alignment of the patella in the trochlea, thus centralizing and normalizing the extensor mechanism, is usually effective.[55] In dislocations the primary treatment is usually nonoperative, but should recurrent dislocations occur, a reefing of the medial structures and sometimes a distal patella tendon realignment can be helpful in stabilizing and minimizing symptoms.

Other procedures, such as a Maquet elevation of the tibial tubercle or a patella osteotomy, lack sufficient scientific evidence to warrant recommendation. Patellectomy might be considered for the end-stage situation where other procedures have failed to relieve symptoms.[56]

Epiphyseal Injuries

In the young athlete the epiphyses of the lower femur and upper tibia may be damaged by macrotrauma. An epiphyseal dislocation must be reduced early, or a severe growth deformity will result. A fracture dislocation, with the fracture going through the articular surface to the epiphyses and displacing only a portion of the articular surface, is even more damaging for the future. It must be anatomically reduced to prevent a growth disturbance of one part of the epiphyseal plate in which a significant malalignment develops as growth occurs. These injuries invariably require surgical treatment.[57]

KNEE BRACING

Prophylactic Knee Bracing

Controversy exists in the literature regarding the efficacy of prophylactic knee bracing in athletes. Although some papers suggest that inappropriately applied braces can increase the incidence of knee injuries, others have shown that bracing can dramatically reduce the incidence of medial collateral ligament injuries. In our experience, gained from association with a professional football team, the advent of protective braces on interior linemen and linebackers reduced not only the incidence of medial collateral ligament injuries but also the severity of the injuries over a study period that lasted more than 12 years. The incidence of anterior cruciate ligament injuries and meniscal injuries was not significantly affected by the application of the knee brace.[6]

Therapeutic Bracing

During the early stages following collateral ligament injury or repair, protective bracing is of value. Either rigid or hinged braces can be used. If hinged braces are employed, they allow flexion movements but avoid varus or valgus stress. These have value for a relatively short period of time (2 to 3 weeks) during the initial healing phase. Lightweight hinged knee braces for treatment of anterior cruciate ligament injuries have become common, but there is little proof of their efficacy. It has been suggested that such braces provide proprioceptive sensations to the athlete, enabling him or her to subconsciously minimize stress on the knee. Other surgeons feel that blocking the knee at 15 to 20 degrees of flexion allows the athlete's hamstring mechanism to engage early and thus protect the knee from anterior subluxation under stress. Many authors are now advocating the use of braces for a relatively short time to allow the healing of bony tunnels and the revascularization and maturation of the transplanted anterior cruciate ligament grafts. Some authors are advocating no bracing whatsoever and stressing the rehabilitation of the musculature in the postoperative phase. Return to activity is based entirely on the severity of the injury and the type of injury. An athlete with a medial collateral ligament sprain or strain can usually return to competitive sports with protective bracing at the 6- to 8-week mark. Most authors hold back anterior cruciate ligament reconstructions for 6 to 8 months, many for 1 year.

THE AGING ATHLETE

The older athlete presents with a problem that is either a result of an injury sustained in the past that eventually has produced the symptoms of an arthritic knee or a new injury that by chance is often associated with an arthritic knee. In the past, surgical treatment of these athletes was avoided, because any open surgical procedure would commonly incapacitate the individual and perhaps make the symptoms worse. However, with the advent of arthroscopic surgery, many of these athletes can be helped with arthroscopic lavage and debridement.[58] This irrigation process is recommended based on grade B evidence.

In more advanced situations a realignment osteotomy through the upper tibia or lower femur can help to transfer weight-bearing stresses from the affected side of the joint to a relatively normal compartment. Although osteotomy carries with it a moderate morbidity and a fairly lengthy rehabilitation process, the change in alignment can benefit appropriately chosen cases and can provide pain-free function for many years.

In the most severe cases, where there is loss of articular cartilage in both compartments, a replacement arthroplasty is generally advised.[59] Older athletes who undergo replacement arthroplasty should avoid contact sports and activities that involve severe or repetitive impact loads on the knee. For example, jogging on hard surfaces, basketball, and volleyball should be avoided. Nonimpact aerobics, treadmill jogging, cycling, swimming, and doubles tennis are more reasonable activities.

HIP INJURIES

Athletic injuries to the hip region may involve the skeleton as well as the surrounding soft tissues. Bony injuries include avulsion fractures, stress fractures, and dislocations. Soft tissue injuries involve strains or sprains and tendinitis.

The anatomical architecture of the hip joint, a bony ball and socket arrangement covered by strong muscles, is not nearly as prone to injury from sporting activities as is the knee joint. However, several lesions, particularly in the younger age-group, must be correctly identified and treated to avoid serious gait abnormalities in later life. Fractures are relatively rare in the athletic age-group, but in the young adolescent before epiphyseal closure, a slipped upper femoral epiphysis is a fairly common problem. Stress fractures can also occur in endurance athletes. Traumatic dislocation of the hip is unusual but does occur in contact sports, such as football.

Slipped Upper Femoral Epiphysis

This problem is commonly seen in young boys who are growing rapidly and in whom the upper femoral epiphysis has not yet fused. The onset of symptoms may be gradual or sudden and often manifests itself by referred pain to the knee and a limp when the adolescent is walking. It is most important to think of a slipped epiphysis when knee pain is the presenting sign in an adolescent. Physical examination will demonstrate a short leg held in external rotation and abduction at the hip. X-rays in two planes should show, to some extent, the femoral epiphysis displaced posteriorly on the neck of the femur. In severe cases a positive Trendelenburg sign is noted. Minor degrees of slip can often be treated by stabilization in situ. Major slips should be identified early, reduced by manipulation, and stabilized with a pin and plate or several transfixing pins.[60] Protected weight bearing is advis-

able for several months until the possible complication of aseptic necrosis can be determined. Return to sport must be restricted until epiphyseal fusion has occurred.

Hip Dislocation

Dislocations of the hip are true orthopedic emergencies. During the time the hip is dislocated, both the blood supply to the femoral head and the adjacent sciatic nerve are compromised. Prompt reduction, within hours, is therefore critical to reduce the risk of permanent pathologic changes. Damage to the articular cartilage, the joint capsule, the supporting ligaments, and denervation or vascular occlusion may lead to traumatic arthritis or avascular necrosis. Dislocations of the hip occur only after excessive trauma and are therefore seen in sports such as football, soccer, and skiing. Posterior dislocations make up the majority of traumatic dislocations, with anterior dislocations accounting for only 8% to 15% of the total number.[61] In posterior dislocations, the femoral head lies posterior to the acetabulum and the patient presents with the lower limb held in flexion and internal rotation. In anterior dislocations, the femoral head lies anterior to the acetabulum, and the patient presents with a typical attitude of abduction and external rotation of the lower extremity. With sports injuries, dislocations are usually not associated with a fracture, and most dislocations can be treated by closed reduction. Before closed reduction is attempted, however, preoperative x-rays should be made to identify the exact extent of the bony trauma. Open reduction of acute dislocations is only indicated when a stable, concentric reduction cannot be achieved by a gentle manipulation with the patient under general anesthesia. An open reduction is frequently indicated when circulatory or neurologic impairment persists following reduction or if interposed soft tissue or osteochondral fragments make a closed reduction impossible. Forceful manipulation under these circumstances might result in further fractures or additional articular trauma. After a closed reduction, the patient can safely start an early mobilization program. Partial weight bearing can start a few days after reduction, and patients can usually be fully weight bearing at 3 months.[62]

Stress Fractures

The key to a more rapid recovery from a femoral neck stress fracture is an early diagnosis, with the primary goal of treatment being to avoid possible associated complications, including avascular necrosis, nonunion, and varus deformity.[63] Unfortunately, it is not uncommon today for an athlete to develop a stress fracture, given the intensity of training associated with some sports.

Stress fractures are the culmination of numerous microfractures that occur at major points of stress. They represent the body's inability to repair the damage done by cumulative and repetitive stresses applied to the bone. The etiology of stress fractures is multifactorial, but in each instance, breakdown is occurring faster than repair. Factors implicated with stress fractures are nutritional status, menstrual status, and most importantly, sudden changes in the level of activity.[64] Therefore a detailed clinical history specifically addressing these factors should raise a high susceptibility for femoral neck stress fractures.

Usually, but not always, the patient presents with pain localized in either the groin area, the anterior thigh, or the knee. This pain exaggerates with activity and exertion. The onset of symptoms is gradual over a 3- to 5-week period. On physical examination there is often a localized tenderness. A painful range of motion with limited hip movements usually exists, and internal rotation of the hip is severely affected. If the history and physical findings suggest a femoral neck stress fracture it should be considered until proven otherwise.

Laboratory tests are generally normal for metabolic and blood count parameters.[65] Distinct findings on conventional radiographs only appear 2 to 4 weeks following the onset of symptoms.[66] If positive findings on conventional x-rays are seen, they are very specific to the diagnosis of stress fractures. Triple-phase 99M technetium bone scans are highly sensitive but unfortunately not very specific. However, bone scans may demonstrate bony changes and possible pathology as early as 48 to 72 hours after the onset of symptoms. MRI has recently been shown to be superior to bone scans in providing an early and accurate diagnosis of stress fractures in young endurance athletes.[67]

Classification of stress fractures is based on the site of the fracture and the degree of fracture displacement, if present. Femoral neck stress fractures are divided into three categories: tension side, compression side, and displaced fractures.[63] The first two categories, both undisplaced femoral neck stress fractures, can be treated with rest. Biomechanically, compression side fractures have a lower risk of displacement than tension side fractures. Treatment consists of bed rest until the patient is pain free. Frequent radiographs need to be obtained, and particular attention should be paid to any signs of widening of the fracture line or displacement of the femoral head. Once a patient is free of pain at rest, he or she can advance from partial to full weight bearing on crutches, to a cane, and then to walking without support, with walking distance gradually increased. The athlete must continue cardiovascular fitness programs to prevent detraining effects.[68] There is no evidence that medication will speed up the rehabilitation process; however, nonsteroidal anti-inflammatories or ice and massage can be implemented for pain relief.

The third category, displaced fractures, are an orthopaedic emergency and must be internally stabilized as soon as possible. As with the undisplaced fractures, the patient is kept in bed until a pain-free range of motion is present, with non-weight-bearing for 6 weeks and progressive weight bearing over the next 6 weeks.

Once again, these suggested treatment protocols are based on *level 3 to level 5* studies, with *grade C recommendations*.

Sprains, Strains, and Bursitis

Sprains, strains, and bursitis around the hip joint are managed as described for injuries of the knee joint. Rest, analgesics, or anti-inflammatories are used as necessary to control symptoms. The return to sport should be postponed until the individual is totally asymptomatic, since the incidence of reinjury is significant if an athlete returns to his or her sport too soon. Return to function also involves appropriate stretching and strengthening exercises.

SUMMARY

Many injuries that affect the hip and knee in athletes are catastrophic and require surgical intervention. For these injuries the treatment is strongly dependent on the experience of the operating surgeon. The surgeon who has had success with one particular operative technique is usually not willing to randomize his or her surgical treatment since the urgency of the situation dictates that there is only one opportunity to obtain the best possible result. Consequently, results of series are reported and compared with the results obtained by other surgeons. This places most of the evidence for treatment in the *level 4 or 5 category*, with *grade C recommendations*. Few of the treatment methods have level 2 evidence, which consists of randomized trials with significantly different responses in various subgroups of treatment. In essence, orthopedic surgery does not lend itself to the high level of scientific criteria demanded of nonsurgical treatment methods.

REFERENCES

1. Kibler WB, Chandler TJ, Stracener ES: Musculoskeletal adaptations and injuries due to overtraining. Exerc Sports Sci Rev 20:99–126, 1992
2. Banerjee SN: Nonsurgical treatment of acute low back pain. In Basmajian JV, Banerjee SN (eds): Clinical Decision Making in Rehabilitation. Churchill Livingstone, New York, 1996
3. Reider B, Sathy MR, Talkington J, et al: Treatment of isolated medial collateral ligament injuries in athletes with early functional rehabilitation. A five-year follow-up study. Am J Sports Med 22(4):470–477, 1993
4. Derscheid GL, Garrick JG: Medial collateral ligament injuries in football. Nonoperative management of grade I and grade II sprains. Am J Sports Med 9(6):365–368, 1981
5. Kannus P: Nonoperative treatment of Grade II and III sprains of the lateral ligament compartment of the knee. Am J Sports Med 17(1):83–88, 1989
6. Jackson RW, Reed SC, Dunbar F: An evaluation of knee injuries in a professional football team—risk factors, type of injuries, and the value of prophylactic knee bracing. Clin J Sport Med 1(1):1–7, 1991
7. Frolke JP, Oskam J, Vierhout PA: Primary reconstruction of the medial collateral ligament in combined injury of the medial collateral and anterior cruciate ligaments. Short-term results. Knee Surg Sports Traumatol Arthrosc 6(2):103–106, 1998
8. DeLee JC, Riley MB, Rockwood Jr CA: Acute straight lateral instability of the knee. Am J Sports Med 11(6):404–411, 1983
9. Veltri DM, Warren RF: Posterolateral instability of the knee. Instr Course Lect 44:441–453, 1995
10. Feagin JA: Principles of diagnosis and treatment. In Feagin JA (ed): The Crucial Ligaments, 2nd Ed. Churchill Livingstone, New York, 1994
11. Jackson RW, Campbell AJ: Diagnosis of partial ruptures of the anterior cruciate ligament (abstract). Orthop Trans 5:441, 1981
12. Marans HJ, Jackson RW, Glossop ND, Young C: Anterior cruciate ligament insufficiency: a dynamic three-dimensional motion analysis. Am J Sports Med 17(3):325–332, 1989
13. Jackson RW, Peters RI, Marczyk RL: Late results of untreated anterior cruciate ligament rupture (abstract). J Bone Joint Surg 62B:127, 1980
14. Shelbourne KD, Nitz P: Accelerated rehabilitation after anterior cruciate ligament reconstruction. Am J Sports Med 18(3):292, 1990
15. Noyes FR, Mangine RE, Barber S: Early knee motion after open and arthroscopic anterior cruciate ligament reconstruction. Am J Sports Med 15(2):149, 1987
16. Falconiero RP, Ditefano VJ, Cook TM: Revascularization and ligamentization of autogenous anterior cruciate ligament grafts in humans. Arthroscopy 14(20):197–205, 1998
17. Passler JM, Schippinger G, Schweighofer F, et al: Complications in 283 cruciate ligament replacement operations with free patellar tendon transplantation. Modification by surgical technique and surgery timing. Unfallchirurgie 21(5):240–246, 1995
18. Harner CD, Hoher J: Evaluation and treatment of posterior cruciate ligament injuries. Am J Sports Med 26(3):471–482, 1998
19. Duri ZA, Aichroth PM, Zorrilla P: The posterior cruciate ligament: a review. Am J Knee Surg 10(3):149–164, 1997
20. Shino K, Horibe S, Nakata K, et al: Conservative treatment of isolated injuries to the posterior cruciate ligament in athletes. J Bone Joint Surg Br 77(6):895–900, 1995
21. Torg JS, Barton TM, Pavlov H, Stine R: Natural history of the posterior cruciate ligament-deficient knee. Clin Orthop 246:208–216, 1989
22. Fanelli GC, Giannotti BF, Edson CJ: The posterior cruciate ligament arthroscopic evaluation and treatment. J Arthroscopic Related Surg 106:673–688, 1994
23. Dandy DJ, Jackson RW: The impact of arthroscopy on the management of disorders of the knee. J Bone Joint Surg Br 57B(3):346–348, 1975
24. Cannon WD Jr, Morgan CD: Meniscal repair: arthroscopic repair techniques. Instr Course Lect 43:77–96, 1994
25. Judy MM, Jackson RW, Nosir HR, Matthews JL: Healing results in meniscus and articular cartilage

photochemically welded with 1,8-naphthalimide dyes. Lasers Surg Med Suppl 9(216):48–49, 1997

26. Northmore-Ball MD, Dandy DJ, Jackson RW: Arthroscopic, open partial, and total meniscectomy. A comparative study. J Bone Joint Surg Br 65B(4):400–404, 1983

27. Schimmer DC, Brillhart KB, Duff C, Glinz W: Arthroscopic partial meniscectomy: a 12 yr follow up and a two-step evaluation of the long term course. Arthroscopy 14(2):136–142, 1998

28. Jackson RW, Rouse DW: The results of partial arthroscopic meniscectomy in patients over 40 years of age. J Bone Joint Surg Br 64B(4):481–485, 1982

29. Wheatley WB, Krome J, Martin DF: Rehabilitation programmes following arthroscopic meniscectomy in athletes. Sports Med 21(6):447–456, 1996

30. Shelbourne KD, Patel DV, Adist WS, Porter DA: Rehabilitation after meniscal repair. Clin Sports Med 15(3): 595–612, 1996

31. Bauer M, Jackson RW: Chondral lesions of the femoral condyles: a system of arthroscopic classification. Arthroscopy 4(2):97–102, 1988

32. Bobic V: Arthroscopic osteochondral autograft transplantation in anterior cruciate ligament reconstruction: a preliminary clinical study. Knee Surg Sports Traumatol Arthrosc 3(4):262–264, 1996

33. Peterson L: Articular cartilage injuries treated with autologous chondrocyte transplantation in the human knee. Acta Orthop Belg 62(S1):196–200, 1996

34. Minas T: Chondrocyte implantation in the repair of chondral lesions of the knee: economics and quality of life. Am J Orthop 27(11):739–744, 1998

35. Frederico DJ, Lynch JK, Jokl P: Osteochondritis dissecans of the knee: a historical review of etiology and treatment. Arthroscopy 6(3):190–197, 1990

36. Jackson RW: Arthroscopic treatment of degenerative arthritis. In McGinty JB, Caspar RB, Jackson RW, Poehling GC (eds): Operative Arthroscopy. Lippincott-Raven, Philadelphia, 1996, pp 405–409

37. Osteoarthritis of the knee. Special focus section. J Knee Surg 3(1):55–63, 1998

38. Garrett WE Jr: Strains and sprains in athletes. Am J Sports Med 26(6S):2–8, 1996

39. Agre JC: 33 Hamstring injuries. Proposed aetiological factors, prevention, and treatment. Sports Med 2(1):21, 1985

40. Puranen J, Orava S: The hamstring syndrome—a new gluteal sciatic. Ann Chir Gynaecol 80(2):212–214, 1991

41. Fritschy D, de Gautard R: Jumper's knee and ultrasonography. Am J Sports Med 16(6):637–640, 1988

42. Johnson DP, Wakeley CJ, Watt I: Magnetic resonance imaging of patellar tendonitis. J Bone Joint Surg Br 78(3):452–457, 1996

43. Stanish WD, Curwin S, Rubinovich M: Tendinitis: the analysis and treatment for running. Clin Sports Med 4(4):593–609, 1985

44. Colosimo AJ, Bassett FH III: Jumper's knee. Diagnosis and treatment. Orthop Rev 19(2):139–149, 1990

45. Duri ZA, Aichroth PM: Patellar tendonitis: clinical and literature review. Knee Surg Sports Traumatol Arthrosc 3(2):95–100, 1995

46. Karlsson J, Sward L, Kalebo P, Thomee R: Chronic groin injuries in athletes. Recommendations for treatment and rehabilitation. Sports Med 17(2):141–148, 1994

47. Mysnyk MC, Wroble RR, Foster DT, Albright JP: Prepatellar bursitis in wrestlers. Am J Sports Med 14(1):46–54, 1986

48. Rothstein CP, Laorr A, Helms CA, Tirman PF: Semimembranosus-tibial collateral ligament bursitis: MR imaging findings. AJR Am J Roentgenol 166(4):875–877, 1996

49. Whitelaw GP Jr, Rullo DJ, Markowitz HD, et al: A conservative approach to anterior knee pain. Clin Orthop 246:234–237, 1989

50. Jackson RW: The role of arthroscopy in patellofemoral arthritis. In Fox JM, DelPizzo W (eds): The Patello-Femoral Joint. McGraw-Hill, New York, 1993, pp 273–277

51. Gedeon P: Les contusions du cartilage articulaire. Thesis, University of Toulouse, France, 1977

52. Repo RV, Finlay JB: Survival of articular cartilage after controlled impact. J Bone Joint Surg 59(A):1068, 1977

53. Ficat P, Hungerford DS: Disorders of the Patello-femoral Joint. Williams & Wilkins, Baltimore, 1977, pp 63–110

54. Bentley G, Dowd G: Current concepts of etiology and treatment of chondromalacia patellae. Clin Orthop 189:209–228, 1984

55. Ogilvie-Harris DJ, Jackson RW: The arthroscopic treatment of chondromalacia patellae. J Bone Joint Surg Br 66B(5):660–665, 1984

56. Blatter G, Jackson RW, Bayne O: Patellectomy as a salvage procedure. In Muller W, Hackenbruch W (eds): Surgery and Arthroscopy of the Knee: 2nd Congress of the European Society, 1988, pp 476–485

57. Salter RB, Harris R: Injuries involving the epiphyseal plate. J Bone Joint Surg Am 45A(3):587–622, 1963

58. Ike RW, Arnold WJ, Rothschild EW, Shaw HL: Tidal irrigation versus conservative medical man-

agement in patients with osteoarthritis of the knee: a prospective randomized study. Tidal Irrigation Cooperating Group. J Rheumatol 19(5): 772–779, 1992

59. Rathjen KW: Total knee arthroplasty. Am J Knee Surg 2(1):58–63, 1998
60. Busch MT, Morrissy RT: Slipped capital femoral epiphysis. Orthop Clin North Am 18(4):637–647, 1987
61. Lavelle DG: Acute dislocations. In Crenshaw AH (ed): Campbell's Operative Orthopaedics Vol. II, 8th Ed. Mosby Year Book, Philadelphia, 1992
62. Schlickewei W, Elsasser B, Mullaji AB, Kurner EH: Hip dislocation without fracture: traction or mobilization after reduction? Injury 24(1):27–31, 1993
63. Fullerton LR Jr, Snowdy HA: Femoral neck stress fractures. Am J Sports Med 16(4):365–377, 1988
64. Myburgh KH, Hutchins J, Fataar AB, et al: Low bone density in an etiologic factor for stress fractures in athletes. Ann Intern Med 113(10):754–759, 1990
65. Lombardo SJ, Benson DW: Stress fractures of the femur in runners. Am J Sports Med 19(4):219–227, 1982
66. Hajek MR, Noble HB: Stress fractures of the femoral neck in joggers: case reports and review of the literature. Am J Sports Med 10(2):112–116, 1982
67. Shin AY, Morin WD, Gorman JD, et al: The superiority of magnetic resonance imaging in differentiating the cause of hip pain in endurance athletes. Am J Sports Med 24(2):168–176, 1996
68. Gross ML, Nasser S, Finerman GAM: Hip and pelvis. In DeLee JC, Drez D Jr (eds): Orthopaedic Sports Medicine Principles and Practice, Vol II. WB Saunders Co, Philadelphia, 1994

Treatment Modalities for Soft Tissue Injuries of the Ankle

D.J. OGILVIE-HARRIS ■ CHONG-HYUK CHOI

Ankle injuries are among the most common injuries seen in sports medicine and can result in considerable morbidity and financial cost. It has been estimated that 25% to 40% may be associated with recurrent instability or prolonged disability.[1,2] These estimates seem higher than usually seen in clinical practice. Ligamentous injuries compose the bulk of all soft tissue injuries around the ankle. For ligament tears, Cass and Morrey[3] classified such injuries into three grades: grade 1 is a mild stretch of the ligament with no laxity, grade 2 is a moderate but incomplete tear of the ligament with minimal laxity, and grade 3 is a complete tear characterized by instability.

Inflammation is usually the result of these acute injuries of the soft tissue around the ankle. The accumulation of inflammatory fluid around an injury site compounds the extent of tissue damage associated with the acute event, delays healing, and may eventually result in some degree of long-term disability. Numerous modes of treatment have been studied for acute soft tissue injuries of the ankle, but the comparative efficacy of these modes in terms of the rapidity of recovery of function and freedom from long-term ankle impairment has not been clearly defined. The main aim of these treatments has been to relieve pain, reduce swelling, restore normal function, and prevent adverse clinical changes from occurring in the acute phase. Published methods of management have included cryotherapy, early ambulation, joint aspiration and local injection of anesthetic, steroids, hyaluronidase, oral proteolytic enzymes, NSAIDs (non-steroidal anti-inflammatory drugs), ultrasound, adhesive strapping, diathermy, primary suture repair, and immobilization.

META-ANALYSIS

We carried out a meta-analysis of the literature to find proper techniques. This is an important issue not only to achieve optimal functional recovery but also in view of the cost implications of treatment.

The Medline and Excerpta Medica databases were both reviewed from 1966 through 1997 inclusive to examine thoroughly the English-language medical and paramedical literature published on soft tissue injuries of the ankle.[4] In total, more than 170 articles were reviewed, including 19 review articles; 19 on the mechanism, pathophysiology, or diagnosis of ankle injuries; 8 letters to editors; and 135 on medical treatment or surgery. Of these 135 articles on treatment modalities, 93 were specific to soft tissue injuries of the ankle (mainly ligamentous injuries). Many articles dealing with treatment modalities for soft tissue injuries in general had to be excluded either because they contained too few ankle injuries in their treatment group or because the results for the specific ankle injury population could not be extracted from the total results. Individual case reports were also not considered in the analysis. Half the cases in a study had to be ankle injuries to be included in this review. Thus 97 articles were characterized and studied. Table 23–1 categorizes the reviewed articles on treatment modalities of soft

TABLE 23–1. Overview of Study Characteristics

| STUDY TYPES | NO. OF STUDIES | NO. OF PATIENTS | NUMBER OF TREATMENTS | | | | | |
			PHARMACOLOGIC TREATMENTS (NO. OF PATIENTS)	SURGICAL REPAIR (NO. OF PATIENTS)	ACTIVE MOBILIZATION (NO. OF PATIENTS)	CRYOTHERAPY (NO. OF PATIENTS)	DIATHERMY (NO. OF PATIENTS)	OTHER TREATMENTS (NO. OF PATIENTS)
Noncomparative	12	637	—	—	618 (1)	—	—	19 (1)
Retrospective	7	359	—	—	359 (7)	—	—	—
Prospective	5	278	—	—	259 (4)	—	—	19 (1)
Comparative	85	8,450	24 (2,494)	18 (2,076)	18 (1,784)	5 (300)	7 (570)	13 (1,226)
Noncontrolled	41	3,780	15 (1,478)	2 (179)	14 (1,191)	2 (203)	6 (530)	2 (199)
Controlled	44	4,670	9 (1,016)	16 (1,897)	4 (593)	3 (97)	1 (40)	11 (1,027)
Retrospective	3	514	—	2 (114)	—	—	—	1 (400)
Prospective	82	7,934	24 (2,494)	16 (1,962)	8 (1,782)	5 (300)	7 (570)	12 (826)
Prospective and randomized	71	7,443	23 (2,433)	13 (1,807)	17 (1,774)	3 (203)	5 (490)	10 (736)
Total no. of studies	97							

tissue injuries of the ankle according to the design employed in the study.

Most papers reviewed were comparative studies, but 12 were noncomparative (Table 23–1). In this analysis, papers were categorized into one of six groups, including pharmacologic treatment, surgical repair, active mobilization, cryotherapy, diathermy, and other treatment modalities. Each paper was analyzed with respect to the 10 characteristics of an ideal study. On each characteristic, the study was given a 0 if it did not meet the criterion and a 1 if it did. The quality score was simply a sum of these points, with a maximum therefore of 10. The 10 characteristics are a revised version of Weiler's list[5] of characteristics of the prototypical ideal study of the use of NSAIDs in sport soft tissue injury. They were altered so that they might be applied to all treatment modalities in this study. These characteristics are as follows:

1. Double-blind. Unless the experimenters and the subjects were blinded as to the treatment being received, unacceptable bias might result.
2. Randomized patients. Unfortunately, with many of the papers analyzed in this study, the method of randomization was not explained. One must question whether the randomization procedure was a suitable one, such as a block randomization. This type tends to decrease the possibility that

an excessive number of patients with similar characteristics will be enrolled in the same treatment group.
3. Placebo controlled. It is essential to provide a control group because tissue injuries will usually heal in the absence of any treatment. Failure to do so will preclude investigators from assessing the true extent of improvement with the treatment.
4. Rigorously controlled interval between injury and beginning of treatment. Because treatment of these injuries generally begins in the acute postinjury stage and because the body will begin healing itself soon after injury, the interval after injury should be similar if comparisons are to be made with other studies. It is known that there is steady improvement beginning soon after injury.
5. Stratification of severity of injuries. It is obvious that grade 1 and grade 3 ankle injuries will heal at entirely different rates, and more severe injuries may naturally be treated more intensively by the clinician. Patients should thus be grouped according to severity of injury if proper comparisons of treatments are to be made. Otherwise, too many severe injuries may be allocated to one treatment modality group.
6. Exclusion of severe injuries. It is important to separate those patients who have experienced more serious injuries (eg, avulsion

or osteochondral fractures). Unless this is done, there will be too much variability in the subject group being compared. Most studies did ensure that such severe injuries were excluded.

7. Consideration that the treatment could harm as well as benefit the injured patient. Significance tests should be two tailed to determine if the procedure or drug is causing any harm.

8. Controls for age, race, size, and gender. This is an important quality because patients with widely varying characteristics may expect different functional results in some cases.

9. Objective signs to be defined before the beginning of the experiment. It is proper to define the criteria to be compared for significance before the experimental results are collected.

10. Specific end points defined. The time to return to work, practice, competition, and so forth should be defined before the beginning of the study also.

Interestingly, a recent publication by Easterbrook et al[6] determined that there is a higher probability of significant experimental results being published than results that show no statistically significant difference. This was particularly evident in observational studies. The report thus warned that conclusions based on a review of published data should be interpreted cautiously. Therefore, in our current review, although comparisons are made between the number of statistically significant vs the number of insignificant studies, one must be cautious to avoid widespread, generalizing conclusions on the bases of these results.

Each of the 97 articles was evaluated in relation to the 10 characteristics of an ideal study and was assigned a quality score. The scores ranged from 0 to 7, with 0 indicating the weakest study possible (Fig. 23–1). The average score for 97 studies was 3.8. Overall, there were 34,065 patients in the studies (Table 23–1). The highest number of criteria met by any one experiment was seven, and six studies possessed this characteristic.

Thirty of the studies were conducted in a double-blind fashion; 71 of them were randomized. It is important to stress the weakness of

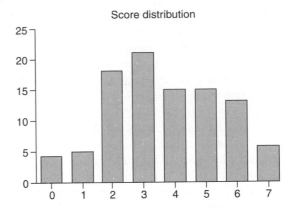

FIGURE 23–1. The number of studies receiving a quality score of 1 to 7. The maximal score was 7; no studies received 8, 9, or 10.

many of the articles that were nonrandomized. In fact, of those that were randomized, only a few articles described the randomization process. Of the 97 studies, 44 stated that a placebo or a control group was used, 43 rigorously controlled the interval between injury and the beginning of treatment, and 6 stratified the severity of injuries. The small number in this latter group illustrates the fact that in many experiments, injuries of varying severity were grouped together, such as grade 1 and grade 2 ankle sprains. In some cases it is difficult to distinguish the difference clinically between slightly differing types of sprains. In 61 studies, however, severe injuries were excluded.

In eight studies the possibility that the treatment (generally pharmacologic) would harm the patient was assessed. In addition, eight studies controlled for age, race, size, and gender. The objective signs to be examined were defined in 78 cases before the beginning of the study—this criterion was the most often fulfilled by investigators. Finally, 11 of the studies defined their end points specifically.

Our analysis of the 97 articles was grouped according to treatment modality deemed to be of primary importance in the study (Table 23–1). For example, a study comparing two NSAIDs to placebo in which one drug was found to be significantly better than another was categorized under the better drug only. In each case, treatment modalities were analyzed in terms of the number of statistically significant study conclusions presented. Of the studies analyzed, however, only a few possessed the main qualities of studies that are most useful: prospective, double-blind, randomized, and placebo controlled. These qualities were most common in the studies on pharmacologic modalities of treatment rather than other modalities. This is because it is relatively easy with medications to provide double-blind study conditions with the use of a placebo medication. For studies comparing mobilization vs plaster casts or cryotherapy vs contrast baths, it is virtually impossible to fulfill all four of these important criteria, especially double-blind, and placebo control. In such studies that are not double-blind, the observer may in fact be blind to the patient's treatment. Thus, although these studies may have fulfilled fewer criteria, it should be recognized that in many cases the cause was the particular types of modalities compared, not poor study design.

PHARMACOLOGIC AGENTS

For the pharmacologic treatment modalities, 24 studies were reviewed. Of these, 23 were prospective randomized and one was non-randomized. Of the 23 prospective randomized studies, 16 also fulfilled the double-blind, placebo-controlled criteria of the most useful studies. Of the four studies published on diflunisal, two were comparative studies of diflunisal vs oxyphenbutazone.[7-10] Both studies indicated a significant improvement in pain relief with diflunisal, and Bernett and Primes[11] also found a significant improvment in tenderness and range of motion with diflunisal. Of the remaining two studies, Aghababian[8] showed no significant difference in resultant pain, swelling, and limitation of motion between diflunisal and acetaminophen with codeine. Finch et al[10] concluded that flurbiprofen provided significantly greater pain relief than diflunisal. In a study comparing the efficacy of clonixin, oxyphenbutazone, and placebo, Viljakka and Rokkanen[12] showed significantly better recovery results with clonixin over placebo, and they estimated better results with clonixin over oxyphenbutazone. Work by Bahamonde and Saavedra[13] and Moran[14] comparing diclofenac with piroxicam and placebo found significantly better results in the diclofenac group.

Five studies were published concerning the use of ibuprofen.[8,15-18] In three of these studies

(one of which was nonrandomized) no significant difference was found between ibuprofen and placebo. McLatchie et al[17] showed that high-dose ibuprofen provided a significantly better improvment in progress than placebo. Sloan et al[18] also showed that ibuprofen administration immediately after injury provided a significant improvement over placebo.

Three studies[19-21] were performed that compared proteolytic enzymes and placebo controls. Calandre et al[20] found a significantly faster rate of symptom relief in the streptokinase-streptodornase group over placebo. In two separate experiments comparing Chymoral (oral proteolytic enzyme) administration to placebo, Brakenbury and Kotowski[19] found a significantly faster rate of resolution in the placebo group, although Craig[21] found no significant difference between the two treatments. Six studies[22-27] compared the efficacy of various topical creams and gels to placebo after injury. Diebschlag et al[23] showed that ketorolac gel provided a significant reduction in posttraumatic ankle pain and swelling over both etofenamate gel and placebo. Dreiser et al[24] also showed a significant reduction in pain could be achieved using nifulmic acid gel vs placebo. Neither treatment produced any improvement in recovery time or long-term resolution of symptoms, however. Although Elswood and MacLeod[25] found no significant improvement using benzydamine cream vs placebo, Linde et al[27] reported that benzydamine cream reduced swelling significantly. Ibuprofen cream was found to reduce the pain after ankle sprain significantly by Campbell and Dunn.[22] Finally, Frahm et al[26] showed that mucopolysaccharide polysulfate–salicylic acid gel significantly reduced pain on ankle movement.

Dreiser et al[28] showed a significant improvement in pain and edema in the flurbiprofen patch group over placebo. Dreiser and Riebenfeld[29] showed that nimesulide had an effect on reduction in pain, functional impairment, and swelling. Recently, Slatyer et al[30] found that piroxicam provided a significant reduction in pain, improvement in physical activity, and reduction in total cost over placebo.

SURGICAL REPAIR, CASTING, AND ACTIVE MOBILIZATION

The modalities of surgical repair, plaster casting, and active mobilization were grouped together because of extensive overlap among these three topics in the literature. In many cases, all three treatments were compared. Fourteen studies were performed that compared surgical repair to nonsurgical (conservative) treatment modalities. In four of these studies, conservative treatment gave significantly better results with respect to decreases in recovery time. Of the remaining 10 studies that showed no significant differences, four found shorter recovery periods in the conservative groups, and three studies found better long-term results and stability with surgical repair. For example, Evans et al[31] showed that although the differences were not significant, the resumption of work activity was earlier by 1 to 2 weeks for patients treated conservatively vs surgically, the residual symptoms were minimal, and functional limitation was rare. Two studies showed no significant difference between surgery and cast groups. In total, 17 studies compared active mobilization and plaster cast immobilization. In 11 of these, active mobilization was significantly better; in 4 it was better, but the difference did not reach significance; and in 2 studies there was no difference. Finally, 13 studies compared different models of active mobilization, including different bandages, ankle supports, and physiotherapy. Two studies stated that better results were achieved with early physiotherapy. Five studies compared different supports (Nottingham, Malleotrain, stabilizing support, semirigid ankle brace, and daily strapping). Four studies showed no significant differences in the supports compared; one interesting study[32] concluded that there was a significantly better result in the elevated control group than the group receiving intermittent pneumatic compression (IPC) or elastic wrap. Karlsson et al[33] found that functional treatment, including physiotherapy and proprioceptive training, as compared with conventional therapy, did not yield significantly better results.

PHYSICAL MODALITIES

Five studies on cryotherapy were reviewed and included three prospective randomized[18,34,35] and two prospective nonrandomized studies.[36,37] In two separate studies,[18,35] cryotherapy was found to be a significantly better treatment than heat. One study[18] comparing one application of ice therapy for 45 minutes in the first 24 hours

after injury showed a trend in favor of the cryotherapy group, although it did not reach significance. Another study[35] showed no significant difference between cryotherapy and controls. Studies have recently shown that cryotherapy acts by reducing blood flow, the inflammatory response, edema production, hemorrhage, and pain sensitivity. One area of difference in these experiments is the defined acute period after injury, which varied among experiments. Hocutt et al[37] in fact showed that cryotherapy initiated on the day of injury provided better resumption of full activities than cryotherapy begun on the following day.

Five prospective studies[38-42] compared diathermy to placebo for the treatment of the acutely sprained ankle. Two of these studies[41,42] concluded that there is a significantly shorter recovery period, with less pain and edema in the diathermy group. Three of these studies[38-40] concluded that there was no significant difference between diathermy and placebo. One study[43] compared pulsed electromagnetic (EM) energy to short-wave diathermy and found pulsed EM therapy to be a significantly better treatment. One study[40] that compared high-voltage pulsed stimulation and ice, compression, and elevation (ICE) to ICE alone found no significant difference. The proposed rationale for diathermy treatment is to reduce the inflammatory response, edema, and pain. Diathermy has been well documented and is an accepted treatment for pain control, but the mechanisms of action of electrical stimulation on edema reduction are unknown. Its action has been postulated to be related to either a muscle-pumping action or an electrophoretic effect.

OTHER MODALITIES

Intermittent pneumatic compression has been shown in two separate experiments to make no significant difference in long-term recovery, but Starkey[44] estimated there was an increased recovery time of 2 days associated with the treatment. Six studies[44-49] focused on aspiration injection treatments, and in two experiments of aspiration of the subtalar joint and injection of local anesthetic, shorter recovery time was reported (only one reached significance). In one study the injection of hydrocortisone provided a significantly faster recovery, and in another study the injection of hyaluronidase showed no significant difference in recovery.

Three studies[50–52] were performed using ultrasound treatments, and in only one of these was there a significantly better response. This response was not compared to a control group, however, but instead to a thermotherapy group. One study using acupuncture revealed a significant improvement in range of movement and pain with treatment.

Axelsen and Bjero[53] showed that there was no significant difference between a low-power laser group and a placebo. In a well-designed study by Borromeo et al,[54] hyperbaric oxygen at 2 atmosphere, compared with air at 1.1 atmosphere, had no significant effect in functional recovery of ankle sprain.

There were 12 noncomparative studies of mobilization and immobilization after ankle sprain. In nine of these studies, active mobilization was studied, and eight of these showed good general results in terms of an earlier return to activities. In two separate experiments, cast immobilization was studied, with a 70% to 80% success rate on average in the two experiments. The experimenter concluded that results were satisfactory with cast immobilization. One study showed that rapid pneumatic compression and cold were a safe and effective treatment for acute ankle sprain.

There were some interesting observations rabout the frequency with which criteria were fulfilled (Table 23–2). Criterion 8 (age, gender, race controls) was only found in three papers. Eight papers examined if the treatments were harmful (criterion 7), and 13 had specific end points (criterion 10). In constructing a study, none of these criteria are particularly difficult to apply.

We gathered data from the literature and performed a meta-analysis of the information. We had hoped to show whether any particular treatment was superior to a placebo or to other treatment based on the statistical analysis of the results contained in these papers. However, a review of the literature indicated that the information we would use to determine outcome was generally not available. There was no standardized method of scoring the severity of ankle injuries. Criteria such as number of days until return to sports are extremely subjective and do not provide definite end points for these studies. Hence, we are unable to perform a statistical analysis despite the fact that there were 34,065 patients entered into the studies.

In many studies of pharmacologic treatment modalities with nonsteroidal anti-inflammatory medication, no significant difference was found between medications, but significant improvement occurred with these medications compared with placebo. In fact, good results were obtained with the use of both diflunisal and diclofenac. No particular drug was shown to be superior to others overall, however. These studies provided reasonable evidence that patient recovery is faster and with less pain when treated with nonsteroidal anti-inflammatories. Although recovery time was shortened with such treatment, there appeared to be no significant difference in the ultimate outcome. Based on this evidence, the use of nonsteroidal anti-inflammatory drugs for acute ankle sprains can be justified if rapid recovery and symptomatic relief are essential.

Conflicting results were obtained in the three studies analyzing the efficacy of proteolytic enzyme treatment. There was no good evidence that proteolytic enzymes produced better overall results than placebo, and as a result they are not recommended for treatment. Topical gels were shown to provide some temporary relief of acute symptoms, but they provided no significant improvement in the final treatment outcome.

The majority of studies comparing surgical repair, plastering, casting, and active mobilization clearly favored active mobilization as the

TABLE 23–2. Number and Percentage of Studies Fulfilling Each Criterion*

CRITERION	NUMBER	PERCENTAGE
1	30	30
2	69	71
3	37	38
4	43	44
5	7	7
6	58	59
7	8	8
8	3	3
9	78	80
10	13	13

*Ninety-eight studies total.

treatment of choice. Nonsurgical treatment seemed to provide more rapid recovery than surgical repair. Studies generally failed to show that surgical repair of injured ligaments provided any significant long-term improvements in symptoms such as instability and pain. Based on this information, one would not recommend surgical intervention. There may be a role for surgical reconstruction in severe ligamentous disruption, but this requires careful individual evaluation and judgment. There was also conclusive evidence that plaster cast immobilization did not help. Active mobilization is the treatment of choice; 15 of 17 studies showed it provided better recovery. Of interest, however, is that in the long term, all conservative treatments seemed to produce satisfactory results.

Studies on the use of cryotherapy showed that treatment generally reduced pain and edema and shortened the recovery period, although not all studies produced a significantly better result with cryotherapy. It had to be applied within the first day or two of injury to be effective. This treatment should remain part of the standard regimen.

Two studies showed diapulse significantly reduced pain, edema, and disability following acute ankle sprains if applied relatively early in the treatment process. Of the diathermy treatment, modalities showed no significant improvements over placebo treatments. Ultrasound was not shown to be particularly effective. Diapulse therefore may have a role in early rehabilitation.

Although it is difficult to determine the efficacy of certain treatment modalities, one study of hyperbaric oxygen therapy showed no significant improvement over air exposure. In one study, low-power laser therapy also made no significant difference in recovery. Although joint aspiration, injection of steroids and hyaluronidase, all proteolytic enzymes, ultrasound, and intermittent pneumatic compression have all been tried, evidence in the literature is insufficient to support their use in either providing more rapid resolution of the injury or improving the overall outcome.

ROLE OF PROPRIOCEPTION IN THE REHABILITATION OF ANKLE INJURIES

Proprioception is a specialized variation of the sensory modality of touch that encompasses the sensation of joint movement (kinesthesia) and joint position (joint position sense).[55] Proprioception and accompanying neuromuscular feedback mechanisms provide an important component for the establishment and maintenance of functional joint stability. Neuromuscular control and joint stabilization are mediated primarily by the central nervous system. Multisite sensory input, originating from the somatosensory, visual, and vestibular systems, is received and processed by the brain and spinal cord. The culmination of gathered and processed information results in conscious awareness of joint position and motion, unconscious joint stabilization through protective spinalmediated reflexes, and the maintenance of posture and balance.

The stability of the ankle joint is maintained with strong ligamentous structures. The ligaments provide neurologic feedback that directly mediates reflex muscular stabilization about the joint. Functional instability of the ankle after a sprain has been classically defined by Freeman[56] as "a tendency for the foot to give way after an ankle sprain." In the ankle sprain, the coupling effect of ligamentous trauma resulting in mechanical instability and proprioceptive deficits contributes to functional instability, which could ultimately lead to further microtrauma and reinjury. Konradsen and Ravn[57] and Lofvenberg et al[58] found a delayed reflex reaction time of peroneus longus muscle to sudden angular displacement and supported the theory that functional instability is induced by a proprioceptive reflex defect. Garn and Newton[59] found significantly greater difficulty detecting passive motion in the ankle with multiple sprains compared with the uninjured ankle, and they demonstrated the need for clinicians to evaluate kinesthetic deficits and to design exercise programs to improve kinesthetic awareness and decrease ankle instability in individuals with multiple ankle sprains. One of the most challenging aspects for the clinician in rehabilitation after an ankle injury is understanding the role of proprioceptively mediated neuromuscular control after joint injury and its restoration through rehabilitation. Regaining joint sense awareness to initiate muscular reflex stabilization to prevent reinjury should be the primary objective once the final stage of rehabilitation is reached. Even though there is still controversy, some authors support proprioceptive rehabilitation in the other direction with "adaptation." They believe that, with repetition, the cerebral cortex can determine the most effective motor pattern for a given task, based on the proprioceptive information of previous attempts.[60]

Mechanoreceptors in the Ankle Joint

Freeman and Wyke[61] demonstrated that tibial, sural, and deep peroneal nerves terminated in mechanoreceptors in the capsule and ligaments of the ankle and felt that functional instability of the foot and ankle was due to motor incoordination, especially peroneus longus and anterior tibialis muscles. They proposed that decreased coordination resulted from articular deafferentiation caused by afferent mechanoreceptor damage that occurred during injury. Mechanoreceptors initiate the afferent loop of proprioceptive feedback to the brain. They are specialized end-organs (neurosensory cells) that convert a physical stimulus into a neurologic signal that can be deciphered by the central nervous system to modulate joint position and movement. Michelson and Hutchins[61a] examined the anterior and posterior talofibular ligament, deltoid ligament, and calcaneofibular ligament from cadaver ankles for mechanoreceptors and classified them according to the four types described by Freeman and Wyke[61] in feline ligaments. Each of the four mechanoreceptor types responds to different stimuli and gives specific afferent information that modifies neuromuscular function. They found three types of mechanoreceptors in the ankle joint. Type II receptors, thought to provide the sensation of the beginning of joint motion, and type III receptors, thought to be activated at the extremes of movement, were predominant.

Training of Proprioception

The training of proprioception should be started as soon as possible after injury for functional restoration. Karlsson et al[33] investigated the effects of early functional treatment, including early full weight bearing and proprioceptive range-of-motion exercise. Even though the final results were similar, they found that early functional treatment resulted in shorter sick leave and facilitated an earlier return to sports. Empir-

ical evidence exists suggesting that proprioceptive training techniques after acute and chronic ankle injuries are highly effective. There are a lot of exercises for proprioceptive training, and these exercises can be classified into two main categories.

Balance Training

Balance training is a major category of proprioceptive exercise. These exercises help to train the proprioceptive system in a mostly static activity. This training includes ankle disk exercise, one-legged standing exercise, and tandem exercises. Balanced board or ankle disk is known as an effective tool for promoting proprioception. This training is started in a sitting position and progresses in a standing, partial weight-bearing position. Tropp et al[62] reported a significant improvement of stabilometric results and subjective "giving way" feeling after 6 weeks of coordination training on an ankle disk. In a study of soccer players with functional instability of the ankle, Gauffin et al[63] found that ankle disk training improved postural control. Sheth et al[64] found that delayed contracture of the anterior tibialis and posterior tibialis muscles favored the correction of excessive ankle inversion in the trap door experiment after ankle disk training. Bahr et al[65] postulated that balanced board training in volleyball players decreased the incidence of ankle injury. Hoffman and Payne[66] presented evidence of decreased postural sway after using the biomechanical ankle platform system. Wester et al[67] reported that 12 weeks of training on a wobble board early after primary stage 2 ankle sprains was effective in reducing residual symptoms following this lesion. Single leg standing is a simple method and a useful testing tool for proprioception. In the initial step of this training method, single leg assistive stork stands are safer. These are accomplished by standing on one leg, concentrating on maintaining the talar neutral position throughout the exercise. This exercise should progress to performing it with eyes closed and on an uneven surface such as a pillow or foam rubber.[68]

Kinetic Chain Exercise

Closed kinetic chain exercises (those in which movement at one joint produces predictable movement at another joint, usually involving axial forces) challenge the dynamic and reflexive aspects of proprioception in the legs and feet. The lower extremities function in a closed chain manner during sports and daily life activities, so these exercises will facilitate the proper neuromuscular program. These exercises include the leg press, squat, circle running, figure of eights, single leg hopping, vertical jumps, lateral bounds, one-legged long jumps, and carioca. Jerosch et al[69] used a one-leg jumping test to document sport-specific skills with various types of braces in athletes with normal ankles and concluded that the tested stabilizing devices seemed to have no negative effect on sports-specific capability.[69]

Test for Proprioception

Although all kinds of exercise for proprioceptive training can be used as a tool for assessment for proprioceptive function, several methods are useful for objective evaluation and reproducibility.

Stabilometry

Freeman et al[2] used a modified Romberg test for quantitative measurements of the proprioceptive deficit. Stabilometry, a measuring system for foot reaction force, is an objective and quantitative method for the study of postural control developed by Tropp et al[62] using the same principles. Tropp et al[70] insisted that the ability to maintain postural equilibrium as demonstrated by stabilometry was reduced among players with functional instability but was not affected by mechanical instability. They believed that coordination and postural control were important for functional instabilty of the ankle. In another study using stabilometry, Tropp[71] suggested that patients who have a chronic ankle instability have peroneal muscle weakness. Friden et al[72] found that when a brace was used, the effect was obvious and none of the parameters studied showed any significant difference compared to the uninjured leg using stabilometry measurements. Leanderson et al[73] investigated postural sway with stabilometry in ballet dancers and concluded that postural stability was impaired for several weeks after an ankle sprain. Isakov and Mizrahi[74] and Jerosch and Bischof[75] found increased postural sway in chronic ankle sprain patients using stabilometry. Recently, instrumented stabilometry techniques have been used

to assess the ability of individuals to incorporate multiple sensory and motor responsive patterns to maintain static and dynamic equilibrium positions.

Position Awareness Test

The evaluation of joint position sense and kinesthesia provides a profile for joint position sensibility in the normal, pathologic, and surgically reconstructed individual. Although there is controversy regarding this test, many authors have used it. Robbins et al[76] examined awareness of foot position in terms of the slope of the weight-bearing surface and found that it declined with age. They concluded that sensitivity to foot position declined with age, mainly owing to loss of plantar tactile sensitivity. They postulated that footwear impairs foot position sense and that this impairment could be improved by ankle taping. Feuerbach et al[77] studied the effect of lateral ankle ligament anethesia on ankle joint proprioception and examined ankle joint position awareness. They suggested that ligament mechanoreceptors contributed little to ankle joint proprioception. Konradsen et al[78] found that passive position sense was impaired by anesthesia but that active position sense was not affected by anesthesia. Gross[79] examined the effects of recurrent lateral ankle sprains on subjects' active and passive judgments of joint position and postulated that joint receptors played a dominant role in joint angle detection and that muscle receptors were more valuable in the perception of joint movement. Lentell et al[80] suggested that a deficit in passive movement sense and anatomic stability were greater concerns than strength deficits when managing the ankle with functional instability.

Muscle Reaction Time

Muscle reaction time means the elapsed time between the sudden sensory input and initiation of contracture of specific muscles by reflex. Konradsen and Ravn[57] investigated peroneal reaction time to sudden ankle inversion and found an increased peroneal reaction time in unstable ankle. These findings supported the theory that functional instability is induced by a proprioceptive reflex, but Konradsen and Ravn reported that the reflex reaction to sudden inversion was initiated at a peripheral level by the inversion motion followed by a reaction pattern mediated by spinal or cortical motor centers and suggested that the reflex reaction time seemed too slow to protect the ankle in case of sudden inversion occurring at the time of heel contact. However, they suggested that afferent input from active calf muscles seemed also to be responsible for dynamic ankle protection against sudden ankle inversion. Lofvenberg et al[58] found the reaction time increased by 15 ms in patients with chronic lateral instability of the ankle and concluded that a delayed proprioceptive response to sudden angular displacement of the ankle could be one of the causes of chronic lateral instability of the ankle and that proprioceptive training should be included in the treatment of acute and chronic ankle disability. Lynch et al[81] reported that speed of inversion moment and plantar flexion angle both caused significant changes in latency responses of the peroneal muscles, with increased speed producing a shorter latency response and increased angle causing a longer latency response; they concluded that there was a loss of protective reflexes with increasing plantar flexion.

Ankle Supports and Proprioception

Ankle orthotics and wrapping have been used for promoting functional stability and have also been suggested to have a proprioceptive benefit even though this is still uncertain. Many studies have supported the positive role of ankle braces for prevention of ankle injury and maintaining stability during exercise. Tropp et al[70] suggested that an orthosis can be used during the rehabilitation period after injury or when an ankle sprain patient is playing on uneven ground. Friden et al,[72] using stabilometry technique, observed that a brace for an ankle injury had an obvious effect and no parameters showed any significant difference compared with the uninjured leg. Calmels et al[82] analyzed the proprioceptive effect of wearing an ankle support and provided information about the prophylactic effect of wearing a flexible support. Feuerbach et al[77] investigated the effect of a rigid ankle orthosis on ankle joint proprioception and concluded that application of an orthosis may increase the afferent feedback from cutaneous receptors in the foot and shank, which may in turn lead to an improved ankle joint position sense. In their

study of postural sway with orthotics, Guskiewicz and Perrin[83] suggested that custom-fitted orthotics might restrict undesirable motion at the foot and ankle and enhance joint mechanoreceptors to detect perturbations and provide structural support for detecting and controlling postural sway in ankle-injured subjects. Jerosch et al[69] found that most of the devices for functionally unstable ankles significantly improved jumping performance. They believed that the stabilizing devices seemed to have no negative effect on sports-specific capability.

In contrast, there are some skeptical reports on ankle supports. Bennel and Goldie[84] investigated the effects of ankle supports on postural control in a one-legged stance test and found that while wearing the tape or brace, subjects were less steady and touched down more frequently. They suggested that postural control was impaired by ankle supports that limited ankle motion. Barrett and Bilisko[85] showed that high top shoes had effects of limiting extreme range of motion, providing additional proprioceptive input, and decreasing external stress, but clinical trials were inconclusive. Robbins et al[86] reported that footwear impaired foot position awareness in both young and old age-groups. In another study,[76] Robbins et al postulated that ankle taping improved proprioception before and after exercise and suggested that ankle taping partly corrected an impaired proprioception caused by modern athletic footwear and that exercise and footwear could be optimized to reduce the incidence of ankle injuries.

Proprioception in the ankle joint has an important role for stabilizing and maintaining the joint during performance and for prevention of further injury. Proprioceptive training should be included in the early stage of rehabilitation programs for early return to daily living and sports activity without anxiety for reinjury and should start with safe and simple techniques and progress to more complex training.

CONCLUSION

This chapter analyzed the current literature and attempted to make specific recommendations about the best treatment for ankle sprains. Early mobilization aided by the use of bandages or strapping seems to provide the best results—a faster recovery rate. We thoroughly recommend early weight bearing as the most important concept in treatment. The use of NSAIDs early in the injury and for short periods of time is of value in achieving an earlier recovery, although use of NSAIDs does not change the overall outcome. Similarly, cryotherapy helps reduce the length of recovery although it does not change the final outcome. Diapulse diathermy seemed to offer improvement in recovery time and in relief of symptoms. Surgery was not shown to provide significant improvement.

Our overall conclusion from reviewing the literature is that ankle injuries have a good prognosis. Looking at the placebo groups in the studies, very satisfactory results are obtained with little treatment. In most cases, long-term prognosis was not altered by treatment, but rather, acute symptoms, pain, and disability could be reduced. Following an ankle sprain, ankles are often weak and have proprioceptive deficits as collateral damage from the original injury. Judicious efforts should be made to regain strength and proprioceptive input. This will aid recovery and minimize the chance for reinjury. Closed chain strength training and balance board exercises are indicated. Sport-specific training programs are the final stage of rehabilitation. Ankle supports probably play a role in early return to sports, as they increase proprioceptive input and limit extreme movement, but their role in pro phylaxis is questionable.

REFERENCES

1. Bahamonde LA, Saavedra H: Comparison of the analgesic and anti-inflammatory effects of diclofenac potassium versus piroxicam versus placebo in ankle sprain patients. J Int Med Res 18:104–111, 1990
2. Freeman MA, Dean MRE, Hanham IWF: The etiology and prevention of functional instability of the foot. J Bone Joint Surg Br 47:678–685, 1965
3. Cass JR, Morrey BF: Ankle instability: current concepts, diagnosis and treatment. Mayo Clin Proc 59:165–170, 1984
4. Ogilvie-Harris DJ, Gilbert M: Treatment modalities for soft tissue injuries of the ankle: a critical review. Clin J Sports Med 5:175–186, 1995
5. Weiler JM: Medical modifiers of sports injuries. The use of non-steroidal anti-inflammatory drugs in sports soft tissue injury. Clin Sports Med 11:625–644, 1992

6. Easterbrook PJ, Berlin JA, Gopalan R, Mathews DR: Publication bias in clinical research. Lancet 337:867–872, 1991
7. Adams ID: Diflusinal in the management of sprains. Curr Med Res Opin 5:580–583, 1978
8. Aghababian RV: Comparison of diflusinal and acetaminophen with codeine in the management of grade 2 ankle sprain. Clin Ther 8:520–526, 1986
9. Andersson S, Fredin H, Lindberg H, et al: Ibuprofen and compression bandage in the treatment of ankle sprains. Acta Orthop Scand 54:322–325, 1986
10. Finch WF, Zanaga P, Mickelson MM, Grochowski KJ: A double-blind comparison of fluriprofen with diflusinal in the treatment of acute ankle sprains and strains. Curr Med Res Opin 11:409–416, 1989
11. Bernett P, Primes P: Diflusinal vs oxyphenbutazone in the management of pain associated with sprains and strains. The Royal Society of Medicine international congress and symposium. Series No. 6. Diflusinal: new perspectives in analgesia. Royal Society of Medicine, London, 51–55, 1979
12. Viljakka T, Rokkanen P: The treatment of ankle sprain by bandaging and antiphogistic drugs. Ann Chir Gynaecol 72:66–70, 1983
13. Bahamonde LA, Saavedra H: Comparison of the analgesic and anti-inflammatory effects of diclofenac potassium versus piroxicam versus placebo in ankle sprain patients. J Int Med Res 18(2):104–111, 1990
14. Moran M: An observer-blind comparison of diclofenac potassium, piroxicam and placebo in the treatment of ankle sprains. Curr Med Res Opin 12:268–274, 1990
15. Dupont M, Beliveau P, Theriault G: The efficacy of anti-inflammatory medication in the treatment of the acutely sprained ankle. Am J Sports Med 15:41–45, 1987
16. Fredburg U, Hansen PA, Skinhoj A: Ibuprofen in the treatment of acute ankle joint injuries: a double-blind study. Am J Sports Med 17:564–566, 1989
17. McLatchie GR, Allister C, MacEwen C, et al: Variable schedules of ibuprofen for ankle sprains. Br J Sports Med 19(4):203–206, 1985
18. Sloan JP, Hain R, Pownall R: Clinical benefits of early cold therapy in accident and emergency following ankle sprain. Arch Emerg Med 6:1–6, 1989
19. Brakenbury PH, Kotowski J: A comparative study of the management of ankle sprains. Br J Clin Pract 37:181–185, 1983
20. Calandre EP, Ruiz-Morales M, Lopex-Gollonet JM, Hernandez MA: Efficacy of oral streptoki-

nase-streptodornase in the treatment of ankle sprains. Clin Orthop 263:210–214, 1991

21. Craig RP: The quantitative evaluation of the use of oral proteolytic enzyme in the treatment of sprained ankles. Injury 6:313–316, 1975

22. Campbell J, Dunn T: Evaluation of topical ibuprofen cream in the treatment of acute ankle sprains. J Accid Emerg Med 11:178–182, 1994

23. Diebschlag W, Nocker W, Bullingham R: A double-blind study of the efficacy of topical ketorolac tromethamine gel in the treatment of ankle sprain in comparison to placebo and etofenamate. J Clin Pharmacol 30:82–89, 1990

24. Dreiser RE, Charlot J, Lopez A, Ditixheim A: Clinical evaluation of niflumic acid gel in the treatment of uncomplicated ankle sprains. Curr Med Res Opin 12:93–99, 1990

25. Elswood R, MacLeod DAD: Treatment of ankle sprains with benzydamine. Practitioner 229:70–71, 1985

26. Frahm E, Elsasser U, Kammereit A: Topical treatment of acute sprains. Br J Clin Prac 47:321–322, 1993

27. Linde F, Hvass I, Jurgensen V, Madsen F: Early mobilizing treatment in lateral ankle sprains: course and risk factors for chronic painful or functional limiting ankle. Scand J Rehab Med 18:17–21, 1986

28. Dreiser RL, Roche R, De Sahb R, et al: Flurbiprofen local action transcutaneous (LAT): clinical evaluation in the treatment of acute ankle sprains. Eur J Rheumatol Inflamm 14:9–13, 1994

29. Dreiser RL, Riebenfeld D: A double-blind study of the efficacy of nimesulide in the treatment of ankle sprain in comparison with placebo. Drugs 46(Suppl 1):183–186, 1993

30. Slatyer MA, Hensley MJ, Lopert P: A randomized controlled trial of piroxicam in the treatment of acute ankle sprain in Australian Regular Army recruits. The kapooka ankle sprain study. Am J Sports Med 25:544–553, 1997

31. Evans GA, Hardcastle P, Frenyo AD: Acute rupture of the lateral ligament of the ankle: to suture or not to suture? J Bone Joint Surg Br 66:209–212, 1984

32. Rucinski TJ, Hooker DN, Prentice WE, et al: The effects of intermittent compression on edema in postacute ankle sprains. J Orthop Sports Phys Ther 14:65–69, 1991

33. Karlsson J, Eriksson BI, Sward L: Early functional treatment for acute ligament of the ankle joint. Scand J Med Sci Sports 6:341–345, 1996

34. Cote DJ, Prentice WE, Hooker DN, Shields EW: Comparison of three treatment procedures for minimizing ankle sprain swelling. Phys Ther 68:1972–1976, 1988

35. Laba E, Roestenburg M: Clinical evaluation of ice therapy for acute ankle sprain injuries. N Z J Physiother 17:7–9, 1989

36. Basur RL, Shephard E, Mouzas GL: A cooling method in the treatment of ankle sprains. Practitioner 216:708–711, 1976

37. Hocutt JE, Jaffe R, Rylander CR, Beebe JK: Cryotherapy in ankle sprains. Am J Sports Med 10:316–319, 1982

38. Barker AT, Barlow PS, Porter J, et al: A double-blind clinical trial of low power pulsed shortwave therapy in the treatment of a soft tissue injury. Physiotherapy 71:500–504, 1985

39. McGill SN: The effects of pulsed shortwave therapy on lateral ligament sprain of the ankle. N Z J Physiother 16:21–24, 1988

40. Michlovitz S, Smith W, Watkins M: Ice and high voltage pulsed stimulation in treatment of acute lateral ankle sprains. J Orthop Sports Phys Ther 9:301–304, 1988

41. Pasilia M, Visuri T, Sundholm A: Pulsating shortwave diathermy: value in treatment of recent ankle and foot sprains. Arch Phys Med Rehabil 59:383–386, 1978

42. Pennington GM, Danley DL, Sumko MH, et al: Pulsed, non-thermal high-frequency electromagnetic energy (diapulse) in the treatment of grade I and grade II ankle sprains. Mil Med 158:101–104, 1993

43. Wilson DH: Comparison of short wave diathermy and pulsed electromagnetic energy in treatment of soft tissue injuries. Physiotherapy 60:309–310, 1974

44. Starkey JA: Treatment of ankle sprains by simultaneous use of intermittent compression and ice packs. Am J Sports Med 4:142–144, 1976

45. Brady TA, Arnold A: Aspiration injection treatment for varus sprain of the ankle. J Bone Joint Surg Am 54:1257–1261, 1972

46. Caro D, Howells JB, Craft IL, Shaw PC: Diagnosis and treatment of injury of lateral ligament of the ankle joint. Lancet 10:720–723, 1964

47. MacCartee CC: Taping treatment of severe inversion sprains of the ankle. Am J Sports Med 5:246–247, 1977

48. McMaster PE: Treatment of ankle sprain: observations in more than five hundred cases. JAMA 122:659–660, 1943

49. Zoltan DJ: Treatment of ankle sprains with joint aspiration, Xylocaine infildraden and early mobilization. J Trauma 17:93–96, 1977

50. Makuloluwe RTB, Mouzas GL: Ultrasound in the treatment of sprained ankle. Practitioner 218:586–588, 1977

51. Moller-Larsen F, Wethelund JO, Jurik AG, et al: Comparison of three different treatments for rup-

tured lateral ankle ligaments. Acta Orthop Scand 59:564–566, 1988

52. Williamson JB, George TK, Simpson DC, et al: Ultrasound in the treatment of ankle sprains. Injuries 17:176–178, 1986

53. Axelsen SM, Bjerno T: Laser therapy of ankle sprain. Ugeskrift for Laeger 155:3908–3911, 1993

54. Borromeo CN, Ryan JL, Marchetto PA, et al: Hyperbaric oxygen therapy for acute ankle sprains. Am J Sports Med 25:619–625, 1997

55. Lephart SM, Pincivero DM, Giraldo JL, Fu FH: The role of proprioception in the management and rehabilitation of athletic injuries. Am J Sports Med 25:130–137, 1997

56. Freeman MA: Instability of the foot after injuries to the lateral ligament of the ankle. J Bone Joint Surg Br 47:669–677, 1965

57. Konradsen L, Ravn JB: Prolonged peroneal reaction time in ankle instability. Int J Sports Med 12(3):290–292, 1991

58. Lofvenberg R, Karrholm J, Sundelin G: Proprioceptive reaction in the healthy and chronically unstable ankle joint. Sportverletzung Sportschaden 10:79–83, 1996

59. Garn SN, Newton RA: Kinesthetic awareness in subjects with multiple ankle sprains. Phys Ther 68:1667–1671, 1988

60. Leisman G: Cybernetic model of psychophysiological pathways: II. Conciousness of tension and kinesthesia. J Manipulative Physiol Ther 12:174–191, 1989

61. Freeman MA, Wyke B: The innervation of the ankle joint: an anatomical and histological study in the cat. Acta Anatomica 68:321–333, 1967

61a. Michelson JD, Hutchins C: Mechanoreceptors in human ankle ligaments. J Bone Joint Surg Br 77:219–224, 1995

62. Tropp H, Ekstrand J, Gillquist J: Stabilometry in functional instability of the ankle and its values in predicting injury. Med Sci Sports Exerc 16:64–66, 1984

63. Gauffin J, Tropp H, Odenrick P: Effects of ankle disk training on postural control in patients with functional instability of the ankle joint. Int J Sports Med 9:141–144, 1988

64. Sheth P, Yu B, Laskowski ER, An KN: Ankle disk training influences reaction times of selected muscle in a simulated ankle sprain. Am J Sports Med 25:538–543, 1997

65. Bahr R, Lian O, Bahr IA: A two fold reduction in the incidence of acute ankle sprains in volleyball after the introduction of an injury prevention program: a prospective study. Scand J Med Sci Sports 7:172–177, 1997

66. Hoffman M, Payne VG: The effects of proprioceptive ankle disk training on healthy subjects. J Orthop Sports Phys Ther 21:90–93, 1995

67. Wester JU, Jespersen SM, Nielsen KD, Neumann L: Wobble board training after partial sprains of the lateral ligaments of the ankle: a prospective randomized study. J Orthop Sports Phys Ther 23:332–336, 1996

68. Losito JM, O'Neil J: Rehabilitation of foot and ankle injuries. Sports Med Rehab 14:533–557, 1997

69. Jerosch J, Thorwesten L, Frebel T: Effect of external stabilizing agents of the ankle joint on sports motor capacities in one legged jumping. Sportverletzung Sportschaden 11(1):27–32, 1997

70. Tropp J, Askling C, Gillquist J: Prevention of ankle sprains. Am J Sports Med 13:259–262, 1985

71. Tropp H: Pronator muscle weakness in functional instability of the ankle joint. Int J Sports Med 7:291–294, 1986

72. Friden T, Zatterstrom R, Lindstrand A, Moritz U: A stabilometric technique for evaluation of lower limb instability. Am J Sports Med 17:118–122, 1989

73. Leanderson J, Eriksson E, Nilsson C, Wykman A: Proprioception in classical ballet dancers. A prospective study of the influence of an ankle sprain on proprioception in the ankle joint. Am J Sports Med 24:370–374, 1996

74. Isakov E, Mizrahi J: Is balance impaired by recurrent sprained ankle. Br J Sports Med 31:65–67, 1997

75. Jerosch J, Bischof M: The effect of proprioception on functional stability of the upper ankle joint with special reference to stabilizing aids. Sportverletzung Sportschaden 8:111–121, 1994

76. Robbins S, Waked E, Rappel R: Ankle taping improves proprioception before and after exercise in young man. Br J Sports Med 29:242–247, 1995

77. Feuerbach J, Grabiner MD, Koh TJ, Weiker GG: Effect of an ankle orthosis and ankle ligament anesthesia on ankle joint proprioception. Am J Sports Med 22:223–229, 1994

78. Konradsen L, Ravn JB, Sorensen AI: Proprioception at the ankle: the effect of anaesthetic blockage of ligament receptors. J Bone Joint Surg Br 75:433–436, 1993

79. Gross MT: Effects of recurrent lateral ankle sprains on active and passive judgements of joint position. Phys Ther 67:1505–1509, 1987

80. Lentell G, Baas B, Lopez D, et al: The contributions of proprioceptive deficits, muscle function, and anatomic laxity to functional instability of the ankle. J Orthop Sports Phys Ther 21(4):206–215, 1995

81. Lynch SA, Eklund U, Gottlieb D, et al: Electromyographic latency changes in the ankle muscu-

lature during inversion moments. Am J Sports Med 24:362–369, 1996

82. Calmels P, Escafit M, Domenach M, Minaire P: Posturographic evaluation of the proprioceptive effect of ankle orthosis in healthy volunteers. Int Disability Studies 13(2):42–45, 1991

83. Guskiewicz KM, Perrin DH: Effects of orthotics on postural sway following inversion ankle sprain. J Orthop Sports Phys Ther 23:326–331, 1996

84. Bennel KL, Goldie PA: The differential effects of external ankle support on postural control. J Orthop Sports Phys Ther 20:287–295, 1994

85. Barret J, Bilisko T: The role of shoes in the prevention of ankle sprains. Sports Med 20:277–280, 1995

86. Robbins S, Waked E, McClaran J: Proprioception and stability: foot position awareness as a function of age and foot wear. Age Ageing 24:67–72, 1995

24

Building on Our Strengths

JOHN V. BASMAJIAN

George Bernard Shaw entitled the preface to one of his plays "The Quintessence of Ibsenism" to usher in the start of the twentieth century. At the start of the twenty-first century, this book has developed into the quintessence of sports medicine rehabilitation thanks to the labors of its authors. When work leading to this volume was first contemplated, the editors had no illusions about the current status of decision making and outcomes in sports rehabilitation, including fitness training. We fully appreciated that we would be dealing with the arts of healing as much (or more than) with its sciences.

Therefore the sparkle of practical scientific rationale and evidence that shine through in the foregoing chapters has been a marvelous bonus. It is true that murky areas are still dominant in the amelioration and rehabilitation of performance problems inhibiting or resulting from disturbances of neuromotor and skeletal systems. Outcomes are unavoidably value laden. They may differ in importance depending on who is judging them—consumer, payer, provider of services, or researchers.

Exploratory research to identify the values of those groups and survey research to determine variations in values are recommended along with flexible approaches for weighing outcomes, promoting dialogue, and obtaining value proxy judgments for children who cannot represent themselves. A broad effort must be made to address (1) boundaries among domains, (2) terminology, and (3) how to consider people's abilities rather than their deficits.

Development of conceptual models of the disablement process and empirical testing of such models are urgently needed. Provisions must be made to gather and relate data across multiple domains. Measurement and analytic tools appropriate to multidomain analysis that use collaborative and interdisciplinary methods are necessary.

OUTCOME MEASURES

The keys to solving many (if not all) problems in health care are to be found in having valid and reproducible methods to measure outcomes of treatment/training programs. The lack of these keys not only has prevented progress but also has kept clinicians and their patients frustrated and in the dark. Recent efforts by physical therapists in North America in this area of study have begun to shed some light on problems.[1-3] Physical rehabilitation outcome measures have three purposes: discriminative, predictive, and evaluative.[3] The last is the most relevant in our context, both for clinicians, trainers, and individual patients and for researchers seeking evidence of the efficacy of a procedure or program in the management of specific disabilities.[4]

Outcome measures and their application themselves require validation, and here progress is being made.[3] Clinicians must rely on evidence from investigators to select appropriate valid measures for a given population. Administrators, too, are deeply involved and must actively promote the use of accurate outcome measures.

STRATEGY AND DESIGN ISSUES

Measures

The conference led by Fuhrer[4] emphasized the importance of obtaining valid, reliable, and sensitive outcome measures for comparing the effectiveness of alternative rehabilitation interventions, systems of care, methods of financing, and consumers' satisfaction and preferences. The conference's report[4] is essential reading for all who help rehabilitate both amateur and professional athletes of all ages and capabilities.

Controlled Studies

Much greater effort is needed to provide evidence for the *effectiveness* and *efficacy* of defined rehabilitative interventions by comparing them to practical service alternatives.

Medical rehabilitation interventions and the service delivery systems of which they are a part are poorly and inconsistently described in reports of outcome studies. Well-documented descriptions of services are also missing for most ongoing clinical databases. Work needs to be done, therefore, to develop theory-based models and classification systems of rehabilitation interventions and practice models that are uniformly applicable to a variety of services and that are related to the outcome goals of medical rehabilitation.[4] There is a need for better data elements, including more details about impairments, broader coverage of outcomes, more refined information about the severity of conditions, and more complete characterizations of interventions and service delivery systems.

MEASUREMENT OF DISABILITY AND HANDICAP

A uniformly useful measure of instrumental activities of daily living appears essential. Developing a measure that can be used for people with various disabling conditions was viewed by the Fuhrer-led conference[4] as being a worthwhile objective. Developing a supplement to scales such as the Functional Independence Measure (FIM) to reflect the cost of resources for supervising cognitively impaired individuals was also deemed beneficial. Shorter and less cumbersome instruments for clinical and research applications are needed, with measurement instruments adapted for cross-cultural use. Translating instruments into other languages is an obvious step in that regard. The instruments then could be validated in these cultures and modified if necessary. Study findings might show that different norms exist for different cultures.[4]

This book was never proposed or written as the final word. In fact, its conception was a deliberate attempt to present the current unsettled state of decision-making processes in sports rehabilitation. As each of the foregoing chapters clearly reveals, for whatever reason, the general state of the art appears to be only moderately successful; however, the *primary* reason for success is rarely a solid base of scientific data and clear reasoning. Our hope is to promote and seek valid improvements, built at least in part by acknowledgment and consideration of the problems raised in this book.

Medical rehabilitation is relatively new to organized health care in industrialized society, although it has been a part of healing efforts since the dawn of civilization in both the West and the East. The burdens of ancient beliefs and practices, including a truly fantastic array of nostrums, have weighed as heavily on rehabilitation as they have on the etiology and pathophysiology of diseases and their acute treatments. Sports rehabilitation is only now emerging as a special field.

DEBONAFIDE EFFECTS VS PLACEBO EFFECTS

In medieval times, to please the patient, desperate physicians would sometimes prescribe or administer a fake potion or manipulation that they knew had no possible benefit. So was born the designation *placebo* (Latin for "I will please") for such a fake treatment. Gradually the term became pejorative.

Modern medicine transferred the term *placebo treatment* to any deliberate use of an inert substance in double-blind studies where one cohort (the placebo group) receives identical-looking capsules of an inert substance (e.g., sugar). It is essential that none of the randomly assigned participants can recognize which capsules are either placebos or the test drug until the official, final code-breaking ceremony.

Similar procedures are attempted with only modest success in investigating other forms of health treatment where physical agents and procedures are the targets. In my early years of biofeedback and pharmaceutical research with my associates and students, I faced these difficulties. We devised complex simulating techniques to mask placebo treatments so neither the patient nor the assessor of results was aware of what treatment individual patients had received.

At that time, I began to reject the concept that placebos were inactive agents because a very large proportion of my patients with quite serious ailments were recovering on placebo drugs and other placebo treatments—at up to 50% of the success rate for patients who had received the investigated drug or therapy.[5-10]

Dissatisfied with the glib designation of these successes as a placebo effect, I began to advocate the replacement term *nonspecific effect* to underline our ignorance of the cause-and-effect sequences. In retrospect, I became convinced that my double-blind studies were research into the power of placebos.

In discussions and debate with an ecobiologist friend, Dr. John Vallentyne (Ph.D.), I was persuaded that in fact "nonspecific" was no more informative than "placebo" to describe the sequence, at least in clinical rehabilitation, general medicine, and applied psychobiologic self-awareness therapies. Why do the placebo therapies in clinical research succeed in significant numbers of patients?

The conclusion that now seems obvious to me is that the process is driven by the same human internal control mechanisms—mind, body, nervous system, and endocrine glands—that keep us alive and usually healthy. The placebo effects are simply a muted form of the internal responses to the more powerful positive responses obtained by appropriate science-proved therapies.

I have coined the term *debonafide effects* for this self-therapeutic phenomenon. It was formed by joining three Latin words: *de, bona,* and *fide,* meaning "derived from," "good," and "faith." The concept of good faith shared by patient and clinician is based on my conviction from my double-blind studies and the many instances in which I have witnessed recoveries where therapies were clearly not present or specific. The single word "placebo" should be retained for drug research use but not "placebo effect."

Both clinicians and clinical researchers should awaken to and even embrace debonafide effects in clinical terminology and for their therapeutic significance. They account for a great number of bona fide therapeutic successes in daily medical practice, clinical research, and also complementary medicine. (Incidentally, Dr. Vallentyne wholeheartedly welcomes the term *debonafide effect.*)

A REVIEW OF THE CONTENTS

The book opens with an essential chapter by Dr. Hart, who, we firmly believe, was the ideal choice. Blending outstanding skills as a sports medicine specialist with wide recognition in rheumatology and clinical epidemiology, he sets the stage. With infinite care to avoid losing any segment of the readers—from the scientifically sophisticated to the clinically naive—he brings us all along as painlessly as possible to an appreciation of evidence-based sports medicine. This chapter will stand for years as the epitome of what this book is all about. Only confirmed Luddites, like their predecessors in the Industrial Revolution, will reject this straightforward review.

Chapter 2 by Demers, Suskin, and McKelvie is a natural follow-up in a book that is deeply concerned with human healing without harm. Skillfully they lay out the cardiovascular benefits and precautions of regular physical activity. Our colleague, Robert McKelvie, holds a Career Scientist Award from the Ontario Ministry of Health for his exemplary clinical research on cardiovascular fitness and disabilities. With his associates, he has reviewed all aspects recorded in the literature. The authors of Chapter 2 emphasize the guidelines of the American College of Cardiology and the American Heart Association. We heartily agree with their recommendations and their conclusion that the data suggest. The cardiac event rate is clearly low among participants in postmyocardial infarction rehabilitation exercise programs, and the event rate has substantially decreased over time.

Also, in logical sequence we encountered nutrition-rich Chapter 3 by Roy and Tarnopolsky. International authorities on nutritional strategies for promoting muscular functional recovery, these distinguished authors explore the existing data and provide practical guidelines and treatment options. We support their strong recommendations for a basic and cost-effective program of protein and carbohydrate supplements followed by therapeutic exercise. They recommend short-term administration of creatine monohydrate both before elective surgery and after, on the basis of good evidence that it will attenuate any decrease in lean body mass and strength.

Chapter 4 is written by one of America's outstanding authorities on the basic science of environmental dehydration and exercise and core temperature. From his vast knowledge of this field, Dr. Bruce Wenger provides us with all that is relevant of the current studies underlining progress in this field of basic and applied science. We are extremely proud of this stellar contribution—and we learned many new ideas. This is a chapter we will read again and again in the future.

The pivotal Chapter 5 by the world-renowned rheumatologist, W. Watson Buchanan, sets the stage for most of the book's other chapters. Inflammation is certainly the central consideration for all activities of amelioration and healing of body tissues. Here, in this authoritative chapter, Buchanan carefully dissects all related factors. This essential service then permits readers of clinically oriented chapters that come later to accept (or reject) their conclusions and recommendations on mechanisms and efficacy of specific therapeutic approaches.

Dr. Lawrence Hart returns with Chapter 6, covering his clinical fields of rheumatology and sports medicine, in which he is recognized as a world leader. With clarity and wisdom, he leads us through the tangled field of conjecture and dogma to an open terrain on which we can make reasonable decisions. This chapter is today the sharpest definition of arthritis and its interaction with sports and exercise regimens. He has covered the world picture, but with our concurrence he avoided citing references to papers he was aware of in languages other than English to avoid confusing the majority of readers. The result is a masterful summary of the field.

In Chapter 7, we turn, with Dr. Larry Leith's guidance, around an unobstructed corner to the psychological and sociologic factors in sports. Indeed, few observers will argue that athletic performances are becoming increasingly more skilled and complex and that this has been complicated with a heavy overlay of temperamental influences. We cannot deny Dr. Leith's endorsement of Kozar and Lord's belief[11] that 80% to 90% of success at elite levels of sport may be

psychological. The section on management of pregame anxiety and nonpharmacologic methods leads to grade A and B recommendations. His coping strategies and training recommendations are excellent, and his review of the total research literature on psychologic and sociologic research provides the reader with an immense resource for sports medicine rehabilitation. The reference list alone will relieve the novice of days of searching for the best sources.

In his follow-up Chapter 8, Mark Tarnopolsky lays out for the reader a road map of the physiologic factors in performance enhancement. This, coupled with Watson Buchanan's chapter on inflammation, helps to explain many of the successes and failures of sports rehabilitation. It is essential reading for all who deal with training, therapy, and surgery of amateur sports and professional rehabilitation of athletes. In particular, Tarnopolsky reports on his major new contributions on the topic of caffeine and carbohydrate loading in endurance exercise. His highly significant research on carbohydrate supplementation is widely recognized. It is a privilege to have his summary in this chapter.

Physical therapy (PT) in the strengthening and healing of people engaged in sports and athletes is the subject of Chapter 9 by Anita Gross and her associates. As a team, they cover the field thoroughly and with an integrity that leaves the editors overwhelmed with gratitude and pleasure. This will become the essential reference for all who have any interest in sports, PT practice, or clinical research. It integrates all aspects of PT involvement with orthopedic, neuromuscular, and cardiovascular-respiratory rehabilitation in amateur or professional sports and recreation. Once more, novice readers are provided with an enormous resource, and old pros will be delighted with the comprehensive summary of all that is relevant.

Again, with Chapter 10, we are guided around a corner to the specific treatment areas examined in this book. Authors Crowther and Grad, respected practitioners of chiropractic, explore the status of their contribution to the healing and health of the bodies of athletes. In a thorough and thoughtful manner, they explore the background and processes used by practitioners who deal with problems of the amateur and professional sporting world. Soberly, they describe clinical applications and the limited research evidence. Proud of their profession and its immense popularity, they still are not satisfied with popular acceptance. Authors like these are on their way to performing and encouraging scientifically acceptable practices and discouraging hearsay evidence. We are proud to have their chapter in this book.

Chapter 11 by the editors of this book is another road map both for those who need information on complementary healing techniques (real or just heavily promoted) and for those who hope to use the methods conscientiously for the care of their patients or family. Of course, the debonafide effect that I described above is ever present. However, people are more interested in results, and certainly the mechanisms of healing are still not absolutely defined. Behavioral medicine is clearly a fundamental factor in both the successes and the failures. A thorough model for a *research protocol* is provided for novice investigators to get started.

The world-famous exercise physiologist Dr. Per-Olaf Åstrand comes next in a lucid Chapter 12 on the mature athlete. It summarizes this eminent author's years of research and contemplation on the factors that determine geriatric motor performance, its rise and fall, and the measures that may be taken for alleviation of problems and their realistic chances for success. I believe that this summary is truly unique.

Following in the footsteps of the geriatrics chapter, Chapter 13 by Dr. Larry Wolfe of Queen's University and Dr. Michelle Mottola of the University of Western Ontario, covers the other extreme—exercise in pregnancy. (They were chosen as authors because of their distinction in their field, not because they are colleagues in our nearby Canadian universities.) Their fully documented chapter is a tour de force. It summarizes all the evidence available in this highly specialized but widely applicable field. The conclusions should be read carefully by all who are involved in sports and exercise classes for women, not to mention the relatives and physicians of this large segment of our population. With proper caution and care, pregnancy is no deterrent for quite vigorous exercise.

Chapter 14 by the senior editor (D.A.K.) was the result of a massive literature search that proved to be a great education for *both* editors. Pediatric sports rehabilitation is itself in its infancy but has generated enormous volumes of

opinions with a thin veneer of evidence-based activities. In this highly specialized field, subspecialties have isolated investigators into narrow chasms, such as childhood obesity treatment. Many useful ideas are explored in this chapter, which will be of interest to all readers.

The following four chapters (15 to 18) focus on practical considerations for both athletes and all who are involved with optimizing their health and performance. First, with their pair of definitive chapters (15 and 16) on neurologic conditions in sports, Drs. Wingerchuk and Dodick of the University of Western Ontario and the Mayo Clinic, respectively, provide significant advice to all professionals working with athletes of all ages who have brain-related performance problems. Then, Drs. Alan Finlayson and Mark Lovell, eminent rehabilitation psychologists, review the current status of treatment standards and outcomes of head injuries in sports with sharp but benign eyes. As two of North America's leading research psychologists who treat and study many types of head injury, they are particularly well suited to write Chapter 17.

This concentration of neuropsychological considerations builds up to the "icing on the cake" provided by Dr. Grimby's superb Chapter 18 on neuromuscular conditions. No one in the world is more appropriate to summarize and analyze the present situation. Chapter 18 is the distillation of a long and productive career in myology that is admired around the world. No one in sports medicine rehabilitation can skip this gem.

With Chapter 19 comes a switch to a series of five practical chapters on rehabilitation management of athletic problems involving regions of the body. These chapters have a major orthopedic underpinning. Although distinguished orthopedists are the main authors, surgical considerations are shadowed by rehabilitation considerations. This section could be considered a handbook of evidence-based rehabilitation management for musculoskeletal problems of the limbs and back and should be of great interest to clinicians who deal with sports and exercise situations. Everyone, regardless of specialty, must read and reread Chapters 19 to 23.

Finally, to echo the opening sentences of both this book and this closing Chapter 24—this book is far from the last word. Increasingly, the various analyses and recommendations will be superseded by fresh data. Meanwhile, however, it will serve the present generation as a principal source of the best available rationale for management of health problems that discourage and disable sports enthusiasts of every kind and every age.

REFERENCES

1. Basmajian JV, Banerjee SN (eds): Clinical Decision-Making in Rehabilitation. Churchill Livingstone, New York, 1996
2. Johnston MV, Keith RA, Hinderer SR: Measurement standards for interdisciplinary medical rehabilitation. Arch Phys Med Rehabil 73:S3, 1992
3. Basmajian JV (ed): Physical Rehabilitation Outcome Measures. Canadian Physiotherapy Association, Toronto, 1994
4. Fuhrer MJ: Conference report: an agenda for medical rehabilitation outcomes research. Am J Phys Med Rehabil 74:243, 1995
5. Basmajian JV: Effects of cyclobenzaprine HCl on skeletal muscle spasms in the lumbar region and back: two double-blind controlled studies. Arch Phys Med Rehabil 60:59–63, 1978
6. Basmajian JV, Kukulka CG, Narayan MG, Takebe K: Biofeedback treatment of foot-drop after stroke compared with standard rehabilitation technique: effects on voluntary control and strength. Arch Phys Med Rehabil 56:231–236, 1975
7. Basmajian JV: Lioresal (baclofen) treatment of spasticity: further experience with double-blind cross-over testing of efficacy in multiple sclerosis. Am J Phys Med 54:175–177, 1975
8. Basmajian JV: Reflex cervical muscle spasm: treatment by diazepam, phenobarbital or placebo. Arch Phys Med Rehabil 64:121–124, 1983
9. Biofeedback and the placebo effect. Psychiatr Ann 13:94–99, 1981
10. Basmajian JV, Gowland CA, et al: Stroke treatment: integrated behavioral-physical therapy, biofeedback versus traditional physical therapy programs. Arch Phys Med Rehabil 68:267–272, 1987
11. Kozar B, Lord R: Psychological considerations for training the elite athlete. In Proceedings of the U.S. Olympic Academy VII. Texas Tech University, Lubbock, Texas. 1983, pp. 78–96

Index

Note: Page numbers in *italics* refer to illustrations; page numbers followed by t refer to tables.